W9-AWI-689

CARDIAC BIOPROSTHESES

Proceedings of the Second International Symposium

CARDIAC BIOPROSTHESES

Printed in the United States of America

First Edition

International Standard Book Number: 0-914316-34-6

Library of Congress Cataloging in Publication Data
Main entry under title:

Cardiac bioprostheses.

"The Second International Symposium on Cardiac Bioprostheses was held in Rome, May 17–19, 1982, sponsored by the University of Padova"—Pref.
Includes bibliographies and index.
1. Heart valve prosthesis—Congresses. 2. Biomedical materials—Congresses. I. Cohn, Lawrence H. II. Gallucci, Vincenzo. III. Università di Padova. IV. International Symposium on Cardiac Bioprostheses (2nd : 1982 : Rome, Italy) [DNLM: 1. Bioprosthesis—Congresses. 2. Heart valve-prosthesis—Congresses. WG 169 C266 1982]

RD598.C343 1982 617'.412 82-17628
ISBN 0-914316-34-6

CARDIAC BIOPROSTHESES

Proceedings of the Second International Symposium

EDITORS

LAWRENCE H. COHN, MD

Professor of Surgery
Harvard Medical School
Department of Surgery
Division of Thoracic and Cardiac Surgery
Brigham and Women's Hospital, Boston, USA

VINCENZO GALLUCCI, MD

Professor of Cardiovascular Surgery
Departments of Cardiovascular Surgery and Cardiology
University of Padova Medical School, Padova, Italy

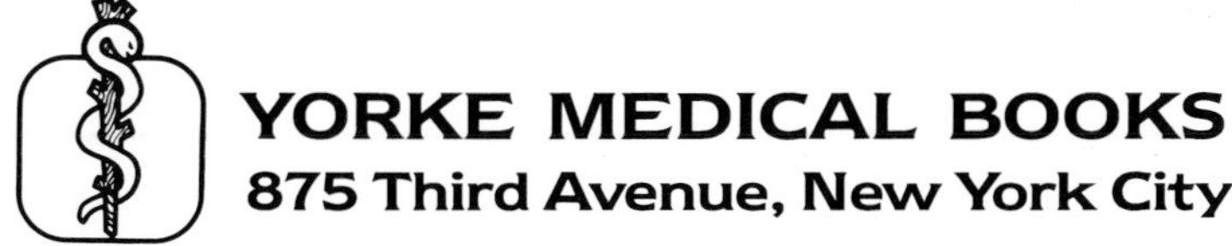

YORKE MEDICAL BOOKS
875 Third Avenue, New York City

PREFACE

Approximately 20 years have gone by since the first reports of homograft aortic valve replacement by Messrs. Donald Ross and Brian Barratt-Boyes, and about 10 years have passed since the first reports began to appear about commercially available, quality-controlled porcine bioprosthetic and bovine pericardial valves. To celebrate these events and to update our global knowledge about tissue heart valves, this international symposium was organized. The first similar international symposium on tissue heart valves was held in Munich, Germany, in 1979, sponsored by the Deutsch Herz Centrum; it was an unqualified success. It was obvious from talking this past year to many colleagues in cardiac surgery, cardiology, pathology and bioengineering that the time was appropriate to come together again to present new ideas and data about these devices which have become an important part of the treatment of patients with valvular heart disease. And so, the Second International Symposium on Cardiac Bioprostheses was held in Rome, May 17–19, 1982, sponsored by the University of Padova.

This symposium was organized on a strictly competitive abstract basis, chosen by an international program committee with four invited honor lectures given by recognized authorities in cardiac surgery and pathology. One hundred and eighty abstracts were submitted, and 45 in 8 categories were accepted. Virtually every major cardiovascular center in the world that has had any meaningful experience with cardiac bioprosthetic valves was represented. We particularly are appreciative of the efforts of the Organizing and Program Committees in helping to make this symposium possible. In addition, discussants for many of the papers were invited from all over the world to add considerable perspective and additional experience to the academic program.

The Proceedings are organized into nine major subdivisions. Section I is a clinical analysis of different cardiac bioprostheses, begun by an Honor Lecture by Mr. Donald Ross. Section II deals with hemodynamics of cardiac bioprostheses. Section III discusses clinical thromboembolism of these valves with an Honor Lecture by Dr. Ake Senning. Section IV discusses pediatric valve replacement, with an Honor Lecture by Dr. Aldo Castaneda. Section V is experimental pathology, emphasizing calcification and *de*calcification of valve bioprostheses. Section VI deals with several papers analyzing explanted valve pathology with the G. P. Morgagni Honor Lecture by William C. Roberts of Bethesda, Maryland. Section VII contains bioprosthetic bioengineering papers, with emphasis on the biophysical elements of tissue heart valve construction that will be of importance in coming years in production of the second generation of these valves. Section VIII is composed of several papers on the long-term follow-up of various bioprostheses from Tampa, Munich, Stanford, Boston, and Detroit, and interesting papers on tricuspid valve replacement. Finally, Section Nine is a summing-up by cardiologist and cardiac surgeon, presenting an overview of the entire proceedings. Thus, we believe that all current aspects of clinical, pathologic and bioengineering data about cardiac tissue valves have been touched upon in this symposium.

We are most grateful for the editorial expertise of Gay Morgulas of Yorke Medical Books, who has single-handedly expedited the publication of these proceedings so that they might reach the medical public in a short (and relevant!) time after the meeting. We thank Barbara Hebert, administrative assistant at the Brigham and Women's Hospital in the Division of Cardiothoracic Surgery who has done a fine job in helping to organize the meeting, insuring accurate manuscripts and receipt of all editorial materials for this book.

Special thanks go to Dr. Victor Ferrans, Head of the Ultrastructural Laboratory of the Section on Cardiac Pathology at the National Heart, Lung and Blood Institute. Dr. Ferrans not only was on the Organizing Committee but he reviewed all the pathology and bioengineering papers in the Proceedings which were of great importance in this meeting. We're grateful to him for his meticulous and efficient editing of these manuscripts.

Finally, we thank Extracorporeal/Hancock, a division of Johnson and Johnson, for their help in underwriting a good deal of the expense of these Proceedings, helping to bring together a distinguished multispecialty group of clinicians and scientists to discuss all aspects of cardiac bioprostheses and assess the "state of the art" with these devices in both congenital and acquired heart disease in 1982.

LAWRENCE H. COHN, M.D.
Boston, Massachusetts
VINCENZO GALLUCCI, M.D.
Padova, Italy

INTERNATIONAL SYMPOSIUM ON CARDIAC BIOPROSTHESES COMMITTEES

Organizing Committee

Vincenzo Gallucci *(Padova, Italy) (Chairman)*
Lawrence H. Cohn *(Boston, U.S.A.)*
Victor J. Ferrans *(Bethesda, U.S.A.)*
Marko Turina *(Zürich, Switzerland)*

Program Committee

Lawrence H. Cohn *(Boston, U.S.A.) (Chairman)*
Neil D. Broom *(Auckland, New Zealand)*
Bernard R. Chaitman *(Montreal, Canada)*
Alain Deloche *(Paris, France)*
Fritz Derom *(Gent, Belgium)*
Carlos M. G. Duran *(Santander, Spain)*
Victor J. Ferrans *(Bethesda, U.S.A.)*
Robert W. M. Frater *(New York, U.S.A.)*
Vincenzo Gallucci *(Padova, Italy)*
Adib Jatene *(São Paulo, Brasil)*
Donald J. Magilligan, Jr. *(Detroit, U.S.A.)*
Philip E. Oyer *(Stanford, U.S.A.)*
Shahbudin H. Rahimtoola *(Los Angeles, U.S.A.)*
Bruno Reichart *(Munich, West Germany)*
Harzell V. Shaff *(Rochester, U.S.A.)*
Gaetano Thiene *(Padova, Italy)*
Marko Turina *(Zürich, Switzerland)*

Invited Discussants

J. Alpert *(Worcester, U.S.A.)*
F. Alt *(Munich, West Germany)*
E. Arbustini *(Padova, Italy)*
H. Bolooki *(Miami, U.S.A.)*
N. D. Broom *(Auckland, New Zealand)*
J. P. Cachera *(Créteil, France)*
A. Carpentier *(Paris, France)*
G. W. Christie *(Auckland, New Zealand)*
L. H. Cohn *(Boston, U.S.A.)*
D. A. Cooley *(Houston, U.S.A.)*
H. DeVivie *(Paris, France)*
C. M. G. Duran *(Santander, Spain)*
V. J. Ferrans *(Bethesda, U.S.A.)*
R. W. M. Frater *(New York, U.S.A.)*
Y. Goffin *(Brussels, Belgium)*
C. Hatcher *(Atlanta, U.S.A.)*
K. Holper *(Munich, West Germany)*
C. Huth *(Tubingen, West Germany)*
A. Jatene *(São Paulo, Brasil)*
R. Karp *(Birmingham, U.S.A)*
D. J. Magilligan, Jr. *(Detroit, U.S.A.)*
T. Martin *(Sheffield, England)*
H. Meisner *(Munich, West Germany)*
M. Morea *(Torino, Italy)*
L. Nunez *(Madrid, Spain)*
P. E. Oyer *(Stanford, U.S.A.)*
G. B. Parulkar *(Bombay, India)*
A. Pierangeli *(Bologna, Italy)*
S. H. Rahimtoola *(Los Angeles, U.S.A.)*
F. Schoen *(Boston, U.S.A.)*
F. Sebening *(Munich, West Germany)*
H. Sievers *(Kiel, West Germany)*
D. Smith *(Leeds, England)*
E. Struck *(Munich, West Germany)*
D. Vrandecic *(Belo Horizonte, Brasil)*
F. Wellens *(Brussels, Belgium)*
S. Westaby *(London, England)*
D. B. Williams *(Rochester, U.S.A.)*
J. T. M. Wright *(Anaheim, U.S.A.)*
G. Ziemer *(Hannover, West Germany)*

CONTENTS

SECTION III. THROMBOEMBOLISM

SECTION IV. PEDIATRIC VALVE REPLACEMENT

SECTION V. EXPERIMENTAL PATHOLOGY

SECTION I

CLINICAL ANALYSIS

1

The Evolution of the Biologic Valve

D. N. Ross

The use of biologic valves as substitutes for diseased heart valves is not a new concept and indeed goes back 20 years, when we inserted the first aortic valve homograft. You will remember that Albert Starr reported his first clinical success with the ball valve in 1961, and by 1962 homografts had been inserted both in the United Kingdom and New Zealand. Since that time, although mechanical valves of one type or another have been in continuous use, homografts have been confined to 2 or 3 centers, and it is only in recent years that there has been a renewed interest in the biologic valve principle.

Enthusiasm for the biologic valve fluctuates as cardiac surgeons are attracted to the obvious advantages of their superior flow characteristics and lack of thromboembolism, but at the same time they are deterred by the questionable durability, possible antigenicity, and the difficulty in achieving a surgically acceptable level of sterility.

Looking at the early 1960s, the recent reemergence of biologic valves presents for me a quiet evolutionary process, rather than a violent revolution, and much to everyone's surprise the biologic valve proponents have demonstrated extraordinary persistence and staying power.

Quite early in my cardiac surgical career, I noted the contrast between the quality of life enjoyed by prosthetic valve patients compared with those with a biologic valve, the latter living a life liberated from the routine of regular visists to the doctors' office and usually without medication of any sort.

The problem is that *quality* of life is difficult to quantitate and does not come to light in statistics. However, I believe we as doctors too readily dismiss the ever-present threat of embolism that hangs like a sword of

---

From the Cardiothoracic Institute, National Heart Hospital, London, England.

Dr. Ross was an honor lecturer at the Second International Symposium on Cardiac Bioprostheses.

Damocles over our patients with a mechanical prosthesis. Added to this are the dangers inherent in anticoagulant therapy—estimated to carry a mortality as high as 1% per year. Although Starr's recent statistics show a fall in the incidence of emboli, there has been a significant concomitant increase in the number of hemorrhagic complications.

Undoubtedly valve durability emerges as the most persistent criticism of aortic homografts, and the same problem applies to all biologic valves. However, we have come to recognize that failure or degeneration in an aortic homograft or any biologic valve is a slowly progressive process very similar to the evolving natural history of, say, rheumatic valve disease. This means there is adequate warning, and plenty of time for a safe, planned second operation, and no one should be ashamed of this admission. As a consequence, *valve-related* deaths are comparatively rare (1% per year) among homograft patients, and the patients are likely to outlive their valves.

In contrast the much vaunted mechanical prosthesis may have the potential to last longer, but it may destroy the patient in the process of establishing its durability. The late deaths occurring in patients with mechanical valves are, however, generally presented as "myocardial failure." In other words, the heart or myocardium is conveniently blamed for the death, and not the valve.

It is evident that, although the mechanical valve may have the potential to last about 100 years, the patient may well die long before then from some form of valve-related sudden death! And this is usually ascribed to myocardial failure. The message I am trying to deliver is that we should not be deflected by the mechanical valve proponents into believing that *valve durability* is the key factor keeping the patients alive. The fact that the valve is fine and unmarked, after the patient is dead, is of little interest to anyone but the manufacturer. It is imperative that we remember that *valve safety* ranks more importantly than durability when related to the clinical scene.

The discrepancies between mechanical valve durability and biologic valve safety are not altogether surprising when one compares the *workshop environment* in which mechanical valves are tested with the harsh biologic realities of their future environment where the blood represents a corrosive saltwater medium, swarming with aggressive macrophages and defensive mechanisms. Also, if we need reminding that mechanical valves can in fact fail, there are innumerable examples in the literature. We recently made a survey of our aortic homograft patients who had survived into the second decade and came up with results that at least attest to the fact that it is a practical and acceptable aortic valve substitute.

There is a steady attrition of homograft valves so that by 10 years about 50% are fully functional, and by 15 years this is reduced to only about 20%. Therefore we cannot expect any homografts to function after 20 years. In contrast to this rather gloomy picture relating to the valve, the same series of patients were analyzed in terms of *patient* rather than *valve* survival, and we now see that well over 70% of these patients are still alive and well at 15 years, some as a result of a planned second operation. I believe we should at present accept the probability of a second operation, and refocus our attention on quality of life and safe patient survival.

Although this is a brief survey of biologic valves, it is worth reviewing the present spectrum of available types. At the same time, we should be absolutely clear that the term "biologic valves" in the strict sense applies only to the homograft, sewn in place freehand in the aortic position or right ventricular outflow, and to the autotransplanted pulmonary valve in the aortic position. All other so-called biologic valves are hybrid creations, partly biologic and partly prosthetic, often including both plastic and metallic components. The resulting product has aptly been described as a bioprosthesis and we have to recognize that once a sewing ring or semirigid stent is incorporated, we lose some of the advantages of the original, fully flexible nonobstructive and nonemoblizing homograft and incur some of the disadvantages of the mechanical prosthesis.

If, however, we accept bioprostheses within the definition of biologic valves, then these may be either homologous, autogenous, or heterologous, i.e., allografts, autografts, or xenografts. Also they are either naturally occurring or man-made productions and may be inserted orthotopically or heterotopically.

We have had some experience with all of these valve types and, although we have few answers, we have accumulated some factual data and have undoubtedly learned something.

The aortic homograft sewn in place freehand is still, in my view, the best all-round aortic valve substitute for men, women, and children. It, and the autotransplanted pulmonary valve, are the only embolism-free replacements that we are aware of, and the patient's quality of life is quite excellent. Also, as I have indicated, sudden valve-related deaths are rare.

The earliest freeze-dried aortic homograft valves have done remarkably well and a few exceptionally well. However, calcific degeneration, starting at about 4 years, has been the main problem. This calcification has been largely *intrinsic,* that is, within valve cusp substance and of course within the aortic wall also. In 1968 on the recommendation of our colleagues in New Zealand, we changed to fresh valves stored in an antibiotic-nutrient medium.

Results with these fresh valves have, on the whole, been better but in the follow-up we have been disconcerted by the development of sudden, unexpected, and on the whole extensive calcification processes occurring in a small number of these fresh valves and as early as 2–3 years. We have also noted that the fresh valve calcification tends to be of an *extrinsic* or granular type, which makes us think of an active surface phenomenon leaving the basic valve structure almost unchanged.

Although there are, no doubt, a number of causes of calcification, one possible explanation is that of an accelerated immunologic rejection process in a few particularly bad tissue matches in these fresh, viable, and therefore antigenically more active valves. Simple wear and tear, on the other hand, seems to be a constant feature in all homografts, and its incidence is probably unchanged with the different methods of valve preservation. It probably relates to many factors, for example, surgical technique, infection, rejection, and turbulence.

I have spent some time on the aortic homograft but I believe it supplies a basic pattern applicable to all so-called biologic valves.

To overcome the possibility of rejection and, at the same time, the problems of valve sterilization and storage, we introduced in 1967 the pulmonary switch operation, or autotransplantation of the pulmonary valve to the aortic valve site, and have performed about 200 operations. These remain, in my view, the only ideal biologic valves so far introduced, but they have a limited application, particularly to isolated aortic valve disease in young people. Undoubtedly, the valve persists as a living structure and certainly they do not calcify or degenerate as far as we can tell.

In 1968, fired with enthusiasm by this living autologous valve experience, we and Ionescu started making valves of autologous fascia lata, taken from the thigh and fixed on a rigid stent. This followed the lead of Senning, who first used living fascial valves inserted freehand.

Our disappointment was rapid, with disasters occurring early, particularly in the mitral and tricuspid areas, where the valves became thickened, stiffened, and encapsulated in tissue overgrowth. Several factors were probably involved in the failure of this living autologous fascia. Among these was the presence of a new set of stresses acting on a living reactive tissue suddenly exposed to an enriched blood medium. These stresses, in turn, gave rise to changes in form, the most interesting being attempts of the fascial mitral valves to revert to a basic bicuspid mitral pattern.

From this chastening fascia lata experience, we clutched with both hands at the dura mater alternative offered by Zerbini in 1974. However, by that time we were cautious and decided to put these dura valves in for not more than 2 years and then to evaluate them, whatever the early results. Consequently, in 1974–1976 we put in 158 dura valves, chiefly in the mitral position.

The results are not good and are still unfolding. Basically, they have been interesting for, although dura valves, sterilized in antibiotic and preserved in glycerol, fail characteristically by detachment of the cusps from their rigid frame, the tissue at 5, 6, or 7 years is still pliable, mobile, nonthickened and, more important, noncalcified, i.e., exactly as it was when first inserted. This lack of calcium, thickening, or thinning has been striking and makes us feel there is a need to reevaluate glycerol as a preserving medium (unless it is the dura that provides the secret, although this seems less likely).

With some reluctance, since we had electively decided to stop the dura valves, we turned to the then commercially available, but clumsy-looking, xenograft for mitral valve replacements.

Our early results with the porcine valve, as will be reported by others, have been very encouraging, but we recognize that the critical testing time and calcification problems may lie just ahead, and these are already disconcertingly evident in children.

Continuing our search for a satisfactory biologic valve, 2 observations derived from this previous experience have influenced our views in planning future biologic *mitral valve* substitutes. These relate to the basic valve design and to the supporting frames or stents.

With regard to design, we noted that aortic homografts lasted longer in the aortic postion than when used inverted in the mitral position. This observation was based on comparable series and also, more importantly, on double valve replacements where a homograft was inserted both as an aortic and a mitral substitute in the same patient for the same period of *time* and subjected to the same biologic and environmental *stresses.*

This may be the result of simple physical factors, like the higher mitral closing pressures acting on an unsupported 3-leaflet aortic type of valve, which lacks the tensioning chordae and papillary muscles present in the normal mitral mechanism. In other words, the 3 cusp structure, the end result of millions of years of evolution, is undoubtedly the wrong design for the mitral area.

Important as these design criteria are, we found on further reviewing our use of inverted human homografts in the mitral area that those mounted in fully flexible supports persisted significantly longer than those on rigid frames, and again this probably applies not only to homografts but to all types of biologic valve.

Therefore, to summarize what we have learned so far, we can say:

1. All homologous and xenograft biologic valves have a limited life-span irrespective of their origin or preparation, but they fail slowly and therefore safely.

2. At present the best *aortic* valve substitute is probably an autologous pulmonary valve or a homologous aortic valve sewn in freehand. We recognize, however, that neither of these valves appeal to busy practicing cardiac surgeons.

3. We remain uncertain how best to sterilize biologic tissue and are unsure whether it should be stored in glycerol or glutaraldehyde or be frozen.

4. We have learned that autografts do not seem to calcify so that some of the factors contributing to calcification may well be a result of rejection, or are immunologically determined.

5. We have been surprised to find that homologous dura mater stored in glycerol seems to retain its physical characteristics and flexibility, and that

calcification is uncommon. It is not clear whether this is due to the dura or the glycerol preservation.

6. We have observed that the tricuspid valve structure is better suited to the aortic and pulmonary position than the mitral.

7. If we are using a mounted 3 cusp valve system, we are convinced it should have a flexible frame or stent.

8. Finally, we need to remind ourselves again, in deciding on a valve type, that patients matter more than simple valve durability.

Putting these observations together should result in the theoretically ideal valve but it will not necessarily be a practical and surgically acceptable one. Consequently, compromise becomes inevitable. For instance, homografts and human dura are both in short supply, particularly in commercially available quantities. This leaves us with autologous or xenograft tissue. There is just not enough autologous tissue to supply the needs of the world's valve surgeons and for this reason we are virtually forced to use xenograft tissue, if we are to have a ready supply of valves of all sizes. This tissue is available in quantity and can be obtained almost sterile. In practice, this implies a porcine valve or one made from xenograft pericardium (unless a superior membrane is found). The porcine valve has perfect commissural supports but some inherent structural disadvantages, including a somewhat immobile right coronary cusp and a relatively thick wall, in relation to the effective valve orifice. On the contrary the man-made pericardial valve offers an unrivaled orifice.

The primary question for all biologic valves, however, relates to the prospect of improving their long-term integrity or durability. I am aware that Barratt-Boyes feels that the repopulation of the valve with host cells could supply one answer. I, on the other hand, feel that, although these "new" cells, if they appear, may be desirable, they may have a more sinister significance, representing a foreign body reaction or rejection phenomenon.

I am increasingly influenced by the probability of rejection, since there does not seem to be a consistent and predictable pattern of degeneration in biologic valves, with some lasting 15 years and others degenerating unexpectedly at 3 years, particularly in young children. The only mechanism I can invoke to explain this random behavior in biologic tissue is an immunologic rejection resulting either from a poor tissue match or varying degrees of tissue incompatibility.

That there is an immune response in the homograft valve has been demonstrated repeatedly in animal work by Mohri and Shumway and it is present even in glutaraldehyde-treated tissue, so that we can no longer ignore it. What we lack at present is firm clinical evidence of a rejection phenomenon in our valve patients or the certain means of predicting the possibility preoperatively. Consequently, if we are to continue to use nonautologous tissue, that is, homografts or xenografts, we must take note of the possibility of rejection and be prepared to deal with it. This may be either by prospective tissue typing, which is hardly practicable; by abolishing the antigenicity of the valve, which is probably not possible; or by long-term low dose immunosuppression, which is not desirable but may be necessary.

Having reviewed the evidence, and trying to submerge my natural prejudices, what valve are we to use: the mechanical or biologic? First there is the vexing question of children requiring a valve. On the available evidence, it is clear we cannot use the present generation of commercial xenografts. Experience with homografts has been much better and I am quite happy to continue with these for aortic replacement and right ventricular outflow reconstruction in children.

For the average adult valve replacement, the patient fortunately now often takes a hand in the decision-making, having read the available evidence, or he has made the choice in the first place by selecting a surgeon with a known preference.

In making our own decisions as surgeons I have come to realize that the mechanical valve is designed almost entirely with the surgeon in mind. It appeals to his vanity and sense of machismo in that it is easy to insert and leaves him with the glowing sense of satisfaction of having put in a permanent replacement—the very best that money can buy!

The biologic valve surgeon, on the other hand, almost has an aura of guilt and furtiveness about him, conscious of his own fallibility and that of his valve, perhaps finding it more difficult and tedious to insert, and constantly aware of his doubts as to whether he is inserting the best valve.

So much for the surgeon. Now, looked at from the patient's point of view, the picture is again different. On the one hand is the mechanical valve patient, tied by an umbilical cord to the hematology laboratory, swallowing pills, and taking precautions against trauma, alcohol, and aspirins, and with the constant threat of embolism hanging over him. The biologic valve patient, on the other hand, is generally leading a trouble-free, doctor-free, and pill-free existence, and enjoying a normal life.

Weighing the pros and cons less emotionally, and more objectively, we have on the one side of the scale the postoperative biologic valve patient, leading a normal life, but facing the almost certain prospect of a 2nd operation at say 10 years, carrying with it a 5% mortality. The chances are he will again have a 10 year trouble-free life-span, bringing him up to 20 years. Adding the 1st operation mortality of 3% to the 5% of the 2nd means a total operative risk of 8–10%. In addition there is about a 1% risk of a valve-related death per patient year. This brings the risk directly relating to the valve operation to 25% and perhaps 30% over a 20 year period.

Looking at the mechanical valve patient, we should again remind ourselves that quality of life does not register statistically. There is little or no risk of a 2nd operation within 20 years but a continuous threat throughout those 20 years from 1) sudden unexplained death, which I believe to be valve-related; 2) embolism; 3) hemorrhage.

Between the Scylla of embolism and the Charybdis of an important or fatal hemorrhagic complication, the patient steers a dangerous course. As one danger recedes, the other looms larger (witness Starr's recent 20 years figure showing a falling incidence of embolism and a 3 times concomitant increasing risk of hemorrhage).

The risk to the patient per year from these 3 complications is, say, 2%, conservatively estimated, making a cumulative risk at the end of 20 years of 40%. More important, this represents a continuing risk factor. Even if we allow for remarkable improvements in anticoagulants and embolism control over this period, it is unlikely the risks will be very much reduced (4.7% per year = 94%).

Having considered all the available evidence, I long ago came down on the side of biologic valves for my patients and I am happy now to let my case rest.

2

Heart Valve Replacement with the Hancock Bioprosthesis: A 5–11 Year Follow-up

V. GALLUCCI, C. VALFRÉ, A. MAZZUCCO, U. BORTOLOTTI, A. MILANO, R. CHIOIN, S. DALLA VOLTA, P. G. CEVESE

Following its introduction into clinical practice in the early 1970s,[1] the glutaraldehyde-preserved porcine bioprosthesis has been widely accepted as a cardiac valve substitute. During the last decade, considerable clinical[2–9] and pathological[10–14] experience with this device has been gained. Insufficient data are currently available to allow a confident assessment of the durability of the porcine bioprosthetic valve beyond 10 years of performance.

The following report presents the experience with patients undergoing heart valve replacement with a porcine bioprosthesis at the Department of Cardiovascular Surgery, University of Padova Medical School; for the purpose of this presentation only patients followed from 5–11 years will be considered.

Patients and Methods

Patient population: The first glutaraldehyde-preserved Hancock porcine xenograft (Hancock Laboratories, Anaheim, CA) was implanted at our institution in March 1970. All patients undergoing heart valve replacement with this device, from 1970–1976, with a follow-up from 5–11 years, were reviewed. The following analysis includes 434 patients (Table I), 200 males and 234 females, 9–68 years old (mean, 53.1 years). Isolated mitral valve

---

From the Departments of Cardiovascular Surgery and Cardiology, University of Padova Medical School, Padova, Italy.

This work was in part supported by Grant No. 80 00449.04 of the Consiglio Nazionale delle Ricerche, Rome, Italy.

TABLE I Summary of clinical data

	MVR*	AVR*	DVR*	mVR*	Total
# patients	257	69	36	72	434
Male/female ratio	93/164	57/12	19/17	31/41	200/234
Age range (yrs)	9–66	17–68	10–65	15–61	9–68
Mean age (yrs)	58.9	43.2	44.8	45.3	53.1
Operative mortality (%)	30(11.6)	10(14.4)	13(36.1)	20(27.7)	73(16.8)
Associated procedures (%)	15(5.8)	10(14.4)	2(5.5)	2(2.7)	29(6.6)

* MVR: mitral valve replacement; AVR: aortic valve replacement; DVR: double Hancock valve replacement; mVR: multiple (porcine plus mechanical) valve replacement.

replacement (MVR) was performed in 257 cases; isolated aortic valve replacement (AVR) in 69; double Hancock valve replacement (DVR) (27 combined mitral and aortic and 9, mitral and tricuspid) in 36; and multiple valve replacement (mVR) using at least 1 porcine valve in association with mechanical prostheses, in 72. A total of 477 bioprostheses were implanted, 353 in the mitral, 100 in the aortic, and 24 in the tricuspid position. Associated surgical procedures were performed in 29 patients (6.7%).

The predominant valvular lesion was regurgitation in 147 patients (33.8%) and stenosis in 287 (66.2%). The etiology of valvular disease was rheumatic in 74.2% of cases, degenerative in 11.3%, infective (endocarditis) in 2%, congenital in 1.6%, and ischemic in 0.4%; 12 patients (2.8%) underwent replacement of a previously implanted mechanical or biologic prosthesis (Table II).

Preoperative functional classification, based on the New York Heart Association (NYHA) criteria, is listed in Table III according to the type of valve replacement: 29 patients were in NYHA class II; 303, in class III; and 102, in class IV.

Surgical technique: All patients were operated on using standard cardiopulmonary bypass techniques, employing a bubble oxygenator and mod-

TABLE II Etiology of valvular lesion

	#	%
Rheumatic	322	74.2
Degenerative	49	11.3
Failed prosthesis	12	2.8
Infective endocarditis	9	2.0
Congenital	7	1.6
Ischemic	2	0.4
Miscellaneous	33	7.7
Total	434	

TABLE III Preoperative and postoperative NYHA functional class

	Preoperative NYHA class				Postoperative NYHA class			
	I	II	III	IV	I	II	III	IV
MVR	—	11	191	55	69	65	17	1
AVR	—	15	44	10	19	13	1	—
DVR	—	1	25	10	4	5	4	—
mVR	—	2	43	27	10	15	4	—
Total	—	29	303	102	102	98	26	1

erate to deep systemic hypothermia. At the beginning of our experience, interrupted aortic cross clamping was employed with topical intrapericardial cooling and coronary arterial perfusion; subsequently, a single aortic cross-clamping time was preferred. Since 1977, cold potassium cardioplegia has been routinely added to the procedure.

The mitral and aortic bioprostheses were implanted using multiple interrupted sutures, buttressed by Teflon pledgets in the presence of a weakened or calcified anulus. Continuous suture was routinely used for tricuspid valve replacement. Valves were oriented so as to avoid obstruction of the coronary ostia in AVR and impingement into the ventricular outflow tract in atrioventricular (AV) valve replacement.

Anticoagulation: All patients were anticoagulated for the first 3 postoperative months, starting soon after removal of the chest drainages. Oral anticoagulant administration was subsequently discontinued in all patients except those with an associated mechanical prosthesis. More recently, long-term anticoagulation was extended also in patients with MVR who had previously sustained embolic accidents and those with giant left atrium and chronic atrial fibrillation and/or evidence of left atrial thrombi at operation.

Definition of valve failure and thromboembolism: The criteria for diagnosis of valve failure were those reported by others.[9,15] Primary valve failure was established at necropsy or reoperation by detection of cusp tears, perforations, or calcification in the absence of an infective process.

Thromboembolic accidents, besides the peripheral or abdominal acute arterial obstructions, were also considered to be either temporary or permanent neurologic events.

Follow-up and postoperative evaluation: The patients included in this investigation were reevaluated during a 6 month period (May–November 1981) either directly or by means of questionnaires compiled by the patient himself or the attending physician. Except for patients who have undergone reoperation, hemodynamic investigation has not been routinely performed. Instead, echocardiographic (ECG) controls are widely employed in the follow-up clinic.

TABLE IV Summary of late mortality and actuarial survival

	MVR	AVR	DVR	mVR	Total
Late mortality	43(3.2 ± 0.5)	11(3.6 ± 1.1)	7(7.4 ± 2.7)	15(5.0 ± 1.3)	78(3.7 ± 0.4)
Thromboembolism					
Overall	32(2.2 ± 0.4)	2(0.6 ± 0.4)	1(1.0 ± 1.0)	5(1.6 ± 0.7)	40(1.9 ± 0.3)
Fatal	7(0.5 ± 0.2)	1(0.3 ± 0.4)	1(1.0 ± 1.0)	3(1.0 ± 0.5)	12(0.5 ± 0.1)
Anticoagulant-related hemorrhage					
Overall	7(0.5 ± 0.2)	—	2(2.1 ± 1.4)	3(1.0 ± 0.5)	12(0.5 ± 0.1)
Fatal	4(0.3 ± 0.1)	—	1(1.0 ± 1.0)	1(0.3 ± 0.3)	6(0.3 ± 0.1)
Primary valve failure	16(1.1 ± 0.3)	8(2.6 ± 0.1)	1(1.0 ± 1.0)	3(1.0 ± 0.6)	28(1.3 ± 0.2)
Endocarditis	4(0.3 ± 0.1)	4(1.3 ± 0.6)	—	1(0.3 ± 0.3)	9(0.4 ± 0.1)

* Data in parentheses expressed as % per patient years.

TABLE V Summary of follow-up results

	MVR	AVR	DVR	mVR	Total
# patients	257	69	36	72	434
Duration of follow-up (patient years)	1,410	300	95	295	2,100
Maximum follow-up (yrs)	11.5	11.6	10.5	10.5	
Range of follow-up (yrs)	4.9–11.5	5.0–11.6	4.9–10.5	4.9–10.5	4.9–11.6
Average follow-up (yrs)	6.2	5.0	4.1	5.6	5.8
Current survivors	152	33	13	29	227
Lost to follow-up*	0.3	0.6	—	0.3	0.8
Survivors at 11 years (%)	64.5	67.4	43.2	41.4	

* Expressed as % per patient years.

Out of the 361 operative survivors, 8 patients were lost to follow-up, i.e., 98% complete 11 postoperative years.

Statistical analysis: Analysis of rates of patient survival, incidence of postoperative thromboembolism and bioprosthetic failure has been expressed by actuarial methods,[16] reporting the 70% confidence limits. Survival actuarial curves include operative mortality. In patients undergoing MVR the actuarial incidence of thromboembolic events has also been separately evaluated for those who were in sinus rhythm (SR) or in atrial fibrillation (AF).

Valve dysfunction has been calculated on the number of prostheses at risk rather than on patients at risk; moreover, separate curves were drawn according to the type of prosthetic replacement performed and the site of insertion.

The chi-square test was employed to determine the statistical significance of the difference between the data of the various groups of patients.

Results

Operative mortality: Operative mortality was 11.6% for MVR patients (30/257), 14.4% for AVR patients (10/69), 36.1% for DVR (13/36), and 27.7% for mVR (20/72) (Table I).

Late mortality and actuarial survival: Of 361 patients discharged from the hospital, 78 died in the late postoperative period (21.6%) (Table IV). This represents an incidence of 3.2 ± 0.5% per patient years for MVR, 3.6 ± 1.1% for AVR, 7.4 ± 2.7% for DVR, and 5.0 ± 1.3% for mVR. The major causes of late death were myocardial failure in 18, noncardiac in 16, systemic or cerebral thromboembolism in 12, hemorrhage in 6, and myocardial infarction in 4.

Operative survivors were reevaluated from 4.9–11.6 years following surgery. Mean follow-up time was 5.8 years and cumulative duration of follow-up was 2,100 patient years (Table V). Reoperation was performed in

TABLE VI Causes of reoperation

	MVR	AVR	DVR	mVR	Total
Primary tissue failure	16(2)*	8(1)	1	3	28(3)
Endocarditis	4(3)	4(3)	—	1(1)	9(7)
Paravalvular leak	3	1(1)	2(1)	2(1)	8(3)
Left atrial thrombosis	2(2)	—	—	—	2(2)

* Operative deaths indicated in parentheses.

47 patients, because of primary tissue failure in 28 (3 operative deaths), endocarditis in 9 (7 operative deaths), paravalvular leak in 8 (3 deaths), and left atrial thrombosis in 2 (2 deaths) (Table VI).

Actuarial survival rates, including hospital mortality, at 11 years postoperatively are as follows: 64 ± 3.7% for MVR, 67 ± 5.9% for AVR, 43 ± 8.3% for DVR, and 41 ± 7.8% for mVR (Fig. 1). The functional classification of 227 current survivors available for evaluation 11 years after surgery is shown in Table III: 102 are NYHA class I; 98, class II; 26, class III; and 1, class IV.

Thromboembolism and hemorrhage: Forty patients sustained a thromboembolic accident: 32 had MVR, 2 AVR, 1 DVR, and 5 mVR; this corresponds to a linearized incidence of 2.2% patient years for MVR, 0.6% for AVR, 1.0% for DVR, and 1.6% for mVR. Seven embolic episodes occurred within the first 6 postoperative months and 33 after the first year (10 of which occurred after the 6th year). Twelve emboli were fatal, with an incidence of 0.5% patient years for MVR, 0.3% for AVR, 1.0% for DVR, and 1.0% for mVR (Table IV). The risk of thromboembolism in the whole population of patients is analyzed in Table VII. The actuarial probability of freedom from emboli at 11 years is 81 ± 3% for MVR, 95 ± 3% for AVR, 95 ± 4% for DVR, and 90 ± 4% for mVR (Fig. 2).

Eight of 32 patients sustaining embolic episodes after MVR were in SR and 24 in AF. The probability of freedom from emboli in patients with MVR and SR -vs- patients with MVR and AF were not statistically significant.

TABLE VII Risk of thromboembolism in patients with porcine bioprostheses

	MVR	AVR	DVR	mVR	Total
Patients at risk	227	59	23	52	361
Patients with SR	57	52	16	32	157
Patients with AF	170	7	7	20	204
Patients with thromboemboli	32	2	1	5	40
Patients receiving anticoagulants	88	7	6	29	130
% patients free of emboli 11 years postoperatively	81 ± 3	95 ± 3	95 ± 4	90 ± 4	90 ± 3

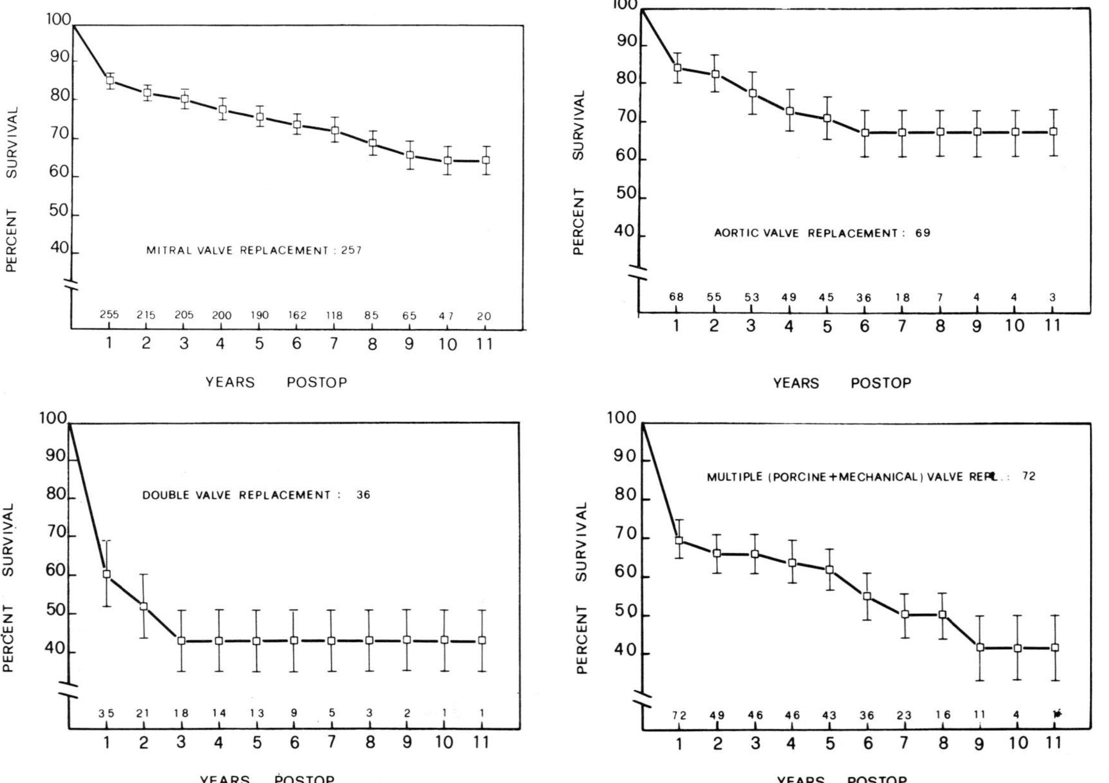

FIG. 1 Overall actuarial survival rates in patients undergoing mitral valve replacement (MVR), aortic valve replacement (AVR), double Hancock valve replacement (DVR) and multiple valve replacement (mVR). Operative mortality is included and number of patients at risk each year postoperatively is shown.

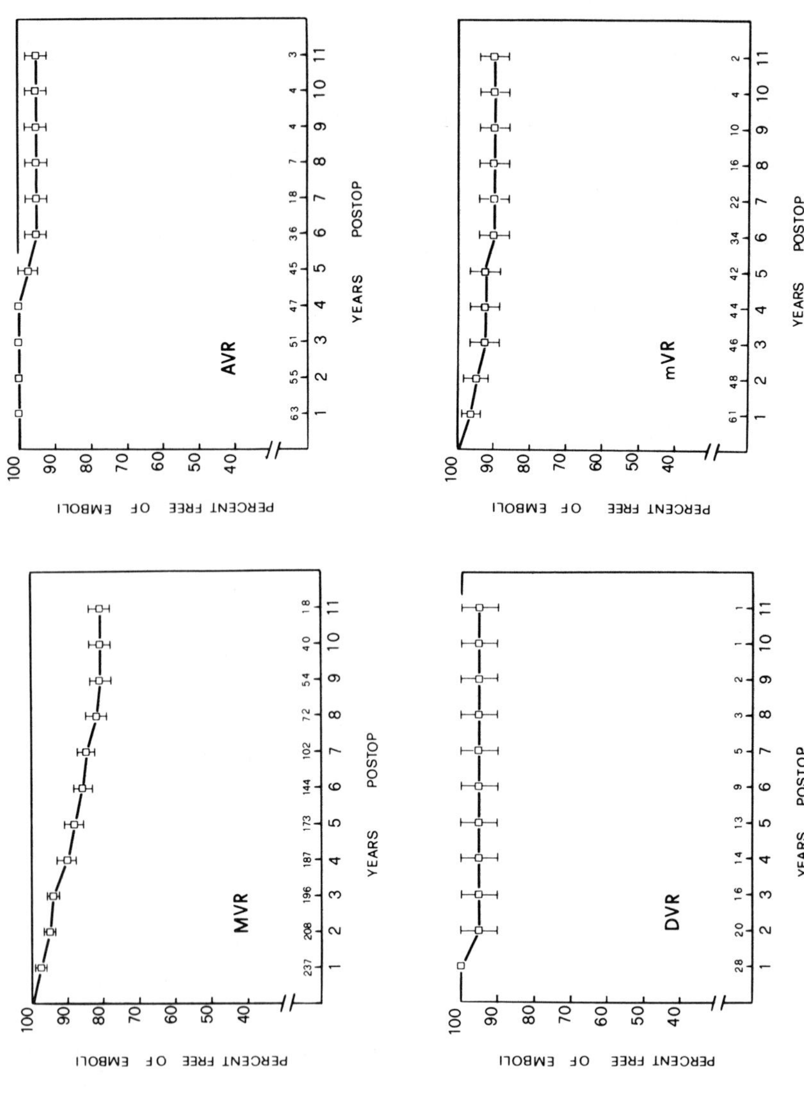

FIG. 2 Actuarial probability of being free of emboli in patients after MVR, AVR, DVR, and mVR. Number of patients at risk is indicated.

Anticoagulant-related hemorrhage was observed in 12 patients and caused death in 6 (because of cerebral hemorrhage in 3 and profuse gastrointestinal bleeding in 3); this corresponds to an overall incidence of 0.5% and 0.3% patient years, respectively (Table IV).

Endocarditis: Endocarditis occurred in 9 patients of this series (4 MVR, 4 AVR, and 1 mVR), most of whom required emergency reoperation. There were 7 operative deaths. The linearized incidence of bioprosthetic infection is 0.3% patient years for MVR, 1.3% patient years for AVR, and 0.3% patient years for mVR patients (Table IV). The morphologic features of infected porcine bioprostheses as well as the microorganisms involved in some of these patients have been reported elsewhere.[17]

Primary tissue failure: Primary tissue failure was observed in 28 patients, who required reoperation; among them, 16 had had MVR; 8, AVR; 1, DVR; and 3, mVR. There were 3 operative deaths (10.7%) (Table VI).

The probability of being free from primary tissue failure at 11 years is 74 ± 6.7% for porcine valves implanted in the mitral position and 66 ± 11% for those in the aortic position (p, NS) (Fig. 3). Including endocarditis, actuarial probability of being free from bioprosthetic dysfunction at 11 years is 72 ± 7% for MVR patients, 57 ± 11% for AVR, 93.7 ± 6% for DVR, and 74.8 ± 11% for mVR (Fig. 4).

The average duration of the explanted devices was 7.2 years for the mitral and 5.8 years for the aortic (p, NS). The mean age of patients requiring reoperation was 43 years, ranging from 11 to 68 years; 3 patients were younger than 15 years of age.

The prevalent mode of failure of both mitral and aortic porcine bioprostheses was the calcification of the cusps, causing stenosis in 12 (10 mitral and 2 aortic) and incompetence in 11 (5 mitral and 6 aortic). Stenosis resulted from calcific deposition and cusp stiffening, whereas incompetence derived from tears and commissural detachment at the site of calcium infiltration (Table VIII).

Comment

Since March 1970, the glutaraldehyde-treated Hancock porcine bioprosthesis has been extensively employed at our institution for heart valve replacement. Previous reports from our center[7,18] emphasized the low incidence of thromboembolic events, the satisfactory performance, and the acceptable rate of bioprosthetic dysfunction at short- and medium-term analysis; such results were confirmed by various other groups.[3,4,6] The fate of the porcine valve beyond 10 years of function is currently not fully assessed and uncertain. Since our experience with this device began quite early, information that is available on a considerable number of patients at risk for bioprosthetic failure 10 or more years postoperatively may help to clarify this issue at least in part.

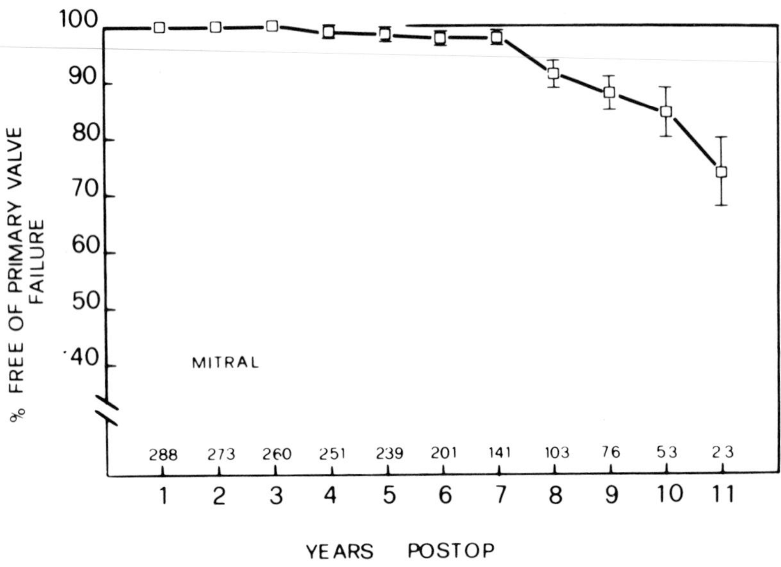

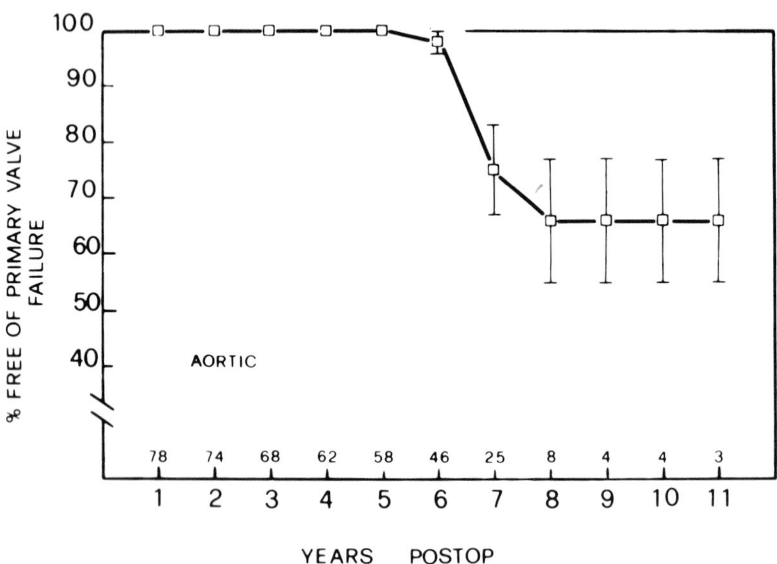

FIG. 3 Actuarial rates of freedom from primary tissue failure in patients with a Hancock valve implanted in mitral or aortic position. Number of valves at risk each postoperative year is shown.

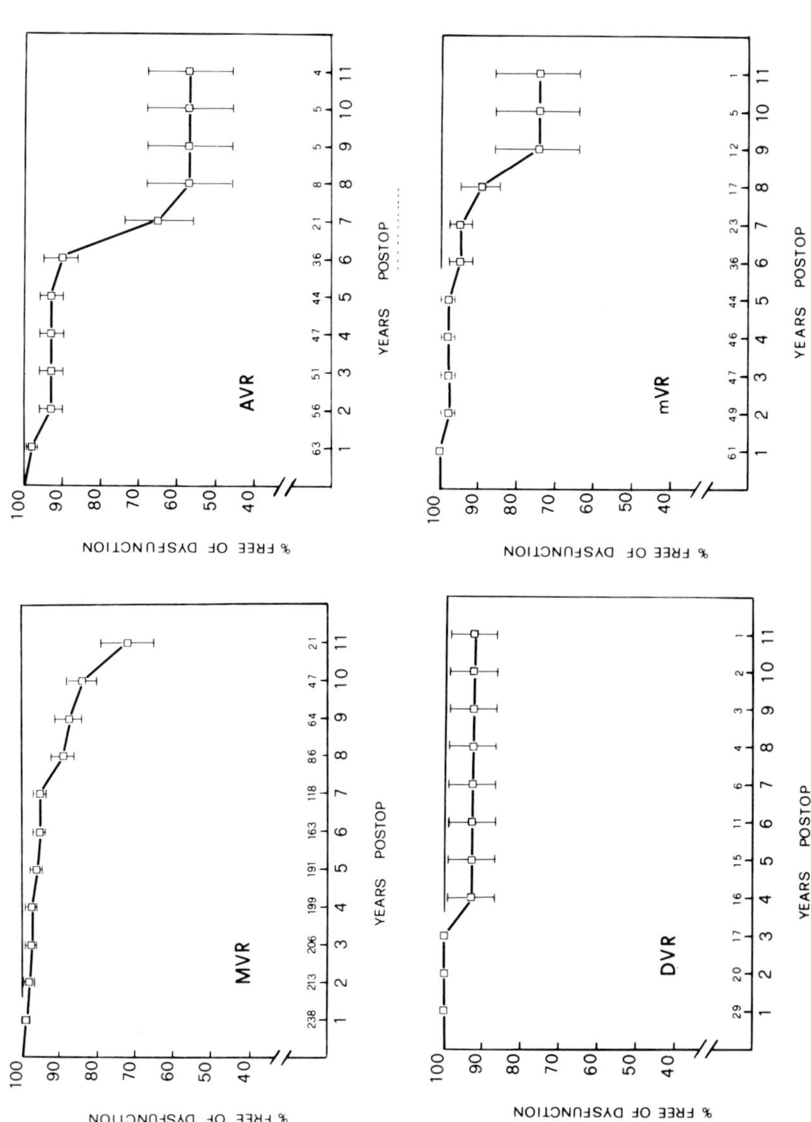

FIG. 4 Actuarial rates of freedom from bioprosthetic dysfunction, including endocarditis, in patients with MVR, AVR, DVR and mVR. Number of valves at risk is indicated.

TABLE VIII Primary tissue failure

	Mitral bioprostheses	Aortic bioprostheses
Bioprostheses at risk	296	80
Range of follow-up (yrs)	4.9–11.5	5.0–11.6
# bioprostheses with primary tissue failure	20	8
Average duration before reoperation (yrs)	7.2	5.8
Range (yrs)	2.8–10.7	3.5–6.6
Bioprostheses free of primary tissue failure at 11 years postoperatively (%)	74 ± 6.7	66.0 ± 11.0

Patient survival: Hospital mortality was quite high in this series and particularly in patients undergoing double or multiple valve replacement. This might be explained by the fact that many patients have been operated at the beginning of our experience and all of them before cold cardioplegia was routinely added to the surgical procedures.[19,20] Long-term survival at 1.1 years postoperatively in patients undergoing MVR or AVR is certainly noteworthy (Fig. 1), since it approximates that reported by Oyer and colleagues[9] at 5 years and by Borkon and associates[21] at 10 years for MVR alone.

Endocarditis: Infection of bioprosthetic valves is rare in our series. All 9 patients underwent reoperation either because antibiotic treatment failed to control the infective process or because endocarditis presented with a rapidly progressing course and early onset of unmanageable cardiac failure. Therefore our results are at variance with those of Gallo et al,[22] who reported 18 patients with bacterial endocarditis on a Hancock valve, 7 of whom were successfully treated without surgery. We cannot confirm the concept that porcine heterografts, once infected, may be quite easily sterilized.[23,24]

Thromboembolism: A low incidence of thromboembolic accidents in patients receiving porcine xenografts is commonly observed in most major clinical series;[3–9,21,22,25] nevertheless, these data are not easily comparable, since the attitude toward long-term anticoagulation in patients with porcine valves varies. Borkon and co-workers[21] reported an incidence of embolism of 2.4% patient years following MVR; most of their patients were not anticoagulated. These data compare favorably with other series in which anticoagulants were more extensively used, such as that of Oyer et al[9] and Cohn et al.[25]

AF is considered a major determinant of atrial thrombosis and systemic emboli.[14,21] In our series it is difficult to assess the importance of AF in this respect, since the probability of being free from emboli at 11 years for patients with MVR and SR was not significantly different from that of patients with MVR and AF. Moreover, at least half of the patients with AF who experienced systemic emboli after MVR were on oral warfarin, although it is difficult to assess the true level of this treatment for some of the patients who were followed at a distance.

Bioprosthesis durability: Long-term durability of the glutaraldehyde-treated porcine bioprosthesis still represents a major concern. Data so far available document good durability of this device up to 6 years after implantation,[13,15] but are not enough to rule out the problem of repeated reoperations, which is now facing many cardiac surgeons.

According to our results, probability of being free of primary tissue failure at 11 years is 74% for mitral and 66% for aortic bioprostheses. Although this difference is not statistically significant, we have the strong impression, as confirmed recently by Lakier and colleagues,[26] that xenografts in the aortic position degenerate earlier than in the mitral. The main cause of primary tissue failure in this series was the occurrence of progressive calcific infiltration that causes cusp stiffening with prosthetic stenosis or commissural detachment and loss of substance with valvular incompetence. This complication was observed not only in patients of the pediatric age group, who are recognized as having an increased tendency to early calcification of the bioprostheses,[27–29] but also in older subjects with no obvious predisposing factor. Other causes of primary tissue failure in this series were much less frequent; this indicates that eliminating or delaying the calcific process, most likely by improving the methods of valve preservation, might be the clue to solving the problem of long-term durability of tissue valves.

Conclusion

Recently, we have drawn a protocol for the treatment of valvular patients, in which the first principle is based on an attempt to preserve the native valve, unless badly damaged by endocarditis, calcification, or gross alterations of the subvalvular apparatus. A second important point is age: the duration of currently available types of porcine valves should go beyond the 10th year, perhaps reach the 15th or longer. If the new modalities of preparation and fixation of the biologic material, the new mounting techniques, and special chemical treatment to prevent mineralization give the expected results, it seems reasonable to extend the indications for porcine bioprostheses implant. This means that our present policy to avoid the use of such devices in young people and to adopt them preferentially in patients older than 55 could be changed, although we would still hesitate to employ them in children.

A third point must also be mentioned: porcine bioprostheses so far are usually not implanted in small anuli, especially the aortic, or in the mitral position when the left ventricle is small. In our early experience a few lethal complications were related either to left ventricular rupture or outflow obstruction due to the size of the valve struts,[19,20] or to important residual transvalvular gradients due to the small inner diameter in aortic bioprostheses less than 23 mm in size. In these cases, if one chooses to implant a biologic valve, excellent results can be obtained with pericardial xenografts, whose long-term behavior is reported to be satisfactory.[30]

A fourth issue is that of anticoagulation and of thromboembolism. There is little doubt about the very low thrombogenicity of bioprostheses, being close to 0 in the aortic position and quite acceptable in MVR and DVR (Table IV). However, it has become customary for many centers to keep the patient on long-term anticoagulant therapy in MVR with AF, giant left atrium, history of previous embolic episodes, or atrial thrombosis found at surgery.[15,22,25] Nevertheless, many of the embolic episodes recorded in our series happened during the first few months after surgery, sometimes with the patient still in the hospital.[7]

Dysfunction of the bioprosthesis, due to primary tissue failure, is an expected event in all cases but it develops rapidly in the young. The main pathologic feature seems to be deposition of calcium, which leads to stiffening, loss of motility, laceration, and even fragmentation.[31] The process is obviously very slow and the occurrence of symptoms of valve failure is gradual, so as to give time for diagnosis and treatment; this is an advantage if compared with the abrupt, often fatal, dysfunction of mechanical devices.[15]

Our experience with glutaraldehyde-fixed porcine bioprostheses is now approaching the 12th year and has definitely been quite interesting, fruitful, and rewarding. It has taught us much about the natural history of these devices and of the patients who carry them. They usually admit to enjoying a better life, both because of the clinical improvement and of the favorable characteristics of these prostheses, such as noiselessness, avoidance of routine anticoagulation, and possibility of bearing children. With time, we have, as has everybody else, understood the limitations of these devices and have relatively restricted their use compared to the initial enthusiasm. We intend to continue to implant them, convinced of the good qualities of these prostheses and expecting even better long-term results from the new products now available, provided the technical and chemical modifications prove efficacious.

References

1. Reis RL, Hancock WD, Yarbrough JW, Clancy DL, Morrow AG: The flexible stent. A new concept in the fabrication of tissue heart valve prosthesis. J Thorac Cardiovasc Surg 62:683, 1971.

2. Carpentier A, Deloche A, Relland J, Fabiani JN, Forman J, Camilleri IP, Soyer R, Dubost C: Six-year follow-up of glutaraldehyde-preserved heterografts. J Thorac Cardiovasc Surg 68:771, 1974.
3. Horowitz MS, Goodman DJ, Fogarty TJ, Harrison DC: Mitral valve replacement with the glutaraldehyde-preserved porcine heterograft. J Thorac Cardiovasc Surg 67:885, 1974.
4. Zuhdi N, Hawley W, Voehl V, Hancock W, Carey J, Greer A: Porcine aortic valves as replacements of human heart valves. Ann Thorac Surg 17:479, 1974.
5. Cohn LH, Lamberti JJ, Castaneda AR, Collins JJ Jr: Cardiac valve replacement with the stabilized glutaraldehyde porcine aortic valve: Indications, operative results and follow-up. Chest 68:162, 1975.
6. McIntosh CL, Michaelis LL, Morrow AG, Itscoitz SB, Redwood DR, Epstein SE: Atrioventricular valve replacement with the Hancock porcine xenograft: A five year clinical experience. Surgery 78:768, 1975.
7. Cévese PG, Gallucci V, Morea M, Dalla Volta S, Fasoli G, Casarotto D: Heart valve replacement with the Hancock bioprosthesis. Analysis of long-term results. Circulation 56 (Suppl II):111, 1977.
8. Davila JC, Magilligan DR Jr, Lewis JW Jr: Is the Hancock porcine valve the best cardiac valve substitute today? Ann Thorac Surg 26:303, 1978.
9. Oyer PE, Stinson EB, Reitz BA, Craig Miller D, Rossiter SJ, Shumway NE: Long-term evaluation of the porcine xenograft bioprosthesis. J Thorac Cardiovasc Surg 78:343, 1979.
10. Spray TL, Roberts WC: Structural changes in porcine xenografts used as substitute cardiac valves. Am J Cardiol 40:319, 1977.
11. Fishbein MC, Gissen SA, Collins JJ Jr, Barsamian EM, Cohn LH: Pathologic findings after cardiac valve replacement with glutaraldehyde-fixed porcine valves. Am J Cardiol 40:331, 1977.
12. Ferrans VJ, Spray TL, Billingham ME, Roberts WC: Structural changes in glutaraldehyde-treated porcine heterografts used as substitute cardiac valves. Transmission and scanning electron microscopy observations in 12 patients. Am J Cardiol 41:1159, 1978.
13. Magilligan DJ Jr, Lewis JW Jr, Jara FM, Lee MW, Alam M, Riddle JM, Stein PD: Spontaneous degeneration of porcine bioprosthetic valves. Ann Thorac Surg 30:259, 1980.
14. Thiene G, Bortolotti U, Panizzon G, Milano A, Gallucci V: Pathological substrates of thrombus formation after heart valve replacement with the Hancock bioprosthesis. J Thorac Cardiovasc Surg 80:414, 1980.
15. Oyer PE, Craig Miller D, Stinson EB, Reitz BA, Moreno-Cabral RJ, Shumway NE: Clinical durability of the Hancock porcine bioprosthesis. J Thorac Cardiovasc Surg 80:824, 1980.
16. Anderson RP, Boncheck LI, Grunkemeier GE, Malbert LE, Starr A: The analysis and presentation of surgical results by actuarial methods. J Surg Res 16:224, 1974.
17. Bortolotti U, Thiene G, Milano A, Panizzon G, Valente M, Gallucci V: Pathological study of infective endocarditis on Hancock porcine bioprostheses. J Thorac Cardiovasc Surg 81:934, 1981.
18. Casarotto D, Bortolotti U, Thiene G, Gallucci V, Cévese PG: Long-term results (from 5 to 7 years) with the Hancock SGP bioprosthesis. J Cardiovasc Surg 20:399, 1979.
19. Thiene G, Bortolotti U, Casarotto D, Valfré C, Gallucci V: Prosthesis-left ventricle disproportion in mitral valve replacement with the Hancock biopros-

thesis: Pathologic observations. In Bioprosthetic Cardiac Valves (F Sebening, WB Klövekorn, H Meisner, E Struck, Eds). Munich, Deutsches Herzzentrum, 1979, p 357.

20. Bortolotti U, Thiene G, Casarotto D, Mazzucco A, Gallucci V: Left ventricular rupture following mitral valve replacement with a Hancock bioprosthesis. Chest 77:235, 1980.
21. Borkon AM, McIntosh CL, Von Rueden TJ, Morrow AG: Mitral valve replacement with the Hancock bioprosthesis: Five to ten year follow-up. Ann Thorac Surg 32:128, 1981.
22. Gallo JI, Ruiz B, Carrion MF, Gutierrez JA, Vega JL, Duran CMG: Heart valve replacement with the Hancock bioprosthesis. A 6-year review. Ann Thorac Surg 31:444, 1981.
23. Magilligan DR Jr, Quinn EL, Davila JC: Bacteremia, endocarditis and the Hancock valve. Ann Thorac Surg 24:508, 1977.
24. Rossiter SJ, Stinson EB, Oyer PE, Craig Miller D, Schapira JN, Martin RP, Shumway NE: Prosthetic valve endocarditis. Comparison of heterograft tissue valves and mechanical valves. J Thorac Cardiovasc Surg 76:795, 1979.
25. Cohn LH, Mudge GH, Pratter F, Collins JJ Jr: Five to eight year follow-up of patients undergoing porcine heart valve replacement. New Engl J Med 304:258, 1981.
26. Lakier JB, Khaja F, Magilligan DJ Jr, Goldstein S: Porcine xenograft valves. Long-term (60−89 months) follow-up. Circulation 62:313, 1980.
27. Kutsche LM, Oyer PE, Shumway NE, Baum D: An important complication of Hancock mitral valve replacement in children. Circulation 60 (Suppl. I):98, 1979.
28. Saunders SP, Levy RJ, Freed MD, Norwood WI, Castaneda AR: Use of Hancock porcine xenografts in children and adolescents. Am J Cardiol 46:429, 1980.
29. Bortolotti U, Thiene G: Calcification of porcine heterografts implanted in children. Chest 80:117, 1981.
30. Ionescu MI, Tandon AP: Long-term clinical and hemodynamic evaluation of the Ionescu-Shiley pericardial xenograft heart valve. In *Bioprosthetic Cardiac Valves* (F Sebening, WP Klövekorn, H Meisner, E Struck, eds) Munich, Deutsches Herzzentrum, 1979, p 199.
31. Ferrans VJ, Boyce SW, Billingham ME, Jones M, Ishihara T, Roberts WC: Calcific deposits in porcine bioprostheses: Structure and pathogenesis. Am J Cardiol 46:721, 1980.

3

A 14-Year Experience with Valvular Bioprostheses: Valve Survival and Patient Survival

A. Deloche, P. Perier, H. Bourezak, S. Chauvaud, P. G. Donzeau-Gouge, G. Dreyfus, J. N. Fabiani, H. Massoud, A. Carpentier, C. Dubost

The introduction of glutaraldehyde[1] in 1968 was associated with improved clinical results when compared to previous techniques of tissue preservation; valvular bioprosthesis became a reasonable alternative to the mechanical valve because of such specific advantages as reduced thromboembolism and fatal complications and because of improved quality of life due to possible freedom from anticoagulant.

Limited valve durability, however, has been a serious concern over the years. It is likely that durability will be further increased in the future as a result of improved techniques of glutaraldehyde preservation and better valve mounting, but limited durability will always be the natural fate of valvular bioprosthesis and the price to pay for their advantages. Limited survival of the valve, however, does not imply limited survival of the patient, since progressive valve deterioration allows reoperation of the patient before the onset of serious complications. This is the point we would like to emphasize, by analyzing long-term results from 5–14 years postoperatively, including the very first patients operated upon with glutaraldehyde-preserved valve tissue.

Patients and Methods

Our experience comprises 443 patients operated upon from 1968–1978 for either aortic valve replacements (AVR), 229 patients, or mitral valve

---

From the Clinique de Chirurgie Cardiovasculaire, Hôpital Broussais, Paris, France.

replacement (MVR), 214 patients. These patients can be separated into 3 groups according to the method of tissue preservation and the technique of valve mounting.

Group I (1968): buffered glutaraldehyde-preserved valves. Porcine valves were preserved in 1% phosphate glutaraldehyde and mounted in a flexible stent in our experimental laboratory. Of 10 patients operated upon, 7 survived the operation.

Group II (1968–1974): oxidized glutaraldehyde-preserved valves. This series comprises 65 porcine valves mounted on a rigid stent and preserved by oxidized glutaraldehyde (0.6%) solution. Of 65 patients operated upon, 55 survived (11 with mitral valves and 44 with aortic valves).

Group III (1974–1978): commercially available valves. In this series, valves were preserved in phosphate-buffered glutaraldehyde solution and mounted in a semirigid stent (Hancock), or on a flexible stent (Carpentier-Edwards). This group comprises 174 aortic valve replacements (82 Hancock and 92 Carpentier-Edwards), and 192 mitral valve replacements (88 Hancock and 104 Carpentier-Edwards). Of 366 patients operated upon, 339 survived (176 with mitral valves and 163 with aortic valves), for a hospital mortality of 7.8%.

Clinical follow-up was achieved by examination of the patient in our hospital or by written questionnaire with return postcard. Criteria for the diagnosis of valve failure were based on 1 or more of the following circumstances: 1) Infective endocarditis resulting in reoperation or death; 2) thrombotic occlusion of the valve necessitating reoperation or resulting in death; 3) periprosthetic leak; 4) tissue failure resulting from either calcification or perforation or both; 5) "intrinsic stenosis" diagnosed on the presence of a transvalvular gradient requiring reoperation without primary tissue alteration.

Results

Group I. This group of 7 patients is particularly important because it represents the longest follow-up available with any glutaraldehyde-preserved tissue valve. Seven patients were followed up to 14 years after implantation. No valves demonstrated evidence of dysfunction during the first 6 years. Two valves failed during the 6th year, 1 from calcification and 1 from cusp perforation.

A 3rd patient reoperated upon 6 years after operation for thrombosis of the left atrium displayed a well-functioning valve that was nevertheless replaced for examination. Histologic study revealed collagen degeneration with areas of hyalinization.

A 4th patient underwent reoperation during the 7th year for a perivalvular leak and died a few months postoperatively.

A 5th valve, in the mitral position, failed 9 years after the operation and displayed cusp perforation.

Two patients are still alive and well with their original aortic valves 14 years after the operation.

Group II: Among the 55 survivors in this group, 6 were lost to follow-up. Eighteen patients died within 13 years following surgery, for a survival rate of 52% at 12 years.

There were 27 cases of valve failure. The actuarial incidence of aortic and mitral valve failure is 32% at 5 years and 68% at 12 years (Fig. 1). Fig. 2 summarizes the various causes of valve failure. Primary tissue failure was

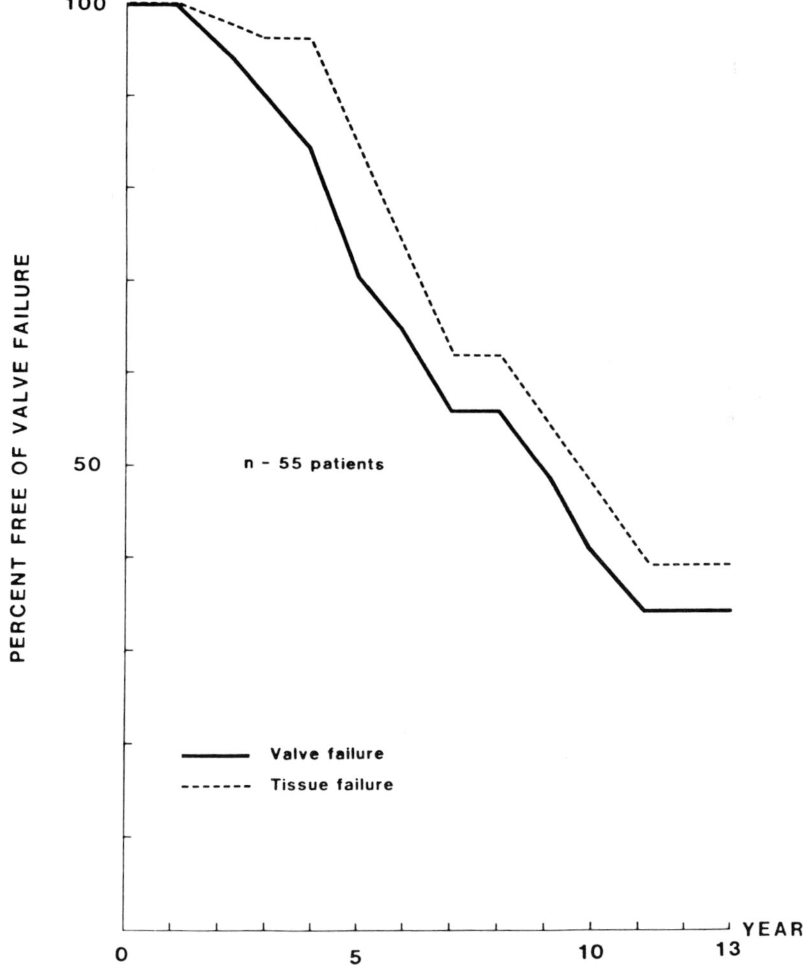

FIG. 1 Actuarial rates of bioprosthesis valve failure and tissue failure (group II).

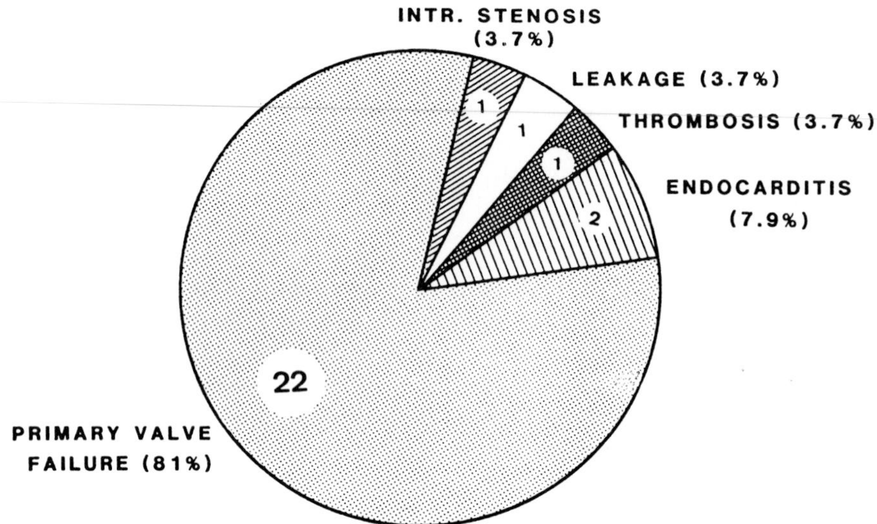

FIG. 2 Summary of the various causes of valve failure (group II).

the most prevalent cause overall (81%) with a similar proportion in both the aortic and the mitral series.

Lesions were primarily calcifications, cusp tears, or perforation. Calcification was more frequent (86%) than expected and probably related to the oxidation process used in association with glutaraldehyde treatment and/or a rigid stent.

Reoperation was performed in 25 patients with a hospital mortality of 28%. Operative mortality rate differed according to the valve location: 50% for the mitral group and 21% for the aortic group. This high mortality rate associated with reoperation in the early series is explained by several factors: poor myocardial preservation and reoperation at a late stage.

Fifty-six percent of the patients are still alive at 12 years, a result that compares favorably with other series of valve replacement in spite of the high mortality associated during reoperation in this series.

Thromboembolic episodes were diagnosed in 3 cases (0.7% per patient year) with 1 instance of thrombosis of the bioprosthesis.

Group III: Among 339 survivors, 37 were lost to follow-up. Actuarial survival rate after MVR expressed as linearized occurrence rate was 4.5% per patient year. The 6 year probability of survival for MVR patients was 73 ± 4.9%. The actuarial survival rate after AVR expressed as linearized occurrence rate was 3.1% per patient year. The 6 year probability of survival for AVR patients was 77 ± 3.7%. The mortality rate related to the bioprosthesis was 0.9% per patient year for MVR, and 0.7% per patient year for AVR.

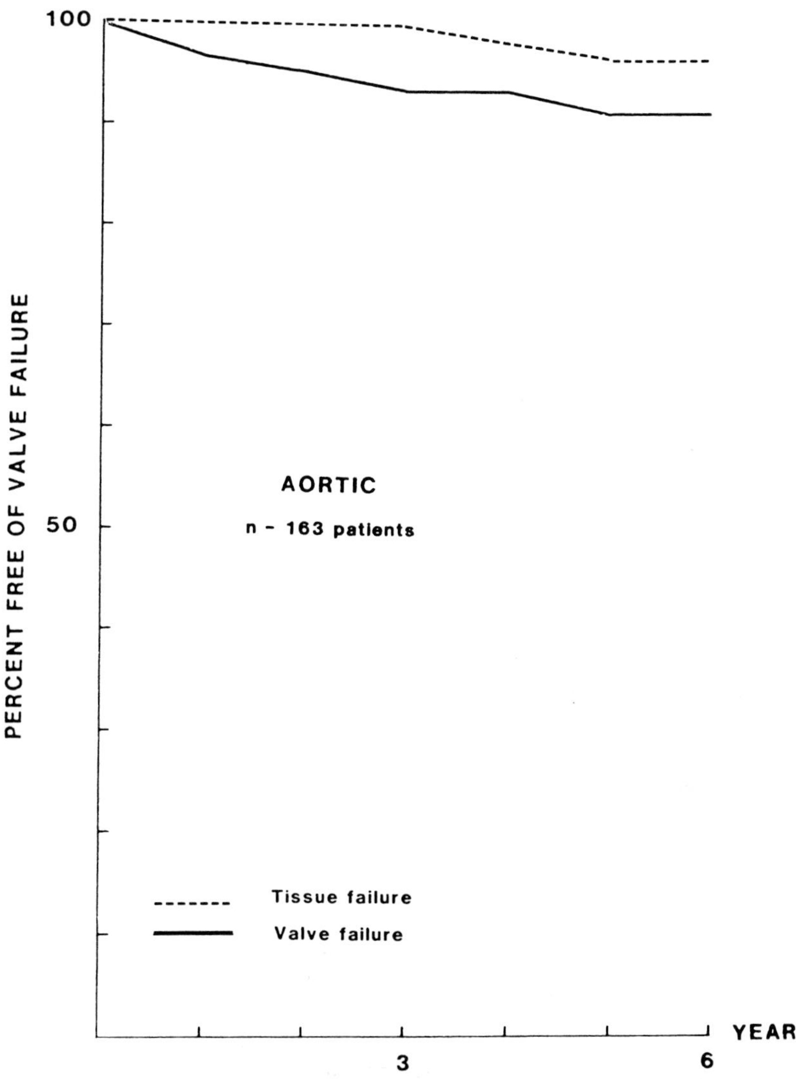

FIG. 3 Actuarial rates of valve failure and tissue failure for AVR patients (group III).

The actuarial incidence of aortic valve failure from all causes among adult patients is shown in Fig. 3. The actuarial probability of remaining free of valve dysfunction for AVR patients was 92 ± 3.6% at 6 years and for MVR patients it was 77 ± 2.7%. Linearized rates of valve failure for AVR and MVR were 1.2 and 2.4% per patient year, respectively. The proportionate contributions to valve failure differed according to valve location. For example, in AVR patients, endocarditis accounted for the majority of failures.

The primary tissue failure incidence was the same in both groups and was not the prevalent cause of valve failure (25%). No differences were observed between the Hancock and Carpentier-Edwards valve series.

The limited number of valves (6) that have failed revealed calcification, cusp perforation, or rupture with focal calcification.

All the primary tissue failure occurred after the third year. No increased tendency toward late bioprosthesis failure can be observed within the constraints of the follow-up period (Fig. 4).

Reoperation for valve failure was necessary in 22 patients with an operative mortality of 13.6% (3/22), and this mortality rate differed from the mode of valve failure, being particularly severe for the endocarditis.

The linearized rate of thromboembolism among MVR patients was 2.4% and among AVR patients, 0.9%/patient/year. Actuarially determined rates of thromboembolism are shown in Figs. 5 and 6. It must be noticed that the risk of thromboembolism was higher during the early postoperative period.

Comment

Continuous research and development of better techniques of valve design and valve preservation in the last 10 years have been associated with significant improvements with the glutaraldehyde-preserved bioprosthesis.[2,3]

The incidence of valve failure was lower in the group of valves treated by glutaraldehyde without oxidation; hence, this technique has been accepted as the method of choice. A valve removed after 6 years and 2 months in the mitral position showed normal function. However, slight collagen degeneration and elastin fragmentation were present due to fatigue lesions. There was a thin layer of fibrin and connective tissue extending over the surface of the cusps and reinforcing the tissue valve. This process of encapsulation could play a significant role in the future of the valve. The use of shock-absorbing flexible stent, as well as production on an industrial scale with accurate selection of the valves and quality control, is critical for improving the durability of valves. When compared clinically, the results obtained with the commercially available valves allows one to predict a 20–30% failure rate at 10 years.

As clearly pointed out in this study, tissue failure is the main concern associated with valvular bioprosthesis. However, it is important to stress that tissue failure should not imply patient death if the reoperation is carried out at the proper stage. Our overall series comprises 32 patients reoperated upon for tissue failure who can be separated in 2 groups: those reoperated upon between 1970 and 1978 with an operative mortality of 35% and those

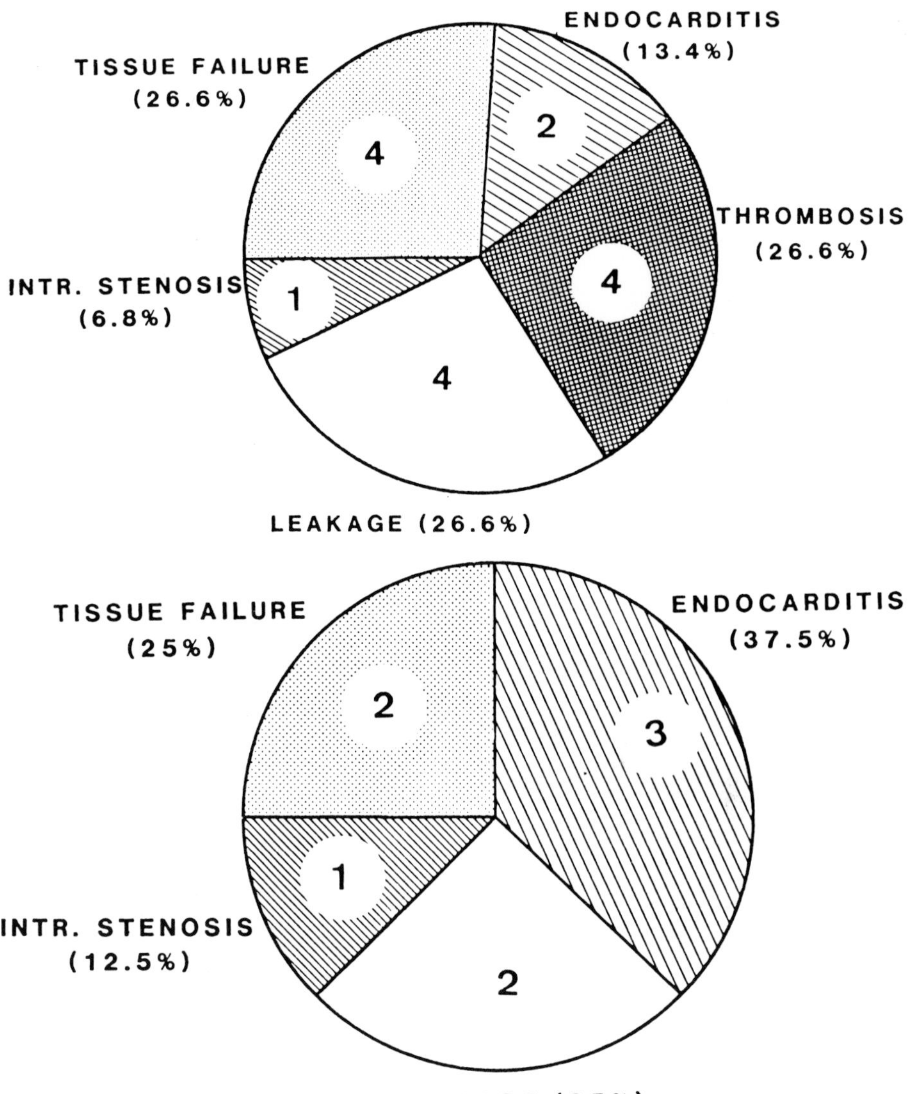

FIG. 4 Various modes of valve failure. (top) In MVR patients (group III), (bottom) in AVR patients (group III).

reoperated upon between 1979 and 1982 with no operative mortality. This is a result of an improved technique and earlier reoperation.

Bioprostheses, like any other artificial valves, are palliative and life-saving, but carries with them a certain risk. Their main advantage over mechanical valves is that of a better quality of life.

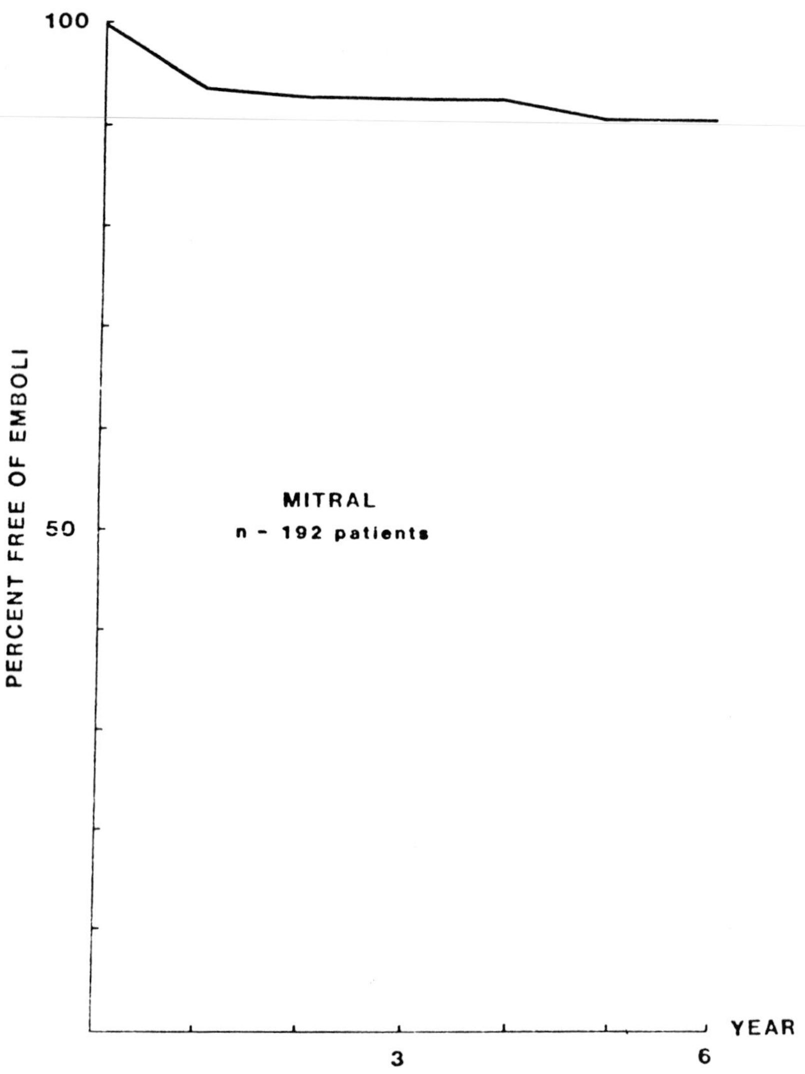

FIG. 5 Actuarial rates of thromboembolism among MVR patients (group III).

Summary

This study concerns the long-term results, from 5–14 years, of an experience that includes the first patients operated upon with glutaraldehyde-preserved tissue. Four hundred forty-three patients were operated on from 1968–1978 for either AVR or MVR.

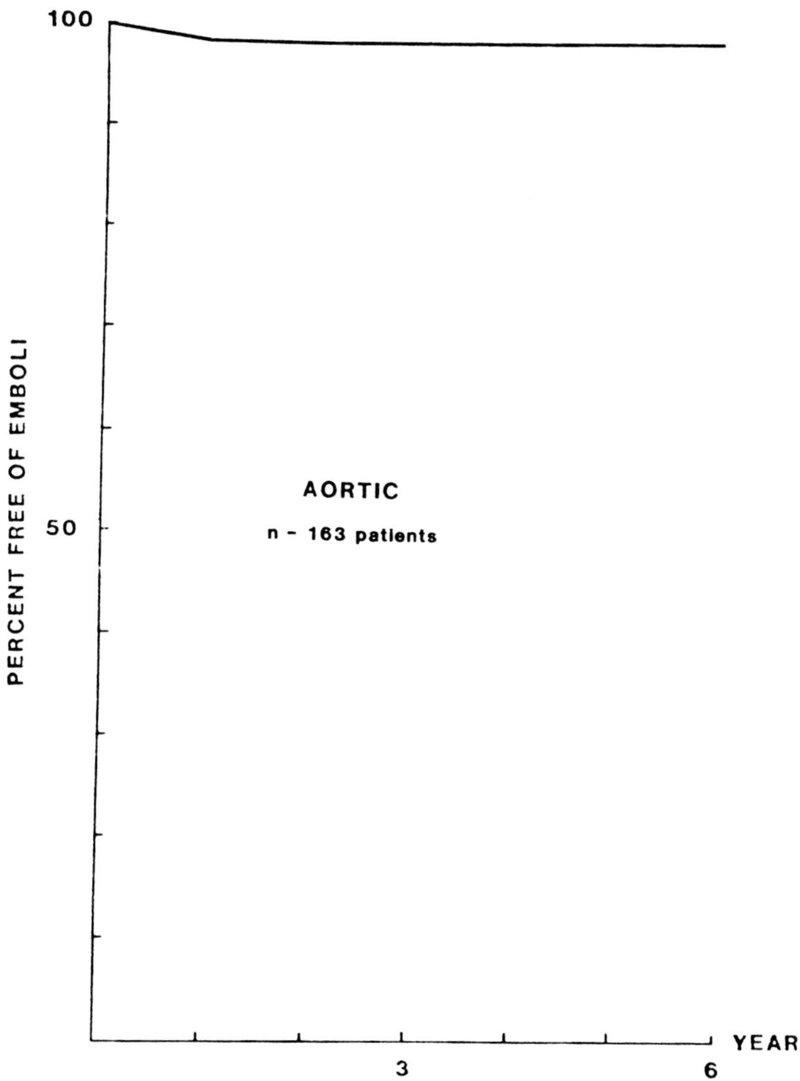

FIG. 6 Actuarial rates of thromboembolism among AVR patients (group III).

These patients can be separated into 3 groups according to the method of tissue preservation: 1) group I (1968): buffered glutaraldehyde-preserved valves (10 patients); 2) group II (1968–1974): oxidized glutaraldehyde-preserved valves (65 patients); 3) group III (1974–1978): commercially available valves (368 patients).

Our overall series comprises 32 patients reoperated upon for tissue failure who can be separated in 2 groups: those reoperated upon from 1970–1979, with an operative mortality of 35%, and those reoperated upon from 1979–1982, with no operative mortality. The latter has occurred as a result of improved myocardial protection and reoperations carried out at an earlier stage.

References

1. Carpentier A, Lamaigre CG, Robert L, Carpentier S, Dubost C: Biological factors affecting long-term results of valvular heterografts. J Thorac Cardiovasc Surg 58:467, 1969.
2. Carpentier A, Deloche A, Relland J, et al: Six-year follow-up of glutaraldehyde preserved heterografts: With particular reference to the treatment of congenital valve malformations. J Thorac Cardiovasc Surg 68:771, 1974.
3. Carpentier A: Valvular xenograft and valvular xenobioprostheses: Past, present, and future. Adv Cardiol 27:281, 1980.

4

A Thousand Porcine Bioprostheses Revisited. Do They Conform with the Expected Pattern?

C. M. G. DURAN, I. GALLO, B. RUIZ, J. M. REVUELTA, A. OCHOTECO

Since the beginning of our unit in 1974, the characteristics of our patient population determined our valvular policy. The distance of patients from the center and the difficulty in maintaining adequate levels of anticoagulation made mandatory a policy of maximum conservative surgery and, when necessary, replacement with bioprosthesis. Although it was assumed that these valves would at some point require replacement, it was thought that a period of time free of concern would balance the limited durability. After 8 years of applying these guidelines, it seemed appropriate to review our experience with porcine bioprostheses.

Patients and Materials

From 1974–1981, 1,292 porcine bioprostheses have been implanted at our institution in 1,114 patients. Of these bioprostheses, 955 were Hancock and 337, Carpentier-Edwards; 59 patients received simultaneously another type of mechanical or biologic prosthesis and were excluded from the study, leaving 1,055 patients with 1,233 bioprostheses. There have been 486 mitral valve replacements (MVR), 391 aortic (AVR), and 178 mitral and aortic replacements (MAVR). Associated procedures, such as conservative tricuspid anuloplasty, coronary bypass, or repair of a congenital malformation were performed in 336 patients (31.8%).

Of the 1,055 patients, 596 patients were male and 459 female. The mean age was of 44.5 years, with a range of 6–72; 59% of the patients were

From the Servicio de Cirugía Cardiovascular and Servicio de Cardiología, Centro Médico "Valdecilla," University of Santander, Santander, Spain.

between 40 and 60 years of age, only 3% were younger than 20, and 10% were older than 60.

Results

The overall operative mortality was of 8.5%. For MVR, it was of 9% (44/486), varying from 7% when isolated to 12% when associated with other types of surgery. For AVR, it was of 5.6% (22/391), varying from 4% when isolated to 8.7% when other surgery was performed simultaneously. For MAVR it was 13.5% whether other surgery was done or not.

All patients were reviewed either directly at the center or through contact with their cardiologist. The follow-up extends from 3–96 months. Seven patients were lost to follow-up (99.2% complete follow-up).

Fifty-four patients (5.5%) have died during the follow-up period. Twenty-five were MVR (5.6%), 17 were AVR (4.6%), and 12 MAVR (7.7%). The primary cause of death has been sudden and unexplained (26 cases), bacterial endocarditis (10 cases), intractable heart failure (5 cases), mitral valve thrombosis (2 cases), 1 of embolism, and 1 of cerebral hemorrhage from anticoagulation. Seven died at reoperation and 2 of noncardiac causes.

There have been 44 thromboembolic accidents in 37 cases. Eleven were peripheral and 33 central with 1 fatal outcome. The linearized incidence for AVR was 0.57% per patient years; for MVR, 2.03%; and for MAVR, 2.59%. It is interesting to note that the incidence of embolism was 9% among the 88 patients with permanent anticoagulation, 8.9% among the 292 with temporal anticoagulation, and 0.4% (2/457) and 0.7 (1/128) when antiaggregates or no antiembolic therapy had been used. No change in these percentages appeared when those patients with AVR were excluded (9.6, 1.6, and 2.1%, respectively).

The vast majority of patients enjoy improved physical capabilities: 74% of the patients were in functional class III or IV preoperatively and 96% were in class I–II postoperatively. Only 3/127 patients remained in class IV postoperatively.

Bacterial endocarditis has been the most common and most serious complication, 34 cases with a 38% mortality (13 cases); for MVR, there were 17 cases with 6 deaths; for AVR, 9 cases with 5 deaths; and for MAVR, 8 cases with 2 deaths. The mortality was higher when bacterial endocarditis appeared in the immediate postoperative period (43%) than during the subsequent follow-up (33%).

Eleven patients were reoperated upon for endocarditis, 3 in the immediate postoperative period with 3 deaths and 8 during the follow-up period with 2 deaths. The difference in mortality between the medical and surgical treatment of this complication is minimal (40 -vs- 45). It is, however, our clinical impression that an earlier, more aggressive surgical treatment of this condition should achieve better results. Excluding the early postoperative endocarditis, the medical treatment carries a mortality of 56% against 25% for the surgically treated.

Reoperations

The total number of patients requiring reoperation during the follow-up, which was extended to 99 months, was 62, an incidence of 6.2%. As already described, 8 were due to bacterial endocarditis with a mortality of 2 cases. These cases were scattered all along the follow-up period and were all Hancock bioprosthetic replacements.

Twenty-two patients were reoperated on without mortality for paravalvular leaks, an incidence of 1.6% for AVR, 2.7% for MVR, and 3.2% for MAVR. Fifteen cases were Hancock (2.1 incidence) and 7, Carpentier valves (2.7 incidence).

Thirty-two patients required reoperation for intrinsic tissue failure (32/1055, or 3%). Thirty were Hancock valves and 2 were Carpentier-Edwards. The operative mortality was 5/32 cases (15.6%).

The causes of valve failure were: 2 cases of mitral valve thrombosis at 3 and 6 months postoperatively, 1 case of mitral stenosis with a small Hancock valve, 9 patients with a rupture of the bioprosthesis appearing from 13–66 months postoperatively and 19 calcifications occurring from 13–80 months postoperatively (Fig. 1)

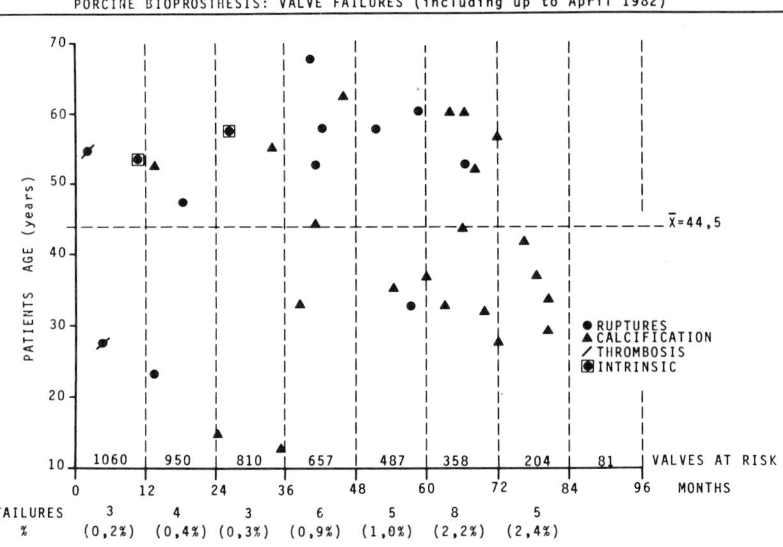

FIG. 1 Intrinsic valve failures. All cases presented relate age of the patient and time of follow-up to reoperation (32 cases) or death (2 cases).

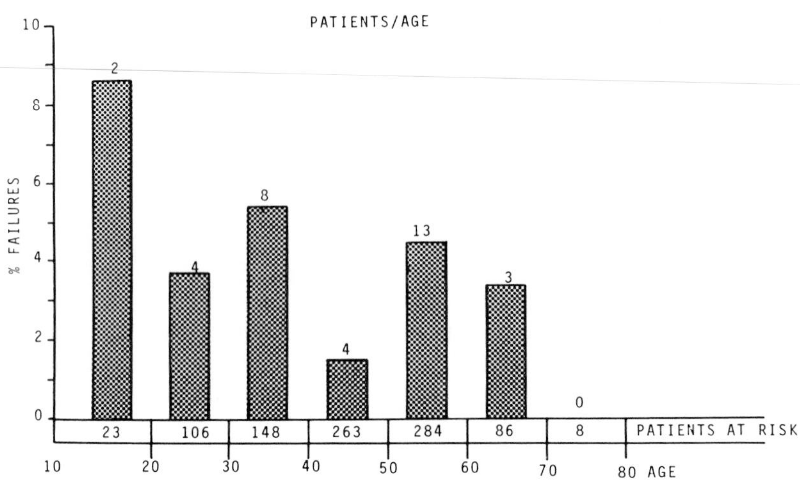

FIG. 2 Number and percentage of intrinsic valve failures per decade.

Intrinsic valve failures by patient's age are shown in Fig. 2. If this incidence is divided into those patients younger or those older than 30 years of age, the incidences are 4.6 and 3.5%, respectively. If the dividing line is at 40 years, the incidence is 3.9 and 1.5%, respectively. The actuarial rate of porcine bioprostheses free of intrinsic valve failures for up to 7.7 years with a total of 1,060 valves at risk is 90.7% (Figs. 3 and 4).

Finally, the overall actuarial survival rate of all patients with a porcine bioprosthesis excluding hospital mortality is 90.5% at 96 months of follow-up (Fig. 5).

Comment

Soon after the use of tissue valves[1–4] began, it became apparent that, although they represented a net improvement in terms of thromboembolism, their durability was limited. The introduction of the frame-mounted glutaraldehyde-preserved bioprosthesis[5–6] meant a very significant advantage, simplifying its insertion and prolonging its durability. However, the decision to use a tissue or a mechanical valve entailed a calculated risk, which even now after a follow-up of nearly 10 years remains difficult to undertake.[7–11] The characteristics of our patient population determined our decision, based on the difficulty of maintaining adequate levels of anticoagulation.

More than 1,000 porcine bioprostheses have been used in our unit from 1974–1982, with almost complete follow-up, since only 7 of 1,055 patients

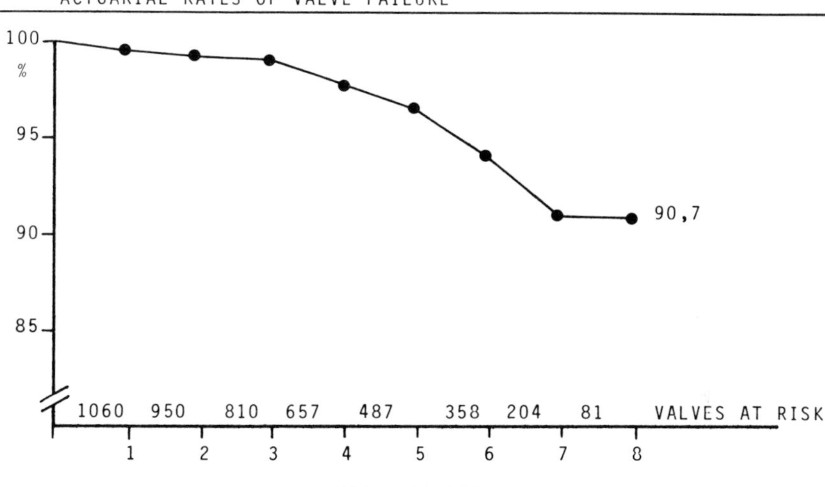

FIG. 3 Actuarial rate of bioprostheses free of intrinsic valve failures.

have failed to report after a last revision 12–27 months postoperatively. One third of the patients included in the study were polyvalvular mostly subjected to a conservative procedure on the mitral and tricuspid valves. Only a few had coronary bypass surgery in a population still dominated by rheumatic sequelae.

The 2 main causes of late death are sudden unexplained death and bacterial endocarditis. This latter complication carries a very high mortality and requires a better prophylaxis and, when suspected, a very prompt and aggressive attitude if better results are to be achieved. The thromboembolic rate confirms previous reports and only stresses the advantage of the bioprosthesis applied to a mostly nonanticoagulated population. Since the beginning, our policy has been only to anticoagulate permanently those patients with a mitral bioprosthesis who had a giant left atrium (relatively common among our patients) and/or large intraatrial (not in the appendage) thrombosis. It has to be stated that these guidelines were often not followed assiduously. The higher incidence of embolism found among the patients on permanent or temporal anticoagulation against those without any anticoagulation or only antiaggregates, in our opinion, is only an argument that the type of patient is a more important factor than the bioprosthesis. A comparative study performed at our center[12] of the incidence of thromboembolic complications between patients with mitral Hancock bioprostheses and mitral anuloplasties failed to differentiate these 2 techniques.

Sixty-two patients (6%) were reoperated upon. The number of reopera-

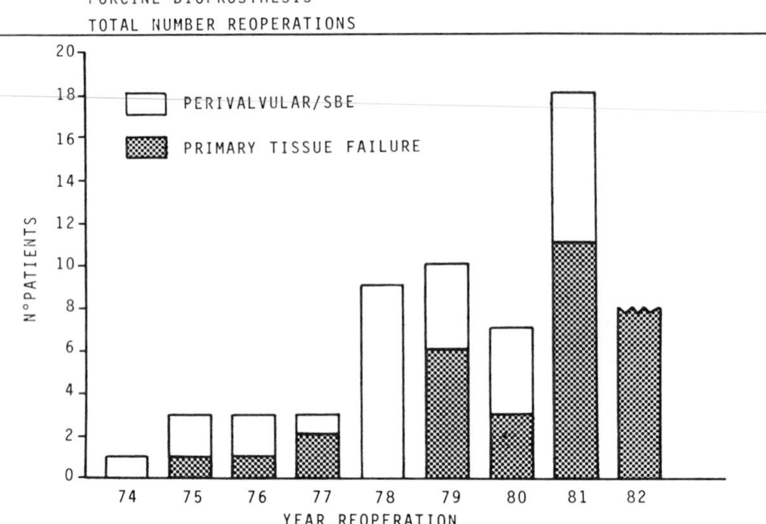

FIG. 4 Number of reoperations performed per year. Broken column corresponds to first 3 months of 1982.

tions have increased progressively and thus gives the initial impression that valves are failing at an increasing rate. In fact, if only those with mechanical failure or calcification are considered ("intrinsic tissue failure"), 34 cases out of 1,060 valves at risk for 96 months have failed, 32 of them being reoperated upon. The actuarial curve shows a 90.7% free of failures, with a plateau

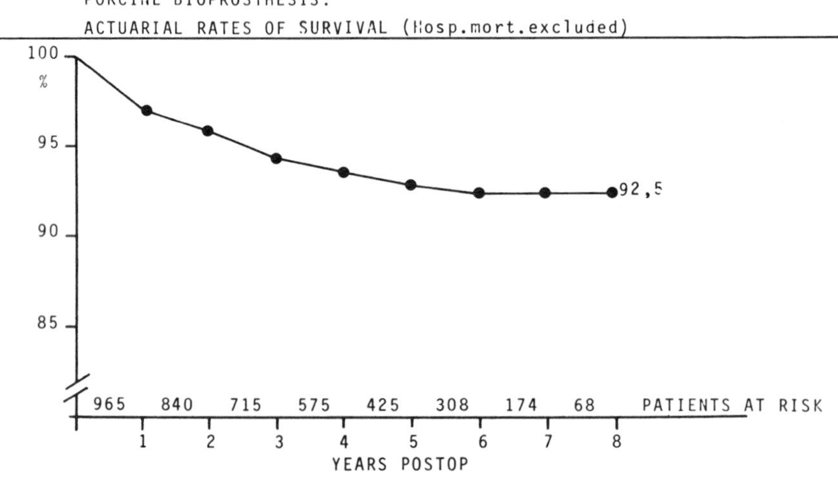

FIG. 5 Actuarial survival rate of all patients with a porcine bioprosthesis, excluding hospital mortality.

in the last year. This period only represents a small number of patients (81 cases) and therefore cannot yet be taken as significant. It is noteworthy in our experience that these valve failures do not seem to appear in a cluster after a certain postoperative date but rather are spread over a period of years. Only a few valves malfunction from manufacturing or surgical error, whereas some others rupture without evidence of calcification from 1–5 years. Others become progressively mineralized and stenotic, eventually rupturing from 4–7 years. A high proportion of valves remain functioning very satisfactorily. What proportion will maintain this level of competence remains to be known. We have not been able to relate clearly the age of the patient and likelihood of failure, excluding the very young. It is evident that bioprosthesis failures have a multifactorial cause where patient, surgeon, and manufacturer are involved.

References

1. Duran CG, Gunning AJ: Total homologous aortic valve in the sub-coronary position. Lancet 2:488, 1962.
2. Ross DN: Homograft replacement of the aortic valve. Lancet 2:487, 1962.
3. Duran CG, Gunning AJ: Heterologous aortic valve transplantation in the dog. Lancet 2:114, 1965.
4. Binet JP, Duran CG, Carpentier A, Langlois J: Heterologous aortic valve transplantation. Lancet 2:1275, 1965.
5. Carpentier A, Blondeau P, Marcel P: Remplacement des valves mitrales et tricuspides par des heterografes. Ann Chirurg Thorac Cardiovasc 7:33, 1968.
6. Reis RL, Hancock WD, Yarbrough JW, Glancy DL, Morrow AG: The flexible stent. A new concept in the fabrication of tissue heart valve prosthesis. J Thorac Cardiovasc Surg 62:683, 1971.
7. Oyer PE, Stinson EB, Reits BA, Craig Miller D, Rossiter SJ, Shumway NE: Long-term evaluation of the porcine xenograft bioprosthesis. J Thorac Cardiovasc Surg 78:343, 1979.
8. Casarotto D, Bortolotti U, Thiene G, Gallucci V, Cevese PG: Long-term results (from 5 to 7 years) with the Hancock SGP bioprosthesis. J Cardiovasc Surg 20:399, 1979.
9. Borkon AM, McIntosh CL, Von Rueden TJ, Morrow AG: Mitral valve replacement with the Hancock bioprosthesis: Five to ten year follow-up. Ann Thorac Surg 32:128, 1981.
10. Cohn LH, Mudge GH, Pratter F, Collins JJ Jr: Five to eight-year follow-up of patients undergoing porcine heart valve replacement. New Engl J Med 304:258, 1981.
11. Gallo JI, Ruiz B, Carrion MF, Gutierrez JA, Vega JL, Duran CMG: Heart valve replacement with the Hancock bioprosthesis. A 6-year review. Ann Thorac Surg 31:444, 1981.
12. Duran CG, Pomar JL, Revuelta JM, Gallo JI, Poveda J, Ochoteco A, Ubago JL: Conservative operation for mitral insufficiency. J Thorac Cardiovasc Surg 79:326, 1980.

5

Clinical Durability of the Pericardial Xenograft Valve: 11 Years' Experience

M. I. IONESCU, A. P. TANDON, N. R. SAUNDERS, M. CHIDAMBARAM, D. R. SMITH

The glutaraldehyde-preserved pericardial xenograft has been used for heart valve replacement since 1971. Previous publications from our institution and other centers have described the clinical[1–7] and hemodynamic[1,3,4,6–14] results and have defined the hydraulic characteristics of the pericardial xenograft.[4,15–18]

Since the follow-up of patients with pericardial valves is now into the 12th year, we have analyzed our results and report the data with particular emphasis on valve durability and thromboembolic risk without the use of long-term anticoagulants.

Clinical and hemodynamic data are also presented from the initial group of patients who received low profile pericardial xenografts during 1981 and 1982.

Patients and Methods

From March 1971 to March 1982, 711 patients received 855 pericardial xenografts for heart valve replacement (305 aortic, 272 mitral, 6 tricuspid, and 128 multiple replacement). Details concerning the patient population are shown in Table I. The mean age for the entire series was 50 years. Preoperatively, the majority of patients (81.2%) were in class III and IV of the New York Heart Association (NYHA) functional classification (aortic 65.6%, mitral 91.7%, and multiple replacement 95.1%).

Twenty-seven percent of all patients had had previous open or closed cardiac surgical operations. Table II shows in percentages the presence of

---

From the General Infirmary at Leeds, Leeds University, and Royal Infirmary, Halifax, England.

TABLE I Patient data

	Aortic		Mitral		Tricuspid		Multiple*	
	#	%	#	%	#	%	#	%
# patients	305	42.9	272	38.3	6	0.8	128	18.0
# valves	305	35.7	272	31.8	6	0.7	272	31.8
Previous cardiac operations	21	7	65	24	1	17	45	35
Concomitant cardiac operations	167(214)†	55	96(142)	35	3(3)	50	54(81)	42
Hospital survivors	286	94	254	93	6	100	116	91
Late deaths (% per annum)	2.9		2.6		—		5.8	
Current survivors	247	81	229	84	6	100	102	81
Months of follow-up, range/mean	3–121/55.4		3–136/50.1		6–118/74.2		3–62/28.3	
Cumulative follow-up years	1,322		961		39		240	

* Sixty-eight patients had mitral and aortic replacement, 26 had mitral and tricuspid, and 16 patients had mitral, aortic, and tricuspid replacement.

† Figures in parentheses denote number of surgical procedures.

TABLE II Factors potentially associated with thromboembolic risk in patients with mitral and multiple valve replacement

Variable	Single mitral replacement (%)	Multiple replacement (%)
Preoperative systemic emboli (5 years preceding the operation)	10.3	8.6
Left atrial thrombus	8	7
Calcified left atrial wall	0.7	1.6
Gross left atrial enlargement	35	38
Chronic atrial fibrillation	74	68
NYHA class III and IV	91.7	95.1
Exclusion of left auricular appendage*	40.8	15.6

* Includes patients with previous closed mitral valvotomy.

factors potentially associated with the risk of thromboembolism in the subgroups of patients with single mitral and multiple valve replacement.

From March 1971 to March 1976 valves were constructed within the hospital and used for single valve replacement only. From April 1976 the pericardial xenografts have been manufactured by Shiley (Irvine, CA) and used for both single and multiple replacements. The technique of valve construction was essentially the same in both hospital-made and Shiley valves. However, the hospital-made valves did not benefit from the accuracy of standardized production. The glutaraldehyde used in the hospital series was a simple dilution of commercially available glutaraldehyde with an unknown and unstable content of monomers and polymers. Moreover, the pericardium was treated prior to glutaraldehyde fixation with sodium metaperiodate and ethylene glycol.

The Shiley pericardial valves are manufactured according to standardized techniques and exacting methods for tissue selection and correct matching of leaflets for uniformity of function. Purified glutaraldehyde[19] is used for tissue fixation without any pressure load.[20] The sodium metaperiodate and ethylene glycol pretreatment is no longer used. The abrasive points in stent design and the quality of Dacron covering have been optimized when compared with the hospital-made valves.

In addition to the standard (ISU) Shiley pericardial xenografts we have implanted, since January 1981, 168 low profile pericardial valves in 131 patients (Table III). The low profile valves differ in some essential respects from the standard pericardial valve. The support stent is made of Delrin, which has a stable molecular memory and therefore is not prone to "creep" deformation. This flexible stent carries a radiopaque marker and is covered with microvel Dacron. The total height of the valve is lower and the implant height is reduced by approximately 30% when compared with the standard valve. The shape of the sewing rim closely conforms with the aortic anulus

TABLE III Types of pericardial xenograft valves used from 1971–1982

Valves replaced	Pts	Total valves	Hospital-made valves*	Shiley-made valves		
				ISU†	LP†	Total
Aortic	305	305	142	111	52	163
Mitral	272	272	68	153	51	204
Tricuspid	6	6	3	1	2	3
Multiple	128	272	—	209	63	272
Total	711	855	213	474	168	642

* Used between 1971 and 1975.
† ISU: standard pericardial xenografts used between 1976 and 1980; LP: low profile pericardial xenografts used during 1981 and 1982.

configuration. The geometry of the valve is improved by changes in tissue-mounting techniques. In vitro evaluation of the low profile pericardial xenograft has shown a reduction in pressure drop of from 10–43% and an increase in effective orifice area of from 10–32% (depending on size) when compared with the standard pericardial valve. Comparative in vitro mechanical fatigue testing using the Rowan Ash (Sheffield, England) life tester[21] has shown the low profile valve to be twice as durable as the standard pericardial valve under identical experimental conditions.

The majority of valves used were of small size: 321 (78.9%) aortic valves had a 23 mm diameter or smaller and 320 (80%) mitral valves had 27 and 25 mm diameters. No effort was made to implant valves larger than could be comfortably accommodated into the respective valve anulus or cardiac chamber.

Surgical Technique

The operative technique for valve replacement has remained constant throughout the study period. For aortic replacement, multiple interrupted mattress sutures have been used in 95% of patients. One continuous suture was used for all tricuspid valves and for 88% of mitral implants. Aortic anuloplastic procedures have not been used in this series. From March 1971 to December 1976, intermittent hypoxia with topical hypothermia for mitral replacement and continuous euthermic coronary perfusion for aortic replacement were the routine procedures. Since January 1977, total body hypothermia (20–28°C) with cold cardioplegia and topical hypothermia were used for all operations. For the past 5 years, in patients with mitral or multiple valve replacement, the left auricular appendage was excluded by ligature when accessible.

Anticoagulant Treatment

Patients with isolated aortic or tricuspid valve replacement did not receive any anticoagulant treatment. Of those with single mitral valve replacement, the initial 68 patients were not given anticoagulants. The remaining 332 patients (204 single mitral and 128 multiple replacement) were treated for 5–6 weeks only, following valve insertion, with warfarin sodium. The prothrombin time of these patients was deliberately maintained at a low level of between 18 and 24 seconds.

Definition of Embolism: Embolism was defined as all new focal neurologic deficits, either transient or permanent, as well as all clinically detectable noncerebral arterial emboli. "Early" emboli were considered as those that occurred within the first 6 postoperative weeks.

Definition of Valve Failure: Pericardial xenograft failure is regarded as 1) the appearance postoperatively of a new regurgitant murmur, unless proved to be perivalvular in origin, 2) confirmed hemodynamic valvular dysfunction necessitating reoperation or causing death, and 3) thrombotic occlusion of the valve.

Hemodynamic Studies

Hemodynamic investigations at rest and during exercise were undertaken in 92 patients. The criteria for selection were the informed consent of the patient and the availability of preoperative investigations. Long-term hemodynamic studies were performed in 80 patients with standard pericardial valves (36 aortic, 29 mitral, 3 tricuspid, and 12 multiple valve replacement) and in 12 patients with low profile valves (6 aortic and 6 mitral). Sequential hemodynamic investigations were undertaken in 13 patients with aortic and 6 patients with mitral valve replacement. In addition to the preoperative investigation, these 19 patients had 3 postoperative studies performed at mean durations of 10, 42, and 69 months following valve insertion.[13] The methodology of hemodynamic investigations has been previously described.[12–14]

All patients were seen by the surgeons and the cardiologists at least once every year in the outpatient clinic of the hospital. At each visit, in addition to a careful history, various clinical and laboratory parameters of valve performance were evaluated. None of the patients was lost to follow-up.

Patient survival and incidence of valve dysfunction and of embolism are expressed both by actuarial analysis and by linearized occurrence rates.[22] Standard statistical formulas have been used for the analysis of data as previously described.[4]

Results

Survival

As shown in Table I, 662 (93.1%) patients were alive when discharged from the hospital; 286 (93.8%) with aortic, 254 (93.4%) with mitral, 6 (100%) with tricuspid, and 116 (90.6%) with multiple valve replacement. The overall late mortality was 3% per annum (2.9 for aortic, 2.6 for mitral, nil for tricuspid, and 5.6 for multiple replacement). The majority of hospital and late deaths were due to cardiac causes. The actuarial survival rate is 73.1 ± 10.6% for patients with aortic replacement at 11 years; 72.4 ± 14.1% for patients with mitral replacement at 12 years and 77.5 ± 8.8% for those with multiple valve replacement at 6 years of follow-up (Fig. 1).

Among long-term survivors, there was significant functional improvement in all patients. According to the NYHA classification, at the latest evaluation 216 (87.5%) patients with aortic replacement were in class 1 and 31 (12.5%), in class II; 184 (80.3%) patients with mitral replacement were in class I and 45 (19.7%), in class II; and 62 (60.8%) with multiple valve replacement were in class I and 40 (39.2%), in class II.

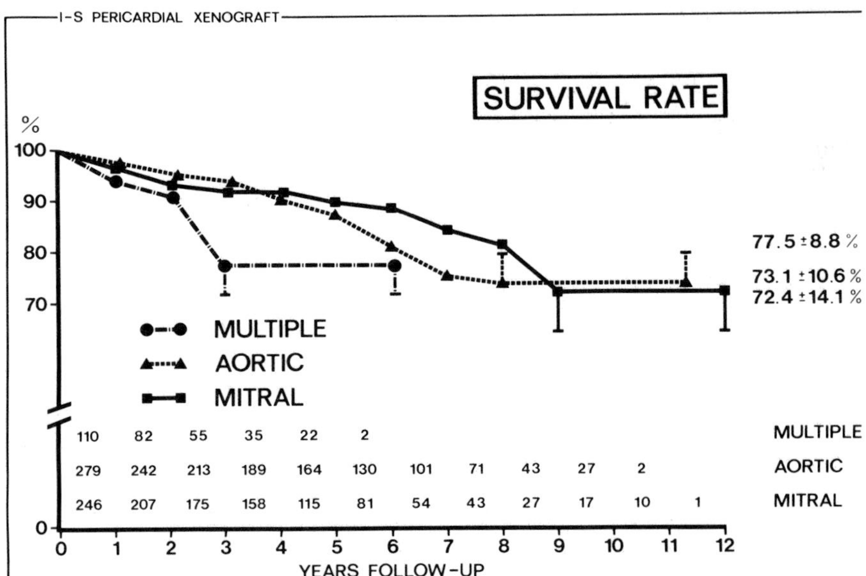

FIG. 1 Actuarial survival curves for patients having heart valve replacement with pericardial xenografts. Individual curves are displayed for the 3 subgroups of patients with aortic, mitral, and multiple valve replacement. The figures above the horizontal axis represent the number of patients at risk for each year of follow-up.

TABLE IV Details of valve dysfunction in 855 valves implanted over a period of 136 months

Valves at risk	# valves	Years of follow-up	Cusp detached	Cusp tear	Calcification	Total	Episodes % per annum
Aortic	407	1,513	4	5	4	13	0.86
Mitral	400	1,201	3*	2	3	8	0.66
Tricuspid	48	118	—	—	—	—	—
Total	855	2,832	7	7	7	21	0.74

* One Shiley-made valve.

Valve Dysfunction

There were 21 pericardial xenograft failures in the entire series (Table IV). Thirteen involved aortic valves (single replacement) and 8, mitral valves (7 in patients with single and 1 from a patient with multiple replacement).

The linearized rate of valve failure was 0.74% per annum for the total number of valves at risk (0.86% for aortic and 0.66% for mitral pericardial xenografts). Three modes of failure have been identified. Seven valves (4 aortic and 3 mitral) sustained partial detachment of a pericardial cusp at the suture line. The first hospital-made valves were constructed with a continuous suture along the scallop-shaped outflow border of the support frame in order to secure the pericardium to the frame. The row of perforations acted as a path of least resistance. Cusp rupture occurred in 7 valves (5 aortic and 2 mitral) in the form of a vertical tear originating at the free margin of the cusp and extending 3–4 mm proximally. Light, diffuse calcification of the pericardium occurred in 7 valves (4 aortic and 3 mitral), rendering the xenografts rigid. The mean age of these 7 patients was 36 years (3 patients were younger than 30 years). The duration of time these 21 valves remained in situ varied from 13–91 months. Of the 21 cases of xenograft failure, 20 occurred in hospital-made valves and 1 affected a Shiley valve in the mitral position where leaflet detachment occurred at 38 months following implantation.

Thrombotic obstruction of the pericardial xenograft has not been encountered in this series.

The actuarial curves of freedom from valve dysfunction related to the 3 groups of patients (aortic, mitral, and multiple replacement) are shown in Fig. 2.

Other Valve-Related Complications

There were 12 episodes of perivalvular leak (5 each in patients with single aortic and mitral replacement and 2 in the multiple replacement group). All

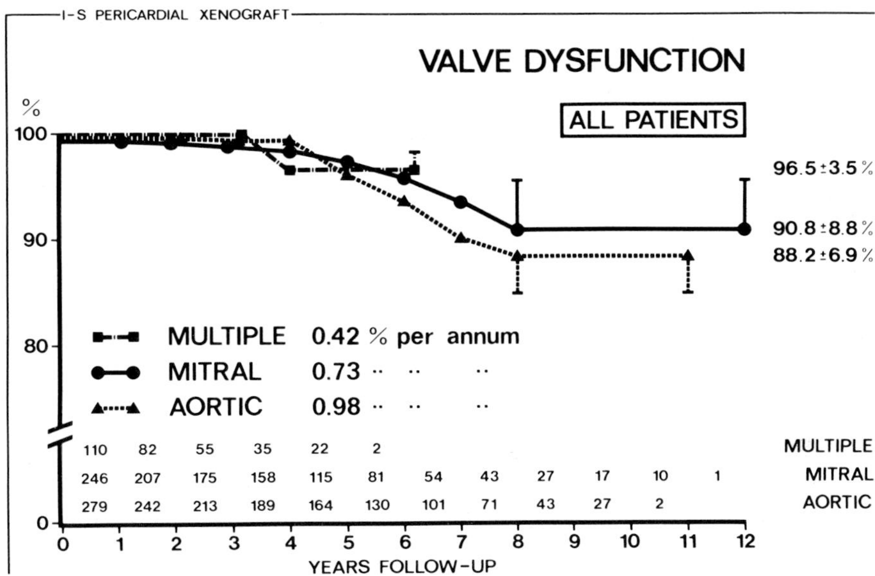

FIG. 2 Actuarial event-free curves for valve dysfunction in patients with pericardial xenograft valve replacement. Individual curves are shown for the 3 subgroups of patients with aortic, mitral, and multiple valve replacement. The numbers along the horizontal axis denote the patients at risk for each year of follow-up.

12 patients were successfully reoperated upon and continue to be well. The actuarial curve of freedom from perivalvular leak is 97.5 ± 1.9% at 5 and 11 years for the aortic, 97.8 ± 1.0% at 1 and 12 years for the mitral, and 97.9 ± 1.5% at 1 and 6 years for the multiple replacement group.

Infective endocarditis occurred in 20 patients (9 with aortic, 5 with mitral, and 6 with multiple valve replacement). Four out of 10 treated only with antibiotics and 6 out of 10 reoperated upon are alive and well (50% survival). The actuarial curve of freedom from endocarditis is 94.7 ± 3.7% at 7 and 11 years for the aortic, 97.1 ± 2.4% at 4 and 12 years for the mitral, and 89.3 ± 8.7% at 4 and 6 years for the multiple replacement group.

Hemodynamic Data

The results of hemodynamic investigations performed in patients with the standard pericardial xenograft (long term and sequential) have been previously reported.[4,11–14] Table V summarizes comparatively the mean values of transvalvular gradients and calculated surface areas (at rest and during exercise) from patients with standard pericardial and with low profile valves.

TABLE V Comparative hemodynamic data (mean values ± SEM) of the standard (ISU) and low profile (LP) pericardial xenograft valves

	Aortic replacement*				Mitral replacement*			
	PSG (mmHg)		XSA (cm^2)		MDG (mmHg)		XSA (cm^2)	
	R	E	R	E	R	E	R	E
ISU	6.4 ± 0.1	9.6 ± 1.6	1.6 ± 0.07	2.0 ± 0.1	6.4 ± 0.5	15.3 ± 0.9	2.0 ± 0.1	2.3 ± 0.1
LP	5.1 ± 0.2	8.2 ± 1.4	1.75 ± 0.2	2.2 ± 0.1	4.8 ± 0.4	13.2 ± 0.6	2.2 ± 0.2	2.4 ± 0.3

* SEM: standard error of the mean; PSG: peak systolic gradient; XSA: calculated xenograft surface area; MDG: mean diastolic gradient; R: rest; E: exercise.

Thromboembolic Complications

Table VI shows the anticoagulant regimen and the number of embolic complications. Eleven embolic events occurred overall. In the single aortic valve replacement subgroup there were 4 early emboli. Six patients with single mitral valve replacement sustained embolic episodes, 4 early and 2 late (at 8 and 67 months) postoperatively.

In the multiple replacement group 1 embolic event occurred on the second postoperative day. With 1 exception (mild residual paresis) all embolic phenomena were transient. Valve thrombosis has not been encountered in our experience with the pericardial xenograft.

The linearized rate of embolization was 0.43% per annum for the entire series (0.30 for single aortic, 0.62 for single mitral, and 0.42 for multiple valve replacement).

The actuarial event-free curves for embolic complications show that 98.5 ± 0.8% of patients with aortic replacement at 11 years of follow-up,

TABLE VI Details of anticoagulant treatment and embolic complications in 711 patients with pericardial xenograft valve replacement

Anticoagulants				# systemic emboli	
Early	Late	Valves replaced	# patients	Early	Late
No	No	Aortic	305	4	—
No	No	Mitral	68	4	1
Yes	No	Mitral	204	—	1
No	No	Tricuspid	6	—	—
Yes	No	Multiple	128	1	—
Total			711	9	2

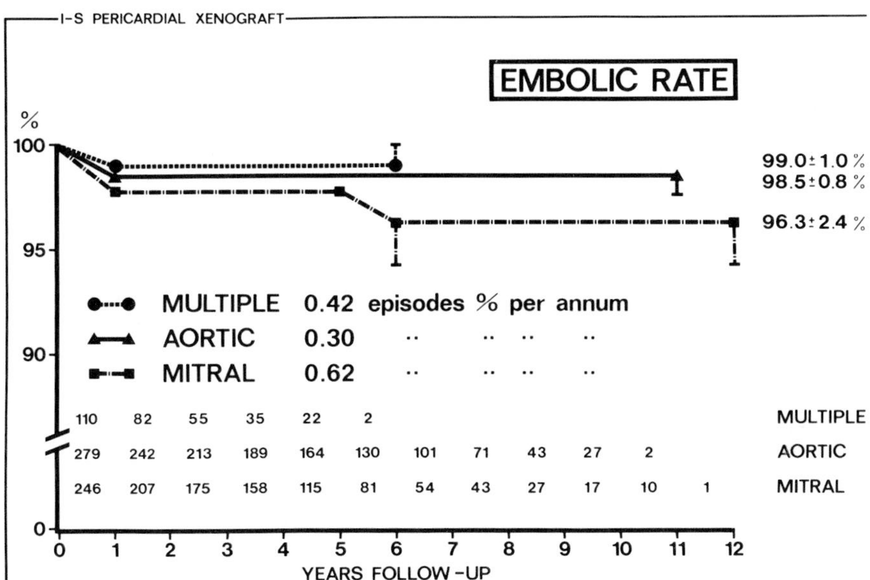

FIG. 3 Actuarial event-free curves for embolic complications in patients having valve replacement with pericardial xenografts. Individual curves are displayed for the 3 subgroups of patients with aortic, mitral, and multiple valve replacement. The figures above the horizontal axis denote the number of patients entering each year of follow-up.

96.3 ± 2.4% of patients with mitral replacement at 12 years of follow-up, and 99.0 ± 1.0% of patients with multiple replacement at 6 years postoperatively are expected to be free from emboli, as shown in Fig. 3.

In this series there was no significant correlation between embolic complications and any of the factors mentioned in Table II with the exception of atrial fibrillation.

In the series of 131 patients who received low profile pericardial xenografts during 1981 and 1982 there have not been any thromboembolic phenomena to date.

Comment

Long-term survival following valve replacement depends on a multitude of factors that are mainly related to patient pathology and, to some extent, to the artificial valve implanted. The actuarial survival rate is therefore a cumulative reflection of many variables. In this series the survival rate is not different from that reported from other institutions with this or other types of tissue valves at similar durations of follow-up.[3,4,23–28]

Long-term durability is undoubtedly the most important single determinant in the evaluation of a heart valve substitute. In our series of 711 patients with pericardial xenografts there were 21 episodes of valve failure (0.82% per annum). In 7 instances (4 aortic and 3 mitral) the pericardium became detached from the support frame due to poor valve construction. These cases have been included in the analysis as valve failures. In 7 other cases cusp tear occurred between 32 and 84 months postimplantation. Due to the small number of cases and their random appearance, no significant conclusion can be drawn. Calcification occurred in 7 patients aged 18 to 53 years (mean, 36) and the implant duration averaged 68 months (49–90 months). Reports of sporadic calcification of other tissue valves in adults have been published.[23–31] It is interesting to note that from the total of 21 valve failures, 20 occurred with hospital-made valves and 1 with a Shiley valve. The follow-up of patients with hospital-made valves extends from 76–136 months and 15 of the 20 failures occurred between 13 and 72 months postoperatively. The follow-up with the Shiley-made valves now extends to a maximum of 76 months and only 1 valve has failed during this time interval. A similarly low failure rate with the Shiley pericardial xenograft valve has been reported by others.[1–3,6,9,32] This significant difference in valve failure observed during the initial 76 months of usage between the hospital-made and the Shiley valves can be attributed to the different techniques of tissue processing and valve manufacture. The Shiley valves are fixed with purified glutaraldehyde without any pretreatment with sodium metaperiodate or ethylene glycol, which are used in the hospital-made valves. Sodium metaperiodate is now known to be an oxidizing agent that is traumatic to the connective tissue. In addition, general improvement in selection and matching of tissue and standardization of valve construction have optimized the overall quality of the pericardial xenograft.

Statistical comparison between actuarial data reported from other institutions is very difficult, but a general impression, concerning trends, can be gained. For tissue valves, the porcine bioprosthesis is a standard against which results can be compared. The Hancock valve has been in use for more than 10 years and a few reports of long-term results have been published.[23–26,28,30] With the exception of Oyer et al,[26] who do not include in the actuarial curve failure due to valve thrombosis, intrinsic stenosis and regurgitant murmurs, we and other authors[23,28,30,32] have used a very similar definition of valve failure for the actuarial analysis. Despite the variability in patient population and methods for data reporting, the trend in the long-term performance of porcine bioprostheses shows a progressively increasing rate of valve failure after 5 years of follow-up. Although the number of patients at risk beyond 5 years is small in all series, and therefore the standard error is larger, there is an obvious disparity in performance after 5 years between the porcine valves on the one hand and the pericardial xenograft on the other.

The failure rate in our entire series of patients with pericardial xenografts has been 0.82% episodes per annum with a slightly lower incidence in the mitral position.

The sustained long-term durability of the pericardial xenograft is probably due to the quality of the tissue and to the functional geometry of the valve. Both contribute to a smoother, more regular opening and closure of the valve without areas of excessive bending or 3-dimensional flexure (Fig. 4), which are damaging to the connective tissue fibers.

Although both porcine and pericardial valves are collagen structures treated with glutaraldehyde, their shape, technique of mounting, hydraulic

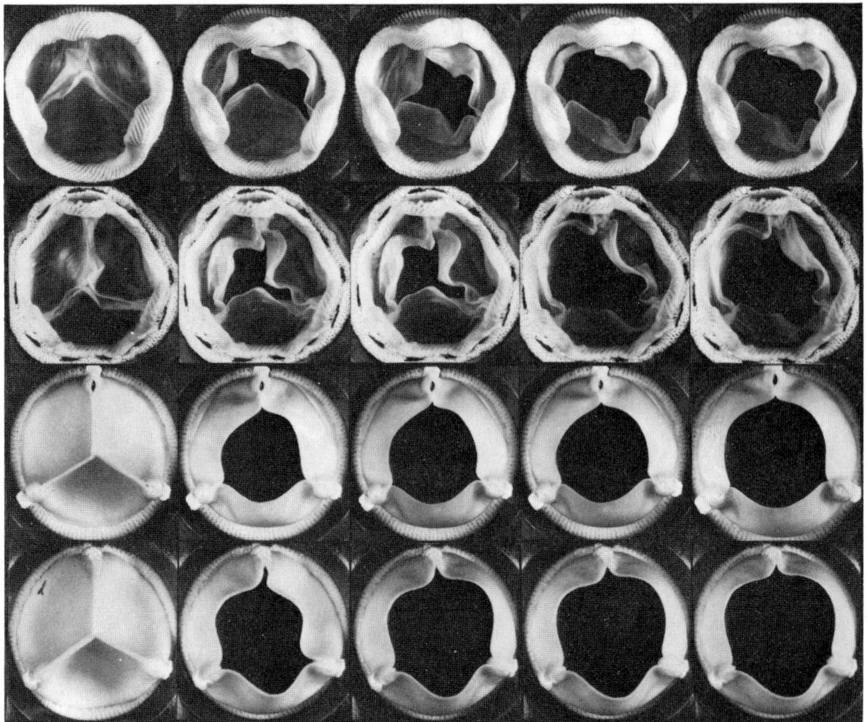

FIG. 4 In vitro comparison of opening characteristics of 4 types of tissue valves. From top: modified orifice Hancock valve; recently modified Carpentier-Edwards valve; standard Ionescu-Shiley pericardial xenograft, and low profile Ionescu-Shiley pericardial xenograft. All valves were manufactured for clinical use and all have the same implantation diameter (25 mm). The valves were tested under identical conditions in a pulse duplicator. The flow rates were for each frame (from left to right): 0, 100, 200, 300, and 400 ml/sec. The opening of the pericardial cusps is synchronous and regular without 3-dimensional flexure. There are no crevices or dead spaces behind the open cusps of the pericardial valves. The low profile valve displays a larger central opening at all flow rates when compared with the other valves.

characteristics, and dynamic function are dissimilar and therefore their long-term performance and mode of failure may be different.

The physicochemical and biologic properties of the natural aortic porcine valve have been profoundly altered by various interventions in order to adapt it for therapeutic means. The porcine "bioprosthesis" has lost all the primordial characteristics of the aortic valve except its shape, which remains unchanged and unchangeable.

The pericardial valve, on the other hand, has been conceived of as an entirely artificial design and therefore its basic shape can be altered in order to optimize its function.

Following extensive in vitro testing, various modifications have been made in the design of the standard valve to further increase its durability, reduce its mass and implant height, and improve its overall hydrodynamic performance. All these goals have been attained by the creation of the low profile valve, which has been under clinical evaluation since January 1981. The implant height has been reduced when compared with the standard pericardial valve and the porcine valves (Fig. 5). This reduction in height along with the introduction of a flexible stent facilitate surgical insertion. The improved geometry of the low profile valve has produced further

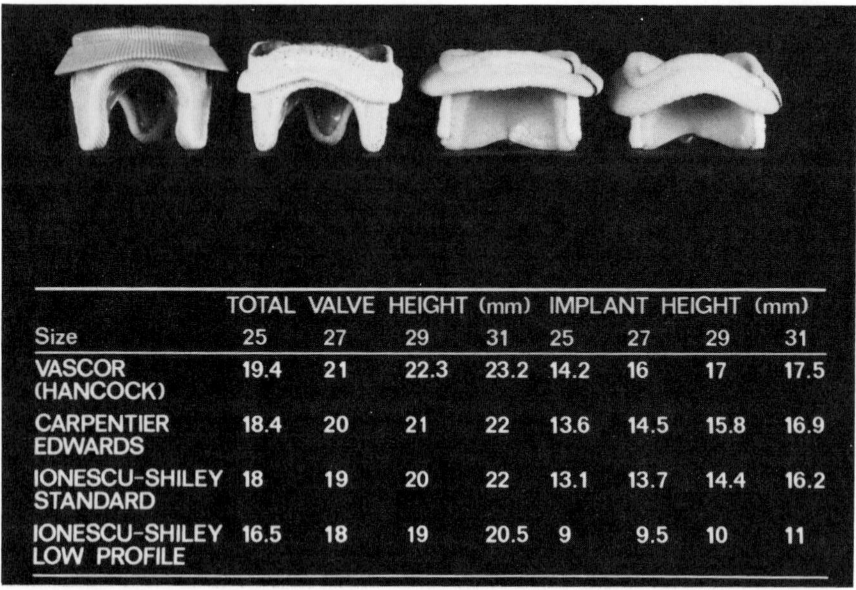

	TOTAL VALVE HEIGHT (mm)				IMPLANT HEIGHT (mm)			
Size	25	27	29	31	25	27	29	31
VASCOR (HANCOCK)	19.4	21	22.3	23.2	14.2	16	17	17.5
CARPENTIER EDWARDS	18.4	20	21	22	13.6	14.5	15.8	16.9
IONESCU-SHILEY STANDARD	18	19	20	22	13.1	13.7	14.4	16.2
IONESCU-SHILEY LOW PROFILE	16.5	18	19	20.5	9	9.5	10	11

FIG. 5 Lateral view of tissue valves. From left: modified orifice Hancock valve, recently modified Carpentier-Edwards valve, standard pericardial xenograft, and low profile pericardial xenograft. All valves were manufactured for clinical use and all have the same implantation diameter (25 mm). The lower panel shows comparatively total valve height and implant height of the valves mentioned.

improvement in its hemodynamic performance. The in vitro mechanical durability of the valve has been considerably extended (Fig. 6). Whether this comparative in vitro increase in durability will be entirely reflected in the clinical situation remains to be demonstrated.

Previously reported results of hemodynamic studies in patients with pericardial xenograft valve replacement from this and other institutions have shown that the performance of the pericardial valve is superior to that of porcine valves.[3,6–8,10–14]

The results of the sequential studies have demonstrated that the initial circulatory improvement is maintained and that there is no change in the essential hemodynamic parameters up to 73 months following the operation.[13] Postoperative hemodynamic studies performed in patients with low profile valves have shown an improvement in both valve surface area and transvalvular pressure gradients when compared with results from patients with the standard pericardial xenograft.

One of the main advantages of tissue valves, especially when used in the mitral position, is their lower propensity for thromboembolism when compared with mechanical prostheses.

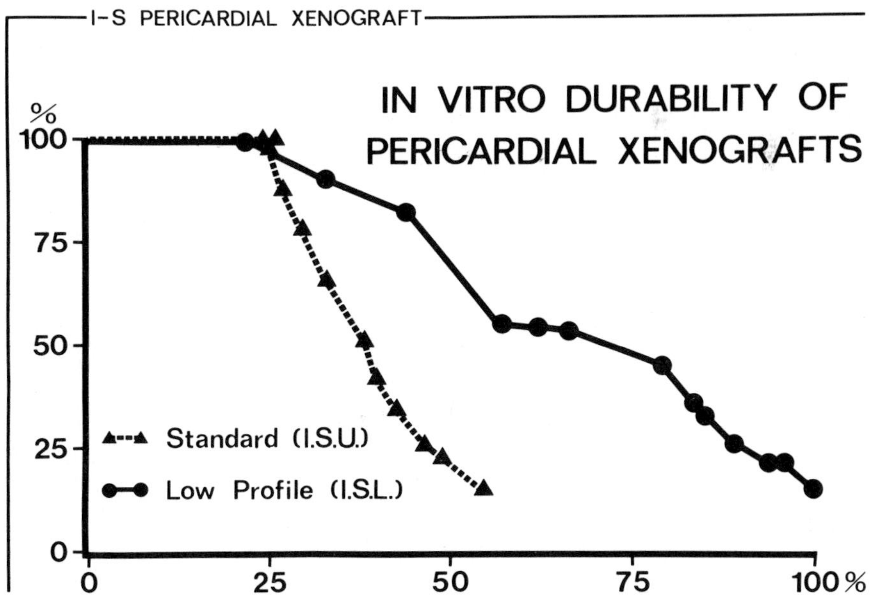

FIG. 6 Graphic presentation of comparative "in vitro" mechanical durability. The testing of 12 standard (ISU) and 13 low profile (ISL) pericardial xenografts was conducted under identical experimental conditions: complete valve opening, 1250 cycles/min, 120 mmHg differential pressure, the test medium was 0.2% glutaraldehyde, and the temperature was 25°C.

TABLE VII Embolic complications and long-term anticoagulant treatment of patients with mitral tissue valves (reported data)

Institution	Years of valve usage	# patients	Emboli % per annum	Long-term anticoagulation
Porcine valves				
Henry Ford Hospital[33]	1971–1975	228	4.7	54% of patients
Stanford University[34]	1971–1978	561	3.1	31% of patients
British Columbia University[35]	1975–1978	261	3.5	45% of patients
Pacific Medical Center[36]	1974–1977	126	5.3	50% of patients
National Institutes of Health, Bethesda[23]	1970–1975	62	3.3	6.5% of patients
Pericardial xenograft				
Leeds General Infirmary	1971–1982	400	0.58	None

This series of patients with pericardial valves is unique because long-term anticoagulation has not been used and also because the follow-up now extends beyond 11 years.

The embolic rate in this series has been extremely low. The linearized rate was 0.43% per annum overall (0.30 for aortic, 0.62 for mitral, and 0.42 for multiple replacement). This compares well with the reported embolic rate in patients with porcine valves whether or not treated with anticoagulants (Table VII). Very low embolic rates in patients with mitral pericardial xenografts (0.2–1.1% per annum) have been confirmed by others.[2,3,6,9,32,37]

Of the 11 embolic events, 9 occurred within 6 weeks of valve replacement. The number of emboli is too small to establish a trend, but there appears to be a considerable difference between the early and late incidence of embolization. We suggest that there may be different etiologic factors operative in early as opposed to late embolism. Although the exact etiology of early embolic phenomena is not known, our experience has indicated that anticoagulant treatment during the initial 6 weeks following mitral valve replacement is advantageous (Table VI).

The reduced propensity for thromboembolism of the pericardial valve is probably related to its design and to the quality of the tissue. The 3 cusps are identical in shape, thickness, and pliability and their degree of inertia is minimal. Consequently, the valve opens and closes synchronously even at low flow rates.[4,15–18] There are no stagnation areas and very little Dacron is exposed to the blood on the outflow aspect of the valve (Fig. 4).

Recent reports support the view that when 1 or more factors associated with an increased risk of thromboembolism, such as atrial fibrillation or enlarged left atrium with or without thrombus, are present, patients with porcine valves should be anticoagulated for life.[24,26,30,35] This recommendation, based on clinical results with the porcine bioprosthesis, probably holds true for that type of valve.

Most of the present knowledge of thromboembolic phenomena in the context of heart valve replacement is based on clinical experience and general impression. There is no scientific evidence available concerning the exact nature or the precise origin of emboli. The patient's cardiovascular and general pathology are certainly responsible for emboli, but only to a certain extent and probably less so following the improvement achieved in cardiac and circulatory performance by valve surgery. For example, the embolic rate after mitral commissurotomy or anuloplasty varies, in recent reports, from 0.34–0.61% per annum, with only 14–21% of patients treated with anticoagulants.[38–41] The implanted artificial valve introduces an additional hazard of thromboembolism that differs with each type of valve substitute. Clinical studies have shown that the risk of thromboembolism is higher in patients with mechanical prostheses than in those with porcine valves.[42–45] Among groups of patients with porcine valves, the embolic risk was not significantly different whether a small proportion of patients (2.3–6.4%) received anticoagulants[23,28] or whether more than half of the patients (50–75%) were given long-term anticoagulants.[33,36] Each type of valve substitute has its specific propensity for thromboembolism and this cannot be reduced below a certain level even under "ideal" conditions of anticoagulation. The endeavor to reduce thromboembolic complications in patients with valve replacement through stringent control of anticoagulation has generated an increased incidence of anticoagulant-related bleeding complications.[23,42,46] The use of anticoagulants therefore introduces an additional risk factor. Theoretically, there is a limit, imposed by the presence of cardiocirculatory pathology, below which the thromboembolic rate cannot be reduced even if the "ideal" valve substitute were available. However, by improvement in materials and in valve design, this limit can be approached either without or with limited anticoagulation and implicitly with a reduced risk of bleeding complications. In our experience the pericardial xenograft represents a great step in this direction.

Conclusion

The analysis of our results with the pericardial xenograft has demonstrated that heart valve replacement can be performed without long-term anticoagulation and with only a minimal risk of embolic complications. Moreover, valve thrombosis or lethal emboli have not been encountered in this series and the potential hazard of anticoagulant-induced hemorrhage was eliminated.

The superior hemodynamic performance of the pericardial xenograft, further improved in the low profile valve, represents an additional advantage, especially in patients with small valve anuli.

Due to the low incidence of valve dysfunction, the pericardial xenograft represents a safe heart valve substitute with a predictable behavior over a period of more than 11 years.

References

1. Becker RM, Sandor L, Tindel M, Frater RWM: Medium term follow-up of the Ionescu-Shiley heterograft valve. Ann Thorac Surg 32:120, 1981.
2. Deac R, Liebhart M, Bratu D, Bradisteanu S, Benedek J: Cardiac valve replacement with pericardial xenograft. In: Cardiovascular Surgery 1980 (W Bircks, J Ostermeyer, HD Schulte, Eds). Berlin, Springer-Verlag, 1981, p 640.
3. Garcia-Bengochea JB, Alvarez JR, Carreno CI, Cendon AA: Resultados clinicos y hemodinamicos a medio plazo con el xenoinjerto de pericardio Ionescu-Shiley. Rev Esp Cardiol 34:283, 1981.
4. Ionescu MI, Tandon AP: The Ionescu-Shiley pericardial xenograft heart valve. In: Tissue Heart Valves (MI Ionescu, Ed). London, Butterworths, 1979, p 201.
5. Ionescu MI, Tandon AP, Mary DAS, Abid A: Heart valve replacement with the Ionescu-Shiley pericardial xenograft. J Thorac Cardiovasc Surg 73:71, 1977.
6. Ott DA, Coelho AT, Cooley DA, Reul GJ: Ionescu-Shiley pericardial xenograft valve: Hemodynamic evaluation and early clinical follow-up of 326 patients. Cardiovasc Dis, Bull Texas Heart Inst 7:137, 1980.
7. Tandon AP, Whitaker W, Ionescu MI: Multiple valve replacement with pericardial xenograft. Clinical and haemodynamic study. Br Heart J 44:534, 1980.
8. Becker RM, Strom J, Frishman W, Oka Y, Lin YT, Yellin EL, Frater RWM: Hemodynamic performance of the Ionescu-Shiley valve prosthesis. J Thorac Cardiovasc Surg 80:613, 1980.
9. Revuelta JM, Pomar JL, Ubago JL, Figueroa A, Ochoteco A, Duran CMG: Pros and cons of the Ionescu-Shiley bioprosthesis. In: Cardiovascular Surgery 1980 (W Bircks, J Ostermeyer, HD Schulte, Eds). Berlin, Springer-Verlag, 1981, p 50.
10. Revuelta JM, Ubago JL, Figueroa A, Ochoteco A, Duran CMG: The problem of the small aortic root: The Ionescu-Shiley pericardial xenograft valve solution. Read at the XV World Congress of the International Cardiovascular Society, Athens, September, 1981.
11. Smith DR, Tandon AP, Hassan SS, Ionescu MI: Long term and sequential hemodynamic investigations in patients with Ionescu-Shiley pericardiac xenograft. In: Cardiovascular Surgery 1980 (W Bircks, J Ostermeyer, HD Schulte, Eds). Berlin, Springer-Verlag, 1981, p 43.
12. Tandon AP, Smith DR, Ionescu MI: Hemodynamic evaluation of the Ionescu-Shiley pericardial xenograft in the mitral position. Am Heart J 95:595, 1978.
13. Tandon AP, Smith DR, Ionescu MI: Sequential hemodynamic studies of the Ionescu-Shiley pericardial xenograft valve up to six years after implantation. Cardiovasc Dis, Bull Texas Heart Inst 6:271, 1979.
14. Tandon AP, Smith DR, Whitaker W, Ionescu MI: Long term haemodynamic evaluation of aortic pericardial xenograft. Br Heart J 40:602, 1978.
15. Gabbay S, McQueen DM, Yellin EL, Becker RM, Frater RWM: In vitro hydrodynamic comparison of mitral valve bioprostheses at high flow rates. J Thorac Cardiovasc Surg 76:771, 1978.
16. Rainer WG, Christopher RA, Sadler TR, Hilgenberg AD: Dynamic behaviour of prosthetic aortic tissue valves as viewed by high-speed cinematography. Ann Thorac Surg 28:274, 1979.

17. Walker DK, Scotten LN, Modi VJ, Brownlee RT: In vitro assessment of mitral valve prostheses. J Thorac Cardiovasc Surg 79:680, 1980.
18. Wright JTM: Hydrodynamic evaluation of tissue valves. In: Tissue Heart Valves (MI Ionescu, Ed): London, Butterworths, 1979, p 29.
19. Woodroof EA: The chemistry and biology of aldehyde treated tissue heart valve xenografts. In: Tissue Heart Valves (MI Ionescu, Ed). London, Butterworths, 1979, p 347.
20. Broom ND, Thomson FJ: Influence of fixation conditions on the performance of glutaraldehyde treated porcine aortic valves. Towards a more scientific basis. Thorax 34:166, 1979.
21. Martin TRP, van Noort R, Black MM, Morgon J: Accelerated fatigue testing of biological tissue heart valves. In: Proceedings of the European Society of Artificial Organs, vol 7 (ES Bucherl, Ed). Geneva, 1980, p 315.
22. Anderson RP, Boncheck LI, Grunkemeier GL, Lambert LE, Starr A: The analysis and presentation of surgical results by actuarial methods. J Surg Res 16:224, 1974.
23. Borkon AM, McIntosh CL, Von Rueden TJ, Morrow AG: Mitral valve replacement with the Hancock bioprosthesis: Five to ten year follow-up. Ann Thorac Surg 32:127, 1981.
24. Cohn LH, Collins JJ: The glutaraldehyde stabilized porcine xenograft valve. In: Tissue Heart Valves (MI Ionescu, Ed). London, Butterworths, 1979, p 173.
25. Lakier JB, Khaja F, Magilligan DJ, Goldstein S: Porcine xenograft valves. Long-term (60–89 months) follow-up. Circulation 62:313, 1980.
26. Oyer PE, Miller DC, Stinson EB, Reitz BA, Moreno-Cabral RJ, Shumway NE: Clinical durability of the Hancock porcine bioprosthetic valve. J Thorac Cardiovasc Surg 80:824, 1980.
27. Thiene G, Bortolotti U, Panizzon G, Milano A, Gallucci V: Pathological substrates of thrombus formation after heart valve replacement with the Hancock bioprosthesis. J Thorac Cardiovasc Surg 80:414, 1980.
28. Williams JB, Karp RB, Kirklin JW, Kouchoukos NT, Pacifico AD, Zorn GL, Blackstone EH, Brown EN, Piantadosi S, Bradley EL: Considerations in selection and management of patients undergoing valve replacement with glutaraldehyde-fixed porcine bioprostheses. Ann Thorac Surg 30:247, 1980.
29. Gordon MH, Walters MB, Allen P, Burton JD: Calcific stenosis of a glutaraldehyde-treated porcine bioprosthesis in the aortic position. J Thorac Cardiovasc Surg 80:788, 1980.
30. Magilligan DJ, Lewis JW, Jara FM, Lee MW, Alam M, Riddle JM, Stein PD: Spontaneous degeneration of porcine bioprosthetic valves. Ann Thorac Surg 30:259, 1980.
31. Platt MR, Mills LJ, Estrera AS, Hillis ID, Buja IM, Willerson JT: Marked thrombosis and calcification of porcine heterograft valves. Circulation 62:862, 1980.
32. Holden MP: The Ionescu-Shiley valve. In Proceedings of Shiley European Cardiovascular Conference—Chamonix, Irvine, Shiley, 1980, p 81.
33. Davila JC, Magilligan DJ, Lewis JW: Is the Hancock porcine valve the best cardiac valve substitute today? Ann Thorac Surg 26:303, 1978.
34. Oyer PE, Stinson EB, Reitz BA, Miller DC, Rossiter S, Shumway NE: Long term evaluation of porcine xenograft bioprosthesis. J Thorac Cardiovasc Surg 78:343, 1979.
35. Jamieson WRE, Janusz MT, Miyagishima RT, Munro AI, Tutassura H, Gerein AN, Burr LH, Allen P: Embolic complications of porcine heterograft cardiac valves. J Thorac Cardiovasc Surg 81:626, 1981.

36. Hetzer R, Hill JD, Kerth WJ, Ansbro J, Adappa MG, Rodvien R, Kamm B, Gerbode F: Thrombo-embolic complications after mitral valve replacement with Hancock xenograft. J Thorac Cardiovasc Surg 75:651, 1978.
37. Cooley DA: Discussion of Becker et al.[1]
38. Gross RI, Cunningham JN Jr, Snively SL, Catinella FP, Nathan IM, Adams PX, Spencer FC: Long-term results of open radical mitral commissurotomy: Ten year follow-up study of 202 patients. Am J Cardiol 47:821, 1981.
39. Halseth WL, Elliot DP, Walker EL, Smith EA: Open mitral commissurotomy. J Thorac Cardiovasc Surg 80:842, 1980.
40. Tandon AP, Lukacs LI, Smith DR, Ionescu MI: Mitral annuloplasty. A long term clinical and haemodynamic study. Thorac Cardiovasc Surg 27:39, 1979.
41. Vega JL, Fleitas M, Martinez R, Gallo JI, Gutierrez JA, Colman T, Duran CMG: Open mitral commissurotomy. Ann Thorac Surg 31:266, 1981.
42. Björk VO, Henze A: Prosthetic heart valve replacement. Nine years' experience with the Björk-Shiley tilting disc valve. In: Tissue Heart Valves (MI Ionescu, Ed). London, Butterworths, 1979, p 1.
43. Hannah H III, Reis RL: Current status of porcine heterograft prosthesis: A 5 year appraisal. Circulation 54 (Suppl 3):27, 1976.
44. Oyer PE, Stinson EB, Griepp RB, Shumway NE: Valve replacement with the Starr-Edwards and Hancock prostheses. Comparative analysis of late morbidity and mortality. Ann Surg 186:301, 1977.
45. Stinson EB, Griepp RB, Oyer PE, Shumway NE: Long term experience with porcine aortic valve xenografts. J Thorac Cardiovasc Surg 73:54, 1977.
46. Pluth JR: Discussion of: Teply JF, Grunkemeier GL, Sutherland HDA, Lambert LE, Johnson VA, Starr A: The ultimate prognosis after valve replacement: An assessment at twenty years. Ann Thorac Surg 32:111, 1981.

6

Long-Term Results of 159 Porcine Valve Implantations

F. Derom, I. Verschuere, L. Berwouts, L. Parmentier

Because of dissatisfaction with the use of mechanical valve prostheses owing to the incidence of thromboembolism and the inevitable bleeding accidents secondary to anticoagulation therapy, the decision was made at the end of 1973 to investigate the possibilities offered by the Hancock porcine bioprosthesis. From that time, all mitral valve replacements (MVR) were done with Hancock porcine valves. Six months later the same decision was made for the replacement of the aortic valve.

Despite the excellent results with these valves concerning embolism and the avoidance of anticoagulants in many cases, there is still some concern about the durability of these bioprostheses.

This report reviews the long-term results with the Hancock mitral or aortic prostheses in 167 patients who had valve implants during a 3-year period from October 1973 to December 1976.

Patients and Methods

From October 1973 to December 1976, 190 patients have been operated on for valvular disease, with 231 Hancock porcine bioprostheses being implanted (Table I).

Mitral valve replacement alone was performed in 86 patients; 65 patients underwent an aortic valve replacement (AVR), and 39 patients needed multiple valve replacement (MR). The ages of the patients were between 16 and 71 years (mean, 49 years).

There was a male preponderance for AVR: 74% male -vs- 26% female, whereas, on the contrary, there was a female preponderance for mitral valve

---

From the Department of Surgery, University Hospital Ghent, Ghent, Belgium.

TABLE I Total experience, 1973–1976

	# pts	# bioprostheses
Mitral	86	86
Aortic	65	65
Mitral-aortic	30	60
Mitral-tricuspid	7	14
Mitral-aortic-tricuspid	2	6
Total	190	231

disease: 64.5% female and 53.5% male. Eighty-five percent of the patients were in NYHA class IV.

The operative mortality in this series was 12%. Most patients died from cardiac failure as a result of poor preoperative cardiac status. The introduction of cardioplegia at the end of 1975 resulted in a significant reduction, to 6%, of the operative mortality in the surgical candidate with a higher risk. There were no valve-related cardiac operative deaths.

There were 167 survivors and follow-up was possible in 159 of them (95%). In all these cases we were able to collect the necessary information from the referring cardiologist, the family physician, or by personal interview. The review was made at the end of 1981, with a minimum follow-up of 5 years and a maximum follow-up of 8 years. The mean duration of follow-up was 4.8 years for AVR, 5.5 years for MVR, and 4.6 years for MR (Table II).

Anticoagulant therapy was not employed routinely, except when there were documented emboli in the past or the presence of arrhythmias. Aortic valve replacement patients were discharged from the hospital without anticoagulation. Actuarial rates of patient survival and valve-related events were derived according to the method of Kaplan and Meier. Linearized occurrence rates were also computed.

TABLE II Follow-up data

	AVR	MVR	MR
# patients	58	74	35
Duration follow-up (yrs)	271	389	159
Maximum follow-up (yrs)	8	8	8
Average follow-up (yrs)	4.8	5.5	4.6
Range of follow-up (yrs)	0.1–8	0.1–8	0.1–8
Current survivors	48	58	28
Lost to follow-up	2 (3.4%)	4 (5.4%)	2 (5.7%)

Results

One hundred and thirty-four of the 159 patients who left the hospital after valve replacement with Hancock bioprostheses were alive at the end of 1981. Late mortality for patients undergoing MVR was 3.75% per patient per year and late mortality for patients undergoing AVR was 2.5% per patient per year.

Actuarial analysis of these results shows that 80 ± 7% of patients after AVR were alive 8 years after the operation and 69 ± 7% were free of complications during those 8 years (Fig. 1). Similar analysis of patients after MVR was 70 ± 6% survival and 58 ± 9% of these patients were complication-free during the 8 years (Fig. 2). Despite more advanced disease, there is not much difference in patients with multiple valvular disease. Actuarial survival at 8 years was 74 ± 8%, and 63 ± 9% of this group was complication-free at 8 years.

Valve-related complications, including endocarditis, valve dysfunction necessitating reoperation, and the incidence of embolic episodes, are shown in (Fig. 3).

There was no incidence of thromboembolism in patients with AVR up to 8 years postoperatively. The risk of endocarditis was estimated at 1% per patient year and reoperation for valve dysfunction was estimated at 1.8% per patient year (Fig. 4).

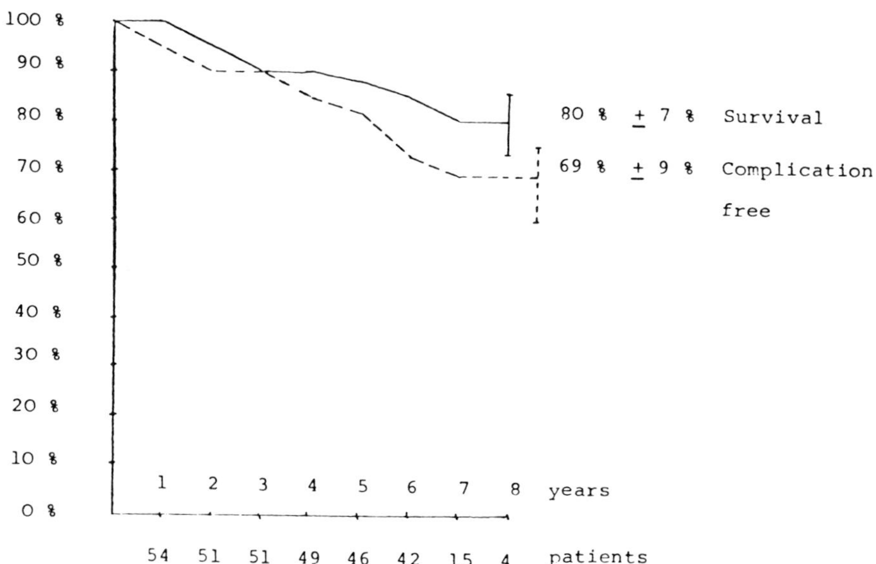

FIG. 1 Actuarial analysis of the aortic valve replacements.

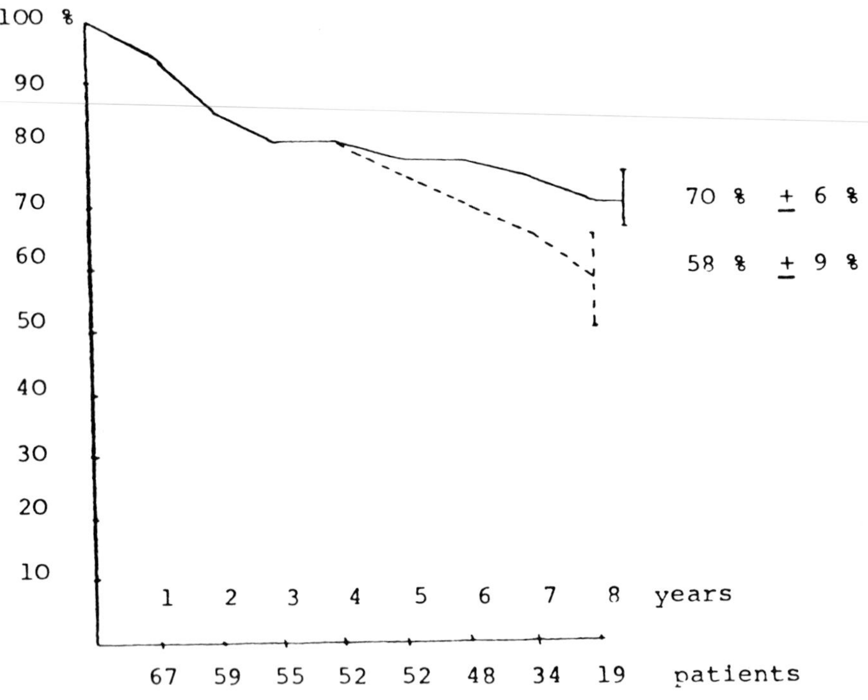

FIG. 2 Actuarial analysis of the mitral valve replacements.

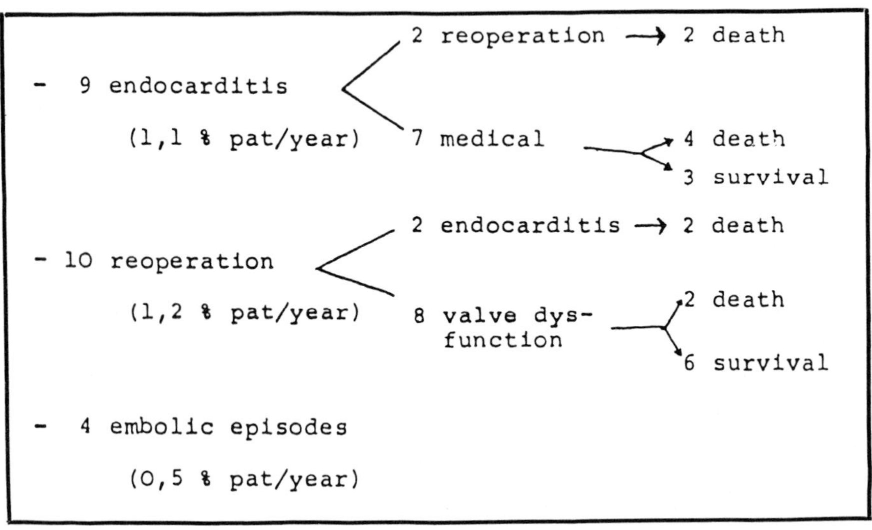

FIG. 3 Late valve-related complications.

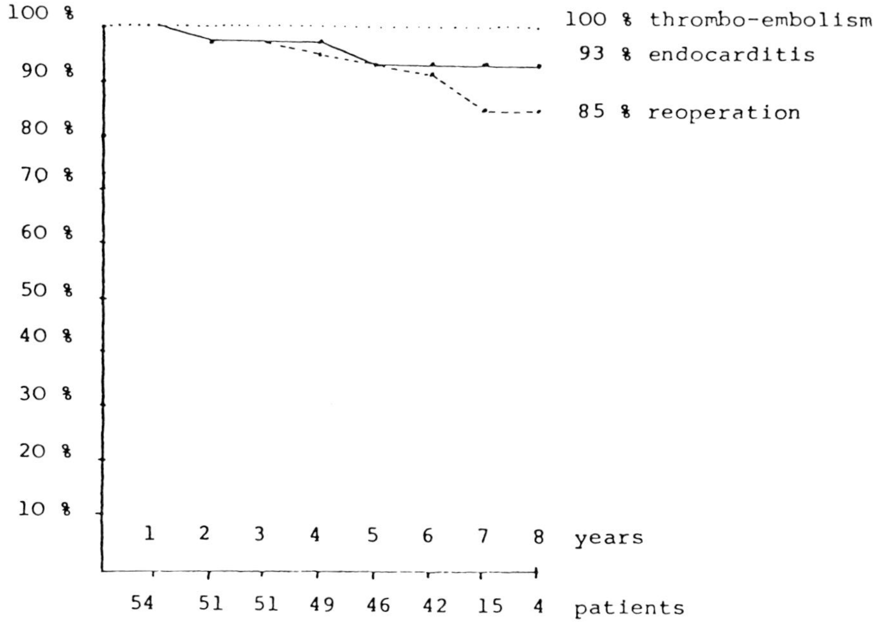

FIG. 4 Actuarial curves for thromboembolism, endocarditis and valve dysfunction in aortic valve replacement.

For MVR, the incidence of thromboembolism was 0.25% patients per year, 0.7% for endocarditis, and 0.7% for valve dysfunction (Fig. 5).

Eight patients had reoperations for valvular dysfunction, with survival and good results in 6 of them. One operative death occurred in a 78-year-old patient. The mortality in our series for patients with endocarditis was prohibitively high. The main reason for this was an excessively long period of medical treatment. Seven of these patients were never offered surgery and 1 underwent surgery only after 6 months of vain medical treatment.

Comment

One of the most significant advantages of the bioprostheses over mechanical valve replacement devices is the very low incidence of thromboembolism without the need of anticoagulants.[1] As a consequence, there is also a very low risk of associated anticoagulant-induced hemorrhage. Another advantage is that valve failure, when it does occur, is slowly progressive rather than sudden and catastrophic.[1] The patient can be carefully investigated for reoperation and the risk should not exceed 10%. In contrast, an acute occlusion or poppet escape is often a very serious complication of the mechanical valves.

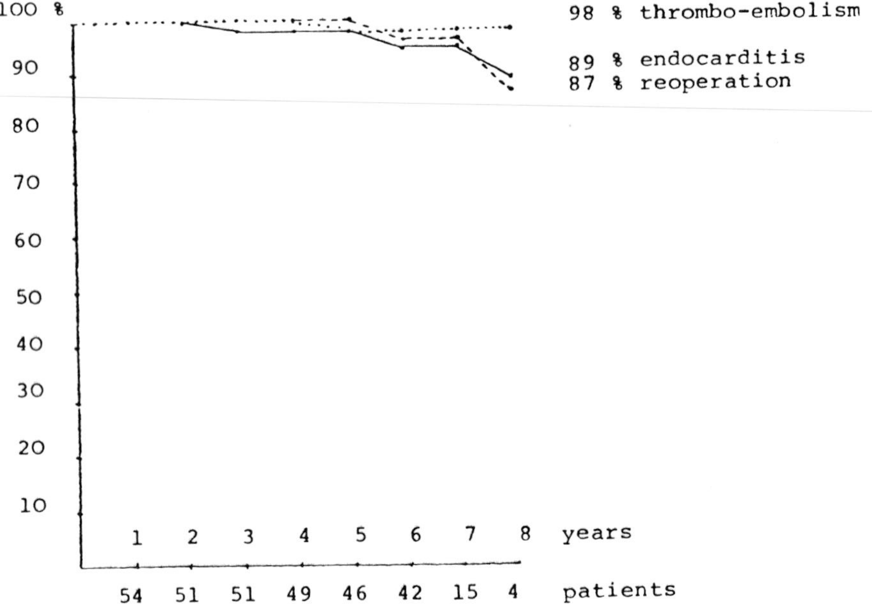

FIG. 5 Actuarial curves for thromboembolism, endocarditis and valve dysfunction in mitral valve replacement.

Fundamentally, there should be no difference in operative risk between bioprosthesis or mechanical valve implantation. MacManus et al[2] reported, after 1260 Starr-Edwards AVR, a mortality rate of 12% and Lepley et al[3] after Björk-Shiley AVR, a rate of 10.2%. Oyer[4] and Cohn et al[5] reported mortality rates of 5.7% and 5.3%, whereas Davila et al[6] Carpentier et al[7] and Casarotto et al[8] described rates of 20%, 13%, and 18.5%, respectively. In our series, operative mortality was 12%. This is a reasonable rate for the years from 1973–1976, especially considering the fact that most patients were in NYHA class IV and that myocardial protection with cardioplegia was not used until after 1976.

Late mortality after AVR in our series was 2.5% per year. Other institutions have reported 4.1%,[4] 3.9%,[5] and 5.7%.[9] After mechanical AVR, yearly deterioration rates were 3%[10] and 6.3[11] per patient year. Our 8-year survival of 80% compares favorably to the 82% 4-year survival after Björk-Shiley AVR[3] or to the 81% 4-year survival after Starr-Edwards 2,400 aortic valve implantation.[12] Björk and Henze[10] reported a 4-year survival of 86% after Björk-Shiley AVR.

After mitral valve implantation, we found a mortality rate of 3.75% per patient year. This is also very low, since other series reported figures of 5.5%[4] and 4.2%.[5] After mechanical mitral valve implantation, yearly mortality rates of 7.5%,[10] 7.9%,[11] and 5.1%[2] have been reported. In summary, in terms of patient survival, our results with Hancock bioprostheses at 8 years are quite good with AVR or MVR.

We noted no thromboembolic complication after aortic valve implantation. Other series with Hancock bioprostheses reported an incidence of 0.5%,[4] 1.3%,[13] and 2.8%[9] per patient year. After mechanical AVR, the risk is definitely higher, reported elsewhere as 5%[2] and 4%.[12] After MVR, we found a thromboembolic risk of 0.25% per patient year. Other Hancock series reported incidences of 0.6%,[12] 2.4%,[14] and 3.1%.[13] For the mechanical valve in mitral position, the risk is 6.8%,[10] 10.9%,[11] 5.8%,[2] and 4.7%,[15] According to our results and follow-up, porcine bioprostheses are definitely advantageous regarding thromboembolism.

No mechanical valve to date can be used safely without anticoagulation therapy. Oyer[11] reported an incidence of 0.7% per patient year of fatal bleedings after Starr-Edwards valve replacement. One patient in this series died of bleeding due to anticoagulant therapy. Anticoagulant therapy was discontinued in our patients with AVR when discharged from the hospital. Despite this early interruption and contrary to the general practice of giving such patients anticoagulants during the first 2 months, no embolism has been observed in our series. The same policy was followed with the few mitral valve patients who were in sinus rhythm when leaving the hospital. Patients with atrial fibrillation usually received a low dosage of anticoagulation therapy after leaving the hospital. The decision of stopping such therapy has been left to the discretion of the referring cardiologist. The advice was given that anticoagulation therapy be stopped when patients returned to sinus rhythm or when there was a marked decrease in heart size. It has been suggested by Hetzer et al[16] that there is no difference in thromboembolic rate with or without anticoagulation in patients with Hancock mitral valve prostheses.

Endocarditis is still a very serious complication after valve replacement. In our series we noted an incidence of 1% per patient year after AVR and 0.7% after mitral valve implantation. Similar incidences were found after mechanical valve replacements. Some reports have suggested that endocarditis occurring on heterograft valves is more easily cured with antibiotics than on prosthetic valves.[17,18] Despite this, high mortality in patients with endocarditis has been reported by Zusman et al.[19] Six of our 9 patients in whom endocarditis occurred during our 5-year follow-up died of their disease. Four of the patients with endocarditis who died were never offered the opportunity of replacing their infected valve and the other 2 patients came to surgery after 2 and 6 months of unsuccessful treatment of their disease.

Conclusions

Based on our experience within the first 8 years, valve dysfunction with the Hancock bioprosthesis is no worse than with mechanical prostheses. Further and longer evaluation of these patients is needed to see if the slope of the degradation curve of these valves remains unchanged. In view of the many advantages of a bioprosthesis and because our long-term results after 8 years are encouraging, we continue to implant porcine bioprosthetic valves at this time in any adult patient.

References

1. Angell WW, Angell JD: Porcine valves. Prog Cardiovasc Dis 23:141, 1980.
2. MacManus Q, Grunkemeier GL, Lambert LE, et al: Non-cloth-covered caged-ball prostheses: The second decade. J Thorac Cardiovasc Surg 76:788, 1978.
3. Lepley D., Felmma RJ., Mullen DC, et al: Late evaluation of patients undergoing valve replacement with the Björk-Shiley prostheses. Ann Thorac Surg 24:131, 1977.
4. Oyer PE: Long-term clinical results of xenograft bioprostheses. Presented at the Symposium on Bioprosthetic Cardiac Valves. Munich, Germany, April 5–7, 1979.
5. Cohn LH, Mee RB, Koster JK, Collins JJ Jr: Long-term follow-up of the Hancock xenograft heart valve: a six-year review. Presented at the 51st. Scientific Session of the American Heart Association. Dallas, Texas, November 1978.
6. Davila JC, Magilligan DJ, Lewis JW: Is the Hancock porcine valve the best cardiac valve substitute today? Ann Thorac Surg 26:303, 1978.
7. Carpentier A, Deloche A, Relland J, et al: Six-year follow-up of glutaraldehyde preserved heterografts. J Thorac Cardiovasc Surg 68:771, 1974.
8. Casarotto D, Bortolotti V, Thiene G, Gallucci V, Cévese PG: Long-term results (from 5 to 7 years) with the Hancock S-G-P bioprostheses. J Cardiovasc Surg (Torino) 20:399, 1979.
9. Pipkin RD, Buch WS, Fogarty TJ: Evaluation of aortic valve replacement with a porcine xenograft without long-term anticoagulation. J Thorac Cardiovasc Surg 71:179, 1976.
10. Björk VO, Henze A: Prosthetic heart valve replacement. Nine years experience with the Björk-Shiley tilting disc valve. In Tissue Heart Valves (M, Ionescu): London, Butterworths, 1979, p 1.
11. Oyer PE, Stinson EB, Griepp RB, et al: Valve replacement with the Starr-Edwards and Hancock prostheses: Comparative analysis of late morbidity and mortality. Ann Surg 186:301, 1977.
12. Starr A, MacManus Q, Grinkemeier G, et al: Clinical results with composite strut (track valve) prostheses. Presented at the American Heart Association meeting, 1977.
13. Duran CG, Pomar JL, Gallo I, et al: Les greffes valvulaires. Problèmes et evolution. Ann Cardiol Angeiol 26:529, 1977.
14. Buch WS, Pipkin RD, Hancock WD, et al: Mitral valve replacement with the Hancock stabilized glutaraldehyde valve. Clinical and laboratory evaluation. Arch Surg 110:1408, 1975.
15. Tandon AP, Sengupta SM, Lukacs L, Ionescu MI: Long term clinical and

hemodynamic evaluation of the Ionescu-Shiley pericardial xenograft and the Braunwald-Cutter and Björk-Shiley prostheses in the mitral position. J Thorac Cardiovasc Surg 76:763, 1978.
16. Hetzer R, Hill JD, Kerth, WJ, Ansbro J, Adappa MG, Rodvien R, Kamm B, Gerbode, F: Thromboembolic complications after mitral valve replacement with Hancock xenografts. J Thorac Cardiovasc Surg 75:651, 1978.
17. Magilligan DJ, Quinn EL, Davila JC: Bacteremia, endocarditis and the Hancock valve. Ann Thorac Surg 24:508, 1977.
18. Rossiter SJ, Stinson EB, Oyer PE, Miller DC, Schapira JN, Martin RP, Shumway NE: Prosthetic valve endocarditis comparison of heterograft tissue valves and mechanical valves. J Thorac Cardiovasc Surg 76:795, 1978.
19. Zusman DR, Levine FH, Carter JE, Buckley MJ: Hemodynamic and clinical evolution of the Hancock modified-orifice aortic bioprosthesis. Circulation 64:189, 1981.

7

Mid- and Long-Term Evaluation of Porcine Bioprosthetic Valves: A 6-Year Experience

G. BLOCH, P. R. VOUHE, H. POULAIN, P. MENU, J. P. CACHERA, P. AUBRY, D. Y. LOISANCE, J. J. GALEY

From January 1975 to December 1981 in the Department of Cardiovascular Surgery of Henri Mondor Hospital, 454 patients underwent isolated or multiple valve replacement using 520 bioprostheses. The majority of the xenografts were Hancock valves, Carpentier-Edwards bioprosthesis, and, more recently, Liotta and Xenomedica bioprostheses. During this period, bioprostheses were used in one-third of all our patients having valve replacement. Children younger than 15 years of age were excluded, as were bioprostheses used for reconstruction of pulmonary outflow tract. Ages ranged from 16–89, with a mean age of 51.2 years and the mean functional class was 2.9, indicating the severity of the preoperative state.

Patients and Results

The patients, 255 men and 199 women, were divided into 3 groups: aortic (AVR), mitral (MVR), and multiple valve replacement (multi VR) (Table I). The overall operative mortality was 7.3%. Since a considerable number of patients were from North and Central Africa, only 275 patients were restudied. The follow-up extended from 3 months to 7 years, with a mean of 2.5 years. The symptomatic improvement was attested to by a mean postoperative functional class of 1.4.

The following rates of valve-related complications were observed (Table II): 1.7% per patient year of thromboembolism; 1.3% per patient year of

---

From the Hôpital Henri Mondor, Creteil, France.

TABLE I Operative mortality and follow-up

	AVR	MVR	Multi VR	Total
# patients	219	168	67	
Overall operative mortality, %	4.6	8.3	13.4	7.3
Current survivors	151	89	35	275
Mean follow-up (yrs)	2.6	2.3	2.6	2.5
Mean functional class (NYHA)	1.3	1.4	1.5	1.4

prosthetic endocarditis; 0.4% per patient year of primary tissue valve degeneration; 1.0% per patient year of paraprosthetic leaks.

At 6 years, 84% of patients are free from any valve failure (Fig. 1). At 6 years, the probability of being thromboemboli-free was 94%. Most emboli occurred in the mitral valve group (emboli-free probability was 85.6% at 6 years) (Fig. 2). After the 2 first postoperative months, long-term anticoagulation was used only for a specific condition, such as chronic atrial fibrillation.

Prosthetic endocarditis was more frequent in the aortic position. Ninety-five percent of patients were free from infection at 6 years (Fig. 3). Valve degeneration was rare and 97% of bioprostheses were functioning well at 6 years (Fig. 4).

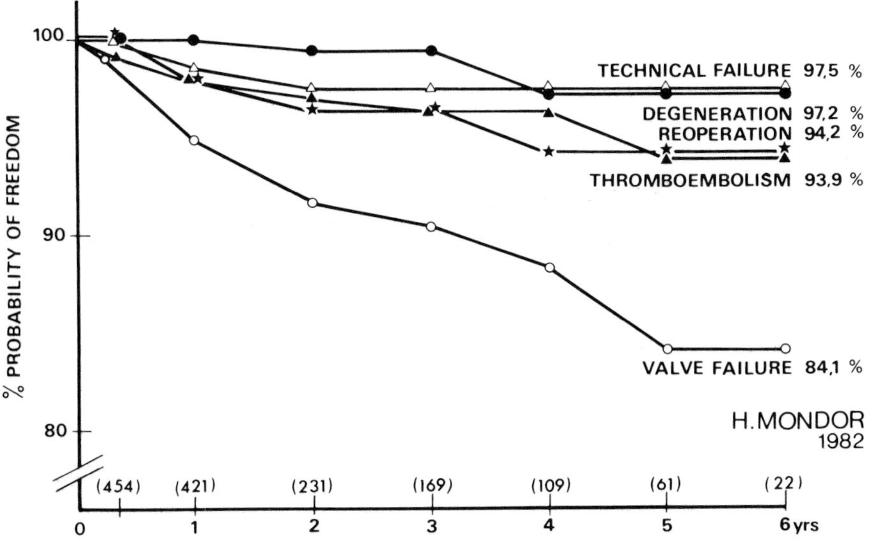

FIG. 1 Valve-related complications. Actuarial curves.

TABLE II Valve-related complications

	AVR*	MVR*	Multi VR*		# valve failure†	# reoperations‡
Thromboembolism	1.0	2.9	2.2	1.7	2(1,4 mo)	1(3 mo)
Endocarditis	1.5	1.0	1.1	1.3	4(2,21,33,50 mo)	3(2,21,46 mo)
Degeneration	0.5	0.5	—	0.4	1(36 mo)	3(20,36,41 mo)
Technical failure	1.3	0.5	1.1	1.0		5(2,4,6,9,16 mo)

* Per 100 patient years.
† Seven patients (1.0/100 patient years).
‡ Twelve patients (1.7/100 patient years).

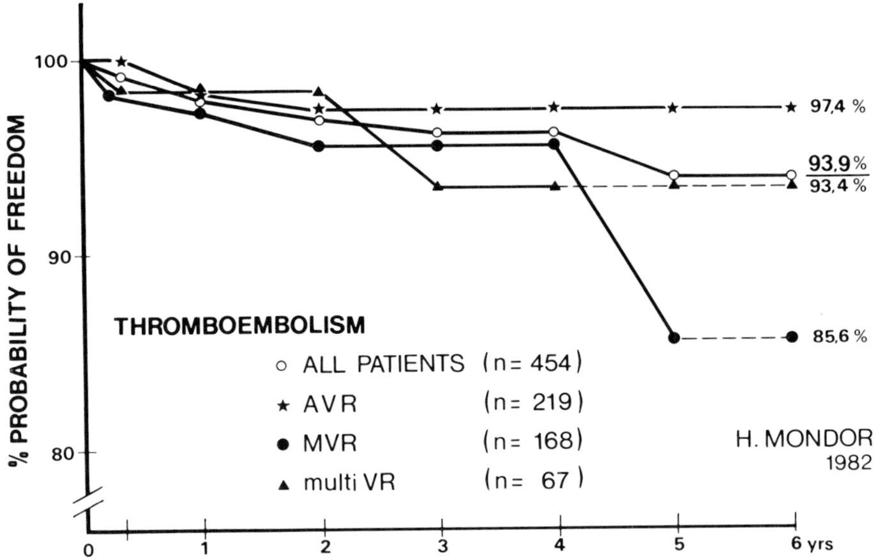

FIG. 2 Complications of thromboembolism. Actuarial curves.

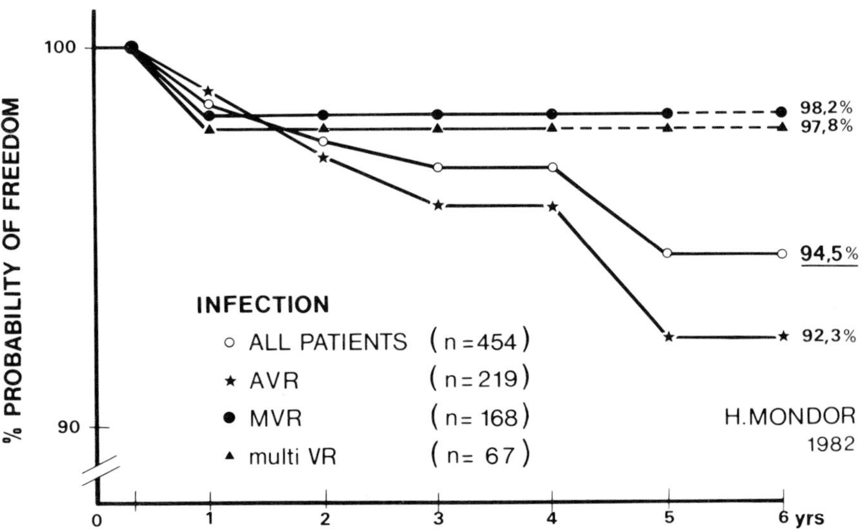

FIG. 3 Complications of endocarditis. Actuarial curves.

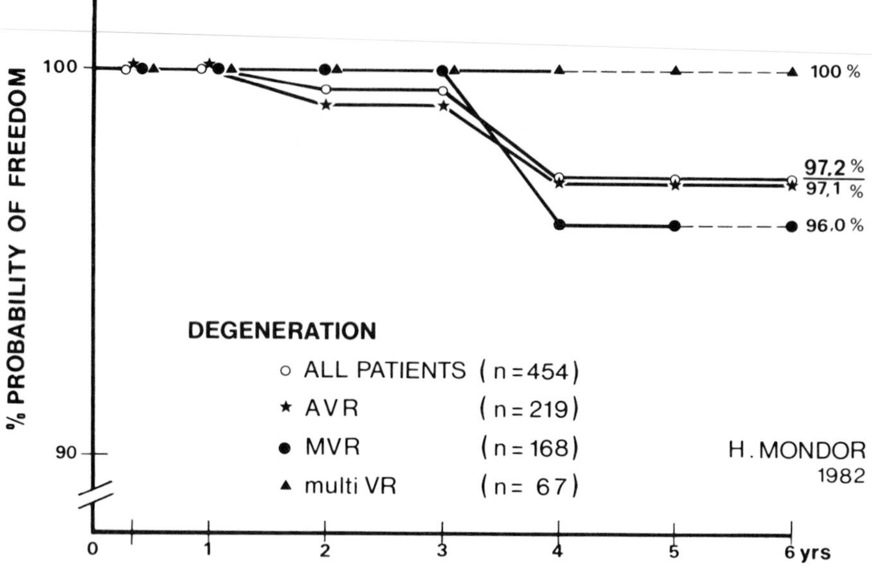

FIG. 4 Primary tissue degeneration. Actuarial curves.

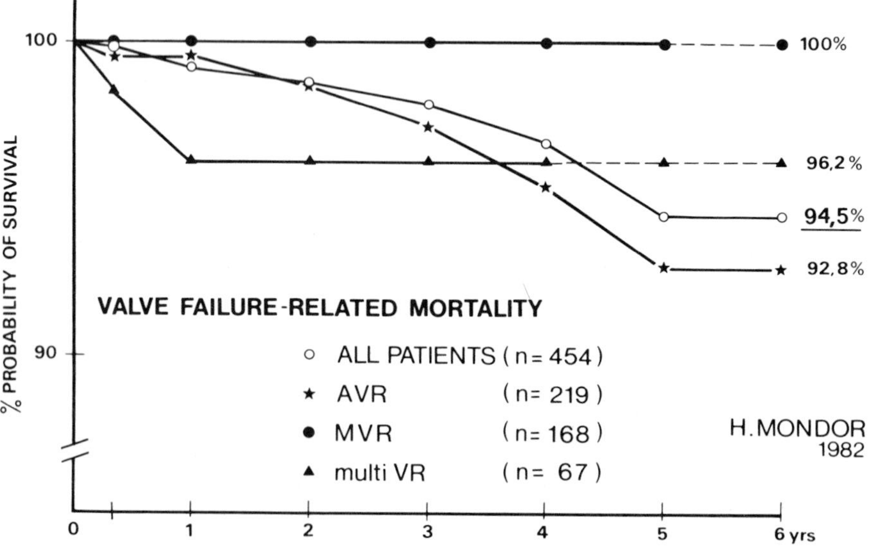

FIG. 5 Valve-related mortality. Actuarial curves.

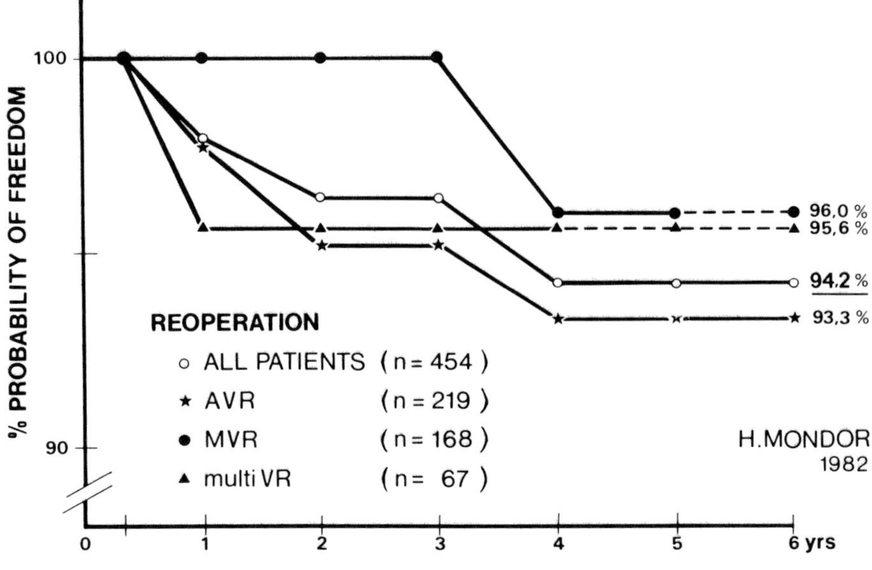

FIG. 6 Rate of reoperation. Actuarial curve.

One percent per patient year died because of a valve failure (Table II). The overall valve-related mortality is 5.5% at 6 years (Fig. 5); the higher rate in the aortic group is due to prosthetic endocarditis.

Reoperation was necessary for 12 patients with valve failures (Table II). Three patients died at reoperation, two for prosthetic endocarditis and the other one for replacement of a degenerated valve. At 6 years, 94% of patients were free of reoperation (Fig. 6).

The overall late mortality was 4.5% per patient year, the cardiac-related mortality, 2.9% per patient year, and the valve-related mortality, 0.7% (Table III). At 6 years, 73% of all patients were alive and 82% were free from cardiac death (Fig. 7).

TABLE III Late mortality

	AVR	MVR	Multi VR	Total
Overall	4.8	3.9	4.4	4.5
Cardiac	2.8	2.4	4.4	2.9
Valve related	1.0	—	1.1	0.7

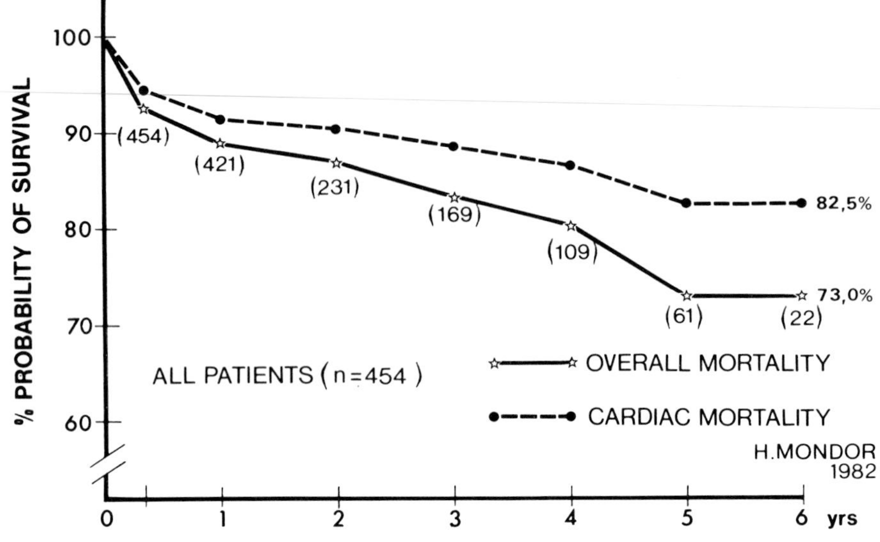

FIG. 7 Actuarial curves of overall and cardiac mortality.

Conclusions

We are aware that the risk of valve degeneration may be higher in the next years. On the other hand, the rate of early valve-related complications is low and bioprostheses remain a valuable alternative in selected patients. The following indications are presently used: patients older than 65 years, specific contraindication to anticoagulants, patients unable to follow long-term anticoagulation for psychologic or geographic reasons, replacement of thrombosed valve, women desiring children, and the patient's own choice after being fully informed.

SECTION II

HEMODYNAMICS

8

Hemodynamic Evaluation of the Hancock Bioprosthesis in the Mitral Position: A 1–7 Years Follow-up

J. L. UBAGO, A. FIGUEROA, T. COLMAN, J. M. REVUELTA, A. OCHOTECO, C. M. G. DURAN

Ideally, serial hemodynamic studies should provide an indication of the time-related general behavior of bioprosthesis. Numerous short-term postoperative hemodynamic studies have been reported in the literature,[1–6] but always averaging the widely different results obtained due to the characteristic flow-dependent orifices of these porcine bioprosthesis.[7,8] In long-term studies it is difficult to determine whether a particular bioprosthesis is functioning correctly in a particular patient unless major dysfunction is present.[9,10] Furthermore, when a comparison is made in a group of patients with early and late hemodynamic studies using the average values of effective orifices and gradients, an impression is conveyed that all biprostheses after 5 years tend to become stenotic even before clinical signs of dysfunction are apparent.[11]

We have developed a method to correlate the area/flow/gradient relationship for each valve size,[12] which makes possible individual evolution of the long-term behavior of the Hancock valve independent of cardiac status at the time of the exploration.

Patients and Methods

Two hundred and thirty-two mitral Hancock bioprostheses in 189 patients were restudied because of a clinical diagnosis of dysfunction in 37 patients and a research protocol in the remaining 152. In 131 patients the

From the Departments of Hemodinamica and Cirugia Cardiovascular, Centro Medico "Valdecilla" and Universidad of Santander, Santander, Spain.

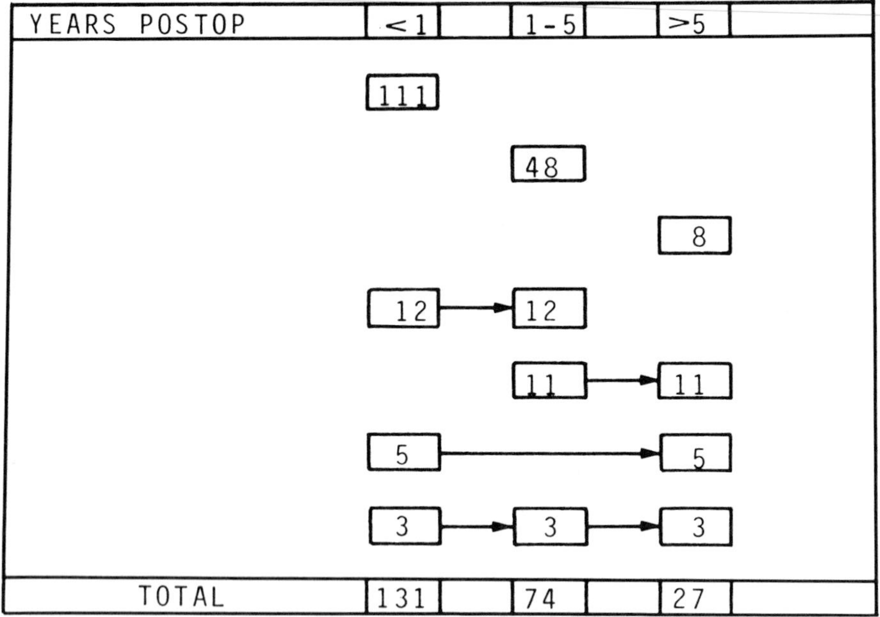

FIG. 1 All Hancock mitral valves recatheterized under 1 year, from 2–5 years, and more than 5 years after surgery. The arrows indicate the sequential studies performed.

follow-up was short-term, less than 1 year, and in 101 it was between 1 and 7 years. Twenty-seven were studied after 5 years of follow-up, 19 had a previous normal postoperative study, and 3 had a total of 3 sequential catheterizations (Fig. 1). In 14 patients the second study was indicated by protocol and with a clinically normal valve.

Forty patients with normal functioning valves under 1 year of follow-up were selected to develop specific gradient/flow/area nomograms for each size of the Hancock mitral bioprosthesis. A standard right and left catheterization was performed with #7 or #8 Cournand and Millar microtip ventricular catheters. Left ventricular cineangiograms were taken in the 30° right anterior oblique projection. In each patient, 0.5–1 ml/kg of 82% meglumine metrizoate was injected in 2 seconds. The electrocardiogram was simultaneously recorded on the film. At the moment of contrast injection, a blank frame appeared on the film and simultaneously a vertical marker was printed every 1/100 second in the pressure tracing. Therefore the angiographic image could be related with the pressure event.

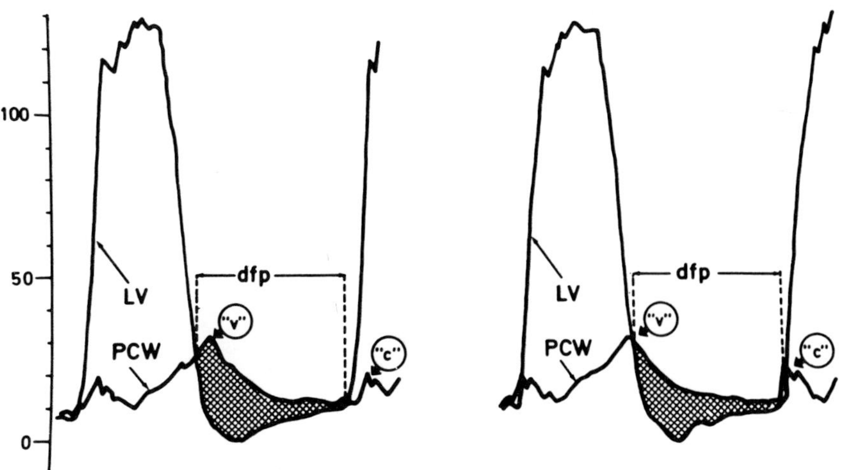

FIG. 2 Simultaneous pressure tracing of left ventricle (LV) and pulmonary capillary wedge (PCW) (left). The wedge pressure is displaced to make the "c" wave coincide with the isovolumetric rising left ventricular tracing (right). dfp: diastolic filling period. Reproduced with permission from Ubago et al.[12]

In order to correct the time delay between the pulmonary wedge and the left atrial pressure, the wedge tracing was moved forward until the "c" wave coincided with the upswing of the left ventricular pressure tracing (Fig. 2).

The atrioventricular emptying period was defined as the diastolic time minus the systolic and diastolic isometric phases and calculated by the interval between the crossing of the ventricular and atrial curves. This emptying period was divided into 3 equal parts: early, middle, and late diastole (Fig. 3a). The gradient was calculated for each part by dividing the corresponding areas, measured by planimetry by the time interval. The partial gradients were expressed as mmHg. The mitral valve gradient was calculated as

$$\frac{\text{area (cm}^2\text{)}}{\text{diastolic filling period (cm)}} \times 10 \text{ (mmHg)}$$

Selecting from the angiogram the first frame of mitral opening corresponding to the pressure tracing selected for study, the same number of markers in the tracing was counted as frames in the cine from the first blank frame (1 msec = 1 cine frame). The partial left ventricular filling volumes that corresponded to each early, middle, and late diastolic period were calculated. Each volume was obtained by subtracting the previous volume (Fig. 3b). The partial diastolic flows were calculated in milliliters divided by their corresponding time intervals in seconds.

The effective orifice of the Hancock valve in each diastolic period was calculated with the formula of Gorlin and Gorlin.[13] The empirical constant

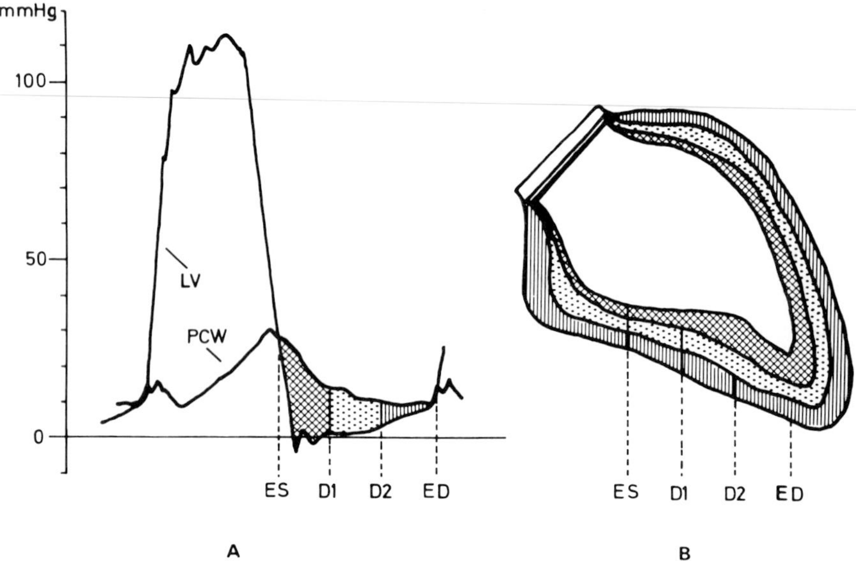

FIG. 3 A. Simultaneous left ventricular (LV) and time-corrected pulmonary wedge (PCW) pressure tracings. ES: end systole; D1: end of early diastole; D2: end of mid diastole; ED: end diastole. B. Left ventricular cineangiographic diastolic shapes. Early diastolic volume: D1−ES. Mid diastolic volume: D2−D1. End diastolic volume: ED−D2. Reproduced with permission from Ubago et al.[12]

of 38 was used because direct measurement of the left ventricular diastolic pressure was available. The mean values and standard deviations of the early, middle, and late diastolic flows and gradients of all patients were plotted together (Fig. 4). These data were placed on Gorlin pressure and flow curves (k = 38).

The early, middle, late, and mean diastolic flows and their corresponding calculated effective orifices were plotted together for all patients with the same Hancock valve size. A relationship between flows and orifices was observed, with larger areas corresponding to larger flows and vice versa; this diagram tended to be a curve (Fig. 5).

When the gradients corresponding to each flow were calculated from this curve, a new flow gradient curve was constructed. By superimposing our flow and gradient data, high correlation coefficients were also obtained. When Gorlin pressure flow curves were superimposed, a graph was constructed for related flows, gradients, and areas for each Hancock valve size (Fig. 6).

Each valve size is represented by a particular curve, all of which cross the fixed orifice Gorlin pressure flow curves, indicating a variability in the effective orifice of the Hancock valve. Therefore all of the Hancock valve

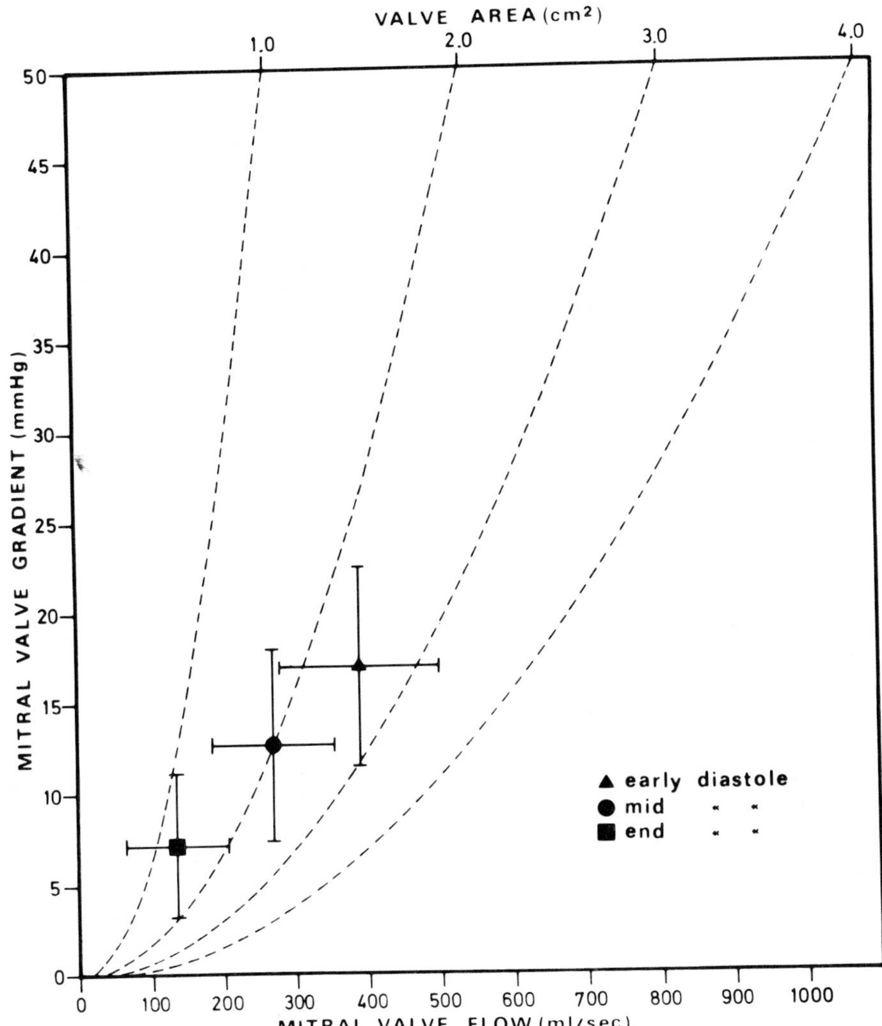

FIG. 4 Mean and standard deviations of early, middle, and late diastolic gradients and flows of the 40 mitral Hancock valves studied. Dotted lines indicate the calculated orifice areas of 1, 2, 3, and 4 cm^2 using the Gorlin formula. Reproduced with permission from Ubago et al.[12]

effective areas increase in response to rises in flow and pressure gradient. These curves mathematically define the behavior of the Hancock valve in relation to the flow that crosses it.

The 101 mitral Hancock prostheses with a follow-up from 1–7 years were studied by calculating the average flow and gradient, which were then

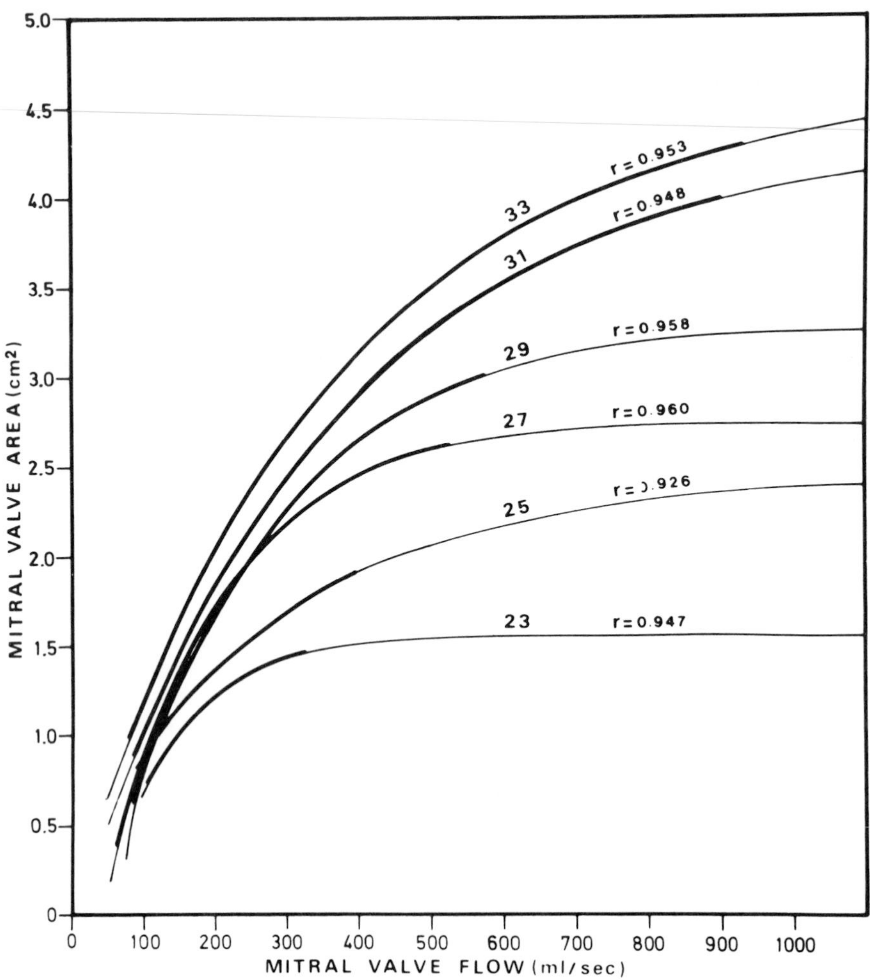

FIG. 5 Hancock mitral xenograft effective orifices related to flows for each valve size. The thick lines correspond to the observed data and the thin lines to the theoretical values at very high flows. Figures on curve indicate the Hancock valve size and the correlation coefficient. Reproduced with permission from Ubago et al.[12]

placed in the Fig. 6 nomogram. If the intersecting point was found to be within the corresponding curve for the valve size, the particular valve was defined as normal functioning for flow and gradient. Similarly, when the average flow and calculated effective orifice were placed in the Fig. 5 nomogram, the function of a particular valve can also be established.

Whenever these values were found outside the nomogram, the valve was considered to be dysfunctioning. In the case of stenosis the flow gradient

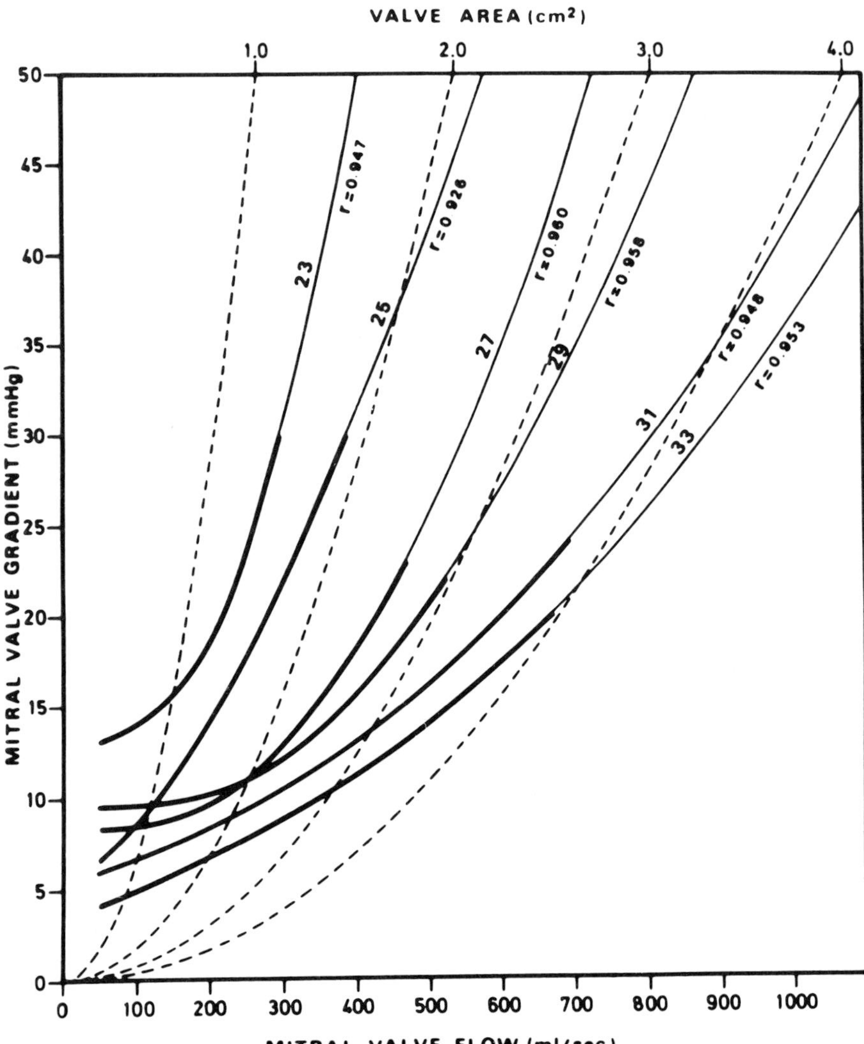

FIG. 6 Flow-gradient relationship for each Hancock valve size. Dotted lines show Gorlin flow pressure curves for different orifice areas. Thick lines correspond to the observed data and thin lines to theoretical values at very high flows. Figures on each curve indicate the Hancock valve size and the correlation coefficient. Reproduced with permission from Ubago et al.[12]

intersection point is displaced toward the left of the nomogram. When regurgitation is present, this point will be situated within the curve but in its higher range. When stenosis is added, it will again move toward the left of the curve (Fig. 7).

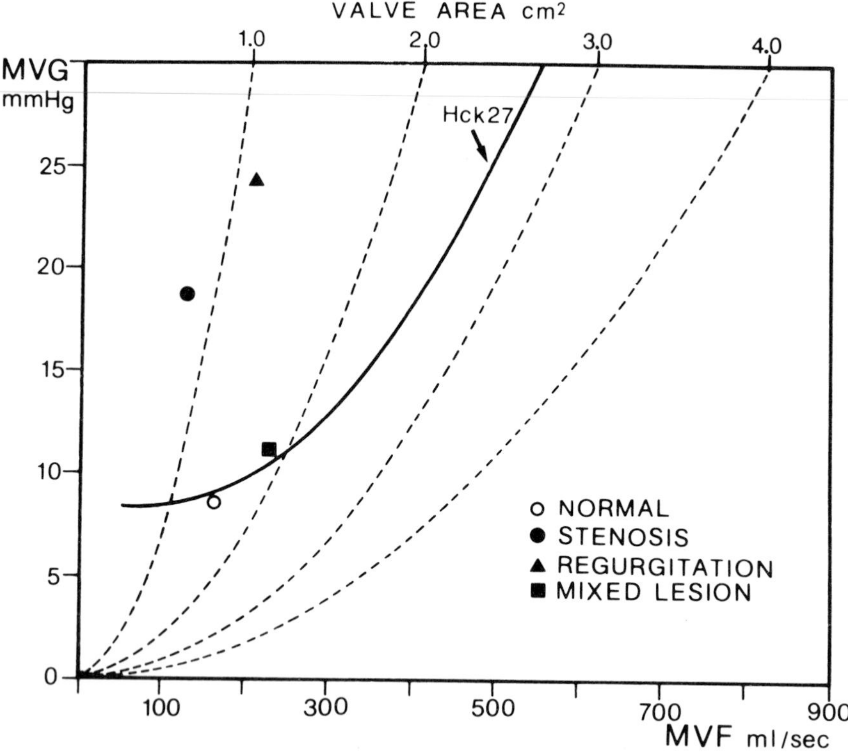

FIG. 7 Typical examples of hemodynamically normal and dysfunctioning Hancock mitral bioprostheses size 27. MVG: mitral valve gradient. MVF: mitral valve flow.

Results

The results in terms of gradient, flow, and effective orifice of the 14 patients with no clinical diagnosis of dysfunction, after more than 5 years of follow-up and a sequential restudy, are shown in Table I. The average effective orifice of the second study was smaller than that found at the early postoperative study (1.26 -vs- 1.40). Similarly the gradients were also higher (12.4 -vs- 9.4). Comparing individually the results of the second against the early postoperative study, it can be observed that in 8 patients the areas have become smaller but in 6 they have become larger. In only 3 patients (#3, 4, and 5), who had an important reduction in area, had the gradients risen. The other 5 patients (#7, 8, 9, 12, and 13) with small reduction in area had similar or lower gradients than in the first study.

Applying the described nomograms to the 232 patients recatheterized, we have found 190 normal valves and 42 dysfunctional (Fig. 8). The dysfunctional valves included 18 with perivalvular leaks; 6 were insufficiencies

TABLE I Hemodynamic data

Pts	Valve size (mm)	Follow-up (mo)	MVG* (mmHg)		MVF* (ml/sec)		MVA* (cm^2)	
			Early	Late	Early	Late	Early	Late
1	23	69	15.0	16.4	76	106	0.51	0.69
2	25	63	16.0	20.4	177	239	1.16	1.51
3	25	66	9.0	27.8	142	111	1.24	0.55
4	27	61	9.2	18.8	152	138	1.32	0.84
5	27	62	10.4	18.5	195	181	1.59	1.10
6	27	90	7.8	7.2	141	169	1.33	1.66
7	27	80	7.9	8.0	138	112	1.29	1.04
8	27	78	7.0	5.3	293	153	2.91	1.60
9	29	81	9.2	8.0	149	116	1.29	1.08
10	29	64	7.6	11.0	109	199	1.04	1.58
11	29	64	10.0	9.5	135	152	1.12	1.30
12	31	69	7.6	7.0	236	195	2.25	1.93
13	31	61	7.4	6.5	102	80	0.99	0.82
14	31	73	8.0	8.6	170	216	1.58	1.94
Mean ±SD		70 ± 9	9.4 ± 2.8	12.4 ± 6.8	158 ± 55	155 ± 47	1.40 ± 0.58	1.26 ± 0.45

* MVG: mitral valve gradient; MVF: mitral valve flow; MVA; mitral valve area.

MITRAL HANCOCK BIOPROSTHESIS: OVERALL RESULTS

TIME POSTOPERATIVE (mos)	0	12	24	36	48	60	72	84	
No POSTOP STUDIES	131	36	20	9	9	19	7	1	232
NORMAL FUNCTION	111	35	17	4	7	9	6	1	190
PERIVALVULAR LEAK	○○○○○ ○○●●● ●●●●●		●	●		○			18
ENDOCARDITIS	●	●	●●	●		●			6
THROMBOSIS	●								1
INTRINSIC: STENOSIS	●								3
INTRINSIC: REGURGITATION	○ ●								
PRIMARY TISSUE FAILURES STENOSIS						○○●●			14
REGURGITATION				●	●	●●	●		
MIXED LESION				●●	●	●●			
TOTAL DYSFUNCTIONS	20	1	3	5	2	10	1	0	42

FIG. 8 Overall results of the 232 Hancock mitral valves recatheterized. Open circles indicate patients without reoperation (hemodynamic diagnosis), black circles indicate patients reoperated upon (hemodynamic and surgical diagnosis).

secondary to bacterial endocarditis, all requiring surgery. One patient had a valve thrombosis and was also reoperated upon; 3 patients had a clinically abnormal behavior since the time of surgery either stenosis or insufficiency, (2 were reoperated again); 14 had a primary tissue failure. Four patients with stenosis are interesting, since none of them had clinical indications for restudy and none was reoperated after the catheterization. Five other patients had massive valvular regurgitation, all requiring surgical therapy, and 5 patients had both a calcified and ruptured prosthesis hemodynamically diagnosed as a mixed lesion.

Comment

Several authors have reported the hemodynamic results of the Hancock mitral valve by showing the mean diastolic gradient and mean effective areas. When all results were grouped by the Hancock valve size, a large scattering of data appeared. Some patients had large areas and some small with the same prosthetic size, and even large valves could have smaller areas than those found in small prosthesis.[1–5]

Similarly, when the valve was restudied long after implantation, a new scatter appeared.[11] The average of these results showed a reduction of the effective orifice, suggesting a time-related progressive and universal stenosis of the mitral Hancock valve. If a similar method is applied to our data, similar results and conclusions result. Furthermore, if the short- and long-term hemodynamic results of each individual patient are compared, the effective orifice calculated in the 2nd study is smaller, equal, or even larger than the calculated area in the 1st postoperative study. This discrepancy between studies performed on apparently normal valves is due to the flow crossing the valve at the time of the study. The isolated reporting of gradients and areas is meaningless and therefore cannot define normality. The diagnosis of dysfunction requires the relationship of flow/gradient, using the specific nomograms described for each valve size.

In sequential studies (Table I) we observed that those patients in whom the calculated orifice had become smaller and theoretically stenotic were of 2 types: those with a parallel reduction in flow and gradient and therefore within the normal curve in the nomogram and those with a rise in gradient without a parallel rise in flow. These latter patients are outside the nomogram and pathologically stenotic.

Applying the nomogram to each of the 232 patients restudied, we have observed 190 absolutely normal valves and 42 dysfunctional. It is interesting to note that among all valves without any clinical diagnosis of dysfunction only 4 were stenotic, 2 being reoperated upon considerably later. The remaining valves were normal.

Our impressions in hemodynamical terms are: 1) some valves show an early dysfunction that is due to either defective construction or surgical error; 2) other valves rupture or calcify, becoming first stenotic and eventually rupturing; 3) many valves remain absolutely normal over a long period of time and do not invariably become stenotic.

References

1. Horowitz MS, Goodman DJ, Fogarty TJ, Harrison DC: Mitral valve replacement with the glutaraldehyde-preserved porcine heterograft. Clinical, hemodynamic and pathological correlations. J Thorac Cardiovasc Surg 67:885, 1974.
2. McIntosh CL, Michaelis LL, Morrow AG, Itscoitz SB, Redwood DR, Epstein SE: Atrioventricular valve replacement with the Hancock porcine xenograft: A five year clinical experience. Surgery 78:1, 1975.
3. Cotter L, Miller H: Clinical and haemodynamic evaluation of mounted porcine heterograft in mitral position. Br Heart J 41:412, 1979.
4. Johnson AD, Daily PO, Peterson KL, LeWinter M, DiDonna GJ, Blair G, Niwayama G: Functional evaluation of the porcine heterograft in the mitral position. Circulation 51 (Suppl I):40, 1975.
5. Lurie AJ, Miller RR, Maxwell KS, Grehl TM, Vismara LA, Hulrey EJ, Mason DT: Hemodynamic assessment of the glutaraldehyde-preserved porcine heterograft in the aortic and mitral positions. Circulation 56 (Suppl II):104, 1977.
6. Cohn LH, Collins JJ Jr: The glutaraldehyde-stabilized porcine xenograft valve. In Tissue Heart Valves (MI Ionescu, Ed). London, Butterworths, 1975, p 173.
7. Gabbay S, McQueen DM, Yellin EL, Frater RWM: In vitro hydrodynamic comparison of mitral valve bioprosthesis. Circulation 60 (Suppl I):62, 1979.
8. Wright JTM: Hydrodynamic evaluation of tissue valves. In Tissue Heart Valves (MI Ionescu, Ed). London, Butterworths, 1975, p 29.

9. Oyer PE, Stinson EB, Reitz BA, Miller DC, Rossiter SJ, Shumway NE: Long-term evaluation of the porcine xenograft bioprosthesis. J Thorac Cardiovasc Surg 78:343, 1979.
10. Hannah H, Reis RL: Current status of porcine heterograft prosthesis: A five year appraisal. Circulation 54 (Suppl III):27, 1976.
11. Lipson LC, Kent KM, Rosing DR, Bonow RO, McIntosh CL, Condit S, Epstein SE, Morrow AG: Long-term hemodynamic assessment of the porcine heterograft in mitral position. Circulation 64:397, 1981.
12. Ubago JL, Figueroa A, Colman T, Ochoteco A, Duran CMG: Hemodynamic factors that affect calculated orifice areas in the mitral Hancock xenograft valve. Circulation 61:388, 1980.
13. Gorlin R, Gorlin SG: Hydraulic formula for calculation of the area of the stenotic mitral valve, other cardiac valves and central circulatory shunts. Am Heart J 41:1, 1951.

9

Hemodynamic Evaluation of the Carpentier-Edwards Standard and Improved Anulus Bioprostheses

C. PELLETIER, B. R. CHAITMAN, R. BONAN, I. DYRDA

After 6 years of experience with the Carpentier-Edwards porcine valve at the Montreal Heart Institute, this bioprosthesis remains the valve substitute of choice in more than 75% of our valve implants. Excellent clinical results have been obtained, with a marked improvement in 86% of the patients and a 93% 5 year probability of remaining free of all valve-related complications.[1] The low rate of thromboembolic complications without permanent anticoagulation is one of the major advantages of tissue valves over mechanical prostheses and justifies their use in selected patients.

Hemodynamic evaluation of the different bioprostheses has been the object of several reports.[2] However, relatively few hemodynamic data are available on the Carpentier-Edwards compared to the Hancock valve, most likely because the Carpentier-Edwards valve became commercially available later. Bioprostheses differ with respect to mounting techniques, sewing ring, and tissue preservation, and several have undergone modifications in recent years. Therefore the clinical and hemodynamic performance of each bioprosthesis requires evaluation on an individual basis. In a previous report we found satisfactory hemodynamic results with the Carpentier-Edwards valve, although it was mildly obstructive in smaller stent sizes.[3] Since then, the anulus of the valve has been modified to increase the effective orifice area of the bioprosthesis. The purpose of the present study is to review our experience with the postoperative hemodynamic evaluation of the Carpentier-Edwards bioprosthesis, and to compare the performance of the improved anulus model available since early 1980 with that of the initial standard anulus valve in use since 1976.

From the Departments of Surgery and Medicine, Montreal Heart Institute and University of Montreal Medical School, Montreal, Quebec, Canada.

TABLE I Sizes of implanted bioprostheses in total series of 837 Carpentier-Edwards valves

Stent size (mm)	Valve replacement					
	Aortic		Mitral		Tricuspid	
	#	%	#	%	#	%
19	12	3	—		—	
21	52	14	—		—	
23	114	30	—		—	
25	109	28	6	2	—	
27	61	16	58	13	1	6
29	28	7	153	35	1	6
31	9	2	156	36	6	35
33	—		62	14	9	53
Total	385	100	435	100	17	100

Patients and Methods

Patient Population

From May 1976 to March 1982, 837 Carpentier-Edwards bioprostheses were implanted in 726 patients, 384 women and 342 men, aged 13 to 77 years at the time of surgery (mean age: 53 years). There were 324 mitral valve replacements (45%), 284 aortic valve replacements (39%), 5 isolated tricuspid valve replacements (0.5%), and 113 multiple valve replacements (15.5%). Coronary bypass grafting was associated with valve replacement in 101 patients (14%), and tricuspid anuloplasty was performed in 41 patients (6%). Among the implanted bioprostheses, there were 629 standard anulus valves (SA, 75%) and 208 improved anulus valves (IA, 25%). The stent sizes of implanted valves in each position are shown in Table I. There were 68 early deaths (30 day mortality, 9.4%). Early mortality was 5.3% with isolated mitral valve replacement (15 deaths), 6.0% with isolated aortic valve replacement (14 deaths), and 16.0% with multiple valve replacement (17 deaths). There were no deaths with isolated tricuspid replacement. There were 22 early deaths in patients with combined coronary and valve surgery. All but 4 patients were followed regularly after surgery. During follow-up, which totaled 1300 patient years 6 patients (0.5% per patient years) underwent reoperation because of dysfunction of the Carpentier-Edwards bioprosthesis (paravalvular leak in 4, primary tissue failure of the valve in 2).

Among the 658 survivors, 71 patients (11%) underwent an elective hemodynamic study 4–15 months following valve implantation (mean, 8

TABLE II Predominant valve disease before surgery in 71 patients studied (74 bioprostheses)

Preoperative valve disease	Valve replacement			
	Aortic		Mitral	
	#	%	#	%
Stenosis	17	45	9	25
Regurgitation	13	34	11	30
Stenosis + regurgitation	8	21	16	45
Total	38	100	36	100

months). Only asymptomatic patients, younger than 65 years of age at the time of surgery, living in the Montreal area were included in the study. The group consisted of 38 men and 33 women, with a mean age of 48 years (range, 23–66 years). There were 35 aortic, 33 mitral, and 3 double valve replacements. Preoperatively, the most common valve lesion was aortic stenosis (45%) among patients who underwent aortic valve replacement and mixed mitral disease (45%) in the mitral replacement group (Table II). Overall, 74 Carpentier-Edwards bioprostheses were studied: 38 aortic valves (32 SA and 6 IA), and 36 mitral valves (26 SA and 10 IA).

Cardiac Catheterization

The technique used for cardiac catheterization and data measurement has been described previously.[3] In summary, gradients across the aortic bioprosthesis were measured by simultaneous recording of central aortic and left ventricular pressures, and gradients across the mitral bioprosthesis were measured by recording direct left atrial pressure by the transeptal technique and left ventricular pressure simultaneously. Peak to peak aortic gradients were determined from 5 systolic periods. Mean aortic gradients were determined by hand planimetry of 5 systolic cycles, and mean mitral gradients, by hand planimetry of 5 diastolic cycles. Cardiac output was measured by the indicator-dilution technique. Pressure and cardiac output measurements were obtained at rest and during moderate supine arm exercise against 50 watts resistance. Valve orifice areas were calculated from the Gorlin formula[4] using mean gradients. A constant of 44.5 was used for aortic bioprostheses and of 31 for mitral bioprostheses. A uniplane left ventricular cineangiogram in the 30° right anterior oblique position and a supra-aortic angiography in the 90° left lateral position were performed. Valvular regurgitation was assessed from the cineangiograms and classified on a scale of 0–3. The ejection fraction was calculated by the area-length method.[5] The Student's t test was used for the statistical analysis of the data.

Results

In 24 patients with predominant aortic stenosis preoperatively, the aortic gradient decreased from 79.8 ± 6.5 mmHg (mean ± SEM; range, 35–178 mmHg) before surgery to 13.1 ± 1.4 mmHg (range, 4–28 mmHg) after valve replacement ($p < 0.001$). In 18 patients with predominant mitral stenosis, the mitral gradient decreased from 17.4 ± 1.7 mmHg (range, 10–37 mmHg) before to 6.4 ± 0.6 mmHg (range, 2–12 mmHg) after operation ($p < 0.001$). The postoperative ejection fraction averaged 61% following aortic valve replacement and 55% following replacement of the mitral valve. Two patients (5%) with an aortic bioprosthesis and 6 patients (17%) with a mitral bioprosthesis had an ejection fraction below 45% at postoperative evaluation. Postoperative cardiac output at rest averaged 5.4 liters/min in patients with aortic and 4.6 liters/min in patients with mitral valve replacement.

Standard -vs- Improved Anulus Bioprostheses

The hemodynamic results of 16 IA bioprostheses were compared to those obtained in 43 SA valves of the same stent sizes. In the aortic position, peak gradient at rest averaged 13.8 ± 2.6 and 12.3 ± 4.4 mmHg for the 21–23 mm size SA and IA valves, respectively, and 9.9 ± 1.9 -vs- 16.3 ± 3.0 mmHg for the 25 mm size SA and IA valves, differences that were not significant. In the mitral position, mean gradients were also similar, averaging 5.8 ± 0.7 -vs- 10 mmHg for the 27 mm size, 7.4 ± 0.9 -vs- 7.3 ± 1.3 mmHg for the 29 mm size, and 5.3 ± 0.4 -vs- 5.3 ± 0.7 mmHg for the 31 mm size SA and IA valves, respectively. In each stent size the average effective orifice area of the SA and IA models were also similar (Fig. 1). In the aortic position, the effective area of the IA tended to be slightly smaller than that of the SA, whereas the opposite occurred in the mitral 27 and 29 mm valve sizes, but the differences were not statistically significant. In the mitral 31 mm size both models had the same average effective area. The effective orifice area was smaller than 1 cm^2 in 3 aortic bioprostheses, 2 among the IA valves (sizes 21 and 23 mm) and 1 in the SA valves (size 23 mm). Overall, no significant difference in pressure gradients or effective areas was found between the 2 models considered by stent size. Individual data for each IA valve did not separate from those of SA valves (Fig. 1). Therefore the results obtained with both the SA and IA valves were considered together for analysis.

Hemodynamic Function at Rest

Resting hemodynamic data for each stent size are given in Table III. The data were grouped by 2 stent sizes, since the difference between adjacent stent sizes was not significant.

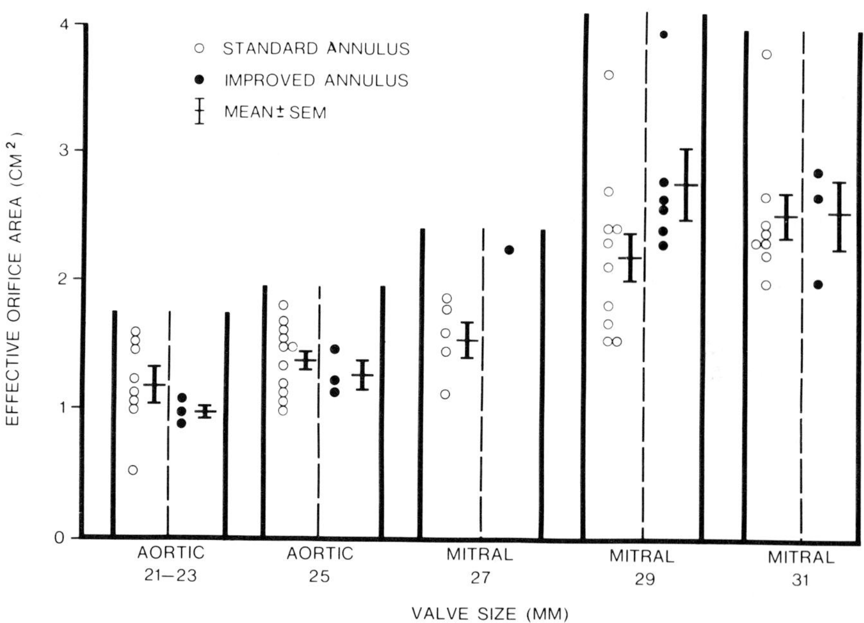

FIG. 1 Comparison of standard and improved anuli effective orifice areas at rest for each valve size. There is no significant difference between the 2 valve models.

In the 38 aortic bioprostheses studied, peak systolic gradient averaged 11.2 ± 1.1 mmHg ($p < 0.001$), and mean systolic gradient averaged 17.3 ± 1.1 mmHg ($p < 0.001$). The difference between peak and mean aortic gradient was significant ($p < 0.001$, Fig. 2). Whereas peak systolic gradient decrease with increasing valve size (21–23 mm: 13.4 mmHg; 25–27 mm: 10.8 mmHg; 29–31 mm: 8.3 mmHg), mean systolic gradient did not correlate to stent size, although it was significantly higher in the 3 groups (Fig. 2).

Mean mitral diastolic gradient averaged 6.4 ± 0.4 mmHg ($p < 0.001$) for the 36 mitral bioprostheses evaluated. The average gradient was 7.1 mmHg in 22 valves of the 27–29 mm stent sizes, and 5.1 mmHg in 14 valves of the 31–33 mm stent sizes.

The calculated effective orifice area at rest averaged 1.43 ± 0.07 cm^2 for aortic valves and 2.38 ± 0.11 cm^2 for mitral valves. The area correlated significantly ($p < 0.05$) with stent size in both the aortic and the mitral position (Fig. 3). The orifice area averaged 1.14 ± 0.09, 1.40 ± 0.06, and 1.95 ± 0.21 cm^2 for each of the 3 aortic stent size groups, respectively, and the average was 2.23 ± 0.15 and 2.64 ± 0.16 cm^2 for the 2 mitral groups.

TABLE III Postoperative hemodynamic data (mean ± SEM) at rest in 74 Carpentier-Edwards bioprostheses

	#	Peak gradient (mmHg)	Mean gradient (mmHg)	Effective area (cm^2)
Aortic				
21 mm	4	8.8 ± 2.5	18.0 ± 2.9	1.15 ± 0.13
23 mm	8	15.8 ± 2.7	22.4 ± 2.8	1.13 ± 0.13
25 mm	14	11.3 ± 1.7	15.9 ± 1.7	1.36 ± 0.07
27 mm	5	9.6 ± 2.7	14.2 ± 1.9	1.50 ± 0.16
29 mm	4	9.8 ± 2.6	18.3 ± 2.9	1.65 ± 0.26
31 mm	3	6.3 ± 3.4	13.7 ± 3.8	2.36 ± 0.20
Total	38	11.2 ± 1.1	17.3 ± 1.1	1.43 ± 0.07
Mitral				
27 mm	6		6.5 ± 0.9	1.68 ± 0.16
29 mm	16		7.4 ± 0.7	2.44 ± 0.17
31 mm	11		5.3 ± 0.3	2.53 ± 0.15
33 mm	3		4.7 ± 0.9	2.99 ± 0.48
Total	36		6.4 ± 0.4	2.38 ± 0.11

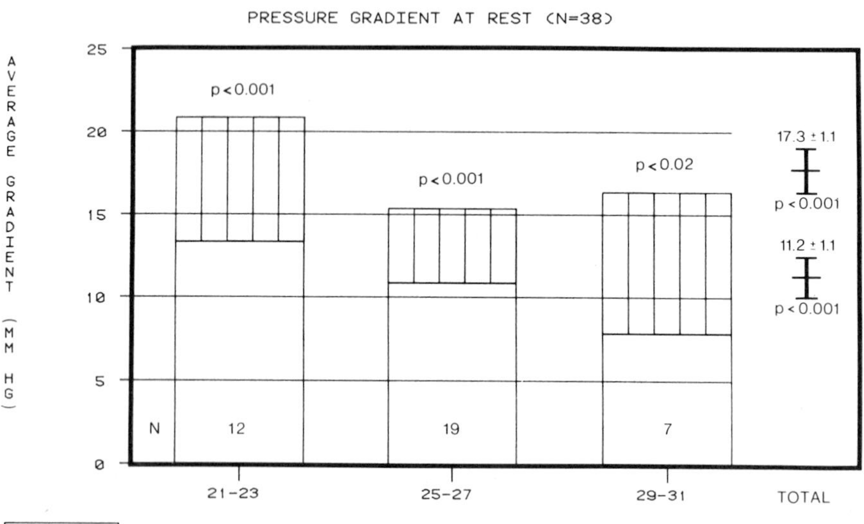

FIG. 2 Average pressure gradients at rest across aortic Carpentier-Edwards bioprosthesis in 38 patients. Comparison of peak and mean gradients shows a significant difference in the 3 groups. Mean ± SEM values for all valves shown at right.

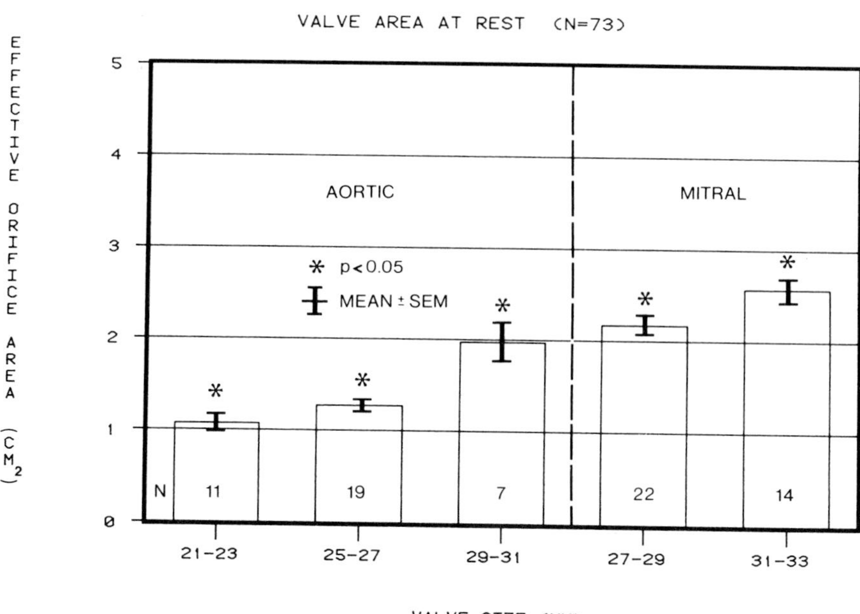

FIG. 3 Average effective orifice area for each stent size of Carpentier-Edwards bioprosthesis. The difference in area between each size group is significant ($p < 0.05$).

The difference in area between each group of stent sizes was significant ($p < 0.05$).

Hemodynamic Results with Exercise

Exercise testing was performed in 65 patients, 34 with an aortic and 31 with a mitral bioprosthesis. A paired comparison of the data at rest and during exercise in the same patient was done. In the aortic valve group, cardiac output increased from an average of 5.5 liters/min at rest to 9.8 liters/min during exercise (78% increase); in the mitral group, it increased from 4.5 liters/min at rest to 7.1 liters/min with exercise (58% increase). During exercise, peak and mean pressure gradients across aortic bioprostheses averaged 17.3 ± 1.4 and 23.2 ± 1.4 mmHg, respectively. Exercise caused an increase in peak aortic gradient in all aortic stent sizes (Fig. 4), the increase averaging 5.1 ± 2.7 mmHg in the 21–23 mm size (not significant), 7.4 ± 1.7 mmHg in the 25–27 mm size ($p < 0.001$), and 2.0 ± 2.5 mmHg in the 29–31 mm size (not significant). Mean diastolic gradient across mitral bioprostheses averaged 13.5 ± 1.0 mmHg during exercise.

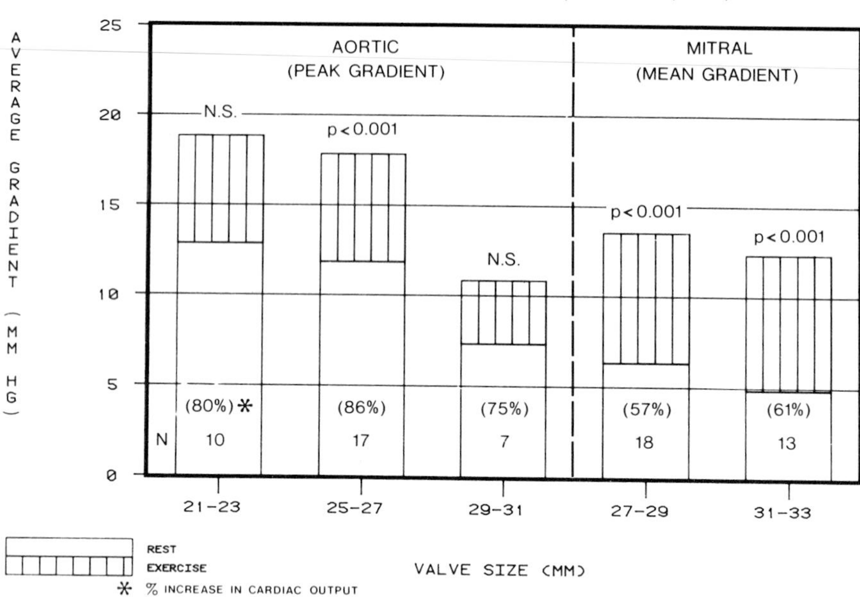

FIG. 4 Paired comparison of pressure gradients across Carpentier-Edwards bioprosthesis at rest and during exercise in 65 patients. Statistical significance for each valve size is shown on top of bar.

The increase in mean mitral gradient was significant ($p < 0.001$) in both stent sizes, averaging 7.2 ± 1.0 mmHg in each (Fig. 4).

The calculated orifice area during exercise increased by an average of 18% with aortic and 21% with mitral bioprostheses. The area increased in all stent sizes from 13.4–27.9%, and the difference was significant for all aortic and mitral sizes, except for the 21–23 mm aortic size (Fig. 5). The increase in area was greater in larger valves, averaging 0.19 ± 0.09 and 0.19 ± 0.06 cm² in the 21–23 mm and 25–27 mm aortic stent size, compared to 0.47 ± 0.19 cm² in the 29–31 mm aortic size, 0.60 ± 0.14 cm² in the 27–29 mm mitral size, and 0.51 ± 0.15 cm² in the 31–33 mm mitral group.

Valvular Regurgitation

There was no valvular regurgitation in 23 of the 38 aortic bioprostheses (60%), and in 29 of the 36 mitral bioprostheses (80%). Trivial regurgitation was observed in 24% and 14% of the aortic and mitral valves, respectively,

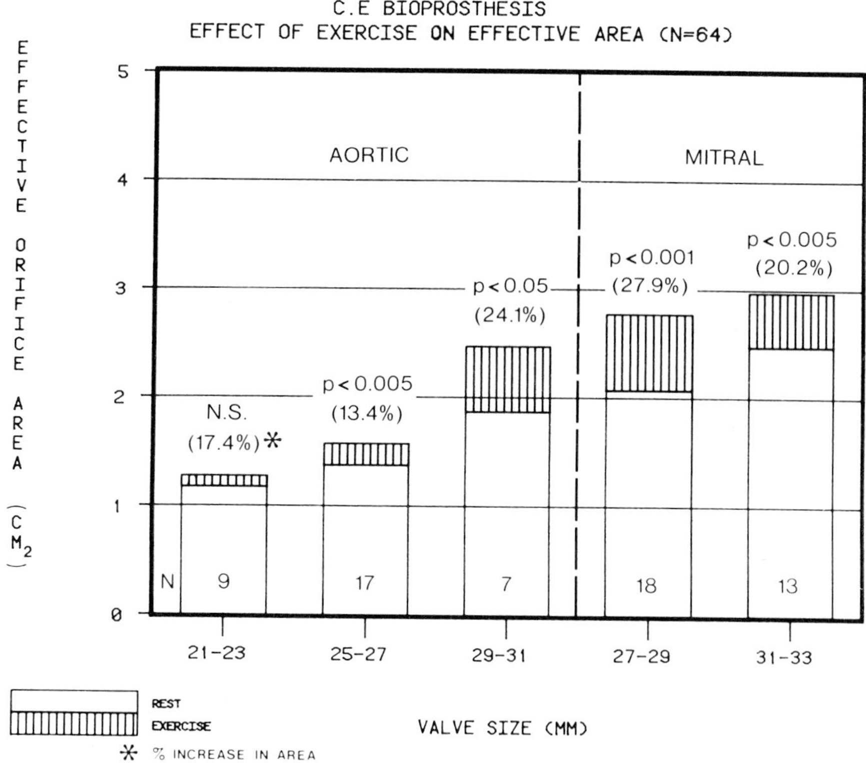

FIG. 5 Paired comparison of effective orifice areas at rest and during exercise in 64 Carpentier-Edwards bioprostheses. There is a significant increase in area with exercise in all but one size group, as shown on top of bar.

and a significant degree of regurgitation was found in 16% of the aortic and 6% of the mitral bioprostheses. However, a grade 2/3 regurgitation was shown in only 1 aortic (3%) and 1 mitral (3%) valve. Since the termination of this study, the latter patient was found to have a paravalvular peak. There were no cases of primary tissue failure of the porcine valve documented among the patients included in the present study.

In our total series of Carpentier-Edwards bioprostheses, 5 other patients required reoperation. These were not included in this study because severe symptoms of congestive heart failure were present at the time of cardiac catheterization. There was a dehiscence of an aortic bioprosthesis in 3 patients, and tissue degeneration of the valve with calcification was discovered in 2 other patients 4½ and 5 years after initial implantation of the bioprosthesis (1 mitral and 1 aortic).

Comment

Since the introduction of glutaraldehyde preservation, there has been a growing interest in bioprostheses.[6] The main characteristic of the Carpentier-Edwards porcine valve is the flexible support design to absorb some of the closing stress imposed on the leaflets. Although excellent clinical results have been obtained with tissue valves, durability and early calcification of the leaflets particularly in young patients remain a major concern.[7-11] The hemodynamic performance of most bioprostheses has generally been satisfactory, but the smaller stent sizes remain mildly stenotic.[3,12-15] In order to improve their function, several modifications have been proposed to increase the inner to outer diameter ratio of the valve. In the Hancock modified orifice valve, the muscle ridge leaflet is removed and replaced by a muscle-free leaflet sewn separately.[16] This muscle shelf is incorporated into the asymmetrical anulus of the Carpentier-Edwards bioprosthesis. In the IA model of the Carpentier-Edwards valve, available since early 1980, the width of the anulus has been reduced to increase the inner diameter and allow a larger heterograft to be mounted on the stent. This IA valve has now been used in 25% of our total Carpentier-Edwards valve implants. Postoperative hemodynamic evaluation of the valve has been performed in 11% of our surviving patients. Only asymptomatic patients were included in the present study; a marked clinical improvement and an important decrease in pressure gradients were shown in these patients at the time of the postoperative evaluation.

No significant difference in pressure gradient or in effective orifice area was found between the IA and the SA bioprostheses. Whereas the effective area of mitral IA valves was slightly larger than that of SA valves, the opposite was seen with aortic valves. Only a limited comparison of the IA to the SA valve was possible because of the relatively few IA valves studied postoperatively. However, individual values of the effective area for IA valves also failed to differentiate from those for SA valves in all but 2 of 16 IA bioprostheses. Therefore data from all valves were grouped for further analysis of the results.

In the aortic position, the average pressure gradient (11 mmHg) and effective orifice area (1.43 cm^2) at rest with the Carpentier-Edwards compare favorably with those of other tissue valves. Average pressure gradients of 16–25 mmHg and effective areas of 1.2–1.4 cm^2 have been reported for the Hancock.[12-15] High gradients with small stent sizes have led to the recommendation that small aortic valves should not be used in the adult.[14] Better results were obtained by Borkon et al.[17] However, in the latter study, 4 of the 9 (44%) 21 mm stent size valve had an effective area smaller than 1 cm^2. A significantly better hemodynamic performance with the Carpentier-Edwards valve compared to the Hancock was also found in the study of Levine et al.[18] The Angell-Shiley bioprosthesis is more stenotic, with a pressure gradient averaging 22 mmHg and an average area of only 1.23 cm^2, even though most valves studied were larger than 25 mm in diameter.[19] The use of a smaller size with this bioprosthesis has been said to be inadequate. There has been a consistent improvement in gradients and effective areas with the Hancock modified orifice valve. Gradients lower than 15 mmHg and areas of 1.5 cm^2 or more have been obtained.[16,20–21] Few hemodynamic data are available for the Ionescu-Shiley pericardial valve. In a study by Becker et al.[22] with intraoperative measurements after implantation of the latter valve, the pressure gradient and surface area average 10 mmHg and 1.5 cm^2. In this study, 4 of the 22 aortic valves (18%) had a surface area smaller than 1 cm^2 compared to 8% in our series.

In the mitral position, the results with most bioprostheses are similar to ours with regard to pressure gradients.[12,19,22,23] However, the average orifice areas reported in these series are smaller than that found in the present one (2.38 cm^2). The smallest area with the Carpentier-Edwards mitral valve was 1.14 cm^2, whereas several cases with an area of 1 cm^2 or less were reported with the Hancock, Angell-Shiley, and Ionescu-Shiley valves.[12,19,22] The most obstructive mitral bioprosthesis appears to be the Angell-Shiley valve, for which only stent sizes larger than 30 mm in diameter were found acceptable.[19]

With exercise, there was a modest but significant increase in pressure gradient across aortic (6 mmHg) and mitral (7 mmHg) bioprostheses. As reported by others,[19] exercise also caused an increase in effective orifice area, ranging from 13–28%. It has been suggested by Johnson et al.[13] that leaflet inertia may be an important determinant of an in vivo effective area of porcine valves. Our findings of a relationship between flow and area support this hypothesis, which is further substantiated by the fact that in nearly all of our patients mean aortic gradient was higher than peak gradient, as a result of a delay in the opening of the aortic leaflets during systole.

Significant valvular regurgitation was found in 16% of aortic and 6% of mitral valves in our study. This compares with the reported incidence of 9–35% with the Hancock valve.[12,13,24] It was not possible to differentiate leaflet degeneration from paravalvular regurgitation in the present study, except in the 1 reoperated patient. Overall, 6 patients required reoperation in our total series of valve implants, an incidence of 0.5% per patient year. In 4 of these patients a dehiscence of the valve was found at surgery.

Conclusions

Substantial clinical improvement and satisfactory hemodynamic performance were obtained in our experience with the Carpentier-Edwards porcine valve, which remains our preferred valve substitute for most patients.

Although primary tissue failure of the valve occurred in only 2 of our patients (0.15% per patient year), long-term durability of the bioprosthesis will not be established until longer follow-up observation is available. Improvement in the hemodynamic function of the valve may be achieved with the new supra-anular design currently under evaluation, since it allows implantation of larger heterografts with a lower stent profile.[25]

References

1. Pelletier C, Chaitman BR, Baillot R, Guiteras Val P, Bonan R, Dyrda I: Clinical and hemodynamic results with the Carpentier-Edwards porcine bioprosthesis. Ann Thorac Surg. 34: (Dec), 1982.
2. Bonchek LI: Current status of cardiac valve replacement: Selection of a prosthesis and indications for operations. Am Heart J 101:96, 1981.
3. Chaitman BR, Bonan R, Lepage G, Tubau JF, David PR, Dyrda I, Grondin CM: Hemodynamic evaluation of Carpentier-Edwards porcine xenograft. Circulation 60:1170, 1979.
4. Gorlin R, Gorlin SG: Hydraulic formula for calculation of the area of the stenotic mitral valve, other cardiac valves, and central circulatory shunts. I. Am Heart J 41:1, 1951.
5. Sandler H, Dodge HT: The use of single plane angiograms for the calculation of left ventricular volumes in man. Am Heart J 75:325, 1968.
6. Carpentier A, Deloche A, Relland J, Fabiani JN, Forman J, Camilleri JP, Soyer R, Dubost C: Six-year follow-up of glutaraldehyde-preserved heterografts. With particular reference to the treatment of congenital valve malformation. J Thorac Cardiovasc Surg 68:771, 1974.
7. Jamieson WRE, Janus MT, Munro AI, Miyagishima RT, Tutassura H, Gerein AN, Burr LH, Allen P: Early clinical experience with the Carpentier-Edwards porcine heterograft cardiac valve. Can J Surg 23:132, 1980.
8. Cohn LH, Mudge GH, Pratter F, Collins JJ: Five to eight-year follow-up of patients undergoing porcine heart-valve replacement. N Engl J Med 304:258, 1981.
9. Magilligan DJ, Lewis JW, Jara FM, Lee MW, Alam M, Riddle JM, Stein PD: Spontaneous degeneration of porcine bioprosthetic valves. Ann Thorac Surg 30:259, 1980.
10. Sanders SP, Levy RJ, Freed MD, Norwood WI, Castaneda AR: Use of Hancock porcine xenografts in children and adolescents. Am J Cardiol 46:429, 1980.
11. Geha AS, Holter AR, Langou RA, Laks H, Hammond GL: Dysfunction and thromboembolism associated with cardiac valve xenografts in adults. Circulation 64 (Suppl II):172, 1981.
12. Lurie AJ, Miller RR, Maxwell KS, Grehl TM, Vismara LA, Hurley EJ, Mason DT: Hemodynamic assessment of the glutaraldehyde-preserved porcine heterograft in the aortic and mitral positions. Circulation 56 (Suppl II):104, 1977.
13. Johnson A, Thompson S, Vieweg WVR, Daily P, Oury J, Peterson K: Evaluation of the in vivo function of the Hancock porcine xenograft in the aortic position. J Thorac Cardiovasc Surg 75:599, 1978.
14. Jones EL, Craver JM, Morris DC, King SB, Douglas JS, Franch RH, Hatcher CR, Morgan EA: Hemodynamic and clinical evaluation of the Hancock xeno-

graft bioprosthesis for aortic valve replacement (with emphasis on management of the small aortic root). J Thorac Cardiovasc Surg 75:300, 1978.

15. Cohn LH, Sanders JH, Collins JJ: Aortic valve replacement with the Hancock porcine xenograft. Ann Thorac Surg 22:221, 1976.
16. Levine FH, Buckley MJ, Austen WG: Hemodynamic evaluation of the Hancock modified orifice bioprosthesis in the aortic position. Circulation 58 (Suppl. I):33, 1978.
17. Borkon AM, McIntosh CL, Jones M, Lipson LC, Kent KM, Morrow AG: Hemodynamic function of the Hancock standard orifice aortic valve bioprosthesis. J Thorac Cardiovasc Surg 82:601, 1981.
18. Levine FH, Carter JE, Buckley MJ, Daggett WM, Akims CW, Austen WG: Hemodynamic evaluation of Hancock and Carpentier-Edwards bioprostheses. Circulation 64 (Suppl II):192, 1981.
19. Rivera R, Infantes C, Delcan JL, Rico M: Clinical and hemodynamic assessment of the Angell-Shiley porcine xenograft. Ann Thorac Surg 30:455, 1980.
20. Craver JM, King SB, Douglas JS, Franch RH, Jones EL, Morris DC, Kopchak J, Hatcher CR: Late hemodynamic evaluation of Hancock modified-orifice aortic bioprosthesis. Circulation 60 (Suppl I):93, 1979.
21. Zusman DR, Levine FH, Carter JE, Buckley MJ: Hemodynamic and clinical evaluation of the Hancock modified-orifice aortic bioprosthesis. Circulation 64 (Suppl II):189, 1981.
22. Becker RM, Strom J, Frishman W, Oka Y, Lin YT, Yellin EL, Frater RWM: Hemodynamic performance of the Ionescu-Shiley valve prosthesis. J Thorac Cardiovasc Surg 80:613, 1980.
23. Tandon AP, Smith DR, Ionescu MI: Hemodynamic evaluation of the Ionescu-Shiley pericardial xenograft in the mitral position. Am Heart J 95:595, 1978.
24. Morris DC, King SB, Douglas JS Jr, Wickliffe CW, Jones EL: Hemodynamic results of aortic valvular replacement with the porcine xenograft valve. Circulation 56:841, 1977.
25. Carpentier A, Dubost C, Lane E, Nashef A, Carpentier S, Relland J, Deloche A, Fabiani JN, Chauvaud S, Perier P, Maxwell S: Continuing improvements in valvular bioprostheses. J Thorac Cardiovasc Surg 83:27, 1982.

10

Hemodynamic Evaluation in Valvular Patients Carrying Low Profile Bioprostheses

J. A. Navia, A. Tamashiro, C. Gimenez, D. Zambrana Vidal, D. Liotta

The low profile bioprosthesis (LPB) for cardiac valve replacement consists of a highly flexible plastic stent supporting a porcine aortic cardiac valve fixed by the glutaraldehyde process. The low profile support, characteristic of this bioprosthesis, was designed according to anatomic findings of the normal porcine aortic valve.[1,2]

This anatomic research demonstrated that the depth of the sinuses of Valsalva, as measured in the lumen of the aortic root from the sinus ridge to the nadir or the aortic anulus, was under 12 mm in 93% of the specimens. On the basis of this finding, a unique low profile support was designed. Three main features have been combined: 1) low profile (reduced height in relation to the frame diameter, 2) wavy shape at the inlet opening, and 3) a wavy conformation of the sewing ring. The wavy shape of the suture ring includes highly flexible commissural struts and allows the commissures of the bioprosthesis to be sewn directly into the anulus of the patient. The functional motion of the patient's anulus during the cardiac cycle is thereby transmitted to the implanted commissures. Once the valve is incorporated into the cardiac tissue of the patient, the likelihood of fracture or fatigue of the flexible struts supporting the commissures is minimized. This is in direct contrast with bioprosthesis mounted on long struts.

Furthermore, low struts avoid protruding components of the bioprosthesis either into the left ventricular cavity or into the ascending aorta. Such bioprosthetic disproportion can easily be demonstrated during double valve

---

From the Cardiovascular Surgical Unit, Hemodynamic Laboratory, Italian Hospital, Buenos Aires, Argentina.

replacement. In addition, low struts minimize blood turbulence and stagnation areas.[2]

The aortic ring of the porcine valve is mounted directly over the inlet opening of the low profile stent. Consequently, during the valve closing time the 3 cusps bulge into the left atrial cavity following mitral valve replacement (MVR) and into the outflow tract of the left ventricle following aortic valve replacement (AVR).

During the valve opening time, the blood flowing through the inlet opening is solely in contact with the endothelium of the porcine aortic valve.

Hemodynamic Methods

The hemodynamic performance of the LPB was studied postoperatively in 40 patients, 18 isolated MVR and 22 isolated AVR in brachial right and left cardiac catheterization, including ergometric testing in a supine position up to 300 kg. The gradient in aortic position was taken by simultaneous recordings of the systolic aortic and left ventricular pressure with a double lumen catheter. For mitral gradients mean pulmonary capillary wedge and left ventricular end diastolic pressure were measured simultaneously. The mean pressure was obtained electronically.

The cardiac output in basal condition and at different times during ergometric testing was measured with the thermodilution method (Cardiac Output Computer 9520, Edwards Laboratories).

Aortograms and/or ventriculograms were performed to document valvular regurgitation with an NIH catheter. The valve orifice areas in the study were calculated from Gorlin and Gorlin formula using mean gradient, a constant of 44.5 for aortic and 31 for mitral bioprosthesis, in order to compare our results with other series.

Hemodynamic Results

Mitral Valve

Twelve patients underwent early postoperative cardiac catheterization (mean, 15 days; range, 8–25 days) and 6 patients underwent late postoperative cardiac catheterization (mean, 26.5; range 12–46 months) after MVR.

The average postoperative mitral valve mean gradient for the early studies (n = 12) was 2 ± 1.7 mmHg at rest and 4.8 ± 2.8 with exercise, with a cardiac output of 5.1 ± 1.1 and 7.1 ± 4.1 liters/min, respectively.

Patients studied in the late postoperative period (n = 6) showed a mean

TABLE I Summary of hemodynamic data: MVR

Postop interval*	Mean prosthetic valve gradient (mmHg)		Cardiac Output (liters/min)		Cardiac index (liters/min/m²)	
	Rest	Exercise	Rest	Exercise	Rest	Exercise
Days						
Mean, 15 (8–25)	2 ± 1.7	4.8 ± 2.8	5.1 ± 1.1	7.1 ± 1.4	3.0 ± 0.6	4.1 ± 1
Months						
Mean, 26.5 (12–46)	2.5 ± 2.6	5.6 ± 3.2	5.2 ± 1.4	7.5 ± 1.4	2.8 ± 0.9	3.8 ± 1.3

* Interval from MVR to postoperative cardiac catheterization. Early catheterization data n = 12; late catheterization data n = 6. LPB mitral sizes 28–30 were used.

TABLE II Mitral valve xenograft

Stent size, (mm)	# pts	Average orifice area (range), cm^2
30	10	3.35 (1.66–4.9)
28	4	3.39 (2.58–4.5)

mitral gradient of 2.5 ± 2.6 mmHg at rest and 5.6 ± 3.2 with exercise, with a cardiac output of 5.2 ± 1.4 and 7.5 ± 4.1 liters/min, respectively (Table I).

LPB sizes 28 and 30 were used in all patients evaluated. The average orifice area (AOA) in cm^2 was performed on 14 mitral patients recatheterized; for size 30 (n = 10) the AOA was 3.35 cm^2 (1.66–4.9) and for size 28, 3.39 cm^2 (2.58–4.5) (Table II).

Hemodynamic data show a small increase during supine exercise with an average increase in cardiac output (Figs. 1 and 2).

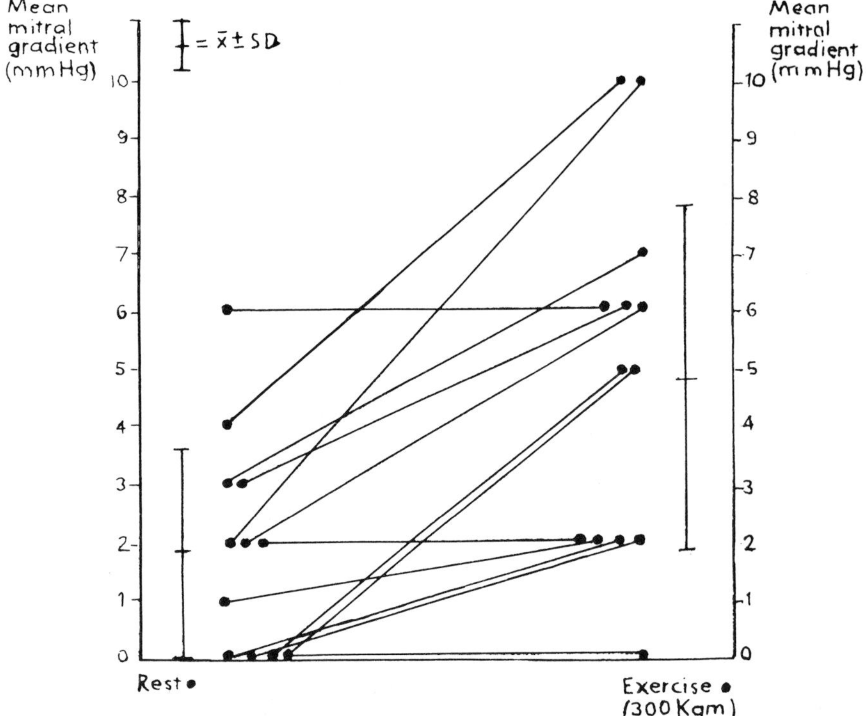

FIG. 1 Average mitral gradient shows a small increase during supine exercise up to 300 kg. Mean, 1.8 mmHg at rest and 4.8 mmHg during exercise.

TABLE III Summary of hemodynamic data: AVR

Postop studies	Valve size	Mean prosthetic valve gradient (mmHg)		Cardiac output (liters/min)		Cardiac index (liters/min/m^2)	
		Rest	Exercise	Rest	Exercise	Rest	Exercise
Days*	23† 24	16.8 ± 9.5	23.7 ± 8.5	5.7 ± 1.3	7.3 ± 1.4	3.4 ± 0.8	4.0 ± 0.7
Mean 15 (8–20)	26† 28	13.5 ± 5.6	16 ± 4.3	5.8 ± 1.5	7.3 ± 1.2	3.4 ± 0.7	4.6 ± 0.1

* Interval from AVR to time of follow-up cardiac catheterization.

† There were 14 patients with valve sizes 23 and 24 and 8 patients with valve sizes 26 and 28.

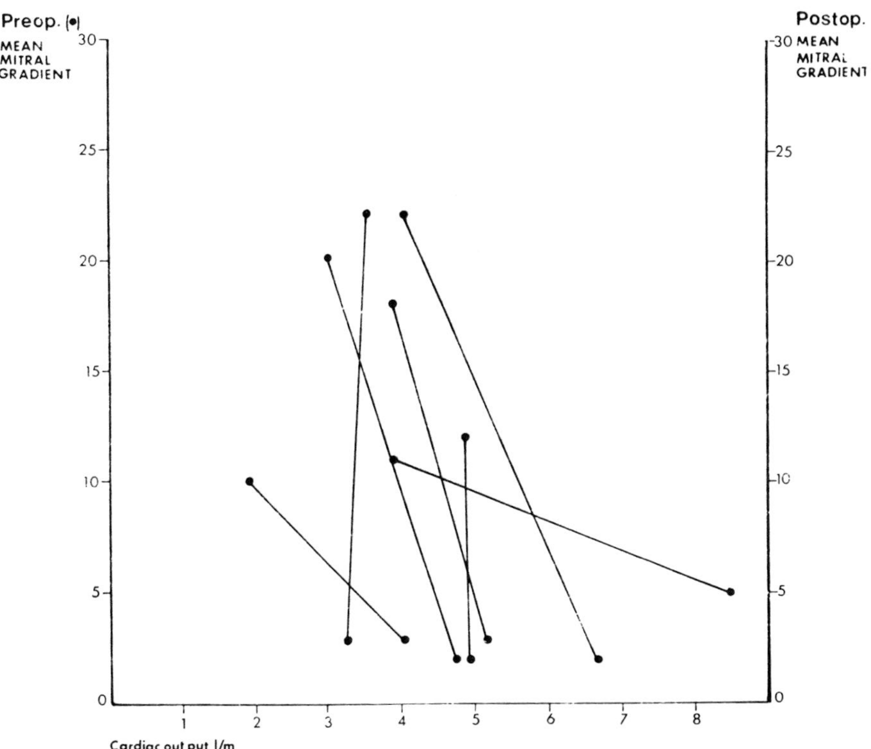

FIG. 2 Pre- and postoperative hemodynamic data, with a sharp reduction in mitral valve gradient after MVR.

Aortic Valve

Twenty-two patients after AVR underwent early postoperative cardiac catheterization in patients carrying LPB sizes 23–24 (n = 14), 26–28 (n = 8) with a mean aortic gradient of 16.8 ± 9.5 at rest and 23.7 ± 8.5 with exercise for 26–28 (Table III). The average effective orifice area for stent size 23 was 2.44 cm² (1.35–2.96); for 24, 2.54 cm² (2.3–2.8); and for 26,

TABLE IV Aortic valve xenograft

	Stent size (mm)	# pts	Average orifice area (range), cm²
A	23	8	2.44 (1.35–2.96)
A	24	4	2.54 (2.3–2.8)
A	26	4	2.25 (1.9–2.5)

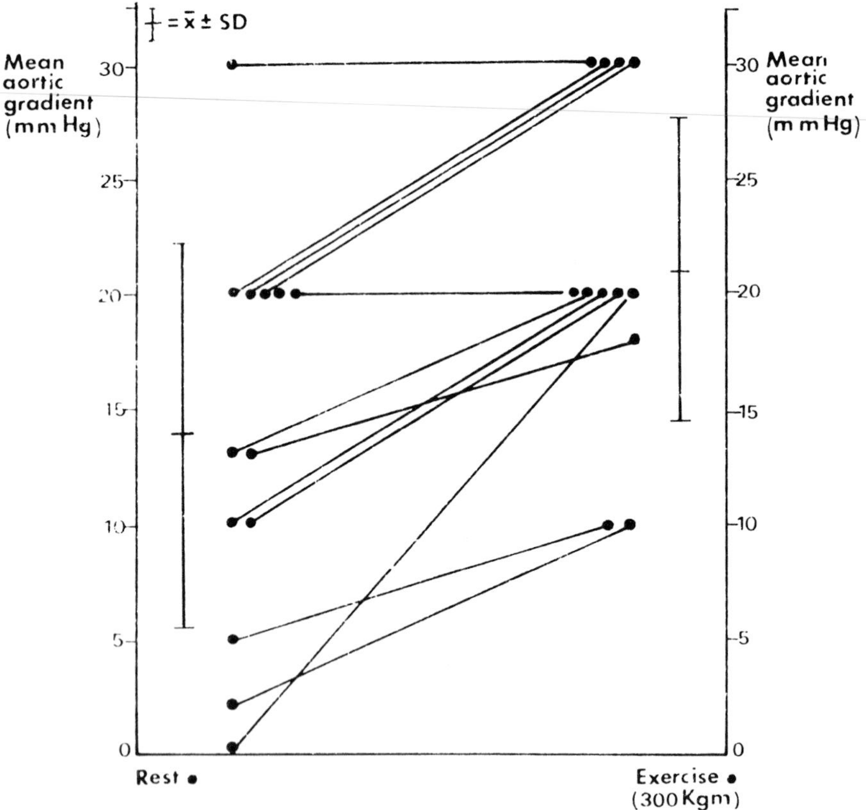

FIG. 3 Mean gradient in aortic valve replacement was 14 mmHg at rest and 21.4 mmHg during ergometric test up to 300 kg.

2.25 cm^2 (1.9–2.5) (Table IV). Between rest and exercise, the mean gradient of size 23 increased from an average 16.6–23.3 mmHg, respectively (Figs. 3 and 4).

Conclusions

The hemodynamic data obtained from the 40 patients studied demonstrate that gradients are quite similar to other series of bioprosthetic valves.[3–6] Hemodynamic results in early and late mitral valve catheterization demonstrate: unchanged LPB effective orifice, at least through the 26.5 months average period after implantation.

Severe or moderate valvular stenosis was not observed in any patient.

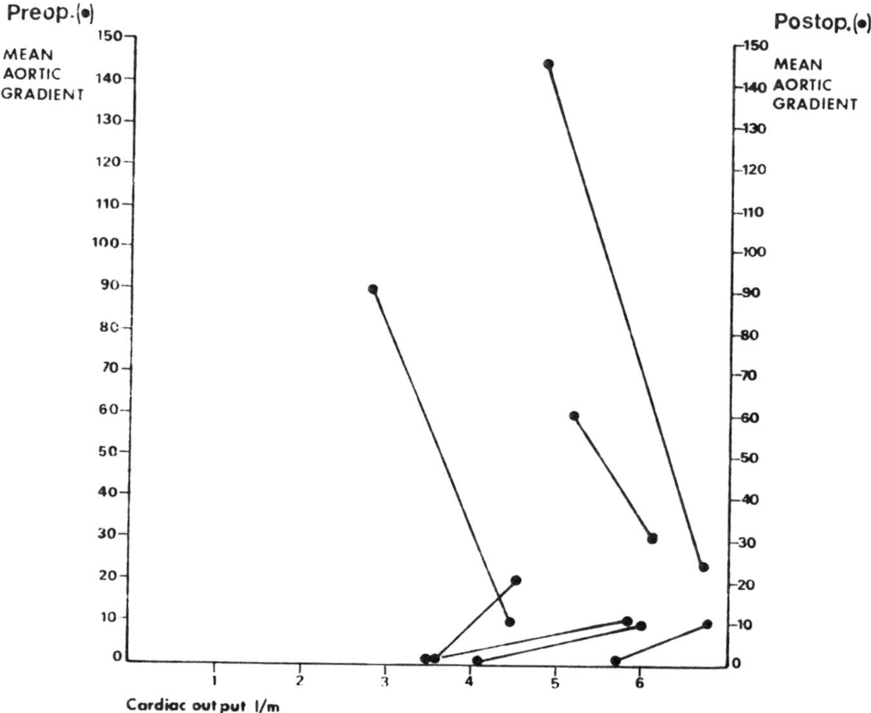

FIG. 4 Pre- and postoperative gradient in patients with aortic stenosis and aortic insufficiency, with a significant increase of cardiac output.

Low profile bioprotheses have an acceptable effective orifice area in the atrial stent sizes 23–24 and the mitral 28–30 evaluated in this study.

Evidences of left ventricle outflow obstruction after MVR and interference with the aortotomy closure after AVR were not observed. The low profile design has been important for obtaining these results.

References

1. Liotta D, Haller J, Pisanu A, Bracco D, Bertolozzi E: Subcommissural implantation of aortic prosthesis with the use of the non-coronary sinus and the fibrous trigones. Cardiovasc Dis, Bull Tex Heart Inst 6:181, 1979.
2. Navia J, Gimenez C, Lima Quintana O, Benito J, Zambrana Vidal D, Tamashiro A, Bertolozzi E, Bracco D, Liotta D: Low Profile bioprosthesis for cardiac valve replacement. Proceedings of the European Society of Artificial Organs, vol. III, Geneva, Switzerland, 1980.
3. Horowitz MS, Goodman DJ, Fogarty TJ, Harrison DC: Mitral valve replacement with the glutaraldehyde-preserved porcine heterograft. Clinical, hemo-

dynamic, and pathological correlations. J Thorac Cardiovasc Surg 67:885, 1974.

4. Craver JM, Franch RH, King SB III, Douglas JS, Jones EL, Hatcher CR, Kopchak J Jr: Late hemodynamic evaluation of Hancock modified orifice aortic valve prosthesis. (Abstr.) Circulation 58 (Suppl II): 191, 1978.
5. Jones EL, Craver JM, Morris DC, King SB III, Douglas JS Jr, Franch RH, Hatcher CR JR, Morgan EA: Hemodynamic and clinical evaluation of the Hancock xenograft bioprosthesis for aortic valve replacement (with emphasis on management of the small aortic valve. J Thorac Cardiovasc Surg 75:300, 1978.
6. Navia JA, Gimenez C, Tamashiro A, Esper R, Haller J, Liotta D: The low profile bioprosthesis: Results with 491 valves implanted in 453 patients for up to 5 years. Tex Heart Inst J 9:141, 1982.

11

Noninvasive Scintigraphic Assessment of Left and Right Ventricular Function in Patients with Bioprosthetic Mitral Valves at Long-Term Risk

B. REICHART, N. SCHAD, G. BOUGIOUKAS, B. M. KEMKES, V. GALLUCCI, U. BORTOLOTTI, A. MILANO

Several authors in the past have documented the safety of porcine bioprostheses for up to 8 years.[1–5] Compared to mechanical valves, these prostheses provide low rates of thromboembolism and hemorrhage secondary to anticoagulation and a favorable outcome with medical therapy for endocarditis; valve failure is usually associated with gradual worsening of the hemodynamic state, so reoperation may be performed on a nonemergency basis.

Yet, ultrastructural investigations using electron microscopy showed that degenerative changes of the valves start soon after implantation and may progress over the postoperative course.[6]

The Cardiovascular Department of the University of Padova started using Hancock porcine bioprostheses stabilized with glutaraldehyde in the early 1970s. This report summarizes the experience with 15 patients who received porcine mitral valve replacement between April 1970 and May 1972 and in whom cardiac performance and valve function were assessed, applying technetium-99m pertechnetate scintigraphy at rest and at peak exercise.

Methods and Materials

The mean age at operation of the 7 men and 8 women was 37.9 ± 10 years, ranging from 29–69 years. According to the NYHA classification,

From the Universities of Munich, City Hospital of Passau, and Herzchirurgische Klinik, Klinikum GroBhadern, Munich, West Germany, and the Cardiovascular Department, University of Padova, Padova, Italy.

12 patients belonged preoperatively to class III and 3, to class IV. Ventriculography verified pure mitral stenosis in 3 patients and pure regurgitation in 1; in 11 cases combined disease was present.

The preoperative cardiac index was 2.61 ± 0.5 liters/min/m^2; the mean pulmonary wedge pressure was elevated to 28.3 ± 10 mmHg, the average pressure gradient across the mitral valve was 23.3 ± 8 mmHg. Pulmonary artery pressure was 20−35 mmHg (mean) in 5 patients, 35−50 mmHg in 4 cases, and ≥50 mmHg in 5 patients. One patient had no preoperative catheter. In 6 patients, 27 mm and 29 mm valve were implanted in each; in two patients, a 33 mm valve; and in 1, a 31 mm valve.

Postoperative Course

At the time of the study (123.8 ± 8 months postoperatively) most of the patients were still improved (Fig. 1). According to the New York Heart Association classification, 7 were class II and 8, class III. Thirteen patients were in atrial fibrillation and 2 in sinus rhythm. Eight patients received anticoagulation and 7 did not. There were no thromboembolic events.

Postoperative RV and LV Radionuclide Studies

Scintigraphic ventriculograms were assessed 123.8 ± 8 months postoperatively after informed consents were obtained from every patient. The studies were performed in 2 steps, at rest and after exercise. The resting part was managed with the patient sitting on a bicycle ergometer in right

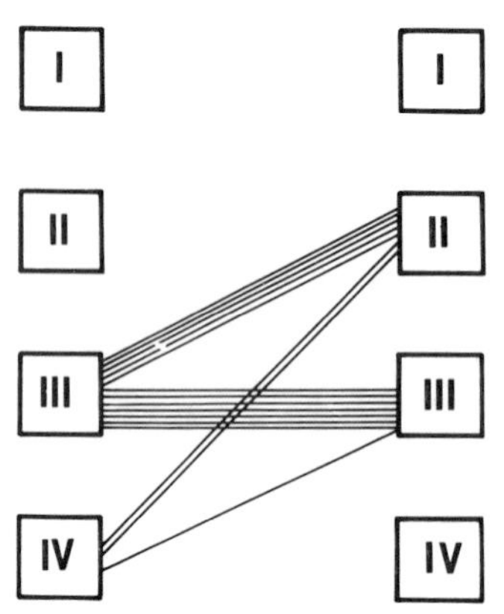

FIG. 1 Pre- and postoperative (123.8 ± 8 months) classification according to the New York Heart Association.

anterior oblique (RAO) view of the heart. Thereafter, the patient exercised through 3–4 levels lasting for 2 minutes each, at the final step bicycling as fast as possible. During exercise, 80% of age-dependent maximum heart rate was achieved.

First pass technique was employed.[7–11] The compact bolus of 18–20 mCi technetium-99m pertechnetate was rapidly injected into a large antecubital vein. Injection was timed by electrocardiograph (ECG), so that the bolus reached the tricuspid valve in systole. During passage of the bolus from the right atrium and right ventricle and through the lungs to the left atrium and the left ventricle, a multicrystal camera (system 77, Baird) defined spatial distributions of radioactivity at a rate of 25 frames/sec at rest or 40 frames/sec during exercise. Since the number of the frames were marked on the recording ECG, each frame was precisely correlated to a corresponding point of the cardiac cycle. Finally, a representative cardiac cycle was created out of frames of 6 to 8 heart beats.

Borderline definition of the left and right ventricle (LV and RV mask) were mathematically established. A border point was fixed wherever the count rate increased steeply over the matrix level of the lungs. Thereafter, nonhomogeneous background of the lungs was subtracted from the ventricular masks. For data assessment, self-established computer programs were employed.

Calculations

The global ejection fraction was calculated in the usual way, dividing the difference between end diastolic and end systolic counts by the end diastolic counts (Fig. 2).

End diastolic volumes (EDV) were assessed by equation (1), derived by Nickel and Schad:[12]

$$< \text{EDV (ml)} = k_1 \cdot \text{NTC} - k_2 \cdot (1 + k_3 \cdot z)^2 > \qquad (1)$$

where NTC is the normalized total count rate; count integral of the ventricles at end diastolic, divided by the maximum count density; k_1, k_2, k_3 are constants; $k_1 = 11.5\ \text{ml} \cdot \text{cm}^{-2}$; $k_2 = 60.8$ m; $k_3 = 0.051\ \text{cm}^{-1}$; z is distance collimator, left or right ventricle. The end systolic volumes (ESV) were derived from equation (2):

$$\text{ESV (ml)} = \frac{\text{ES} - \text{counts}}{\text{ED} - \text{counts}} \cdot \text{EDV (ml)} \qquad (2)$$

The cardiac output was calculated by multiplying the stroke volume by the heart rate.

The rapid filling rate is the volume after rapid diastolic filling of the left ventricle divided by the corresponding time (Fig. 3); the volume of rapid filling was calculated by analogy with EDV measurements.

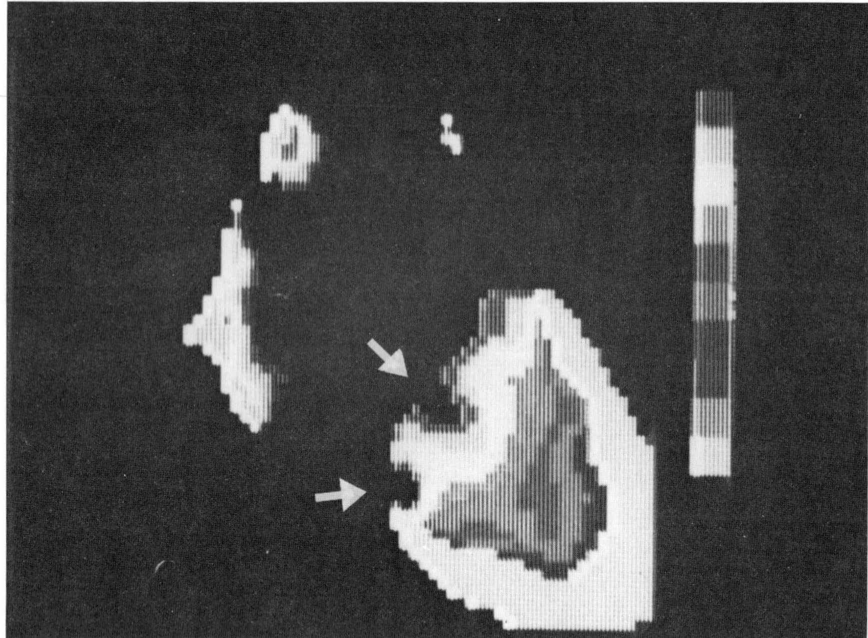

FIG. 2 Scintigraphic ejection fraction image (RAO view of the heart); the left ventricular global ejection fraction is subdivided into 10 regions; the brightest tint on the outside symbolizes the highest number of 100%; the lowest numbers are situated at the inflow and outflow tract of the left ventricle. The struts of the bioprosthesis (white arrows) are marked by two black spots.

The time a radionuclide bolus needs to travel from the right to the left atrium is called mean pulmonary transit time (PTT) (Fig. 4). This time is influenced by the right and left ventricular function, the pulmonary vascular resistance, and, finally, the functional status of the mitral valve.

Data were averaged and statistical differences obtained by using paired and unpaired Student's *t* test.

Results

Table I summarizes the left ventricular volumes on an average 123.8 ± 8 months (range, 112–140 months postoperatively). While the heart was beating at a rate of 85.1 ± 6 min^{-1} at rest, EDV and ESV measured 130.6 ± 44 and 64.8 ± 38 ml; stroke volume was calculated for 63.3 ± 15 ml and cardiac index, for 3.29 ± 1.04 liter/min/m^2. The ejection fraction (EF) was 51.4 ± 13%.

```
PL. DT CRCTD PAT                DP RCRD NUM   1333
CT  INT  1.080 AC  INT         1.080 Y-NM    14645

   1301      14645
   1302      13961
   1303      12655
   1304      11132
   1305       9748
   1306       8570
   1307       7937
   1308       7990
   1309       8423
  >1310       8861
   1311       9362
   1312      10170
   1313      11145
   1314      11708
   1315      11799
   1316      11789
   1317      11946
   1318      12572
   1319      13351
  >1320      13515
   1321      12897
```

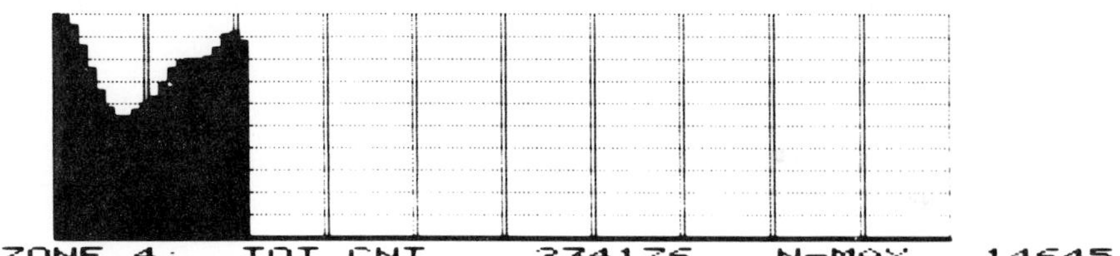

FIG. 3 Volume-curve of the left ventricle at rest. The volume of the rapid diastolic filling divided by the corresponding time equals the rapid filling rate (ml/min).

At peak exercise, heart rate rose to 150.5 ± 24 beats/min, cardiac index increased accordingly, since neither EDV nor ESV changed. EF remained unchanged.

Right ventricular volumes are listed in Table II. As on the left side, no changes were found at peak exercise in regard to EDV, ESV, and EF.

The left ventricular volumes of 14 patients, with a bioprosthesis in mitral position for 10 years or more, are compared in Table III with the mean values of 19 healthy volunteers presented by Scholz et al.[14] Only measurements at rest are presented, since Scholz et al did not perform exercise tests. As one may see from heart rates (79.6 ± 16 -vs- 85 ± 16, p = NS) both groups are comparable. There were no statistical differences in any of the data presented, including EDV, ESV, stroke volume, cardiac index, and

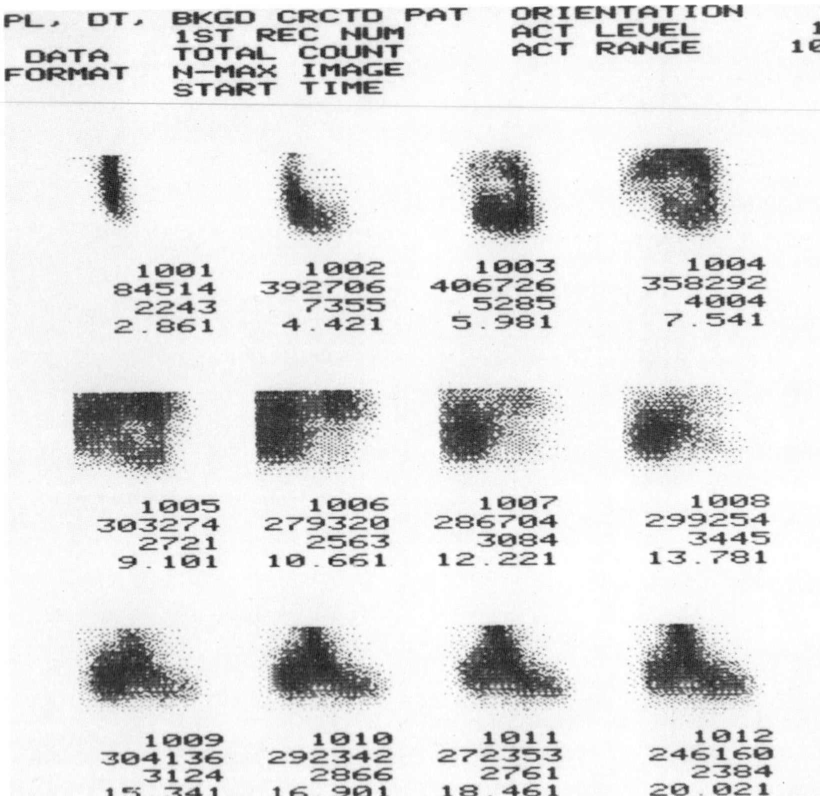

FIG. 4 So-called 12 image view which demonstrates, after borderline definition and background subtraction, the travel of a compact technetium-99m pertechnetate bolus from the superior vena cava (upper panel, first frame), the right atrium (upper panel, second frame), through the lungs, to the left atrium (panel in the middle, third and fourth frames and the left ventricle (lower panel). The pulmonary transit time (PTT) measures the travel of the bolus from the right to the left atrium.

TABLE I Left ventricular volumes assessed by scintigraphic technique 123.8 ± 8 months postoperatively.

	Rest	Exercise	Statistics
HR* (min^{-1})	85.1 ± 16	150.5 ± 24	$p < 0.05$
EDV (ml)	130.6 ± 44	130.6 ± 46	NS
ESV (ml)	64.8 ± 38	67.7 ± 42	NS
SV (ml)	63.3 ± 15	61.2 ± 17	NS
CI (liters/min/m^2)	3.29 ± 1.04	5.50 ± 1.45	$p < 0.05$
EF (%)	51.4 ± 13	50.3 ± 14	NS

* HR: heart rate; EDV: end diastolic volume; ESV: end systolic volume; SV: stroke volume; CI: cardiac index; EF: ejection fraction.

TABLE 2 Right ventricular volumes 123.8 ± 8 months postoperatively

	Rest	Exercise
EDV* (ml)	129.7 ± 22	126.9 ± 19
ESV (ml)	63.8 ± 22	59.5 ± 15
EF (%)	50.5 ± 12	50.9 ± 10

* See Table I for explanation of abbreviations.

EF. However, EDV and ESV and therefore stroke volume and EF did not change at peak exercise (Table I). Statistical differences ($p \leq 0.05$) were obtained measuring the heart rate (85.1 ± 16 -vs- 150.5 ± 24 min^{-1}), and matching the cardiac index (3.29 ± 1.04 -vs- 5.50 ± 1.45 liters/min/m^2). Compared with the physiologic response of healthy volunteers at peak exercise[15] in whom EDV would be expected to increase by 10%, ESV to decrease by 32%, and therefore stroke volume to rise by 36%, our patients had a limited, heart rate dependent reaction to physical activity. This may be explained by an increased left ventricular stiffness, since right ventricular volumes did not change at the same time (Table III).

Functional Status of the Bioprosthesis in Mitral Valve Position

The function of the bioprosthesis was assessed applying the mean PTT and the rapid filling rate (RFR). In patients with severely stenosed mitral valves, PTT and RFR should both be prolonged, at least at peak exercise. As already mentioned, this did happen in 2 patients. In the remaining 13 PTT decreased at peak exercise in all cases (7.4 ± 1.4 -vs- 4.2 ± 0.8 sec), rendering adequate mitral valve function.

TABLE III Comparison of left ventricular data

	Normal volunteers*	Pts. with mitral valve replacement	Statistics
HR† (min^{-1})	79.6 ± 16	85.1 ± 16	NS
EDV (ml)	121.0 ± 21	130.6 ± 44	NS
ESV (ml)	45.0 ± 20	64.8 ± 38	NS
SV (ml)	77.0 ± 20	63.3 ± 15	NS
CI (liters/min/m^2)	3.3 ± 0.8	3.29 ± 1.04	NS
EF (%)	65.0 ± 7	51.4 ± 13	NS

* The normal mean values of 19 subjects were presented by Scholz et al.[14]
† See Table I for explanation of abbreviations.

TABLE IV Comparison of mean pulmonary transit time at rest

	Normal volunteers*	Pts with mitral valve replacement	Statistics
Rest	6.5 ± 1.2	7.4 ± 1.4†	NS
Exercise	—	4.2 ± 0.8†‡	—

* The normal mean values of 19 subjects are derived from the study of Scholz et al.[14]
† Pulmonary transit time not measurable in 2 patients.
‡ Rest/exercise $p < 0.05$.

PTT at rest was not significantly different from the mean values of 19 volunteers by Scholz et al[14] (7.4 ± 1.4 -vs- 6.5 ± 1.2 sec) (Table IV). RFR increased in 13 patients at peak exercise, 201.9 ± 76 -vs- 400.2 ± 148 ml/sec, which are within normal ranges.

The PTT at rest was unmeasurably long in 1 patient and in another at both rest and peak exercise. The data on the remaining 13 patients are shown in Fig. 5. PTT measured 7.4 ±1.4 sec at rest and decreased in all cases on an average to 4.2 ± 0.8 sec.

The rapid filling rate of the left ventricle responded to exercise matching: at rest 201.9 ± 76 ml/sec, it increased in 13 patients at peak exercise to 400.2 ± 148 ml/sec (Fig. 6). Again, RFR was unmeasurable in the already mentioned 2 persons.

Comment

As reported by several authors,[1–5] tissue valve failure almost always occurs gradually. Although changes in symptomatology might require surgery within a month, sudden catastrophes, well-known in prosthetic valve patients, are uncommon. Therefore decision-making for reoperation requires clinical examination, invasive studies in the catheterization laboratory, and reproducible and quickly available, noninvasive methods, particularly with the bioprosthesis in the mitral position. Echocardiographic[13] and phonocardiographic[3] methods have been developed and are now being evaluated. Scintigraphic access to ventricular function may be performed under near physiologic conditions with a patient sitting upright at both rest and peak exercise conditions, which are difficult to obtain applying echocardiographic or phonocardiographic techniques.

Employing noninvasive radionuclide techniques, RAO view can only be achieved by recording the successive first pass of a compact technetium pertechnetate bolus through the heart chambers. Information is drawn from

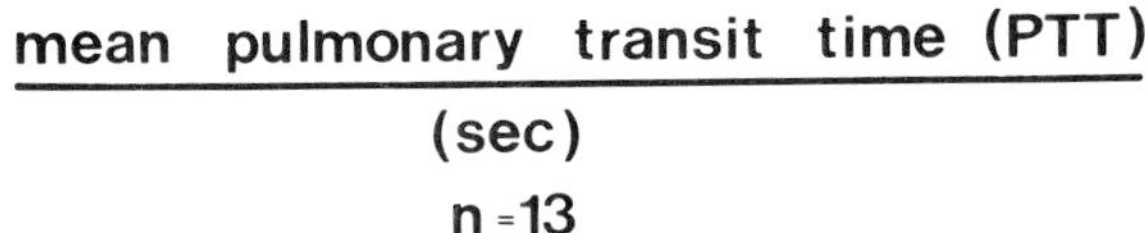

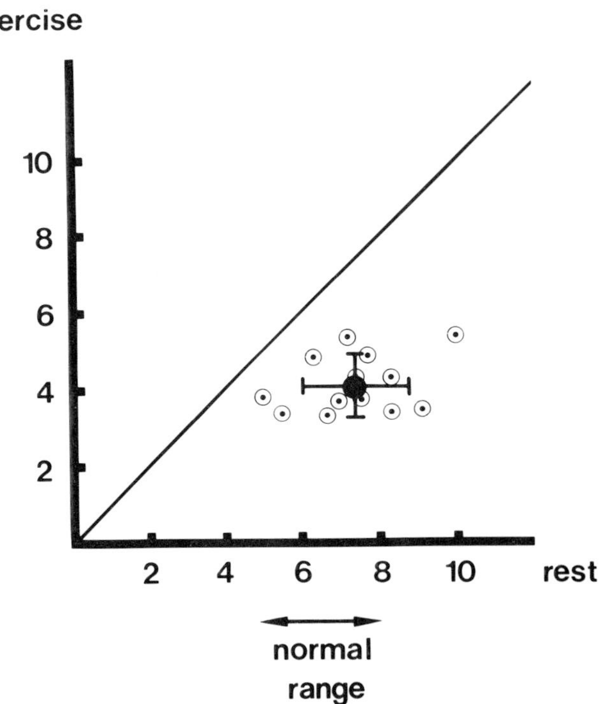

FIG. 5 Mean pulmonary transit time (PTT) of 13 patients. PTT was 7.4 ± 1.4 s at rest and decreased in each case on an average of 4.2 ± 0.8 s. In 2 other patients PTT was unmeasurable, in 1 patient at peak exercise and in the 2nd at both rest and peak exercise.

the left ventricular washout phase of the radionuclide bolus, when the right ventricle is practically emptied from activity. In contrast, pool technique, where all 4 chambers are simultaneously filled, would result in complete superimposition of the right ventricle over the left ventricle in the RAO view.

Scintigraphy gives a 3-dimensional look at ventricular function, which is not biplane, as in conventional contrast ventriculography, and which makes application of the Sandler and Dodge formula[14] unnecessary. Therefore global EF was simply assessed by dividing the difference between end diastolic and end systolic counts by the end diastolic counts. This approach was

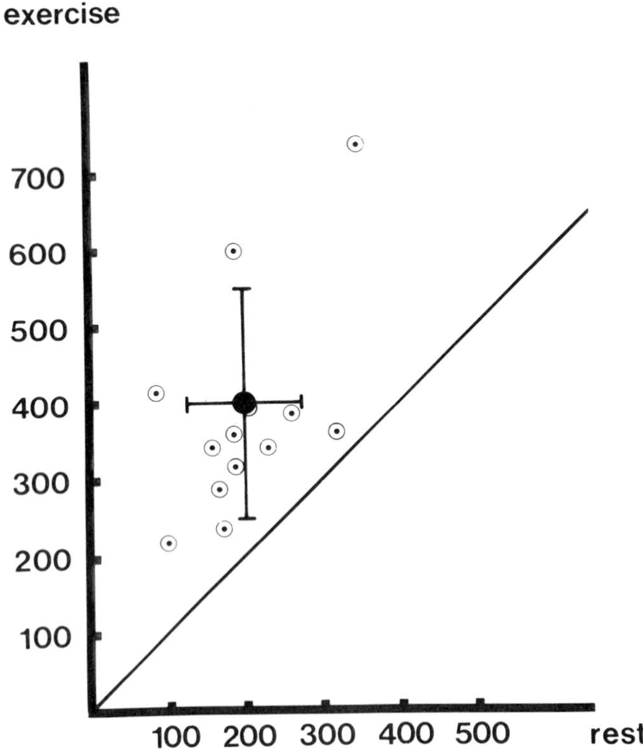

FIG. 6 Rapid filling rate (RFR) of 13 patients increased at peak exercise from 201.9 ± 76 to 400.2 ± 148 ml/s; RFR was unmeasurable in 2 patients (see Fig. 5).

validated in 35 patients with coronary artery disease, who had both contrast and scintigraphic ventriculography (correlation factor $r = 0.9$).

The volumes of end diastole and after rapid diastolic filling were calculated according to the equation of Nickel and Schad.[12] The integral of counts within the ventricle is proportional to the volume. Only the proportionality constant is unknown and depends on the tracer concentration. If the count integral is divided by the maximum count density, the resulting NTC rate is independent of the concentration. The equation was validated in 71 patients, in whom end diastolic volumes were calculated according to the Sandler and Dodge formula (contrast ventriculograms) and by means of the Nickel and Schad formula. The comparison of both methods resulted in a correlation factor of r = 0.95.

Conclusions

Technetium-99m pertechnetate scintigraphy is an effective diagnostic tool in evaluating tissue valves at long-term risk. At 112–114 months post-operatively, 13 of the 15 porcine valves examined in mitral position seemed to function adequately. Two bioprostheses proved stenotic at 112 and 136 months.

References

1. Casarotto D, Bortolotti U, Thiene G, Gallucci V, Cevese PG: Long-term results (from 5 to 7 years) with the Hancock S-G-P bioprosthesis. J Cardiovasc Surg 20:399, 1979.
2. Cohn LH, Mudge GH, Pratter F, Collins JJ Jr: Five to eight-year follow-up of patients undergoing porcine heart valve replacement. N Engl J Med 304:258, 1981.
3. Magilligan DJ, Lewis JW, Jara FM, Lee MW, Alam M, Riddle JM, Stein PD: Spontaneous degeneration of porcine bioprosthetic valves. Ann Thorac Surg 30:259, 1980.
4. Oyer PE, Miller DC, Stinson EB, Reitz BA, Moreno-Cabral RJ, Shumway NE: Clinical durability of the Hancock porcine bioprosthetic valve. J Thorac Cardiovasc Surg 80:824, 1980.
5. Durability assessment of the Hancock porcine bioprosthesis: A multi-center retrospective analysis of patients operated prior to 1975. Anaheim, Hancock Laboratories, 1980. p 1.
6. Ferrans VJ, Spray TL, Billingham ME, Roberts WC: Structural changes in glutaraldehyde-treated porcine heterografts used as substitute cardiac valves. Am J Cardiol 41:1159, 1978.
7. Jones RH, Rerych SK, Newman GE, Scjolz PM, Howe WR, Oldham HN, Goodwich JK, Sabiston DC: Non-invasive radionuclide procedures for diagnosis and management of myocardial ischemia. World J Surg 2:811, 1978.
8. Jones RH, Newman GE, Rerych SK, Scholz PM, Upton MT, Sabiston DC: Rest and exercise radionuclide angiography in surgical patients. World Federation of Nuclear Medicine and Biology, Second International Congress, Washington, D.C., Sept. 17–21, 1978, p 95.
9. Schad N: Non-traumatic assessment of left ventricular wall motion and regional stroke volume after myocardial infarction. J Nucl Med 18:333, 1977.
10. Schad N, Nickel O: Radionuclide angiography in coronary heart disease: Where do we stand? Cardiovasc Radiol 1:27, 1978.
11. Nickel O, Schad N: Image analysis of the heart action recorded with a high speed multi-crystal gamma camera. Med Prog Technol 5:1, 1978.
12. Nickel O, Schad N, Andrews EJ, Fleming JW, Mello M: Scintigraphic measurement of left ventricular volumes from the count density distribution. In press.

13. Alam M, Madruzo A, Magilligan DJ, Goldstein S: M-mode and two-dimensional echocardiographic features of porcine valve dysfunction. Am J Cardiol 43:502, 1979.
14. Scholz PM, Rerych SK, Moran JF, Newman GE, Douglas JM, Sabiston DC, Jones RH: Quantitative radionuclide angiography. Cathet Cardiovasc Diagn 6:265, 1980.
15. Upton MT, Rerych SK, Newman GE, Bounous EP, Jones RH: The reproducibility of radionuclide angiographic measurement of left ventricular function in normal subjects at rest and during exercise. Circulation 62:125, 1980.
16. Sandler H, Dodge HT: Use of single plane cine angiocardiograms for the calculation of left ventricular volume in man. Am Heart J 75:325, 1968.

12

Orifice View Roentgenography for Evaluation of the Orifice Area of Bioprosthetic Valves

P. D. STEIN, H. N. SABBAH, G. M. FOLGER, JR, D. T. ANBE

In view of the prevalence of degeneration of bioprosthetic valves[1] it has become increasingly important to assess the functional status of these valves in patients. Two-dimensional echocardiography has not been able to show the valve with sufficient detail to measure the functional area of the orifice, although echocardiography is useful for assessing thickening, fluttering, or abnormal motion of the leaflets.[2] Measurement of the orifice has remained dependent upon hemodynamic calculations by means of the Gorlin equation[3] or modifications of that equation. Even though this technique is a cornerstone for hemodynamic evaluations, it has limitations, including the necessity of crossing the valve, the requirement for an accurate measurement of the pressure gradient (which in the case of mildly stenotic valves may be small and subject to error), and the simultaneous accurate measurement of cardiac output. In this study, a roentgenographic method for evaluation of the functional orifice area[4–6] was applied to bioprosthetic valves. The technique permits a direct measurement of the functional orifice area from contrast roentgenograms. The orifice can be seen directly en face, thereby giving a qualitative impression as well as a quantitative assessment of the valve area.

Methods and Materials

Selection of Patients

Orifice view roentgenograms of good quality were obtained in 11 patients with porcine bioprosthetic valves (models 242 and 342, Hancock

---

From the Henry Ford Hospital, Detroit, Michigan.

Supported in part by U.S. Public Health Service, National Heart, Lung and Blood Institute Grant HL23669-03.

Laboratories, Anaheim, CA). All of the valves had a muscular shelf beneath the right coronary cusp. In 5 patients, the valves were in the aortic position and in 6 they were in the mitral position.

All of the patients were catheterized for clinical reasons. Usually this related to an assessment of cardiac symptoms, particularly chest pain or dyspnea, or an evaluation of associated cardiac abnormalities. Only 1 patient (patient 9) was catheterized because of dysfunction of the bioprosthetic valve (Table I), and severe regurgitation of the valve in the mitral position was confirmed at cardiac catheterization. Subsequent examination of the surgically excised valve showed no stenosis or stiffening of the leaflets. Contrast injections in 3 (patients 4, 7, and 8) showed a "whiff" of prosthetic valve regurgitation. None of the other patients showed identifiable dysfunction of the valves.

All of the patients with prosthetic valves in the aortic position had grade 2/6 systolic ejection murmurs. None had an audible early diastolic murmur. Among the patients with prosthetic valves in the mitral position, only those with mitral regurgitation (1 severe and 2 mild) had a systolic murmur. None had a diastolic murmur.

The average duration of insertion of the bioprosthetic valves in these patients was 4 years (range, 11 months to 7 years 8 months). Relevant clinical features of these patients are shown in Table I.

Technique of Orifice View Roentgenograms of the Aortic Valve

Orifice view aortograms were obtained in 4 patients on 35 mm cine at 60 frames/s and in 1 patient on 105 mm film at 12 frames/s. The tip of the catheter was positioned in 1 of the sinuses of Valsalva. The use of standard angiographic catheters with side holes near the tip is preferred. Catheters with side holes located a significant distance from the tip, such as a pigtail catheter, do not give satisfactory results because they fail to make the primary injection sufficiently close to the sinuses of Valsalva. The contrast material, sodium and meglumine diatrizoate 75% (Hypaque-M), 30–40 ml, was injected at a rate to allow opacification of the region of the aortic valve for 2 or more cardiac cycles. This was usually in the range of 10–12 ml/s, depending upon the heart rate. The functional orifice of the valve is shown by the radiolucent jet of unopacified blood as it passes through the opacified aorta.

The aortic valve usually tilts toward the right, and only somewhat anteriorly[3,4] (Fig. 1). It has not been necessary therefore to compensate for the anterior tilt. The technique for positioning the patient to show the aortic valve en face is depicted in Fig. 2. Siemens (Pandoros-optimatik) angiographic equipment was used. The "U" arm, on which the image intensifier and camera were mounted, was rotated to a lateral projection, and the angiographic table was turned counterclockwise 40° to give a craniocaudal

TABLE I Clinical characteristics of patients

Pt	Valve position	Age (yrs)	Sex*	Duration of insertion (mo)	Prosthetic murmurs*	Prosthetic regurgitation (angiography)	Reason for catheterization*	Findings at catheterization*
1	Aortic	29	M	87	Grade 2/6 ejection	0	Chest pain	Normal coronaries
2	Aortic	16	M	11	Grade 2/6 ejection	0	VSD	VSD
3	Aortic	61	M	36	Grade 2/6 ejection	0	DOE	Poor LV function
4	Aortic	44	M	44	Grade 2/6 ejection	1+	DOE	Good LV function
5	Aortic	53	M	29	Grade 2/6 ejection	0	Chest pain	Normal coronaries
6	Mitral	49	F	30	0	0	Chest pain	Coronary disease
7	Mitral	57	F	36	Grade 2/6 pansystolic	1+	Pleural effusion, DOE	Pulmonary hypertension
8	Mitral	61	F	55	Grade 2/6 systolic	1+	Recent endocarditis, mild AI, coronary disease with bypass graft	Mild AI, patent bypass graft
9	Mitral	56	M	72	Grade 3/6 pansystolic	4+	Increased murmur	Prosthetic insufficiency
10	Mitral	50	F	92	0	0	Chest pain	Normal coronaries
11	Mitral	16	F	36	0	0	Evaluate LV function	Poor LV function

* M: male; F: female; DOE: dyspnea on exertion; LV: left ventricle; AI: aortic insufficiency; VSD: ventricular septal defect.

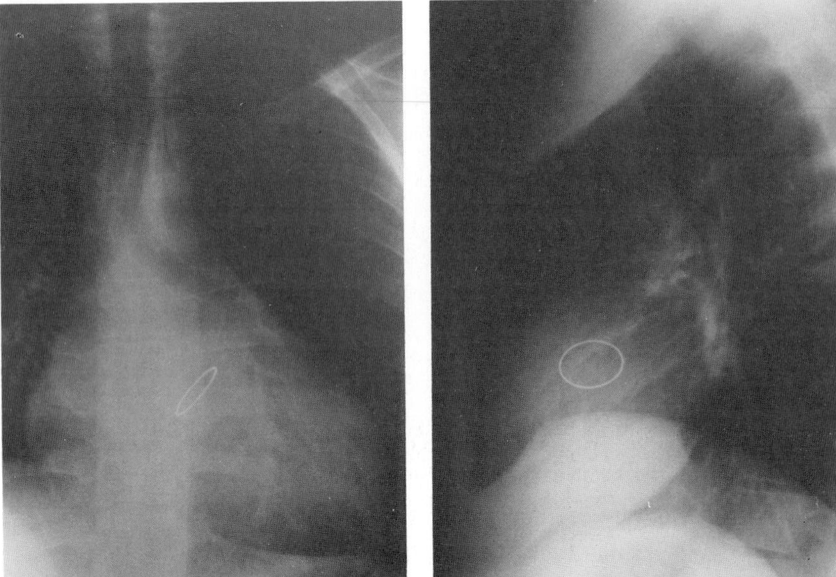

FIG. 1 Plain chest roentgenogram in the posteroanterior projection (left) and lateral projection (right) of patient 1 with a bioprosthetic valve in the aortic position. The anulus tilts prominently toward the right. There is only a small anterior tilt.

projection. In this position, the x-ray beam travels in a direction approximately from the right axilla to the left iliac crest. In most patients, the table should be angulated 45°,[4,5] but some equipment, including the Siemens "U" arm and table, may be limited to a somewhat smaller angle. In any particular patient, because the valve ring is radiopaque, the projection can be modified if necessary to show the valve ring as a perfect circle, thereby eliminating any error due to distortion of the projected image.

Technique for Orifice View Roentgenography of the Mitral Valve

Orifice view roentgenograms of bioprosthetic valves in the mitral position were obtained on 35 mm cine at 60 frames/s in 5 patients and on 105 mm film at 12 frames/s in 1 patient. The mitral valve usually tilts toward the right and anteriorly[6] (Fig. 3). To show the mitral valve en face in most patients, the x-ray beam should be projected obliquely across the heart in a craniocaudal projection with the tube elevated 25° cranially from a true lateral.[6] The patient should be rotated with his right side up 60°.[6] To accomplish this projection with a U arm and rotating table, the table was angulated obliquely in a craniocaulal direction by rotating it 25° in a counterclockwise direction. The U arm was rotated 30° from the vertical in a

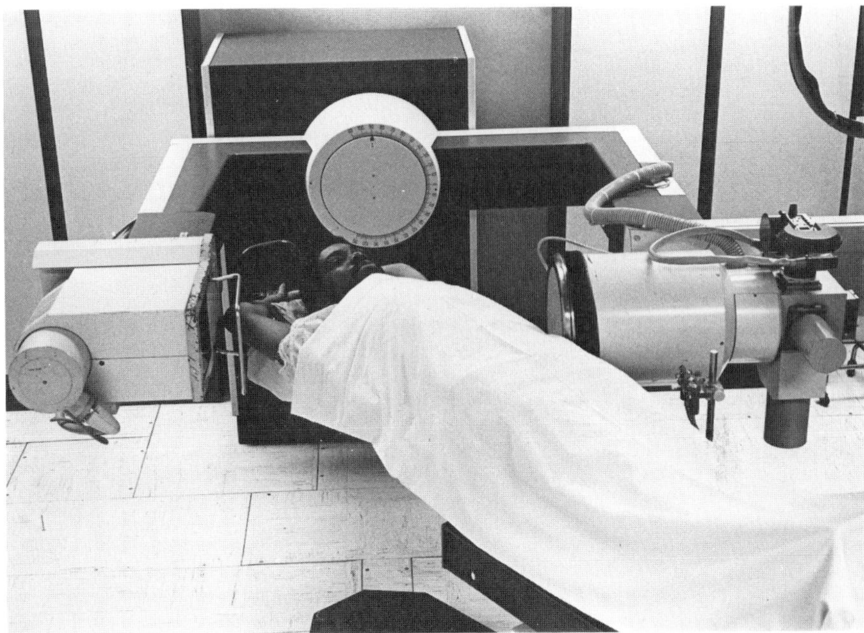

FIG. 2 Position for visualization of the orifice of the aortic valve. Typically, the table should be rotated 45°counterclockwise, although it may not be possible to achieve this rotation due to limitations of the equipment. Visualization of the orifice will be adequate in most patients if the table is rotated somewhat less than 45°.

clockwise direction (toward the patient's left side) (Fig. 4). We showed previously that in 80% of patients, this projection would permit measurement of the cross-sectional area of the mitral valve with less than 10% error due to distortion of the projected image.[6] As with the aortic valve, modification of this projection can be made, if necessary, to show the ring of the prosthetic valve as a perfect circle. This would eliminate any error due to distortion of the projected image. The rate of injection of contrast material was the same as described with orifice view aortograms. The orifice of the mitral valve is shown as unopacified blood flows through the valve into the opacified left ventricle. Pigtail catheters may be useful for these injections.

Calculation of Orifice Area from Orifice View Roentgenograms

The frame on the orifice view aortogram or ventriculogram that showed maximal valve opening was identified and the area of the orifice was measured by planimetry. The image was corrected for magnification on the basis of the known outside diameter of the anulus of the valve, which was clearly visible on the film. If the diameter of the anulus is not known, a calibrated

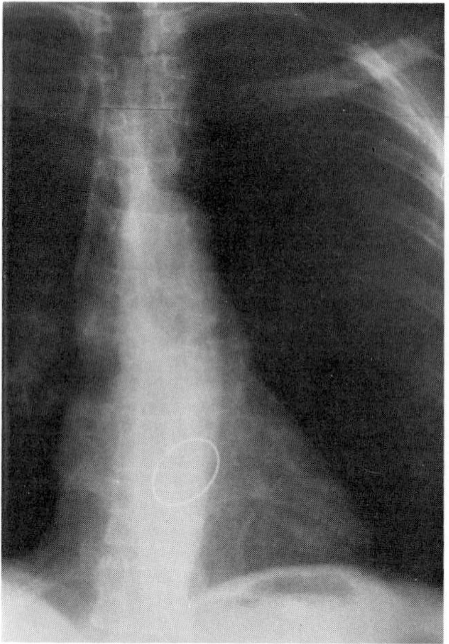

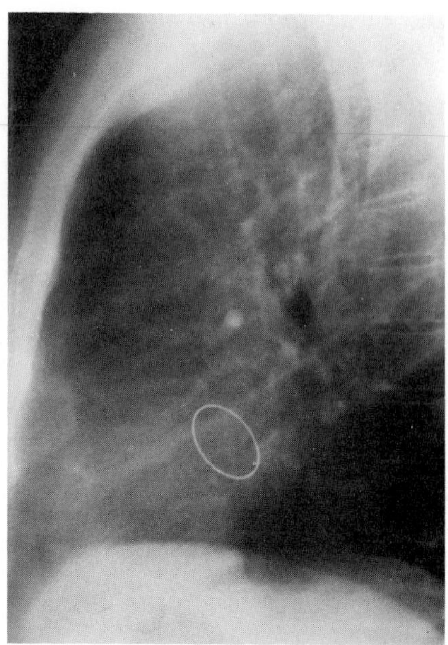

FIG. 3 Plain chest roentgenogram in the posteroanterior projection (left) and lateral projection (right) of patient 10 with a bioprosthetic valve in the mitral position. The anulus of the valve tilts prominently toward the right and anteriorly.

grid can be positioned perpendicular to the x-ray beam at the level of the valve. Only patients with films of satisfactory quality were included. Five patients had unsatisfactory visualization of the valve orifice on orifice view roentgenograms. In 4 of these patients, the valve was in the mitral position and 3 of 4 had severe mitral regurgitation. In 1 patient with a bioprosthetic valve in the aortic position, the orifice view aortogram was also unsatisfactory, and that patient had severe aortic regurgitation.

Results

The areas of the valve orifices, measured from the orifice view roentgenogram, corresponded with values calculated by the Gorlin equation as shown in Table II. The orifice areas, determined by both methods, agreed within 0.5 cm^2 in 4 of 5 patients in whom sufficient hemodynamic data were obtained for calculation of the valve area by the hydraulic equation. The pressure gradients across these valves are shown in Table II. The stroke volume in the 10 patients in whom it was measured was 49 ml or greater, which suggests that a reasonably full opening would have been achieved by these valves.

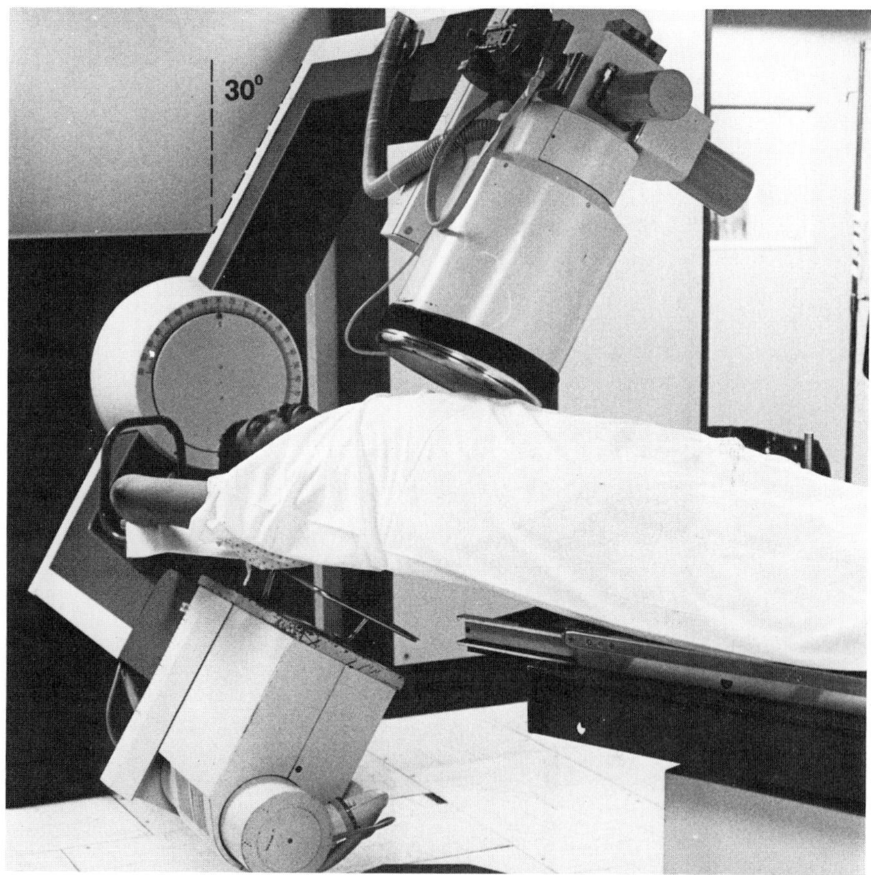

FIG. 4 Position of patient for showing the orifice of the mitral valve. The table is rotated counterclockwise 25°. The U arm is rotated 30° clockwise from vertical.

An example of an orifice view aortogram of a normal aortic bioprosthetic valve is shown in Fig. 5. Among the 5 patients with bioprosthetic valves in the aortic position, the orifice areas as measured on the orifice view aortograms ranged from 1.4–2.3 cm^2 (Table II). The approximate orifice area, estimated by the manufacturer, ranged from 3.8–4.49 cm^2. The ratio of the orifice area of the aortic valves, as measured on the orifice view aortograms, to the nominal orifice area, as specified by the manufacturer, averaged 0.39 (range, 0.33–0.47) (Table II). The orifice area, as shown on orifice view aortograms, was also correlated with the area inscribed by the tissue anulus diameter, which has been termed by some as the implantation area (Fig. 6). The average value of the ratio of the orifice area of the aortic valves to the area inscribed by the tissue anulus diameter was 0.31 (range, 0.24–0.35).

TABLE II Hemodynamics and roentgenographic measurements

Pt	Valve position	Tissue anulus diameter (mm)	Valve area by orifice view (cm^2)	Valve area by Gorlin equation (cm^2)	Pressure* gradient (mmHg)	Stroke volume (ml)	Orifice view area/specified area	Orifice view area/tissue Anulus area
1	Aortic	29	2.3	—	2	82	0.47	0.35
2	Aortic	25	1.4	1.7	30	120	0.37	0.28
3	Aortic	29	1.6	—	—	49	0.33	0.24
4	Aortic	25	1.5	1.8	18	73	0.39	0.30
5	Aortic	27	1.6	2.6	14	115	0.38	0.28
6	Mitral	29	1.3	—	—	—	0.27	0.20
7	Mitral	29	1.4	1.7	9	83	0.29	0.21
8	Mitral	35	2.0	1.5	10	76	0.28	0.21
9	Mitral	31	2.8	—	0	61†	0.49	0.37
10	Mitral	27	1.2	—	0	99	0.29	0.21
11	Mitral	31	1.7	—	5	51	0.30	0.22

* Pressure gradient refers to the peak systolic pressure in the case of the aortic valve, and mean diastolic pressure gradient in the case of the mitral valve.

† Flow across the mitral valve would be larger due to mitral regurgitation.

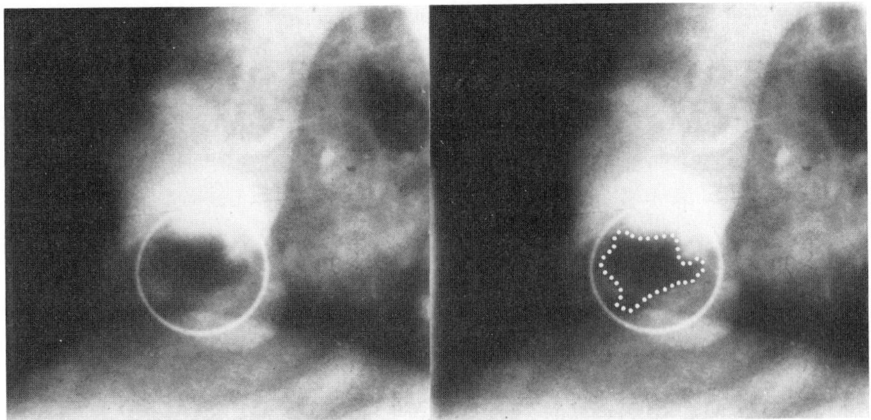

FIG. 5 (left) Orifice aortogram of patient 1. (right) The functional orifice is outlined by dots.

An example of an orifice view aortogram of a bioprosthetic valve in the mitral position is shown in Fig. 7. Among the 6 patients with bioprosthetic valves in the mitral position, the orifice area, as measured from orifice view roentgenograms, ranged from 1.2–2.8 cm^2 (Table II). The approximate area of the orifice, as estimated by the manufacturer, in these valves ranged

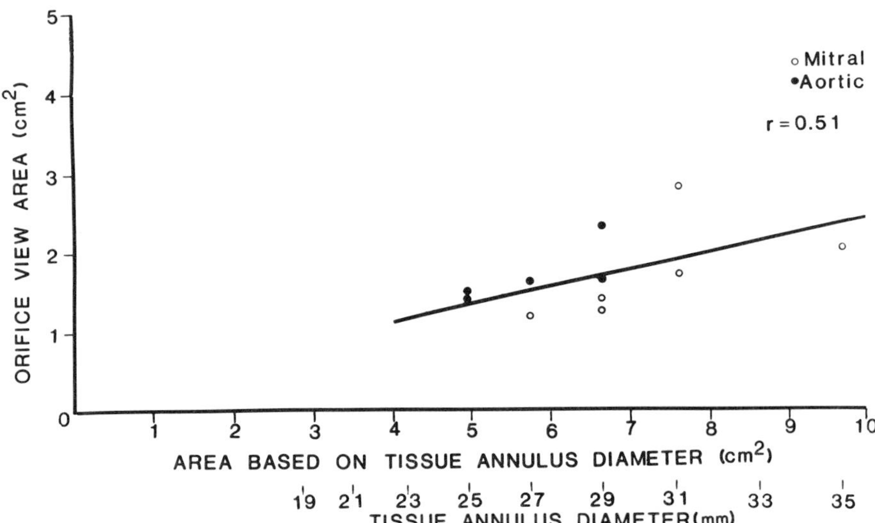

FIG. 6 Relationship of functional orifice area, as shown on orifice view roentgenograms, to the area inscribed by the tissue anulus diameter. The correlation coefficient (r) was 0.51.

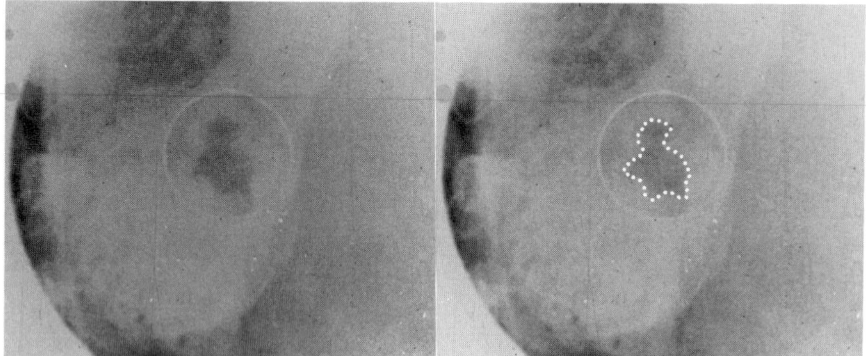

FIG. 7 (left) Orifice roentgenogram of the mitral valve of patient 11. (right) The functional orifice area is outlined by dots.

from 4.2–5.7 cm^2. The average ratio of the orifice area, as shown on orifice view roentgenograms, to the specified orifice area of these valves was 0.32 (range, 0.27–0.49). The area inscribed by the tissue anulus diameter of these valves (the implantation area) ranged from 5.8–9.7 cm^2 (Fig. 6). The average ratio of the orifice, as shown on orifice view roentgenograms, to the area inscribed by the tissue anulus diameter was 0.24 (range, 0.20–0.37).

Comment

The areas of the orifices of these valves in the aortic position, as measured by orifice view aortograms, were comparable to the calculated areas of the orifices in our patients in whom hemodynamic evaluations were also made. The areas of the orifices shown on orifice view aortograms also corresponded closely to the average orifice areas calculated on the basis of pooled data of hemodynamic measurements by several other investigators in patients with essentially normally functioning unmodified (model 242) Hancock porcine bioprosthetic valves[7–11] (Table III). The average orifice areas shown at cardiac catheterization of the 25, 27, and 29 mm aortic valves were 1.5, 1.6, and 1.6 cm^2, respectively.[7–11] Average areas shown on the orifice view aortograms of these valves were 1.5, 1.6, and 2.0 cm^2, respectively. An in vitro assessment of the orifice area of a 29 mm Hancock model 242 aortic valve based upon the Gorlin equation showed an area of 1.7 cm^2.[12]

We assessed the orifice area of a 29 mm model 242 Hancock porcine aortic valve in vitro by orifice view (en face) motion pictures. The hemodynamic system and method for obtaining these films have been described previously.[13] For these studies, we obtained films at 200 frames/s. A

TABLE III Effective orifice area of Hancock model 242 aortic valve

Anulus diameter (mm)	Orifice view area (cm^2)	Postoperative hemodynamic area* (cm^2)	In vitro orifice view area* (cm^2)	In vitro hemodynamic area* (cm^2)
25	1.5	1.5	—	1.6
	n = 2	n = 32		n = 1
27	1.6	1.6	—	—
	n = 1	n = 7		
29	2.0	1.6	1.7	—
	n = 2	n = 2	n = 1	

* Postoperative hemodynamic measurements were based upon the Gorlin equation and were from Lurie et al,[7] Cohn et al,[8] Jones et al,[9] Morris et al,[10] and Johnson et al.[11] In vitro measurements of the valve area from orifice view motion pictures were our own measurements presented in this article. In vitro hemodynamic measurements were based upon the Gorlin equation and are from Wright.[12]

mixture of glycerin and saline with a viscosity of 0.04 poise was used. The stroke volume was 77 ml, aortic pressure was 100/45 mmHg, and the rate was 76 beats/min. The maximal opening was 1.7 cm² (Fig. 8).

Regarding the valves in the mitral position, the areas of the orifices shown on orifice view roentgenograms were comparable to the areas calculated by the Gorlin equation in the 2 patients in whom the data were obtained. The observed areas shown on orifice view roentgenograms of the valves in the mitral position also were comparable to the orifice areas calculated by the

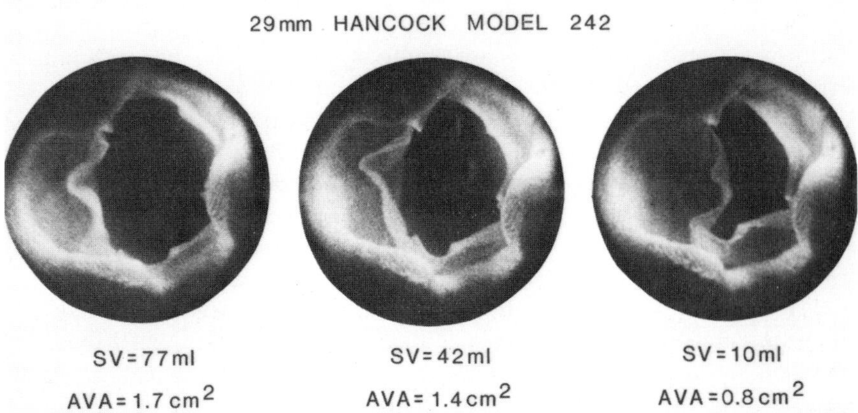

FIG. 8 Frames from in vitro motion pictures showing maximal opening of a 29 mm Hancock model 242 aortic bioprosthetic valve. At a stroke volume (SV) of 77 ml, during maximal opening, the aortic valve area (AVA) was 1.7 cm². At smaller stroke volumes, the maximal opening was less.

TABLE IV Effective orifice area of Hancock model 342 mitral valve

Anulus diameter (mm)	Orifice view area (cm^2)	Postoperative hemodynamic area* (cm^2)	In vitro orifice view area* (cm^2)	In vitro hemodynamic area* (cm^2)
27	1.2 n = 1	1.7 n = 15	—	1.6 n = 1
29	1.4 n = 2	2.2 n = 20	1.8 n = 2	1.9 n = 1
31	2.3 n = 2	2.0 n = 30	1.7 n = 1	2.0 n = 2
33	—	2.7 n = 8	—	1.9 n = 1
35	2.0 n = 1	2.6 n = 17	—	—

* Postoperative hemodynamic measurements were based upon the Gorlin equation and were from Lurie et al,[7] Cotter and Miller,[14] Johnson et al,[15] Horowitz et al,[16] and Duran et al.[17] In vitro orifice view measurements and in vitro hemodynamic assessments of the area were from Walker et al[18] and Wright.[19]

Gorlin equation in patients catheterized by others following valve insertion. Pooled data from several investigators showed average orifice areas for the 27, 29, 31, 33, and 35 mm valves of 1.7, 2.2, 2.0, 2.7, and 2.6 cm^2, respectively[7,14–17] (Table IV). In vitro hemodynamic calculations of the orifice areas as well as en face motion pictures of the valves in the mitral position also showed comparable areas[18,19] (Table IV).

The extent that normal aortic valves[20] and normal mitral valves open[21] depends upon the flow across the valve and this is also true of stent-mounted valves.[17,20] This was also demonstrated on the in vitro motion pictures that we obtained in this study. With stroke volumes of 77, 42, and 10 ml, the opening areas were 1.7, 1.4, and 0.8 cm^2, respectively (Fig. 8). When the stroke volume or rate of flow across the valve is abnormally low, a small orifice due to incomplete opening is shown on the orifice view roentgenogram. When interpreting the significance of a small visualized orifice, it is useful therefore to know the stroke volume. The stroke volume in the 10 patients in this study in whom it was measured was $\geq$49 ml.

In one study[22] in which hemodynamic assessments were made intraoperatively of Hancock valves in the aortic and mitral positions, the calculated orifice areas were greater than observed in our patients or by others during cardiac catheterization months after operation.[7–11,14–17] These investigators speculated that the smaller orifices reported at postoperative cardiac catheterization may have been due to subclinical stiffening of the valves that occurred after insertion.[22] The orifice areas that they measured intraoperatively, however, also were larger than shown in vitro by others[12,18,19] as well as by us, using fresh, unimplanted valves.

The advantages of orifice view roentgenography are that the valve orifice can be seen with sufficient clarity to permit a measurement of the area of the orifice by planimetry. The technique is suited to normal as well as abnormal valves. It is not necessary to cross the valve, and in patients in whom the valve cannot be crossed, or in whom sufficiently accurate hemodynamic measurements cannot be made, orifice view roentgenograms are particularly useful. In patients with heavily calcified natural aortic valves, it was possible to estimate the area of the orifice by the area circumscribed by calcium,[23,24] thereby allowing the method to be totally noninvasive. The normal aortic valve may be somewhat triangular or circular[4] depending in part upon the stroke volume and rate of ejection[20] (Fig. 9). Porcine aortic bioprosthetic valves inserted in the mitral position would show the same roentgenographic configuration as the aortic valve. If a valve is stenotic, the size and configuration of the deformity can be visualized[5,25,26] (Fig. 10).

In patients with natural valves, particularly aortic valves, the technique of orifice view roentgenography has enabled us to identify those, particularly children with congenitally stenotic conditions, whose valves would be improved by valvuloplasty. Conversely, on the basis of such films, we have identified, prior to thoracotomy, conditions in children that would require valve replacement rather than valvuloplasty. Orifice view roentgenography also occasionally has been useful for the identification of patients who would require a particularly large or a particularly small bioprosthetic valve for an appropriate fit of the anulus. An example of strikingly enlarged aortic valve with a dilated anulus that was shown by orifice view aortography was in a patient with Ehlers-Danlos syndrome.[27]

The evaluation of bioprosthetic valves is particularly suited to the technique of orifice view roentgenograms because the metal anulus of the prosthetic valve can be used to assist the physician in positioning the x-ray beam perpendicularly to the valve. In applying the technique to patients with natural valves, it is necessary to employ a projection that, in most patients, would produce the least distortion of the projected image. The variability of the orientation of the aortic[4,5] and mitral[6] valves was described previously, as well as the position required for visualization of the orifice and the amount of error that might result from an unusual orientation of the valve. In patients with bioprosthetic valves, any variability of the ideal projection due to an uncommon orientation of the valve can be compensated for by adjusting the projection to show the metal anulus of the prosthetic valve as a circle.

Orifice view roentgenography was shown to be useful in a patient with a stenotic degenerated bioprosthetic valve in the mitral position.[28] A 0.46 cm^2

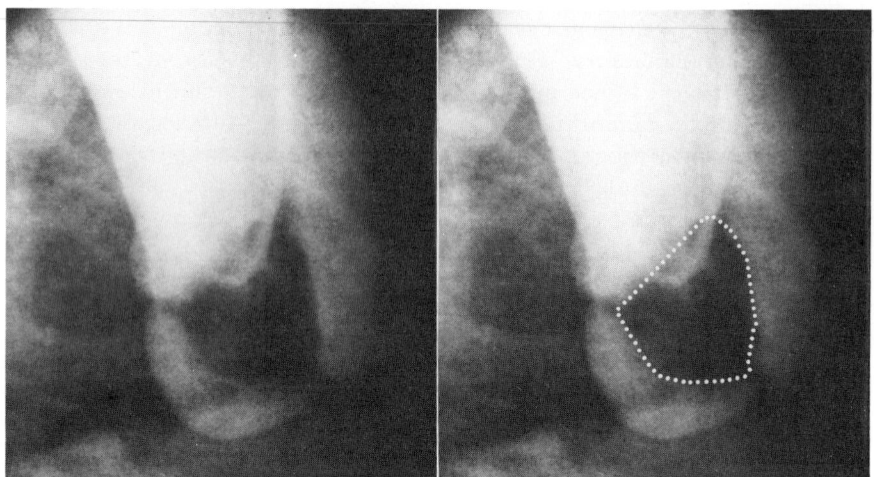

FIG. 9 (left) Orifice aortogram of a patient with a normal natural aortic valve. (right) The orifice is outlined by dots.

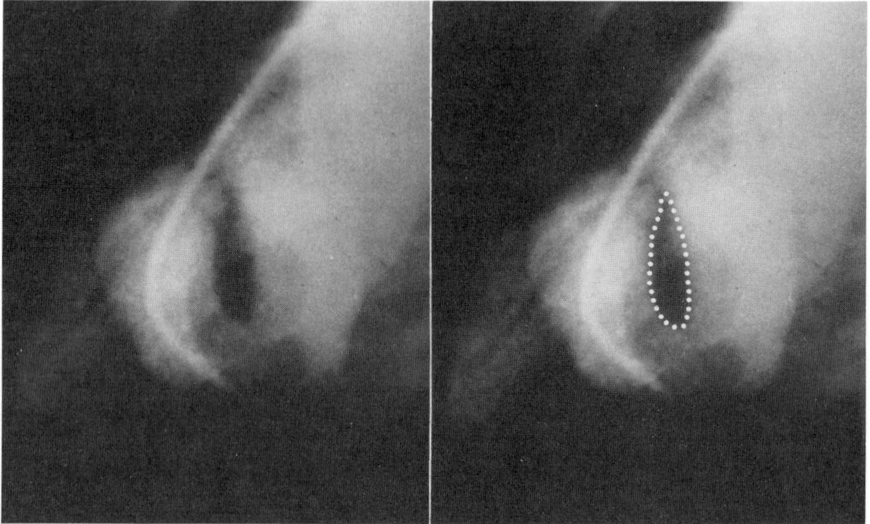

FIG. 10 (left) Orifice aortogram of a patient with a congenitally bicuspid aortic valve. (right) The stenotic orifice is outlined by dots.

orifice was shown by the orifice view roentgenogram and confirmed on measurement of the orifice of the excised surgical specimen.

In conclusion, orifice view roentgenograms showed the functional orifice of bioprosthetic valves in the aortic and mitral positions with sufficient detail to permit a measurement of the orifice areas. The areas of the orifices of the valves of 11 patients corresponded well to hemodynamic measurements obtained by others as well as by us at cardiac catheterization. The areas shown on orifice view roentgenograms also corresponded well to measurements of the orifice obtained by motion pictures in vitro. The functional area of the orifices of the valves in the aortic position was 39% of the predicted orifice area, based upon the manufacturer's estimate of the valve area, and in the mitral position the functional orifice was 32% of the nominal orifice.

References

1. Magilligan DJ Jr, Lewis JW Jr, Jara FM, Lee MW, Alam M, Riddle JM, Stein, PD: Spontaneous degeneration of porcine bioprosthetic valves. Ann Thorac Surg 30:259, 1980.
2. Alam M, Madrazo AC, Magilligan DJ, Goldstein S: M mode and two dimensional echocardiographic features of porcine valve dysfunction. Am J Cardiol 43:502, 1979.
3. Gorlin R, Gorlin SG: Hydraulic formula for the calculation of the area of the stenotic mitral valve, other cardiac valves, and central circulatory shunts. Am Heart J 41:1, 1951.
4. Stein PD: Roentgenographic method for measurement of the cross-sectional area of the aortic valve. Am Heart J 81:622, 1971.
5. Stein PD, Sabbah HN: Orifice-view roentgenography for evaluation of the aortic valve. Am J Roentgenol 125:847, 1975.
6. Stein PD, Sabbah HN: Orifice-view roentgenography of the mitral valve. Am J Roentgenol 125:854, 1975.
7. Lurie AJ, Miller RR, Maxwell KS, Grehl TM, Vismara LA, Hurley EJ, Mason DT: Hemodynamic assessment of the glutaraldehyde-preserved porcine heterograft in the aortic and mitral positions. Circulation 56 (Suppl II):104, 110, 1977.
8. Cohn LH, Sanders JH Jr, Collins JJ Jr: Aortic valve replacement with the Hancock porcine xenograft. Ann Thorac Surg 22:221, 1976.
9. Jones EL, Craver JM, Morris DC, King SB III, Douglas JS Jr, Franch RH, Hatcher CR Jr, Morgan EA: Hemodynamic and clinical evaluation of the Hancock xenograft bioprosthesis for aortic valve replacement (with emphasis on management of the small aortic root). J Thorac Cardiovasc Surg 75:300, 1978.
10. Morris DC, King SB III, Douglas JS Jr, Wickliffe CW, Jones EL: Hemodynamic results of aortic valvular replacement with the porcine xenograft valve. Circulation 56:841, 1977.
11. Johnson A, Thompson S, Vieweg WVR, Daily P, Oury J, Peterson K: Evaluation of the in vivo function of the Hancock porcine xenograft in the aortic position. J Thorac Cardiovasc Surg 75:599, 1978.
12. Wright JTM: A pulsatile flow study comparing the Hancock porcine xenograft aortic valve prostheses models 242 and 250. Med Instrum 11:114, 1977.

13. Sabbah HN, Stein PD: Mechanism of early systolic closure of the aortic valve in discrete membranous subaortic stenosis. Circulation 65:399, 1982.
14. Cotter L, Miller HC: Clinical and haemodynamic evaluation of mounted porcine heterograft in mitral position. Br Heart J 41:412, 1979.
15. Johnson AD, Daily PO, Peterson KL, LeWinter M, Didonna GJ, Blair G, Niwayama G: Functional evaluation of the porcine heterograft in the mitral position. Circulation 51 (Suppl I):40, 1975.
16. Horowitz MS, Goodman DJ, Fogarty TJ, Harrison DC: Mitral valve replacement with the glutaraldehyde-preserved porcine heterograft: Clinical, hemodynamic and pathological correlations. J Thorac Cardiovasc Surg 67:885, 1974.
17. Duran CG, Ubago JL, Gallo JI, Colman T, Figueroa A: Clinical and hemodynamic evaluation of the Hancock valve bioprosthesis. In: Proceedings of the Symposium on Bioprosthetic Cardiac Valves. (F Sebening, WP Klövekorn, H Meisner, E Struck, Eds). Munich, Deutsches Herzzentrum, 1979, p 233.
18. Walker DK, Scotten LN, Modi VJ, Brownlee RT: In vitro assessment of mitral valve prostheses. J Thorac Cardiovasc Surg 79:680, 1980.
19. Wright JTM: Hydrodynamic evaluation of tissue valves. In: Tissue Heart Valves. (MI Ionescu, Ed). London, Butterworths, 1979, p 29.
20. Stein PD, Munter WA: New functional concept of valvular mechanics in normal and diseased aortic valves. Circulation 44: 101, 1971.
21. Chandraratna PAN, Sabbah HN, San Pedro S, Stein PD: Echocardiographic assessment of the mitral valve in non-calcific mitral stenosis. In: Non-Invasive Cardiovascular Diagnosis: Current Concepts. (E Dietrick, Ed). Baltimore, University Park Press, 1978, p 373.
22. Levine FH, Carter JE, Buckley MJ, Daggett WM, Akins CW, Austen WG: Hemodynamic evaluation of Hancock and Carpentier-Edwards bioprostheses. Circulation 64 (Suppl II):192, 1981.
23. Stein PD: A new roentgenographic assessment of anatomic deformity in calcific aortic stenosis. Am Heart J 84:321, 1972.
24. Stein PD: Assessment of calcific aortic stenosis by measurement of area circumscribed by calcium on plain film orifice-view roentgenograms. Chest 65:518, 1974.
25. Folger GM Jr, Sabbah HN, Anbe DT, Stein PD: Orifice-view aortography in patients with congenitally deformed aortic valves: Determination of aortic valve area. Cathet Cardiovasc Diagn 6:135, 1980.
26. Folger GM Jr, Sabbah HN, Stein PD: Evaluation of the anatomy of congenitally malformed aortic valves by orifice-view aortography. Am Heart J 100:152, 1980.
27. Simon AP, Stein PD: Aortic insufficiency in Ehlers-Danlos syndrome. Angiology 25:290, 1974.
28. Smuckler AL, Kahl FR: En face demonstration of a prosthetic mitral valve orifice during left ventriculography. Cathet Cardiovasc Diagn 7:403, 1981.

SECTION III

THROMBOEMBOLISM

13

Alterations in Valvular Surgery: Biologic Valves

Å. SENNING

It has been fascinating to follow the development of valvular heart surgery during the time I have been working as a surgeon. In 1956, Murray et al[1] reported that although experimentally fresh aortic homologous valves showed shrinking changes under the microscope, they retained their form and function during the 9½ months that they were experimentally implanted. He operated upon 3 patients with aortic insufficiency who survived up to 6 years with valves in the descending aorta.

In the late 1950s experimental work was performed in construction of prostheses to replace heart valves. In 1960 Harken et al[2] reported the implantation of ball valves in the subcoronary position to replace the aortic valve, and later in the next year Starr et al[3] used a modified ball valve in the mitral position. All recognized the risk of thromboembolism and all interest was directed to tissue valves. The first successful orthotopic valve replacement with a fresh aortic valve allograft was performed in 1962 by Ross[4] and a little later by Barratt-Boyes.[5] This was the beginning of a new era in cardiac valve replacement.

Fascia Lata

Having worked with organ transplantation, I felt that allografts or homografts would be slowly destroyed by immunologic factors. In the same year I began replacing the aortic valve with autogenous fascia lata, which was taken sterile at the time of operation, eliminating the problems of

---

From the Surgical Clinic A, University Hospital, Zurich, Switzerland.
Dr. Senning was an honor lecturer at the Second International Symposium on Cardiac Bioprostheses.

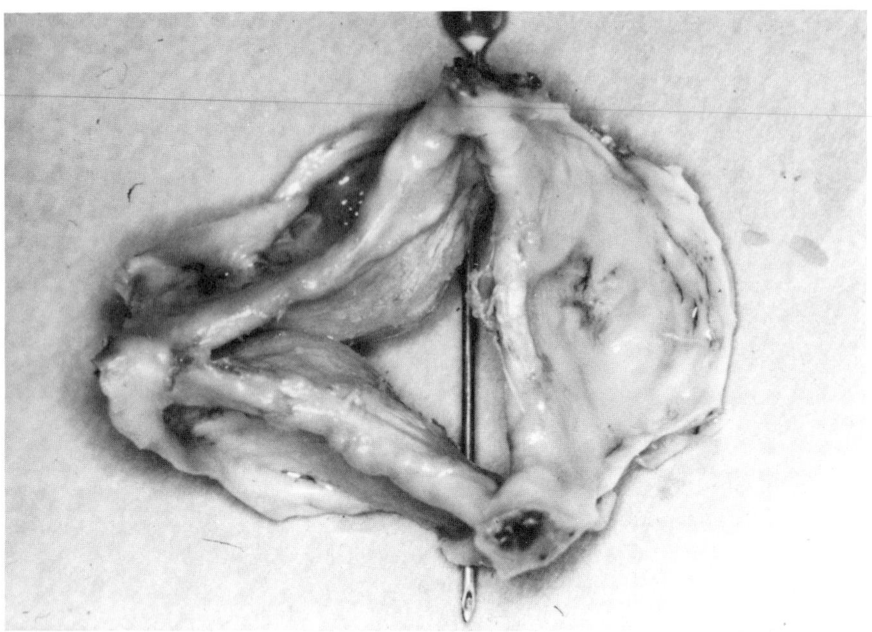

FIG. 1 Aortic valve replacement with fascia lata 6 years postimplantation. All 3 leaflets became thick and stiff, their bases aneurysmatic; free ends were stretched. Valve became incompetent and had to be replaced.

sterilization, preservation, immunologic reactions, and thromboembolism. But unexpected histologic changes occurred. Three years postoperatively, a valve could be thin and flexible but there were strong individual variations in the reaction on the valve and many valves became thickened and began to leak after 4 years (Fig. 1). The fascia was rapidly covered with protein and cellular elements, and within time most of the valves became covered with thick layers of fibrotic tissue, especially on the ventricular side. The collagen fibers became stretched and some broke, causing aneurysmatic dilation of the bottom of the cusps followed by traction of the free edges of the valves with incompetence as a consequence. Tissue calcification was generally found about 8 years postoperatively. With increased valvular changes, the rate of late bacterial endocarditis increased and after 12 years it was 28%.

After 5 years, 15% of the valves had to be replaced; after 10 years, only 40% of the patients had a functioning fascia lata valve. Therefore we stopped using fascia lata aortic valve replacement in 1970. Eighteen patients are still alive 12–20 years postoperatively with their original fascia aortic valve, and 13 have no or minimal dysfunction.

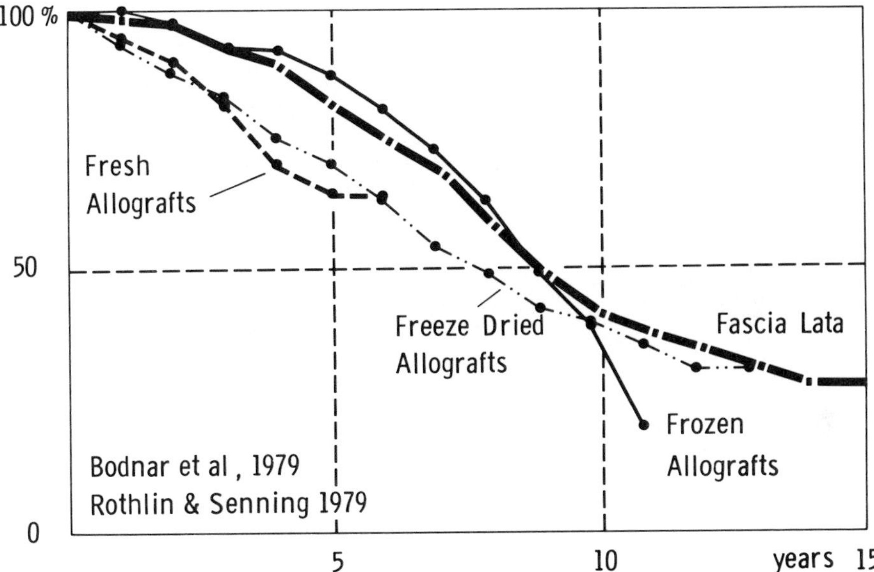

FIG. 2 Cumulative and comprehensive complication-free performance of valves in aortic position. Operative mortality excluded (according to Bodnar et al, 1979; Rothlin and Senning, 1979).

Mitral Allografts

Having heard many optimistic reports on the results of aortic allograft replacement, I erred in performing mitral allograft replacements in 13 patients; the mitral valve was excised from a person who died 24 hours before and placed orthotopically unstented in the mitral position of the patient. It was technically difficult to adjust the allograft in the mitral position, and there were 3 hospital deaths. One patient was reoperated on early and only 6 survived 4–14 years. All valves were finally completely destroyed.

In our cases we could observe degeneration of the collagen tissue with covering and ingrowing fibrous tissue, chondromatous transformation, and calcification and destruction of the valve, again causing mitral insufficiency.

Aortic Allografts

Valve replacement with aortic allografts was still in vogue and some surgeons, e.g., Ross[6] and Barratt-Boyes et al[7] reported excellent results. It was believed that differences in sterilization and preservation techniques

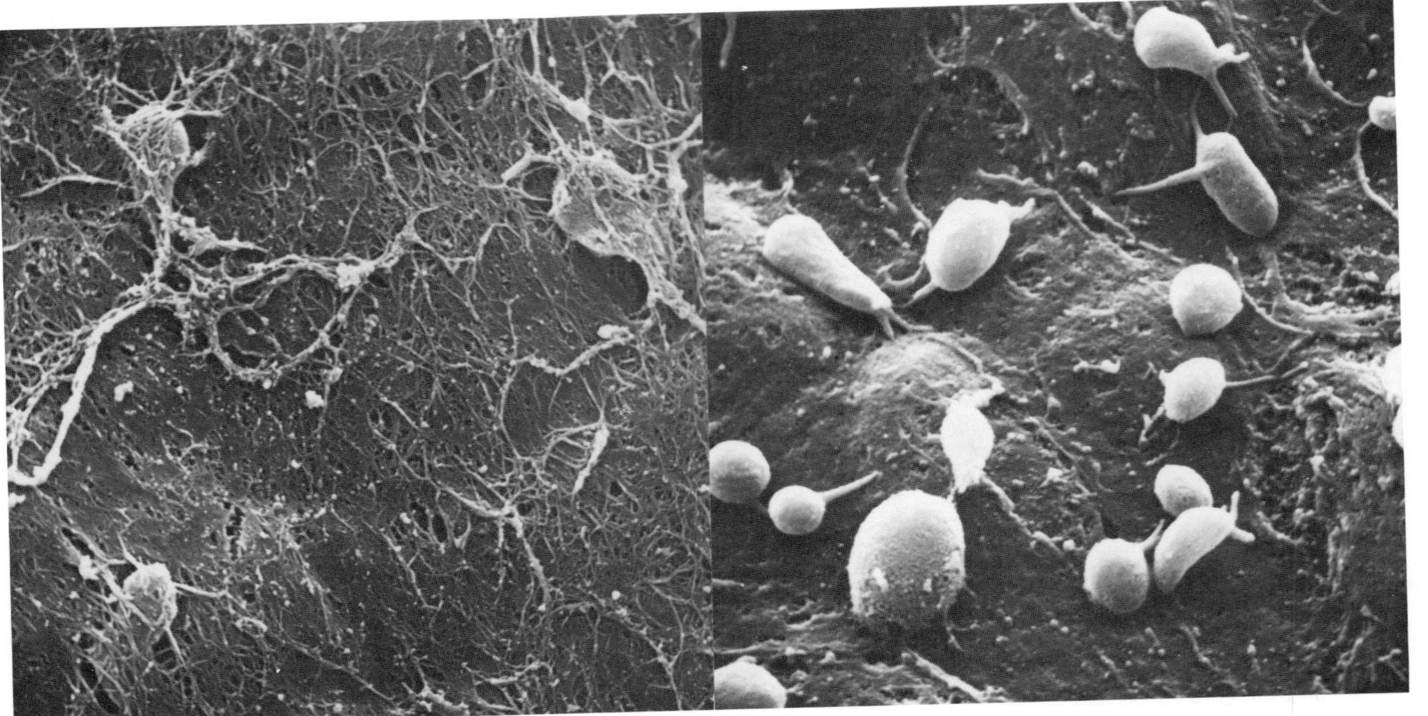

FIG. 3 Experimental pulmonary valve replacement. Left: 60 s after implantation of bioprosthesis, surface of leaflets is covered by loosely attached platelets (×17,000). Right: 1½ h after implantation, macrophages are incorporated in the valve surface (×25,000).

had negatively influenced the long-term performance of homograft valves, explaining the disappointing results in other follow-up studies.[8–10]

Bodnar et al[11] in Ross's group compared freeze-dried, frozen, and fresh homografts (Fig. 2) and found that finally degeneration affects homograft valves more or less to the same degree, irrespective of the method used for sterilization and preservation, and is the cause of limited durability. If cells in the transplanted valves are living at implantation or not seems irrelevant, as the viability of the valvular cells declines rapidly after implantation and the valve will not be incorporated as a living tissue capable of tissue maintenance and repair. The cusps with time become thin and often calcified. Compared to the fascia lata valve replacement, the allografts do not seem to have a distinct advantage.

Bioprostheses

Legal hindrance made allografts unavailable in France. Binet et al[12] in 1965 tried instead xenograft valves taken from a calf, conditioned in organo-mercurial salt to stabilize the tissue and make it less antigenic. The 4 year follow-up of their first series of 90 patients showed, that only 10% of valves functioned normally. O'Brien and Clarebrough[13] in 1966 used xenografts tanned with formaldehyde but around 40% of these valves were incompetent after 3 years. Carpentier et al[14] had found that dissolution of the cross-linkage of the collagen occurred in the cusp treated with formaldehyde, so he started using glutaraldehyde to get a more stable cross-linkage of the collagen, as well as a good sterilization. Carpentier[15] also introduced the term "bioprosthesis" for chemically stabilized biologic tissue valves.

There has been continuous research work to refine bioprostheses since 1968, when the first implantation was performed. As a result, commercially available valves now show far better results. In contrast with other grafts, according to Carpentier,[15] the durability of the bioprostheses depends upon the "unfailing" stability of the biologic material and not upon the regeneration by the host cells. When completely denaturized, the biologic material should cause no immunologic problems and the danger of valvular thromboembolism minimized. Although this so-called "unfailing stability of the biologic tissue" is postulated, our canine experiments and the changes seen by scanning electron microscopy (SEM) in the excised valves of human beings are very similar to the alterations of the fascia valves. Surface alterations seem to progress as in fascia lata, only slower. The covering of the leaflet surface with connective tissue seems identical.

Immediately after implantation, the surface of the leaflets of the bioprosthesis are covered by a protein layer followed by loosely attached platelets (Fig. 3). Microthrombi already appear on the surface of the valve

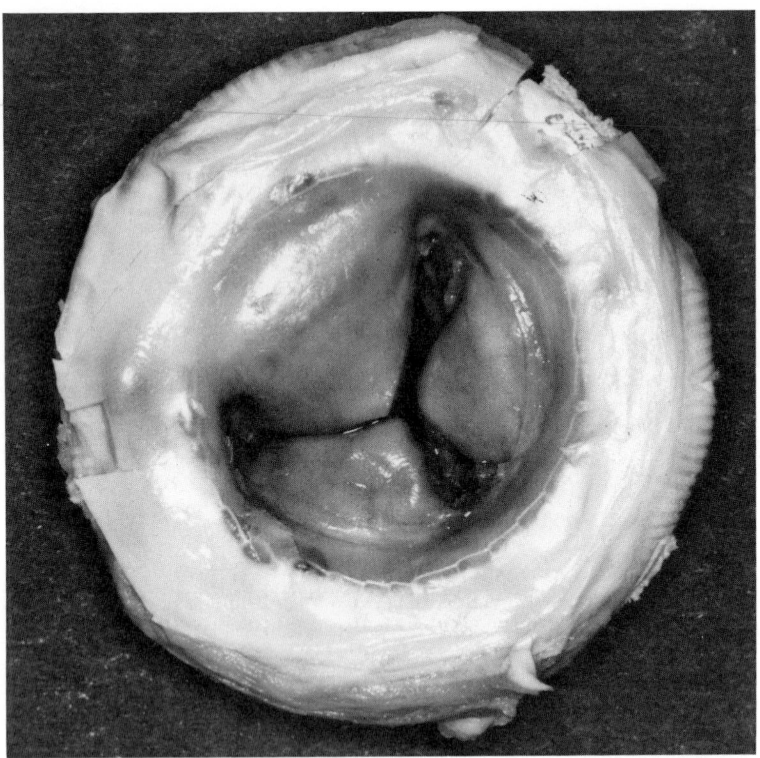

FIG. 4 TVR with Hancock bioprosthesis #33, in a 34-year-old woman, 17 months postimplantation. Excessive connective tissue overgrowth, causing leaflet stiffness. Thrombotic material is on all 3 commissures.

12 minutes after implantation. They reach their maximum after 3–4 weeks. There is no doubt that at this time platelet inhibitors or anticoagulation are of protective value. In the following weeks fibers of connective tissue are formed mainly on the less mobile part of the valves. The running suture fixing the xenograft on its supporting ring (stent) becomes completely covered by connective tissue and the tissue continues to grow onto the leaflets in the direction of the free edge. This tissue gives on the one side a certain support to the leaflet and protects it from tears caused by collagen degeneration. It can cover completely also the stent, making its surface smooth. On the other side, this overgrowth of connective tissue occasionally can cause valve stiffness (Fig. 4). In a SEM picture of a valve, implanted 26 months in the mitral position, collagen overgrowth arises in layers. We can count at least 7 different layers (Fig. 5). Further on and over the middle part of the same leaflets inflow side, (Fig. 6) we can see 2 different fiber types, which

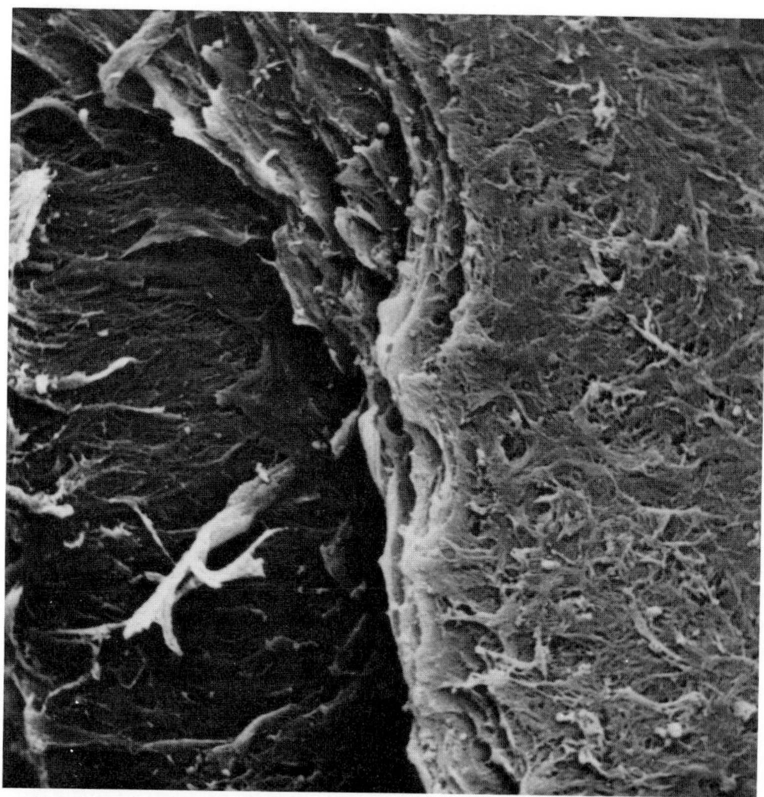

FIG. 5 MVR with Hancock bioprosthesis #33, in a 30-year-old man 26 months postimplantation. Collagen overgrowth arises in layers. At least 7 different layers can be counted (×240).

can be recognized as younger collagen fibers and older ones that are completely incorporated on the leaflets' surface. Next to this natural overgrowth, degeneration of the collagen can occur, leading to leaflet tears, calcification, and perforation. Calcification occurred mainly in the free edge of the leaflets (Fig. 7). As Ferrans et al[16] has pointed out in the last symposium on bioprostheses in Munich 1979, calcification can occur either in the collagen fibrils or in the interfibrillary spaces around the fibers or both. In contrast to mechanical valves, thrombosis of the bioprostheses occurs very seldom, although anticoagulation is generally not given. In our material of more than 500 bioprostheses implanted, less than 1% per patient year has been replaced due to thrombosis. The tissue changes described look very alarming and it can be expected that the fate of the bioprostheses will be the same as that of the fascia lata valves. If we look at a comparison of the

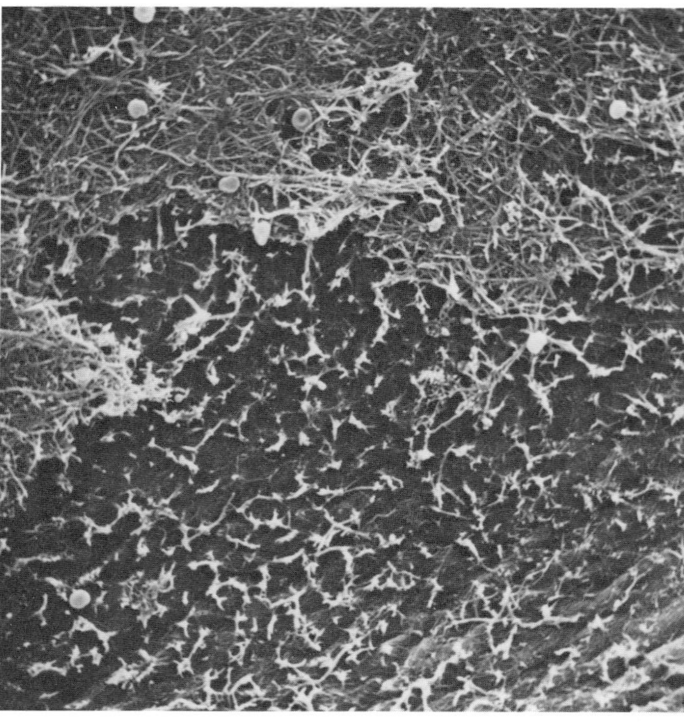

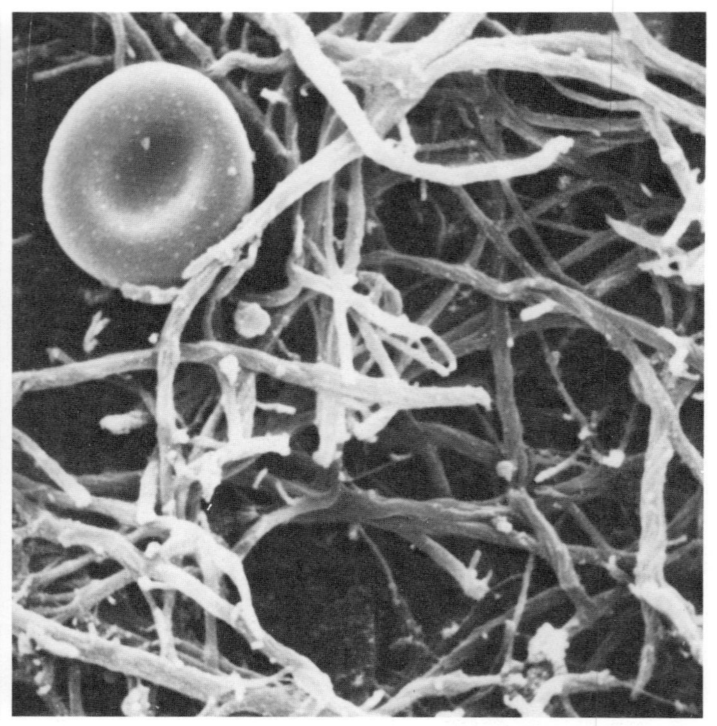

FIG. 6 MVR 20 months postimplantation, same patient as Fig. 5. Left: collagen overgrowth over middle part of inflow side of leaflet. On upper part younger collagen from host covers leaflets surface; on lower part older connective tissue of host adheres on leaflets surface. Right: higher magnification of parts of picture on left. (left ×600, right ×6,000).

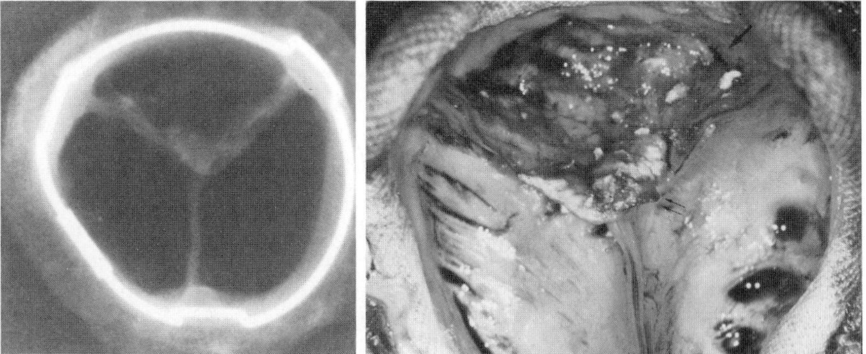

FIG. 7 Calcification on free edge of porcine bioprosthetic valve. (left) Radiograph (right) Gross pathology (arrows point to free edge calcium).

fascia lata valve and the experimental series of Carpentier et al,[14] their course is practically the same and only 80% of their patients survived 6 years. Carpentier's later series[15] with commercially available valves, though, showed a much more favorable outcome (Fig. 8).

Geha et al[17] found that in 325 adult patients only 2 valves were destroyed by primary tissue failures and 6 were caused by endocarditis between 1 and

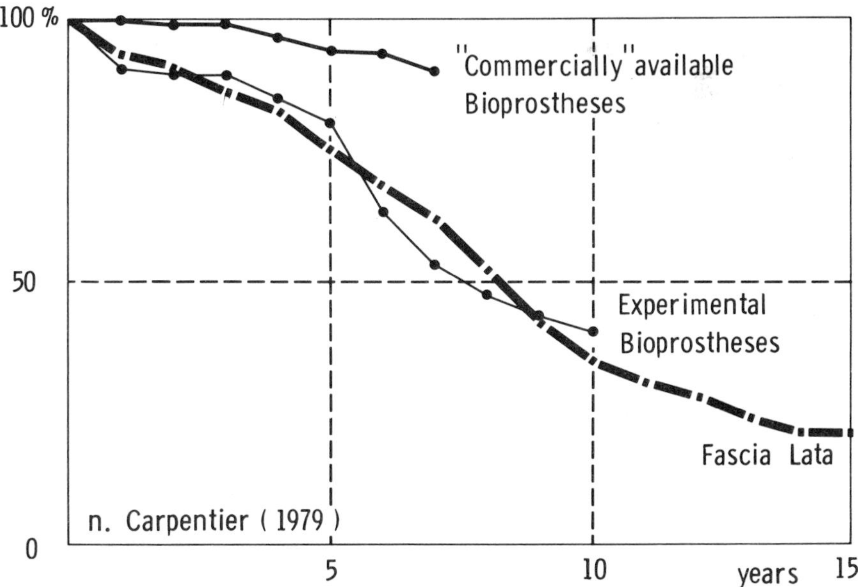

FIG. 8 Comparative valve durability (actuarial curve) of fascia lata valve in aortic position and of experimental series, commercially available bioprostheses. Operative mortality included (Carpentier, 1979; Rothlin and Senning, 1979).

3 years after insertion. On the other hand, in their series of children 23% of cardiac valves had to be replaced 21–41 months postoperatively. There was no thromboembolism in patients with MVR and sinus rhythm who had antiplatelet agents or warfarin and there were no emboli in AVR.

Oyer and co-workers[18] follow-up data on 1,285 patients with Hancock prosthesis indicated that the actuarial probability of valve dysfunction was 5% at 5 years for AVR, 7% for MVR, and 5% at 4 years for AVR-MVR. There seems to be no propensity for late failure due to tissue disruption and their follow-up data further indicated that overall xenograft cardiac valve performance in older adults remains excellent up to 85 months postoperatively. Magilligan et al[19] found that for 624 valves at risk with 100% follow-up the percentage free of prosthesis failure was 97% at 5 years and 80% at 8 years. The incidence of degeneration of the valves did not increase in linear fashion with time but seems to decline. Instead of 16 expected degenerated valves in 1980, only 5 occurred. Magilligan et al have a higher frequency of thromboemboli but they have not been using antiplatelet agents, as have Geha et al[17] in two-thirds of their patients. It is plausible that the platelet-collagen reaction, the first step in the thrombosis, may play a role in adhesion of the platelets to the tissue surface and subsequent degeneration.

Considerable favorable experience has now been reported with the pericardial bioprosthesis by Ionescu et al.[20]

As man during the last 6,000–7,000 years has learned to fabricate better qualities of leather by improving tanning of the collagen, the same improvement has happened with cardiac bioprostheses. Exposing the valve to formaldehyde after the tanning with glutaraldehyde has resulted in improved sterility and a still lower antigenicity. We have calculated a durability of the bioprostheses of about 10 years, but it is possible that in the future this can be prolonged. The fibrotic overgrowth must not have a deleterious effect if it is not too abundant and can possibly serve to grow over and invade degenerated areas to repair them, thus preventing wear and tear.

The modern bioprosthesis has good hemodynamic performance. Thromboembolism, anticoagulant bleeding, and hemolysis, the main complications of the mechanical prosthesis, are today practically nonexistent in patients with normal cardiac output and sinus rhythm treated with antiplatelet drugs. The individual negative reaction on tissue valves can perhaps be eliminated when antigenicity has been completely abolished. In any case we cannot compare the long-term results of valve replacements with bioprostheses made today with earlier series.

In older patients the bioprosthesis is ideal for valve replacement. The accelerated degeneration and calcification in young individuals, especially small children, and patients under dialysis are still unsolved problems. We can hope that they will be solved in the near future.

References

1. Murray G, Roschlau W, Laugheed W: Homologous aortic valve-segment transplants as surgical treatment for aortic and mitral insufficiency. Gariner Med Res Inst, S. 466, 1956.
2. Harken DE, Soroff HS, Taylor WJ, et al: Partial and complete prostheses in aortic insufficiency. J Thorac Cardiovasc Surg 40:744, 1960.
3. Starr A, Edwards ML, McCord CW, Griswold HE: Aortic replacement. Clinical experience with a semi-rigid ball valve prosthesis. Circulation 27:779, 1963.
4. Ross DN: Homograft replacement of the aortic valve. Lancet 2:487, 1962.
5. Barratt-Boyes BG: Homograft aortic valve replacement in aortic incompetence and stenosis. Thorax 19:131, 1964.
6. Ross DN: Surgical reconstruction of the aortic valve. Lancet 2:571, 1963.
7. Barratt-Boyes BG, Roche ABG, Whitlock RML: Six years review of the results of freehand aortic valve replacement using an antibiotic sterilized homograft valve. Circulation 55:353, 1977.
8. Copeland JG, Griepp RB, Stinson EB, Shumway NE: Long-term followup after isolated aortic valve replacement. J Thorac Cardiovasc Surg 74:875, 1977.
9. Anderson ET, Hancock EW: Long-term followup of aortic valve replacement with fresh aortic homograft. J Thorac Cardiovasc Surg 72:151, 1976.
10. Kouchoukos NT: Tissue valve replacement: The choices, the results. Adv Cardiol 22:101, 1977.
11. Bodnar E, Waind HW, Martelli V, Ross DN: Long-term performance of 580 homograft and autograft valves used for aortic valve replacement. Thorac Cardiovasc Surg 27:31, 1979.
12. Binet JP, Duran CG, Carpentier A, Langlois J: Heterologous aortic valve transplantation. Lancet 2:1275, 1965.
13. O'Brien MF, Clarebrough JK: Heterograft aortic valve transplantation for human valve disease. Aust Med J 2:228, 1966.
14. Carpentier A, Blondeau P, Marcel P: Remplacement des valves mitrales et tricuspides par des heterogreffes. Ann Chir Cardiovasc 7:33, 1968.
15. Carpentier A: Valvular xenografts and valvular xenobioprosthesis: Past, present and future. Adv Cardiol 27:281, 1980.
16. Ferrans VJ, Boyce St.W, Billingham ME, et al: Calcific deposits in porcine bioprostheses: Structure and pathogenesis. Am J Cardiol 46:721, 1980.
17. Geha AS, Hammond GL, Laks H, Stansel HC, Glenn WW: Factors affecting performance and thromboembolism after porcine xenograft valve replacement. J Thorac Cardiovasc Surg 83:337, 1982.
18. Oyer PE, Stinson EB, Reitz BA, et al: Long-term evaluation of the porcine xenograft bioprosthesis. J Thorac Cardiovasc Surg 78:343, 1979.
19. Magilligan DJ, Lewis JW, Jara FW, Lee MW, Alam M, Riddle JM, Stein PD: Spontaneous degeneration of porcine bioprosthetic valves. Ann Thorac Surg 30:259, 1980.
20. Ionescu MI, Tandon AP: Long-term clinical and hemodynamic evaluation of the Ionescu-Shiley pericardial xenograft heart valve. In: Bioprosthetic Cardiac Valves (F Sebening, WP Klövekorn, H Meisner, E Struck, Eds). Munich, Deutsches Herzzentrum, 1979, p 199.

14

Early and Late Results of Porcine Bioprostheses Versus Mechanical Prostheses in Aortic and Mitral Position

C. MINALE, P. BARDOS, N. P. BOURG, B. J. MESSMER

Both of the 2 available types of valve substitutes, mechanical and biologic prostheses, have advantages and disadvantages. With mechanical valves, there is more consistent durability associated with a certain degree of morbidity; with biologic valves, there is low morbidity but at the cost of a hypothetically shorter durability.

Experience with mechanical prostheses is large enough to extrapolate the results but, in contrast, the bioprostheses have been employed for a relatively short time[1-6] and the final outlook for these valves is not yet clarified.

In 1976, we began implantation of glutaraldehyde-fixed porcine bioprostheses in patients with single, double, and triple valve disease at our institution and during the same period we continued to implant conventional mechanical prostheses in comparable series of patients.

After a 6 year experience with porcine bioprostheses and mechanical prostheses we present an analysis of each type of valve, restricted to the isolated aortic or mitral valve replacement to evaluate the precise role of each type of prosthesis in each of the 2 positions.

Patients and Methods

Between June 1976 and December 1981, 526 consecutive patients underwent isolated mitral or aortic valve replacement. Of these, 322 received a porcine bioprosthesis and 204 received a mechanical valve. To limit bias, in comparing the 2 categories of prostheses, all patients requiring associated procedures, such as aortocoronary bypass, aortic aneurysm resection, left ventricular aneurysmectomy, were excluded from this study.

From the Department of Cardiovascular Surgery, University of Aachen School of Medicine, Aachen, West Germany.

TABLE I Mitral valve replacement: patient data

	Bioprostheses	Mechanical prostheses
# of patients	220	35
# prostheses	222	36
Male	67	8
Female	153	27
Average age (yrs)	51 ± 0.8	53 ± 1.4
Range	22–74	34–71
65 years or older	14	6

Mitral Valve Disease

In 220 patients a porcine bioprosthesis was implanted and in 35 patients a mechanical (Björk-Shiley) valve. Patient data are summarized in Table I. For mitral valve replacement, the bioprosthesis was favored except in those patients who requested a mechanical device to avoid the possible reoperation. Preoperative diagnoses with relative details and functional class are shown in Table II and Fig. 1.

Postoperatively, all patients received warfarin for a minimum of 2 months. Long-term anticoagulation was prescribed for patients with mechanical prostheses and for all patients with atrial fibrillation.

Aortic Valve Disease

In the aortic position, 102 patients received a porcine bioprosthesis and 169 patients had a mechanical valve. Patient data are summarized in Table III.

TABLE II Mitral valve replacement: preoperative diagnosis and details

	Bioprostheses		Mechanical prostheses	
	#	%	#	%
Mainly stenosis	85	39	12	34
Mainly incompetence	18	8	1	3
Combined	117	53	22	63
Total	220		35	
Reoperation	20	9	11	33
After commissurotomy	13	6	10	29
After valve replacement	7	3	1	4
Acute infective endocarditis	5	2	1	3
Total	25		12	

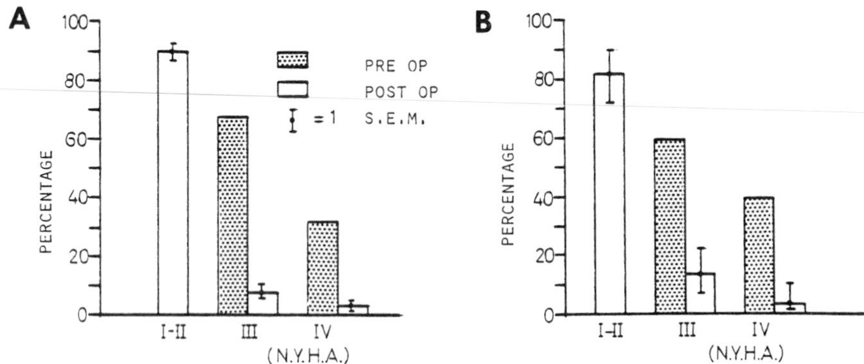

FIG. 1 Mitral valve replacement with bioprostheses (A) and with mechanical prostheses (B). Pre- and postoperative functional class (NYHA) patient distribution.

Bioprostheses were preferred in adults younger than age 40 years and in patients older than age 70. In addition, severe renovascular hypertension and hemorrhagic diathesis were indications for implantation of a bioprosthesis. Bioprostheses were, however, only used when the aortic anulus allowed a minimal size of 27 mm. For sizes 25 and lower, mechanical valves were used. Preoperative diagnosis with relative details and functional class are shown in Table IV and Figure 2.

Anticoagulation was prescribed for 2 months postoperatively for patients with bioprostheses and indefinitely for patients with mechanical prostheses.

Surgical Technique

All patients underwent operation with cardiopulmonary bypass, moderate hypothermia (28°C) and reduced flow perfusion (1.6 liters/min^{-1}/m^{-2} body surface area [BSA]). Membrane or bubble oxygenators were employed interchangeably. Myocardial protection was afforded by cold cardioplegic

TABLE III Aortic valve replacement: patient data

	Bioprostheses	Mechanical prostheses
# patients	102	169
# valves	102	169
Male	89	110
Female	13	59
Average age (yrs)	45 ± 1.6	54 ± 1.0
Range	18–68	21–72
65 years or older	8	34

TABLE IV Aortic valve replacement: preoperative diagnosis and details

	Bioprostheses		Mechanical prostheses	
	#	%	#	%
Mainly stenosis	17	17	51	30
Mainly incompetence	37	36	25	15
Combined	48	47	93	55
Total	102		169	
Reoperation after valve replacement	0	0	5	3
Acute infective endocarditis	6	6	3	2

cardiac arrest. After the ascending aorta was cross clamped, a single dose of Cardioplegin[7] (120 ml/m^{-2} BSA) at 4°C was injected either in the aortic root or directly in both coronary orifices.

In the mitral position, both types of prostheses were secured on the valve anulus with 14–20 interrupted 2-0 Tycron mattress sutures, generally buttressed with Teflon felt pledgets placed on the ventricular side of the mitral anulus. Only in a small sample of patients at the beginning of our series were no Teflon pledgets employed in securing the valve.

In the aortic position, the bioprosthesis was secured by means of 10–15 interrupted 2-0 Tycron mattress sutures buttressed with Teflon felt pledgets, placed on the ventricular side of the aortic anulus. The mechanical prosthesis was secured generally with 20–30 interrupted 2-0 Tycron stitches.

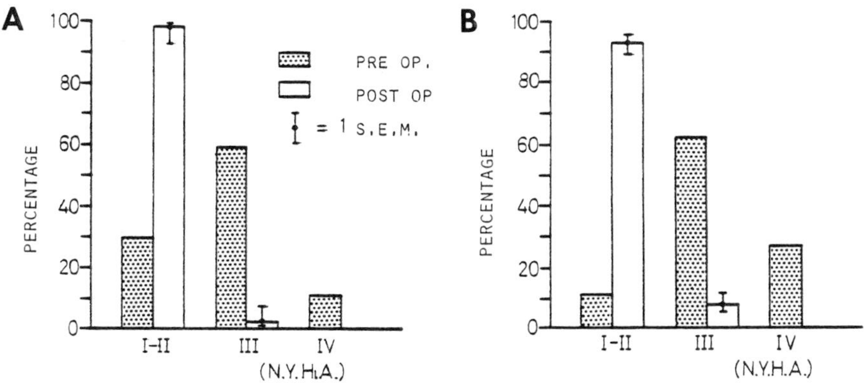

FIG. 2 Aortic valve replacement with bioprotheses (A) and with mechanical prostheses (B). Pre- and postoperative functional class (NYHA) patient distribution.

Follow-up

Only patients operated upon until December 31, 1980, were included in the follow-up study in order to have a reasonable minimal observation time. Follow-up information has been obtained mainly by interviewing the patients in our outpatient clinic at regular intervals. For patients living at a far distance, a questionnaire was sent to the patient and to the referring physician.

All late deaths of unclear origin were attributed to valve-related cause. Thromboembolic complications include all new focal neurologic defects, either transient or permanent, unless they were proved to be of other origin, as well as peripheral arterial emboli.

All hemorrhagic episodes sustained by patients under anticoagulant therapy were attributed to the valve prosthesis.

Valve failure was considered every time a new regurgitant murmur and/or disappearance of the normal metallic click, in the case of the mechanical valve, was discovered. Need for reoperation was not essential for the definition of valve failure. Paravalvular leak and prosthesis endocarditis are not included under valve failure but are considered separately. Details of follow-up are listed in Tables V and VI.

Statistics

Continuous variables are presented with ± 1 standard error of the mean (SEM). The value of categorial variables are expressed as the mean value with its 70% confidence limit band.[8] Proportion and percentage differences were tested against the O hypothesis by means of the Pearson chi-square test[9] for a $2 \times K$ contingency table. In sample size less than 10 the Fischer's exact test was used.[10] Survival rates probability are expressed with the actuarial or life table method according to Kaplan and Meier.[11] Operative mortality is included in these curves.

Complication-free rates of surviving patients are estimated with the

TABLE V Mitral valve replacement: follow-up

	Bioprostheses	Mechanical prostheses
# patients	138	30
# patients lost to follow-up	5 (3.6%)	0
Duration (patient year)	262	99
Average (yrs)	2 ± 0.09	3.3 ± 0.25
Range (yrs)	0.18–4.5	0.5–5.1
Current survivors	120	29

TABLE VI Aortic valve replacement: follow-up

	Bioprostheses	Mechanical prostheses
# patients	57	129
# patients lost to follow-up	6 (10%)	7 (5%)
Duration (patient year)	72	295
Average (yrs)	1.5 ± 0.1	2.5 ± 0.3
Range (yrs)	0.15–5	0.1–5.1
Current survivors	49	115

cumulative complication-free rate method of Grunkemeier et al.[12] Since the total and the average postoperative follow-up time is different in each group to be compared, late mortality and morbidity are presented as "linearized occurrence rate."[13] In this way, the occurrence rate of an event is not considered as an absolute value, but related to the observation time of a patient or a valve at risk.

Results

Patient Survival

Hospital mortality (30 days) was 0.9% and 0 for mitral valve replacement with bio- and mechanical prostheses, respectively, and 1.9 and 1.2% for aortic valve replacement with bio- and mechanical prostheses, respectively (Tables VII, VIII). Late mortality, expressed as linearized rate, was 3.0 and 1.0% ($p = 0.2$) for mitral valve replacement with bio- and mechanical prostheses, respectively, and 2.6 and 2.3% ($p = 1$) for aortic valve replacement with bio- and mechanical prostheses, respectively (Tables VII, VIII).

Actuarially calculated patient survival rates, which include the operative mortality rate, are shown in Figs. 3 and 4. No significant difference was observed between patients having bio- or mechanical prostheses either in the mitral ($p = 1.0$) or aortic positions.

TABLE VII Mitral valve replacement: mortality

	Bioprostheses		Mechanical prostheses		
	#	%	#	%	Significance
Early mortality	2/220	0.9	0/35	0	$p = 0.6$
Late mortality	8/133	3.0*	1/30	1.0*	$p = 0.2$

* Linearized values (% per patient year).

TABLE VIII Aortic valve replacement: mortality

	Bioprostheses		Mechanical prostheses		
	#	%	#	%	Significance
Early mortality	2/102	1.9	2/169	1.2	p = 0.6
Late mortality	2/58	2.6*	7/130	2.3*	p = 1.0

* Linearized values (% per patient year).

Complications

Late complications include thromboembolism, bleeding, endocarditis, perivalvar leakage, and valve failure. The incidences for these in our experience are shown in Tables IX and X.

In the mitral position we noted a higher incidence of thromboembolism, 5.2% per patient year -vs- 2.0% per patient year with mechanical than with bioprostheses. Although the difference in thromboembolic complications was not statistically significant (p = 0.07), it must be noted that this is probably due to the relatively small number of patients with mechanical prostheses in the mitral group. Patients with a bioprosthesis in the aortic position showed a significantly higher (p = 0.001) occurrence of endocarditis than those who had a mechanical valve (4% per patient year -vs- 0.3% per patient year).

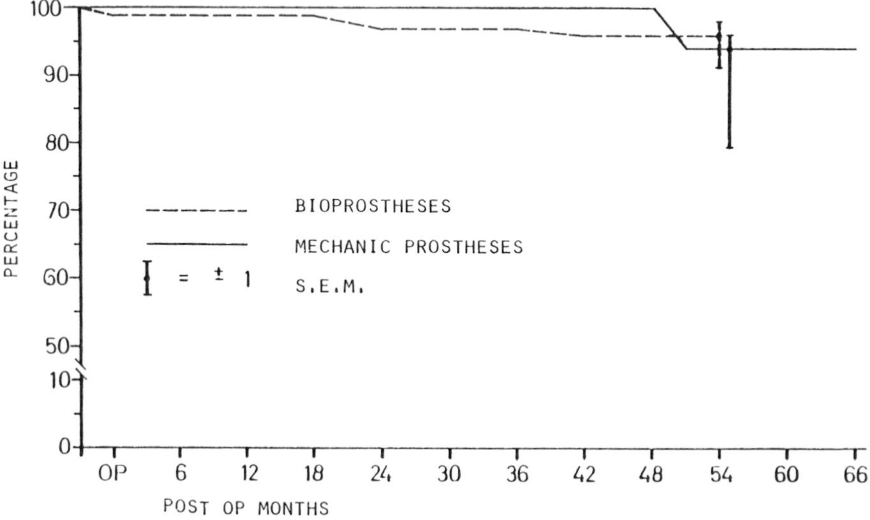

FIG. 3 Mitral valve replacement. Actuarial overall survival with bioprostheses and with mechanical prostheses.

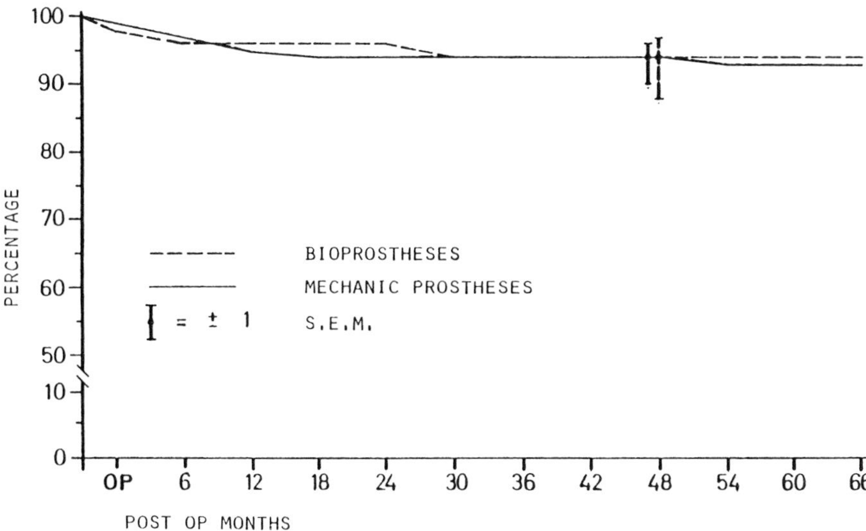

FIG. 4 Aortic valve replacement. Actuarial overall survival with bioprostheses and with mechanical prostheses.

No perivalvular leakage was noted after aortic valve replacement, whereas this complication was observed in 2 cases after mitral valve replacement, at the beginning of our experience, when no buttressed sutures were employed. The event-free rates among patients surviving after mitral valve replacement was, however, significantly higher (p = 0.04) in the bioprosthesis group than in the mechanical prosthesis group (Fig. 5). The percentage of complication-free survivors after aortic valve replacement was the same in the 2 groups of patients (p = 1.0) (Fig. 6). More than 95%

TABLE IX Mitral valve replacement: late complications

	Bioprostheses			Mechanical prostheses			
Variable	#	%	70% CL*	#	%	70% CL*	Significance
Thromboembolism	5	2.0†	0.7–4.0	5	5.2†	1.5–13.0	p = 0.07
Hemorrhage	2	0.8†	0.2–2.7	4	4.2†	0.7–11.0	p = 0.02
Endocarditis	1	0.4†	0.1–2.3	1	1.0†	0.2–9.0	p = 0.42
Valve failure	0	0.0†	0.0–1.9	0	0.0†	0.0–8.0	
Perivalvular leak	2	0.8†	0.1–2.5	1	1.0†	0.2–9.0	p = 1.0
Actuarial 5 year complication-free survival		87.0	81.0–90.0		69.0	53.0–78.0	p = 0.04

* CL: confidence limit.

† Linearized value (% per patient year).

TABLE X Aortic valve replacement: late complications

Variable	Bioprostheses			Mechanical prostheses			Significance
	#	%	70% CL*	#	%	70% CL*	
Thromboembolism	0	0.0†	0.0–5.1	3	0.9†	0.2–3.0	p = 0.32
Hemorrhage	1	1.3†	0.3–6.4	9	3.0†	1.4–5.5	p = 0.39
Endocarditis	3	4.0†	1.4–8.9	1	0.3†	0.1–2.5	p = 0.001
Valve failure	0	0.0†	0.0–5.1	0	0.0†	0.0–2.2	
Perivalvular leak	0	0.0†	0.0–5.1	0	0.0†	0.0–2.2	
Actuarial 5 year complication-free survival		90.0	83.0–94.0		82.0	77.0–85.5	p = 1.0

*CL: confidence limit.
† Linearized value (% per patient year).

of patients of each group improved their functional status of at least 2 classes (Figs. 1 and 2).

Neither long-term anticoagulation nor sinus rhythm are able to prevent thromboembolic complications (Tables XI and XII). Moreover, patients without anticoagulant therapy and/or with chronic atrial fibrillation have no significantly higher thromboembolism rates than others. This statement is valid for both bio- and mechanical prostheses. This means that if the common factor, such as no anticoagulation or atrial fibrillation, is excluded, the

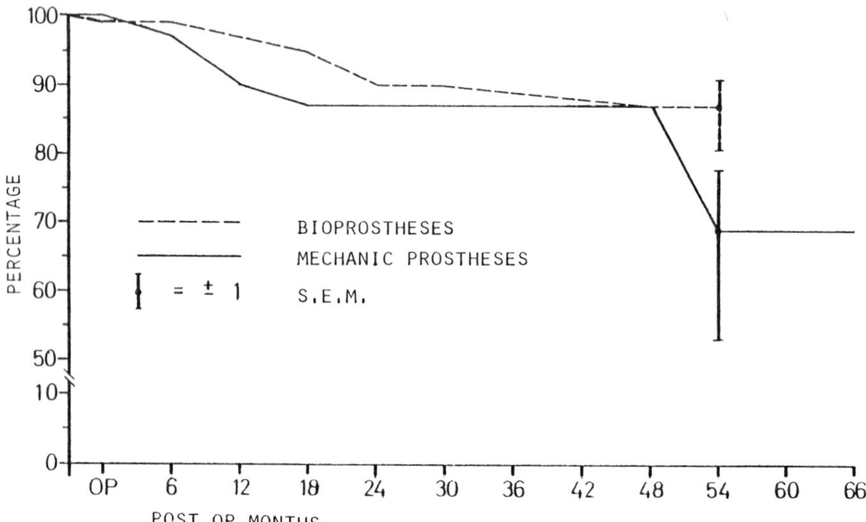

FIG. 5 Mitral valve replacement. Actuarial cumulative complication-free survival with bioprostheses and with mechanical prostheses.

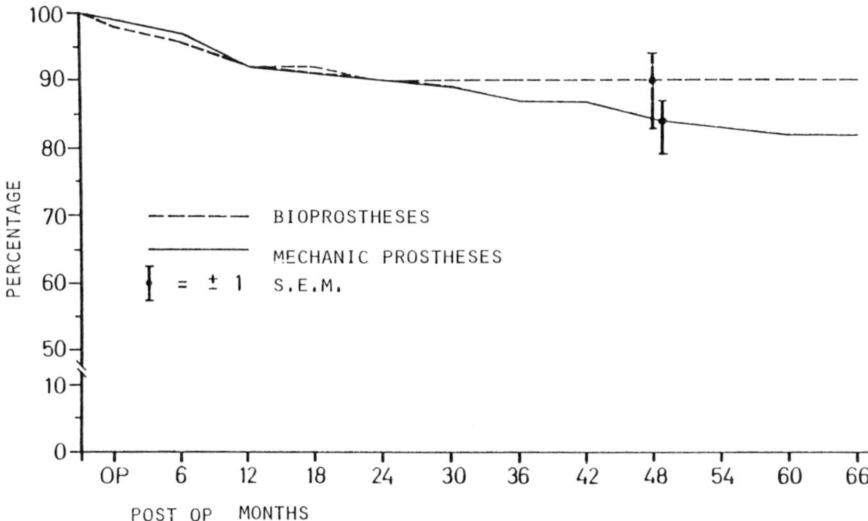

FIG. 6 Aortic valve replacement. Actuarial cumulative complication-free survival with bioprostheses and with mechanical prostheses.

prosthesis remains the main risk factor and its intrinsic characteristics are determinant for the difference of thromboembolic complication incidence.

Comment

The 5 year mortality for significant heart valve disease ranges between 25 and 75%,[14,15] depending upon the type of the vitium and upon the residual function of the myocardium. Many authors[16,17] have demonstrated a significant improvement of myocardial function after valve replacement. Yet the 2 categories of available valve substitutes have still some unresolved problems, relating mainly to late complications.

Mechanical valves include the great advantage of durability, but at the same time the great disadvantage that patients must be anticoagulated adequately and indefinitely. But even under these optimal conditions, the risk of thromboembolic complications is not excluded and hemorrhagic complications are frequent.

Other aspects are hemolysis with consequent anemia and valve noise. For these reasons many people tried to find an alternative. Since 1968, when Carpentier et al[18] implanted clinically the first glutaraldehyde-fixed porcine xenograft, the interest for "bioprosthesis" has grown tremendously. In the meantime different models became commercially available. The initial experience with this new type of valve substitute showed promising middle-

TABLE XI Mitral valve replacement with bioprosthesis: relation between risk factors and thromboembolic complications

Variable	Patients #	Patients %	Thrombo-embolism #	Thrombo-embolism %	70% confidence limit	Significance
Anticoagulation	71	57	4	5.6	3–99	p = 0.21
No anticoagulation	54	43	1	1.9	0.4–6	
SR*	57	45	1	1.7	0.3–6	p = 0.16
AF*	68	55	4	5.9	3–10	
SR + anticoagulant	20	28	1	5.0	1–15	p = 1.0
AF + anticoagulant	51	72	3	6.0	2.7–11	
SR no anticoagulant	37	69	0		0–7	p = 0.09
AF, no anticoagulant	17	31	1	6.0	1.2–18	

* SR: sinus rhythm; AF: atrial fibrillation.

term results, mainly concerning the low thrombogenicity, the possible avoidance of anticoagulants, and the favorable hemodynamic characteristics. However, one aspect of the bioprostheses was negative: the durability. Many innovations have been introduced in the methods of preparation, fixation, shipping, and different types of stents in order to improve the durability of the valve. Nevertheless, when implanting a bioprosthesis, one must keep in mind the fact that the patient may require reoperation after 10 to, at most, 20 years. Today the need for reoperation does not represent a significant risk if in the meantime the myocardial function has improved.[19]

Early and late survival are not significantly different with bio- and mechanical prostheses, either in the aortic or mitral position. Our results agree with those reported in the literature.[1,3,5,20–25]

TABLE XII Mitral valve replacement with mechanical prosthesis: relation between risk factors and thromboembolic complications

Variable	Patients #	Patients %	Thrombo-embolism #	Thrombo-embolism %	70% confidence limit	Significance
Anticoagulation	26	86.5	4	15.4	8–26	p = 0.6
No anticoagulation	4	13.5	0		0–38	
SR*	9	30.0	1	11.0	2–32	p = 0.18
AF*	21	70.0	3	14.3	6–26	
SR + anticoagulant	8	30.0	2	25.0	9–49	p = 0.63
AF + anticoagulant	18	70.0	2	11.0	4–24	
SR, no anticoagulant	3	75.0	0			
AF, no anticoagulant	1	25.0	0			

* SR: sinus rhythm; AF: atrial fibrillation.

Thromboembolic complications occur more frequently with mechanical than with bioprostheses in the mitral as well as in the aortic position, even though there are more anticoagulated patients in the mechanical than in the bioprosthesis groups. We noted no significant difference between aortic patient groups. This may be due to the better dynamic characteristics to which the prosthetic valves are exposed in the aortic position. The high flow velocity and the favorable anatomic situation of the pre- and postprosthetic compartments prevent thrombus formation.

Thromboembolic complications after implantation of a bioprosthesis occur mainly during the first 4 months postoperatively; afterward, the frequency decreases rapidly. During this early phase the Dacron sewing ring is not yet completely endothelialized and a fibrin apposition is possible. For this reason anticoagulation seems to be essential during this period. Thereafter neither anticoagulation nor sinus rhythm seems to influence the occurrence of this complication.

Hemorrhagic complications are generally related to the anticoagulant therapy. Bleeding rate reported in the literature[26–33] averages 1.5% per patient year with bioprosthesis and 3.5% per patient year with mechanical prostheses.

Prosthetic endocarditis is a serious problem for it is responsible for an average mortality of 57%.[34] In the present series, 2 cases of prosthetic endocarditis have been encountered in the mitral position, 1 each in a bio- and a mechanical prosthesis. Both valves were replaced and the infection could be eliminated. Moreover, we had 4 cases of prosthetic endocarditis in the aortic position, 3 with the bioprostheses and 1 with the mechanical prosthesis. Two patients with bioprostheses died during conservative management and 1 survived. The patient with mechanical prosthesis could be treated conservatively. This means that if a sepsis occurs on a bioprosthesis, a short medical management should be tried. If this fails, the bioprosthesis should be replaced immediately since it can be destroyed, resulting in irreversible heart failure. In our series of patients we noted a higher incidence of endocarditis on bioprostheses than on mechanical prostheses among aortic patients. Generally, however, there is no significant difference, as demonstrated by Rossiter et al.[34] Among 1,347 patients with mechanical prostheses and 837 with bioprostheses, he noted endocarditis occurrence of 2.5 and 1.9%, respectively. The difference was not statistically significant. The aortic prostheses were, however, 2.5 times more involved than the mitral prostheses.

The durability of mechanical prostheses is excellent. Bioprostheses, however, have a higher failure rate within 10 years after implantation[5] and perhaps 100% after 15–20 years. Factors influencing the durability are primarily the patient's age[35] and conditioning methods. It has been demonstrated that durability is reduced in young patients and especially in children.[35] Fixation methods, employing relatively high pressure during glutaraldehyde preservation, destroys the architecture of the collagen fibers of the valve.[36] Some laboratories are now employing low-fixation pressures of less than 4 mmHg. In our series, there were no bioprosthetic valve failures and, moreover, the event-free probability considering all complications was higher with bioprosthetic than mechanical valves.

Conclusions

Bioprostheses offer the advantage of a lower morbidity than mechanical prostheses. The survival rate of the patient is the same for both types of valve substitutes. For the patient this means a superior quality of life, without being limited in the choice of profession, in sports activity, in bearing children. Moreover, the patient is not conditioned to live as a chronic sick person, obligated to consult his physician continuously for anticoagulant treatment. Bioprostheses offer also advantages to older people, in whom a cerebral insult is always possible and anticoagulation could be deleterious. The only limitations for bioprostheses are represented by anticoagulation during the first 3–6 months after implantation and a hypothetically higher susceptibility to endocarditis. If endocarditis occurs, the valve should be replaced without hesitation if one would expect a complete recovery without a high risk.

The durability of the bioprosthesis is another limiting factor that is, however, overwhelmed by the advantages. The risk of reoperation is low if in the meantime the cardiac conditions have improved.

References

1. Carpentier A, Deloche A, Relland J, Fabiani JN, Forman J, Camillieri JP, Soyer R, Dubost C: Six year follow-up of glutaraldehyde preserved heterografts. J Thorac Cardiovasc Surg 68:771, 1974.
2. Hannah A, Reis RL: Current status of porcine heterograft prostheses. A 5 year appraisal. Circulation, 54 (Suppl III):27, 1976.
3. Angell WW: A nine year experience with the Angell-Shiley xenografts and a comparative literature review of the porcine bioprosthesis versus mechanical prosthesis. In: Bioprosthetic Cardiac Valves (F Sebening, WP Klövekorn, H Meisner, F Struck, Eds). Munich, Deutsches Herzzentrum 1979, p 81.
4. Carpentier A: From xenograft to valvular xenobioprosthesis. In: Bioprosthetic Cardiac Valves (F Sebening, WP Klövekorn, H Meisner, F Struck, Eds). Munich, Deutsches Herzzentrum, 1979, p 1.
5. Oyer PE, Stinson EB, Rossiter SJ, Miller DC, Reitz BA, Shumway NE: Extended experience with Hancock xenograft bioprosthesis. In: Bioprosthetic Cardiac Valves, (F Sebening, WP Klövekorn, H Meisner, F Struck, Eds). Munich, Deutsches Herzzentrum, 1979, p 47.
6. Struck E, Meisner H, Schmidt-Habelmann P, Sebening F: Cardiac valve replacement with Hancock and Carpentier-Edwards bioprostheses. In: Bio-

prosthetic Cardiac Valves, (F Sebening, WP Klövekorn, H Meisner, F Struck, Eds). Munich, Deutsches Herzzentrum 1979, p 61.

7. Kirsch U, Rodewald G, Kalmar P: Induced ischemic arrest. Clinical Experience with Cardioplegia in open heart surgery. J Thorac Cardiovasc Surg 63:121, 1972.
8. Clopper CJ, Pearson ES: The use of confidence or fiducial limits illustrated in the case of the binomial. Biometrika 26:404, 1934.
9. Graf H, Henning W, Stange H, Eds: Formeleund Tabellen der mathematischen Statistik. Berlin, Springer Verlag, 1966.
10. Mainland D, Ed: Elementary Medical Statistics. Philadelphia, W. B. Saunders, 1963.
11. Kaplan EL, Meier P: Non-parametric estimation from incomplete observation. J Am Stat Assoc 53:457, 1958.
12. Grunkemeier GL, Lambert LE, Bonchek LI, Starr A: An improved statistical method for assessing the results of operation. Ann Thorac Surg 20:289, 1975.
13. Anderson RP, Bonchek LI, Grunkemeier GL: The analysis and presentation of surgical results by actuarial methods. J Surg Res 16:224, 1974.
14. Olesen KH: The natural history of 271 patients with mitral stenosis under medical treatment. Br Heart J 24:349, 1962.
15. Rapaport E: Natural history of aortic and mitral valve disease. Am J Cardiol 35:221, 1975.
16. Krayenbuehl HP, Turina M, Hess AM, Rothlin M, Senning Å.: Pre and post-operative left ventricular contractile function in patients with aortic valve disease. Br Heart J 41:204, 1979.
17. Schwarz F, Flameng W, Schaper J, Hehrlein F: Correlation between myocardial structure and diastolic properties of the heart in chronic aortic valve disease: Effect of corrective surgery. Am J Cardiol 42:895, 1978.
18. Carpentier A, Lemaigre G, Robert L, Carpentier S, Dubost C: Biological factors affecting long-term results of heterograft valves. J Thorac Cardiovasc Surg 58:467, 1969.
19. Wideman FE, Blackstone EH, Kirklin JW, Karp RB, Kouchoukos NT, Pacifico AD: Hospital mortality of re-replacement of the aortic valve: Incremental risk factors. J Thorac Cardiovasc Surg 82:692, 1981.
20. Cevese PG, Gallucci V, Morea M, Dalla Volta S, Fasoli G, Casarotto D: Heart valve replacement with the Hancock bioprosthesis: Analysis of long term results. Circulation 56 (Suppl 2):111, 1977.
21. Davilla JC, Magilligan DJ, Lewis JW: Is the Hancock porcine valve the best cardiac valve substitute today? Ann Thorac Surg 26:303, 1978.
22. Cohn LH, Mee RB, Koster JK, Collins JJ: Long-term follow-up of the Hancock xenograft heart valve: A six year review. Presented at the 51st Scientific Session of the American Heart Association, Dallas, Texas, November 15th, 1978.
23. Buch WS, Pipkin RD, Hancock WD, Fogarty TJ: Mitral valve replacement with the Hancock stabilized glutaraldehyde valve: Clinical and laboratory evolution. Arch Surg 110:1408, 1975.
24. McIntosh CL, Michaelis LL, Morrow AG, Itscoitz SB, Redwood DR, Epstein SE: Atrioventricular valve replacement with the Hancock porcine xenograft: A five year clinical experience. Surgery 78:768, 1975.
25. Rivera R, Infantes C, Zuardo JA: Resultados clinicos en las substituciones valvulares pro bioprotesis de Angell-Shiley. Presented at the VI Jornadas Internacionales de Actualizacion Cardiovacular, Madrid, Spain, December 4th, 1978.
26. Lepley D, Flemma RJ, Mullen DC, Singh H, Chakravarty S: Late evaluation of

patients undergoing valve replacement with the Björk-Shiley prosthesis. Ann Thorac Surg 24:131, 1977.
27. Björk VO, Book K, Cernigliaro C: The Björk-Shiley tilting disc valve in isolated mitral lesions. Scand J Thorac Cardiovasc Surg 7:131, 1973.
28. Oyer PE, Stinson EB, Griepp RB, Shumway NE: Valve replacement with the Starr-Edwards and Hancock prostheses: Comparative analysis of late morbidity and mortality. Ann Surg 186:301, 1977.
29. McManus Q, Grunkemeier GL, Lambert LE, and Starr A: Non cloth-covered caged-ball prosthesis: The second decade. J Thorac Cardiovasc Surg 76:788, 1978.
30. Isom WO, Spencer FC, Glassman E, Tieko P, Boyd AD, Cunningham JN: Long-term results in 1375 patients undergoing valve replacement with the Starr-Edwards cloth covered ball prosthesis. Ann Surg 186:310, 1977.
31. Pipkin RD, Buch WS, Fogarty TJ: Evaluation of aortic valve replacement without long-term anticoagulation. J Thorac Cardiovasc Surg 71:179, 1976.
32. Housmann LB, Pitt WA, Mazur JH, Litchford B, Gross SA: Mechanic failure (leaflet disruption) of a porcine aortic heterograft. J Thorac Cardiovasc Surg 76:212, 1978.
33. Hetzer RH, Hill JD, Kerth WJ, Ansbro J, Adappa MG, Rodvien R, Kamm B, Gerbode F: Thromboembolic complications after mitral valve replacement with the Hancock xenograft. J Thorac Cardiovasc Surg 75:651, 1978.
34. Rossiter SJ, Stinson EB, Oyer PE, et al: Prosthetic valve endocarditis. Comparison of heterograft tissue valve and mechanical valves. J Thorac Cardiovasc Surg 76:795, 1978.
35. Magilligan DJ Jr, Lewis JW Jr, Jara FM, et al: Spontaneous degeneration of porcine bioprosthetic valves. Ann Thorac Surg 30:259, 1980.
36. Broom ND, Thomson FJ: Influence of fixation conditions on the performance of the glutaraldehyde-treated porcine aortic valves: Toward a more scientific basis. Thorax 34:166, 1979.

15

Mitral Bioprostheses in 202 Patients with Chronic Atrial Fibrillation, Giant Left Atrium, and Atrial Thrombi: Long-Term Results with No Anticoagulation

N. Spampinato, P. Stassano, C. Gagliardi, L. B. Tecchia, D. Pantaleo

In some situations long-term anticoagulation therapy is rarely effective, safe, or even feasible. Among the many positive factors related to bioprostheses, such as low thrombogenicity, favorable central flow, and the absence of noise, the lack of need for anticoagulation has represented the main reason for the elective use of bioprostheses.[1–4]

However, patients in chronic atrial fibrillation, with giant left atrium, left atrial thrombi, and previous embolic accidents, are often treated with lifelong anticoagulation, after bioprosthetic mitral valve replacement (MVR), for fear of increased thromboembolic accidents.[3,5,6]

Considering that the majority of patients undergoing operation for MVR in our country remain in atrial fibrillation postoperatively, the mandatory use of long-term anticoagulation in these patients would obviously nullify the main practical advantage of the bioprostheses.

We have reviewed our experience with bioprosthetic MVR in patients with chronic atrial fibrillation, giant left atrium, atrial thrombi, history of previous systemic embolization, not treated with long-term anticoagulation, in order to evaluate the incidence of postoperative thromboembolic events.

Patients and Methods

Between January 1976 and June 1981, 402 bioprosthetic MVR operations have been performed in our institution. Two hundred and two patients (50.2%) were in atrial fibrillation, 31 had a giant left atrium, and in 39

From the Department of Cardiac Surgery, 2nd Medical School, University of Naples, Naples, Italy.

large thrombi were found in the left atrium. The patients' ages ranged between 19 and 68 years (mean age, 44.2 years). Forty patients were in NYHA functional class II (19.8%), 109 in functional class III (53.9%), and 53 (26.2%) in functional class IV. Rheumatic disease was responsible for 90% of the valvular lesions.

There were 130 isolated MVR, 14 MVR associated with tricuspid anuloplasty, 58 mitral and aortic valve replacements, 1 triple valve replacement. The patients were operated on using a bubble oxygenator, hemodilution, moderate hypothermia (25–28°C), and cold cardioplegic cardiac arrest. Interrupted buttressed horizontal mattress sutures were used for implantation.

Fifty-one patients (from January 1976 to October 1978) did not receive any anticoagulation whatsoever, not even as a temporary measure. Since November 1978, the patients have been anticoagulated with warfarin starting on the third postoperative day and gradually discontinuing the therapy after the third postoperative month.

Results

Hospital mortality was 9.9% (20 patients). Follow-up ranged between 4 and 63 months and included 154 patients (mean, 23.3 months) for an equivalent of 503 patient years. Follow-up was obtained by direct interview with the patient or the attending physician or both.

The definition of thromboembolic event included all peripheral emboli and all new neurologic deficits, which were classified as major whenever they lasted for several days or produced a permanent impairment; or minor when symptoms were transient and resulted in complete recovery.

Ten patients died between 17 days and 15 months postoperatively. Two deaths occurred from system embolization and 1 from cerebral hemorrhage under anticoagulation therapy. The functional results were judged to be good in 127 patients (82.5%) (I and II functional class), modest in 25 (16.2%) (III functional class), and bad in 2 (1.3%) (IV functional class).

There were 7 major embolic accidents, including the 2 with fatal outcome (2.1% per patient years), 5 in the group with no anticoagulation—all within the first 6 months—and 2 in the group on the 3 month anticoagulation regimen after 7 and 11 months.

Transient ischemic attacks were suspected in 8 patients (2.3% per patient year).

Comment

Analyzing our results after bioprosthetic MVR in patients with chronic atrial fibrillation without long-term anticoagulation, we have found an acceptable incidence of thromboembolism.

In the group of patients which did not receive any postoperative anticoagulation, not even as a temporary measure, thromboembolic accidents occurred during the first 6 months after implantation.[7] Temporary (3–6 months) anticoagulation reduces greatly the incidence of early embolization. After 1 year, it is very rare to record systemic emboli even in the patient with chronic atrial fibrillation.[6]

Furthermore, an incidence of 0.7–1.2% per patient year of anticoagulation-related hemorrhages has been reported in patients with mechanical or biologic valves.[1,8]

Therefore weighing the risk of a poorly managed anticoagulation therapy against the incidence of thromboembolic accidents, we believe that patients with bioprosthetic MVR who remain in chronic atrial fibrillation can be safely and advantageously managed with temporary (3 month) anticoagulation.

References

1. Oyer PE, Stinson EB, Reitz BA, Miller DC, Rossiter SJ, Shumway NE: Long-term evaluation of the porcine xenograft bioprosthesis. J Thorac Cardiovasc Surg 78:343, 1979.
2. Jamieson WRE, Janusz MT, Miyagishima RT, Munro AI, Tutassura H, Gerein AN, Burr LH, Allen P: Embolic complications of porcine heterograft cardiac valves. J Thorac Cardiovasc Surg 81:626, 1981.
3. Cevese PG, Gallucci V, Morea M, Dalla Volta S, Fasoli G, Casarotto D: Heart valve replacement with the Hancock bioprosthesis. Analysis of long-term results. Circulation 56(Suppl II):111, 1977.
4. Cohn LH, Sanders JH, Collins JJ: Actuarial comparison of Hancock porcine and prosthetic disk valves for isolated mitral valve replacement. Circulation 54(Suppl 3):60, 1976.
5. Becker RM, Sandor L, Tindel M, Frater RWM: Medium-term follow-up of the Ionescu-Shiley heterograft valve. Ann Thorac Surg 32:120, 1981.
6. Gallo JI, Ruiz B, Carrion MF, Gutierrez JA, Vega JL, Duran CMG: Heart valve replacement with the Hancock bioprosthesis: A 6-year review. Ann Thorac Surg 31:444, 1981.
7. Spampinato N, Gagliardi C, DeAmicis V, Stassano P, Covino E: Incidence of thromboembolism on bioprosthetic cardiac valves not treated with anticoagulants. In: Bioprosthetic Cardiac Valve (F Sebening et al, Eds). Munich, Deutsches Herzzentrum, 1979, p 121.
8. Borkon AM, McIntosh CL, Von Rueden TJ, Morrow AG: Mitral valve replacement with the Hancock bioprosthesis: Five-to ten-year follow-up. Ann Thorac Surg 32:127, 1981.

16

Thromboembolism and Anticoagulation after Isolated Mitral Valve Replacement with Porcine Heterografts

R. Hetzer, T. Topalidis, H. G. Borst

The most appealing aspect of biologic valves—if not the only one in the presently available types—is the lower thrombogenicity and the reduced need for anticoagulation. Whereas it has been fairly accepted that, due to an almost negligible thromboembolic risk, patients with a bioprosthesis in the aortic position do not need permanent anticoagulation, this has remained a controversial topic for the mitral valve group, particularly in those patients with chronic atrial fibrillation.[1,2]

In this study our patients with single mitral valve replacement using a porcine xenograft were followed with particular regard to thromboembolic events and anticoagulation complications, and probable risk factors were analyzed.

Patients and Methods

This study is based on 254 unselected patients receiving a porcine xenograft valve (Hancock) in the mitral position between 1977 and the end of 1981. Included are 14 patients with concomitant direct coronary revascularization (aortocoronary saphenous vein grafts) and 16 patients with repair of associated tricuspid incompetence.

There were 183 women and 71 men, ranging in age from 14–70 years, with a mean of 53.8 years.

Hospital mortality (30 days postoperative) was 9.8%, more than half of the fatal outcomes being due to cardiopulmonary failure following surgery for end stage mitral disease.

From the Division of Thoracic and Cardiovascular Surgery, Surgical Center, Hannover Medical School, Hannover, West Germany.

Of 229 patients who were discharged from the hospital, 223 (97.4%) were followed up to April 1982, the individual follow-up period ranging from 4–63 months, with a mean of 25 months (total follow-up 546 patient years). Follow-up information was obtained from hospital records and questionnaires sent to patients or their physicians or both. Questions were asked relative to the patient's physical and rehabilitation status, medication, prothrombin levels, and symptoms that might suggest thromboembolism or anticoagulation-related hemorrhage. Whereas only spontaneous hemorrhages were accepted as "anticoagulation-related," all new and otherwise unexplained ischemic symptoms, cerebral or peripheral, were considered "embolic."

There were 14 late deaths. Four were not related to cardiovascular disease, 2 were due to thromboembolism and to anticoagulant hemorrhage. Six patients died from chronic cardiac failure and 2 suffered sudden death. There were no autopsy resports available on these latter 8 patients. However, since they were all anticoagulated, it could not be decided whether embolism or hemorrhage played any role in their death. They were not included in either the embolism or the hemorrhage group.

Out of the total of 254 patients, 203 (79.9%) were in chronic atrial fibrillation (AF) or changing rhythm. Only 51 patients were in a stable normal sinus rhythm (NSR). Anticoagulation with coumarin preparations (Marcumar) was started in all as soon as oral intake was possible after surgery. Prothrombin level was monitored by the Quick test, aiming at 15–25% of normal.

In 47 of the long-term survivors (35 in AF, 12 in NSR) anticoagulation was discontinued 2–6 months after operation, and 182 patients (147 in AF, 35 in NSR) were kept permanently on anticoagulants. These decisions were made following both our recommendations and the cardiologists' or attending physicians' beliefs.

Results

Thromboembolism and Anticoagulation Hemorrhages

Ten patients suffered thromboembolism, severe in 7 instances, including 2 deaths (8 cerebral, 1 coronary, 1 peripheral), 3 were minor and transient (all cerebral). Sixty-three patients had hemorrhagic complications, 19 were severe requiring hospitalization (central nervous system, 5; visceral, 7; soft tissue, 7), 1 was fatal (intracranial), and 44 patients had repeated minor bleeding troubles. Within the permanent anticoagulation group, 45% of the patients said they were substantially limited in their activities by this medication.

Eight of the 10 emboli occurred within 3 months after the operation, 6 within the first postoperative month, 9 emboli occurred while the patient was under anticoagulation, 5 of these were seemingly well anticoagulated according to laboratory tests. Within the first 3 months, thromboembolic incidence was calculated to be 13.3/100 patient years; beyond that time it was as low as 0.4/100 patient years (Fig. 1).

Severe bleeding episodes were independent of the time after operation; in our anticoagulated patients it was 4.4/100 patient years (Fig. 1, Table I). In one-third of the patients prothrombin level records indicated major shifts to ineffectively high (>30%) and dangerously low (<10%) values.

"Atrial" risk factors for thromboembolism. Three findings were considered potential factors of increased thromboembolic risk: atrial fibrillation, a history of preoperative embolism, and thrombus in the left atrium at the time of surgery (Fig. 2, Table II).

All emboli occurred in patients with chronic AF; there was none in the stable NSR group. Patients with a history of emboli before operation and those with thrombi in the atrium suffered emboli at a higher rate. The probability of embolism was particularly high in patients with a combination of all these findings. Almost every fourth patient of this group suffered an embolism. Both patients with embolism later than 3 months after the operation had 2 and all 3 of these factors. In patients with AF alone the embolic incidence was relatively small, 2.4%.

Since most embolic events occurred within the first 3 postoperative months, a calculation of incidence of thromboembolism and hemorrhage was undertaken, differentiating between the whole observation time and the time beyond 3 months after operation (Table I). This shows a higher rate of hemorrhagic events in all patient groups under anticoagulation and the embolic rate in the nonanticoagulated group was even less than in the

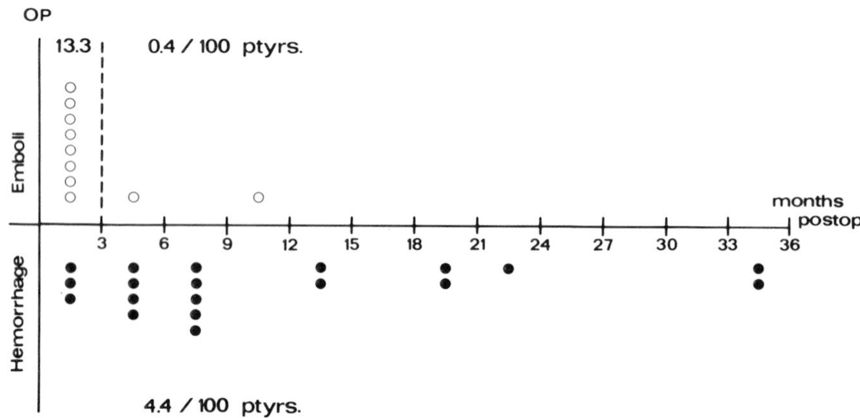

FIG. 1 Time and incidence of thromboembolism (above) and anticoagulation-related hemorrhage (below).

TABLE I Incidence of thromboembolism and severe anticoagulation hemorrhage

Group	Total postoperative period					Later than 3 months postoperatively			
	All pts	AC*	No AC*	NSR*	AF*	All pts.	AF	AF, no AC	AF + AC
Patients	254	254	47	51	203	220	182	35	147
Years	546	431	115	112	434	473	345	84	279
Thromboembolism†	10	9	1	0	10	2	2	0	2
Per 100 patient years	1.8	2.1	0.9	0.0	2.3	0.4	0.6	0.0	0.7
95% CL*	0.8–3.4	0.9–3.9	0.0–5.0	0.0–3.3	1.0–4.3	0.1–1.4	0.1–2.4	0.0–4.3	0.1–2.4
Hemorrhage†	19	19	—	2	17	16	15	—	15
Per 100 patient years	3.5	4.4	—	1.8	3.9	3.4	4.3	—	5.4
95% CL	2.3–5.9	2.7–7.0	—	0.2–6.4	2.3–6.4	2.0–5.4	2.3–7.3	—	3.1–8.5

* AC: Anticoagulation; NSR: normal sinus rhythm; AF: atrial fibrillation; CL: confidence limit.
† Thrombolism -vs- hemorrhage 73 months postoperatively: $p < 0.05$.

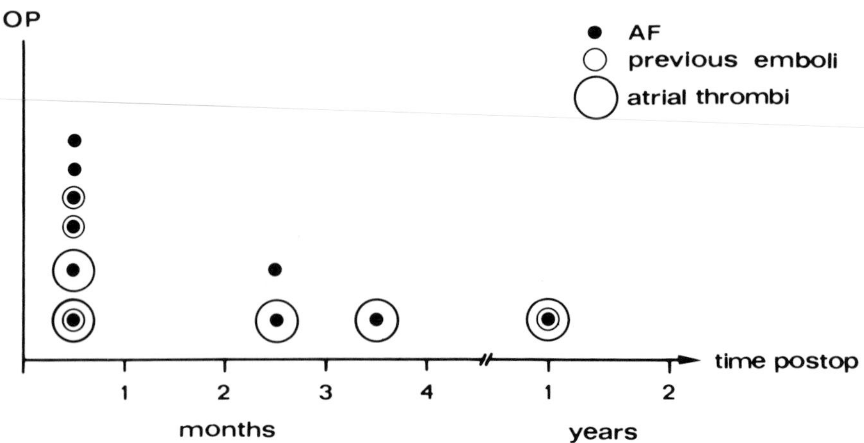

FIG. 2 Time of thromboembolism and "atrial" risk factors. All emboli occurred in patients with atrial fibrillation (AF), 4 also had a history of embolism and 5 had atrial thrombi at time of operation, 2 patients had all 3 factors.

anticoagulated patients. In fact there was only 1 embolism in a nonanticoagulated patient. This picture becomes even more striking in the time period after 3 postoperative months. Hemorrhagic events by far exceeded the embolic rate.

Even in the patient group with chronic AF, the hemorrhagic rate was more than 5 times higher than the embolic incidence (5.4 -vs- 0.7/100 patient years). Interestingly, in our series, patients in chronic AF and no anticoagulation did not suffer either emboli or bleeding, whereas in the chronic AF group and anticoagulation 2 emboli and 15 severe hemorrhages occurred, accounting for a total incidence of events of 6.1/100 patient years.

The probability of freedom from thromboembolism and anticoagulation hemorrhage was calculated by actuarial methods[3] (Figs. 3, 4). These curves show freedom from thromboembolism of 95.5% from 1 year on for all patients (Fig. 3). Freedom from hemorrhage becomes less at a continuous rate, at 3 years only 72% of the anticoagulated patients are free from embolism plus hemorrhage.

The differences in risk become even more evident when looking at the time after 3 months postoperatively, even in the debated AF group. Whereas thromboembolism was very low regardless of anticoagulation, in the same range as in patients following mitral reconstruction, the anticoagulated patients are continuously threatened by hemorrhage and this risk by far exceeds the embolic risk.

Whereas freedom from embolism was 98.3 and 100% with and without anticoagulation, respectively, at 24 months 12.8% of anticoagulated patients had suffered an episode of severe hemorrhage. Multiple episodes of

TABLE II Influence of "atrial" factors on thromboembolism

Factor	Factor present						Factor not present					
	# pts	Yr	TE*	%	/100 pt yr	95% CL*	# pts	Yr	TE	%	/100 pt yr	95% CL
AF	203	434	10	4.9	2.3	1.0–4.3	51	112	0	0	0	0.0–3.3
Preoperative TE	47	101	4	8.5	4.0	1.1–9.9	207	445	6	2.8	1.3	0.4–2.9
Clot in atrium	31	67	5	16.1	7.5	2.5–16.6	223	479	5	2.2	1.0	0.32–2.3
AF + TE + clot in atrium	9	16	2	22.2	12.5	1.6–38.4						
AF without TE and clot in atrium	127	281	3	2.4	1.1	0.2–2.9						

* TE: thromboembolism; CL: confidence limit.

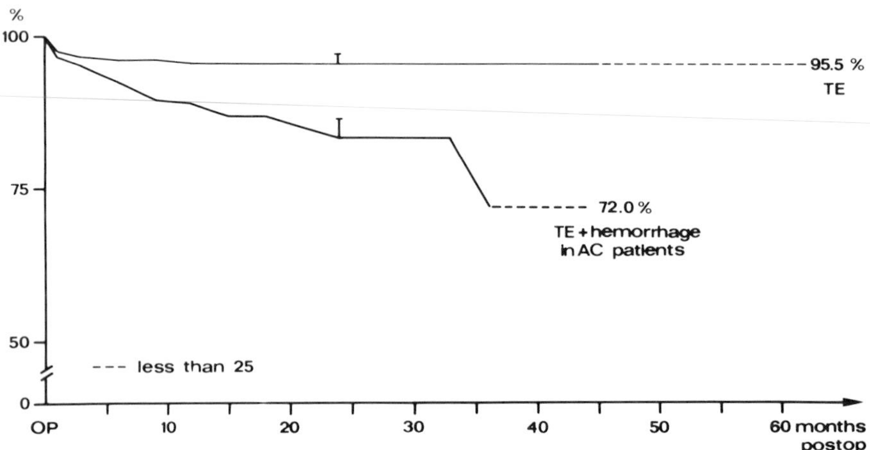

FIG. 3 Freedom from thromboembolism (TE) and anticoagulation (AC) hemorrhage, actuarial method calculation.

minor bleeding and the limitations of physical activity further reduce the quality of life in these patients.

Comments

Although commercially available bioprostheses have at least partly achieved the goal of biologic valve substitutes, i.e., nonthrombogenicity, thromboembolism still occurs at a certain rate and in some patient groups. This has led to considerable confusion and controversial opinions and, often unsupported, statements as to which patients need to be anticoagulated and for how long. The ongoing discussion, which is mostly due to the complete lack of large, prospective comparative studies, becomes apparent from the reviews of Cohn,[1] Angell,[4] and Borst[5] and, in particular, in the panel discussion closing the Symposium on Bioprosthetic Cardiac Valves in Munich, 1979.[2]

It has been generally accepted that patients with biologic prostheses in the aortic position and in the mitral position in patients with NSR have a very low thromboembolic risk in the long-term and therefore do not require permanent anticoagulation.[1–4,6,7] Some authors have denied this need for patients in AF as well, whereas others advocate permanent anticoagulation for this group.[1,2,5,8–10] Since in the Central Europe mitral disease clientele the proportion of patients who come to surgery with AF is large, in our series four-fifths of the total group, the question of anticoagulant recommendation for this subset is highly important. Furthermore, it has been

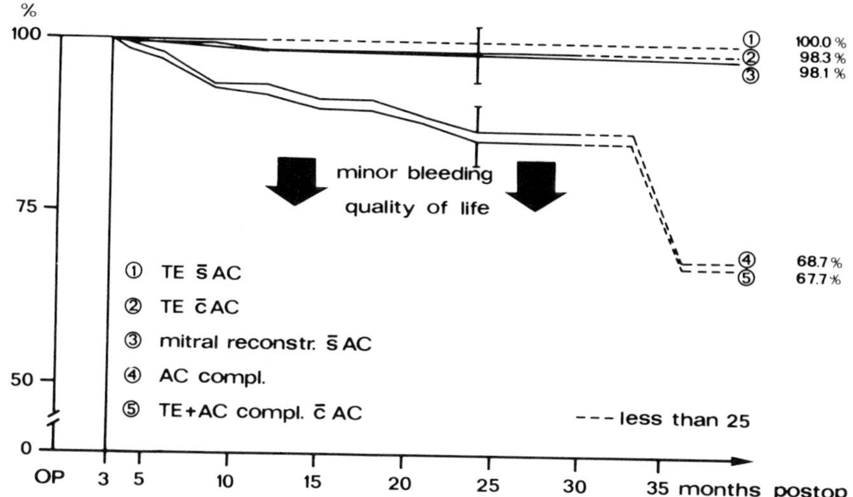

FIG. 4 Freedom from thromboembolism (TE) and anticoagulation (AC) hemorrhage (complications) in patients with chronic atrial fibrillation later than 3 months postoperatively, actuarial method calculation (overall thromboembolism curve of 124 patients after mitral reconstruction is included for comparison—curve 3). (At 24 months 1: 100%; 2: 98.3%; 3: 98.1%; 4: 87.2%; 5: 85.7%).

questioned whether the use of biologic valves is justified in these patients if they are to be permanently anticoagulated anyway.

Our study is a retrospective analysis of thromboembolism and anticoagulant-related hemorrhages following a broad variety of anticoagulant regimens, partly due to inconsistent recommendations from us and partly following the individual opinion of the attending physicians. As a consequence, due to different numbers and somewhat different severity of disease in the various groups, this study does not claim statistical reliability as to the comparison of alternative treatment.

The definition of "thromboembolism" is somewhat controversial in a retrospective analysis. All symptoms suggesting new and otherwise unexplained ischemia were considered "embolic." Thus, thromboembolism may be overrated in comparison to anticoagulant hemorrhages where only severe and spontaneous bleeding was entered into the calculation.

Two patients with late "sudden death" that could have been embolic complications were not included, since both patients were also anticoagulated and the chances of embolism, hemorrhage, and arrhythmia appear to be equivalent. Even if these patients are considered embolic, this would not alter the final conclusions.

Six of the 10 emboli occurred during the first postoperative month, 8 within the first 3 postoperative months. The remaining 2 emboli occurred at 4 and 12 months after operation. The relatively high incidence of thromboembolism early after operation and the decrease of this rate to very low values in the long range have been observed by several authors.[2,4,8,11–13]

The general opinion has been that the cloth-covered sewing ring and the implantation sutures are quite thrombogenic until they are covered by a "nonintima," which supposedly takes several weeks. The biologic leaflet surface seems to be nonthrombogenic unless altered by degenerative or endocarditic processes. In our total experience with bioprostheses, valve thrombi were observed in 6 valves with prosthetic valve endocarditis and in 2 valves with early degeneration.

With the large difference of thromboembolic rate early and late in mind, calculation of embolic incidence in linearized manner (i.e., per 100 patient years) over the total postoperative period appears to yield somewhat meaningless data. It is quite interesting to see that the reported rates of thromboembolism for porcine mitral bioprostheses, ranging from 1.8–5.4/100 patient years, on the whole become smaller the longer the follow-up.[1,4,5]

Probability of freedom from thromboembolism as calculated by actuarial methods ranges from 83–95% at 3–5 years after mitral valve replacement with porcine xenografts;[1,4] in our series this was 95.5%. Beyond 3 months after operation, this curve is almost identical to those calculated for the total postoperative time following biologic aortic valve replacement[1,4] and in a series of 124 patients after mitral reconstruction without anticoagulation followed at our department (Fig. 4).

The contribution of a significantly distended left atrium and its sequelae—i.e., AF, stagnant flow, and turbulences—to thromboembolism has been reported for the natural diseased mitral valve,[7] for mechanical valves,[14] and for bioprostheses.[1,2,5,11,13] The size of the left atrium relative to the cardiac output would certainly be a good parameter to compare with thromboembolic incidence. However, at present we do not know of any reliable method to quantify the left atrium. Therefore the factor "large left atrium" as used by us in an earlier study[11] and by others[13] was not evaluated in this series, since it appears to be an incomparable indicator, open to individual judgment and bias.

A history of thromboembolism before operation and the finding of thrombi in the atrium at the time of operation at least indicate a higher propensity to build up atrial thrombi, be this related to a large atrium or not.

In any case, in our series all emboli occurred in patients with chronic AF, in 8.5% of patients who also had a history of emboli, in 16.1% of patients who had atrial thrombi, and in almost one-quarter of the patients who had all 3 findings. By contrast, only 2.2% of patients with AF alone suffered an embolus. These data are very similar to the results of the Pacific Medical Center Study in 1977.[11] Interestingly, both patients who suffered an embolus later than 3 months postoperatively had 2 and 3 of the factors.

Aside from the risk that comes from a distended, fibrillating left atrium there seem to be individual coagulation patterns that impose a higher risk of thrombus formation early[16] and late[17] after operation. Pursuing such studies may well help to identify patients at a higher thromboembolic risk in the future.

In this series we are faced with a disastrously high incidence of severe anticoagulant-related bleeding complications. This does not take into account the many minor bleeding troubles, the limitation of activities, and the quality of life that many of the anticoagulated patients have to accept.

The incidence of hemorrhages is higher than the ones reported in most other valve patient follow-up studies,[4,8,10–12] which could imply a low quality of anticoagulant surveillance in our area.[18] However, such hemorrhages even occur under in-hospital day by day coagulation testing and under seemingly well-controlled prothrombin levels. To make the picture even worse, 9 of 10 emboli occurred while the patients were under anticoagulation.

When looking at the actuarial curves of freedom from thromboembolism and hemorrhage in anticoagulated and nonanticoagulated patients in the crucial group with AF later than 3 months after operation, there was no event whatsoever in the nonanticoagulated group and a frighteningly high rate of 6.1/100 patient years in the anticoagulated patients with a relationship of embolism to hemorrhage of 1:7.5.

Even if there were a certain number of emboli in the nonanticoagulated patients, as one should expect in a large series, this would have to be estimated at such a high range to outnumber the bleeding complications that therefore the number would appear unrealistic, according to our data.

In summary we would conclude from this review that the risk of thromboembolism after mitral valve replacement with porcine xenograft is highest in the immediate postoperative period and decreases within the following months. Later than 3 months after operation, it is quite small and is limited to patients with a higher tendency to build up thrombi in the atrium. Besides these "atrial factors," a very low cardiac output or leaflet destruction either by degeneration or prosthetic valve endocarditis may be causes of thrombus formation on the valve.[11,19]

On the other hand, some first attempts to characterize patients with a higher embolic risk by detailed coagulation studies have pointed out promising new aspects. The fact that the majority of emboli in our series occurred under anticoagulation, regardless of whether this was seemingly well-controlled or not, would support Duran's assumption that some patients may have a tendency toward thrombi on the valve unaffected by conventional anticoagulation.[2]

Chronic anticoagulation with coumarin preparations appears to be a potentially dangerous treatment with a continuously high incidence of severe complications that significantly exceeds the embolic rate in the vast majority of patients, even in those with AF. This medication does not exclude embolism, is difficult to control under outpatient conditions, and substantially limits the quality of life, and, in our opinion, it actually deprives the patient of the single most important advantage of having a biologic valve, i.e., not to need anticoagulation.

Besides closure of the left auricle in all cases with mitral valve replacement, at present and until we know some more about the individual risk factors of thromboembolism, we would start heparin ("low dose," 15,000 U/day for 8–10 days) as soon as there is no surgical bleeding. We would recommend coumarin preparations for 3 months after operation, which should be discontinued by then as a rule, including those patients with AF. Longer anticoagulant treatment appears to be justified only in patients with accumulation of several "atrial" risk factors.

References

1. Cohn LH: Bioprosthetic cardiac valves—anticoagulation or not? In: Bioprosthetic Cardiac Valves (F Sebening, WP Klövekorn, H Meisner, E Struck, Eds). Munich, Deutsches Herzzentrum, 1979, p 107.
2. Panel discussion on thromboembolism and anticoagulant therapy. In: Bioprosthetic Cardiac Valves (F Sebening, WP Klövekorn, H Meisner, E Struck, Eds). Munich, Deutsches Herzzentrum, 1979, p 384.
3. Grunkemeier GL, Starr A: Actuarial analysis of surgical results: Rationale and method. Ann Thorac Surg 24:404, 1977.
4. Angell WW: A nine year experience with the Angell-Shiley xenograft and a comparative literature review of the porcine bioprosthesis versus the mechanical prosthesis, In: Bioprosthetic Cardiac Valves (F Sebening, WP Klövekorn, H Meisner, Struck E, Eds). Munich, Deutsches Herzzentrum, 1979, p 81.
5. Borst HG, Papagiannakis N, Beddermann C, Oelert H: Cardiac valve replacement. Problems solved and unsolved. Thorac Cardiovasc Surg 27:76, 1979.
6. Cohn LH, Lamberti JJ, Castaneda AR, Collins JJ Jr: Cardiac valve replacement with the stabilized glutaraldehyde porcine aortic valve: Indications, operative results and followup. Chest 68:162, 1975.
7. Szekely P: Systemic embolism and anticoagulant prophylaxis in rheumatic heart disease. Br Med J 1:1209, 1964.
8. Cevese PG, Gallucci V, Morea M, Dalla Volta S, Fasoli G, Casarotto D: Heart valve replacement with the Hancock bioprosthesis. Analysis of long-term results. Circulation 56 (Suppl II):111, 1977.
9. Edminston WA, Harrison EC, Duick GF, Pamassus W, Lau FYK: Thromboembolism in mitral porcine valve recipients. Am J Cardiol 41:508, 1978.
10. Jamieson WRE, Janusz MT, Miyagishima RT, Munro AL, Tutassura H, Gerein AN, Burr LH, Allen P: Embolic complications of porcine heterograft cardiac valves. J Thorac Cardiovasc Surg 81:626, 1981.
11. Hetzer R, Hill JD, Kerth WJ, Ansbro J, Adappa MG, Rodvien R, Kamm B, Gerbode F: Thromboembolic complications after mitral valve replacement with Hancock xenograft. J Thorac Cardiovasc Surg 75:651, 1978.
12. Oyer PE, Stinson EB, Reitz BA, Miller DC, Rossiter S, Shumway NE: Long-term evaluation of porcine xenograft bioprosthesis. J Thorac Cardiovasc Surg 78:343, 1979.

13. Roux JJ, Jouven JC, Talmondi T, Antypas G, Rapuzzi A, Malmejac C, Houel J: Early thromboembolic complications of porcine xenografts. In: Bioprosthetic Cardiac Valves (F Sebening, WP Klövekorn, H Meisner, E Struck, Eds). Munich, Deutsches Herzzentrum, 1979, p 125.
14. Matloff JM: Discussion to Hetzer et al.[10]: J Thorac Cardiovasc Surg 75:1978.
15. Cohn LH, Sanders JH, Collins JJ Jr: Actuarial comparison of Hancock porcine and prosthetic disc valves for isolated mitral valve replacement. Circulation 54 (Suppl III):56, 1976.
16. Plauth G, Barthels M, Oelert H, Poliwoda H: Veranderungen des Gerinnungspotentials nach implantation biologischer Klappen in aorten und mitral Position. In: Hamolyse bei Herzfehlern und Angiopathien (R Schreiber, Ed). Munich, Muller and Steinicke, 1981, pp 227–231.
17. Vollmer I, Welsch U, Wenzel E, Stapenhorst K: Anticoagulatory therapy after valve replacement with xenografts, a hemostasiological study. Thorac Cardiovasc Surg 28:12, 1980.
18. Struck E, Meisner H, Schmidt-Habelmann P, Sebening F: Cardiac valve replacement with Hancock and Carpentier-Edwards bioprostheses. In: Bioprosthetic Cardiac Valves (F Sebening, WP Klövekorn, H Meisner, E Struck, Eds). Munich, Deutsches Herzzentrum, 1979, p 61.
19. Hetzer R, Hill JD, Kerth WJ, Wilson AJ, Gerbode F: Thrombosis and degeneration of Hancock valves: Clinical and pathological findings. Ann Thorac Surg 26:317, 1978.

17

Preoperative Determinants of Return to Sinus Rhythm after Valve Replacement

A. BETRIU, B. R. CHAITMAN, A. ALMAZAN, P. GUITERAS VAL, C. PELLETIER

It is well known that atrial fibrillation adversely affects cardiac output and increases the risk of thromboembolism. Although restoration of sinus rhythm appears to be the best protection against the hazard of atrial fibrillation, a normal sinus mechanism after cardioversion is maintained in less than one-half of patients.[1–4] This figure may be higher in patients undergoing prosthetic valve replacement if a near normal hemodynamic state can be achieved after surgery.[5] To date, few data are available on the success of valve replacement to restore and maintain sinus rhythm. Characterization of factors determining such success is relevant, since preoperative atrial fibrillation is an important consideration in deciding the choice of valve device. Therefore the present study was undertaken to identify baseline preoperative variables influencing the return to sinus rhythm after valve replacement.

Methods

Patient Population

From June 1976 to December 1980, a consecutive series of 685 patients underwent bioprosthetic valve replacement at the Montreal Heart Institute. Thirty-day operative mortality was 9% (62 patients) and 34 patients died during the follow-up. Of the 589 survivors, 148 patients were in atrial fibrillation before surgery and had a minimum 6-month follow-up. There

---

From the Departments of Medicine and Cardiovascular Surgery, Montreal Heart Institute and the University of Montreal Medical School, Montreal, Quebec, Canada.

were 61 men and 87 women whose mean age was 55 (range, 23–78) years. The etiology of valvular disease was rheumatic in 141 patients, congenital in 6, and traumatic in the remaining patient. Associated coronary artery disease ≥50% was present in 25 patients.

Surgical Procedure

Operation was performed via a median sternotomy. Standard cardiopulmonary bypass and total body hypothermia (24°C) were used. Crystalloid cold cardioplegia and topical hypothermia were used for myocardial protection. All patients received a Carpentier-Edwards bioprosthesis.

Ninety-four patients received a mitral valve, 12 an aortic valve, and 42 had a multiple valve procedure (26 patients underwent mitral and aortic replacement, 13 had mitral valve replacement combined with tricuspid anuloplasty, and 3 patients had mitral and aortic valve replacement associated with tricuspid anuloplasty. Concomitant aortocoronary bypass graft surgery was performed in 13 patients; 10 had a single, 2 a double, and 1 patient had 3 bypass grafts.

Data Collection and Analysis

After hospital discharge, the patients were periodically seen at the cardiac valve clinic, the visits being scheduled at 2, 6, and 12 months following surgery and every 12 months thereafter. Mean follow-up was 18 months, ranging from 6–60 months. Sinus rhythm was restored and maintained throughout follow-up in 52 patients (group 1). The group 1 patients were all converted to sinus rhythm within 6 months after operation, 38 spontaneously and the remaining 14 patients following cardioversion. The remaining 96 patients (group 2) stayed in (76 patients) or reverted to atrial fibrillation after an initially successful cardioversion (20 patients).

Both groups were compared with regard to the following: age, sex distribution, length of follow-up, duration of atrial fibrillation prior to surgery, left atrial size, cardiothoracic ratio, left and right atrial pressures, left ventricular end diastolic pressure, location of replaced valve, stent diameter, prevalence of previous mitral commissurotomy, associated tricuspid anuloplasty, prevalence of coronary artery disease, and incidence rate of thromboembolism (Table I).

Duration of atrial fibrillation was assessed from previous electrocardiographic tracings and/or clinical records. The preoperative left atrial size was measured by M mode echocardiography as the maximal left atrial dimension in early diastole.

Data are expressed as mean ± standard deviation. Comparison between groups of continuous variables was made by the Student's *t* test (2 tailed) for unpaired data. Chi-square analysis was used for 2 × n comparisons. A

TABLE I Intergroup comparison of baseline variables

	Group 1*	Group 2†	x^2	*t*	p
Patient age (yr)	54 ± 12	55 ± 11		1.2	NS‡
Female/male ratio	1.8	1.2	1.0		NS
Extent of follow-up (mo)	15 ± 10	18 ± 12		1.6	NS
Duration of atrial fibrillation (<1 yr)	86%	5%	64.3		<0.001
Prior mitral commissurotomy	21%	43%	7.5		<0.001
Tricuspid anuloplasty	6%	14%	2.5		NS
Coronary artery disease	25%	12%	3.7		NS
Thromboembolism	0	5%	2.8		NS
Left atrial size (mm)	52 ± 10	60 ± 15		2.6	<0.025
Cardiothoracic index (%)	56 ± 7	61 ± 9		3.5	<0.001
Left ventricular end diastolic pressure (mmHg)	13 ± 7	14 ± 6		0.6	NS
Left atrial pressure (mmHg)	22 ± 7	24 ± 7		1.1	<NS
Right atrial pressure (mmHg)	7 ± 3	9 ± 4		2.5	<0.5
Diameter of stent					
Mitral	30.4 ± 1.7	30.0 ± 1.3		0.7	NS
Aortic	28.0 ± 1.4	23.6 ± 3.0		1.8	NS

* Group 1: sinus rhythm after surgery.
† Group 2: atrial fibrillation after surgery.
‡ NS: not significant.

probability (p) value of 0.05 or less was considered statistically significant. The predictive value of preoperative variables in determining return to sinus rhythm was determined.

Results

Clinical Variables

The mean age of both groups (54 ± 12 years in group 1 and 55 ± 11 in group 2), the sex distribution (female to male ratio: 1.8 in group 1 and 1.2 in group 2), and the length of follow-up (15 ± 10 in group 1 and 18 ± 12 months in group 2) were similar, and all were not significant.

The duration of atrial fibrillation prior to surgery could be determined in 96 patients, 35 in group 1 and 61 in group 2. Atrial fibrillation of less than 1 year was found in 30 group 1 patients (86%) and only 3 group 2 patients (5%) ($p < 0.001$).

No differences between the 2 groups were found with regard to both the location of the replaced valve and the diameter of stent, assessed in patients who had a single valve replacement. Previous mitral commissurotomy was found to be more prevalent among group 2 patients (43 -vs- 21%; $p < 0.001$). Associated tricuspid anuloplasty was carried out in 3 group 1 patients (6%) and in 14 group 2 patients (14%), a nonsignificant difference. The incidence of coronary artery disease was similar in both groups (6 group 1 patients and 9 group 2 patients). There were 5 thromboembolic episodes, all confined to group 2 patients (atrial fibrillation).

Laboratory Variables

Ninety-six patients had a preoperative echocardiogram (36 group 1 and 60 group 2 patients). The mean left atrial diameter of group 1 patients was significantly lower than group 2 patients (52 ± 10 -vs- 60 ± 15; $p < 0.025$). The preoperative chest x ray cardiothoracic ratio was lower in group 1 patients (0.56 ± 0.07 -vs- 0.61 ± 0.09; $p < 0.001$).

The left ventricular end diastolic pressure and the mean left atrial pressure were similar in both groups (13 ± 7 -vs- 14 ± 6 mmHg and 22 ± 7 -vs- 24 ± 7 mmHg, respectively; nonsignificant), whereas right atrial pressure was higher in group 2 patients (9 ± 4 -vs- 7 ± 3 mmHg; $p < 0.025$).

The predictive value of the preoperative variables in determining return to sinus rhythm are summarized in Table II. The best predictor of return to sinus rhythm was the duration of atrial fibrillation before surgery. The probability of return to sinus rhythm was 91% for patients presenting with atrial fibrillation of *less than 1 year's* duration before surgery and 8% for patients in whom atrial fibrillation was longer than 1 year.

Comment

Atrial fibrillation, a complication of virtually every form of heart disease, is undesirable for a number of reasons. Its mere presence may be disquieting to the patient, since the ventricular rate, even when controlled at rest, is often inappropriately rapid with exercise or emotional stress. Furthermore, the absence of atrial contraction can be of major hemodynamic significance. The lack of atrial kick reduces ventricular filling, which results in a fall in cardiac output, and incomplete atrial emptying favors thromboembolism. Closure of the atrioventricular valves may also be adversely affected on a beat to beat basis. Although prevalence of thromboembolic phenomena in patients with bioprosthesis is lower than that reported with artificial mechanical valves,[6–11] the hemodynamic burden imposed by lacking atrial contraction on valve closure may be more significant in prostheses of biologic origin, since they behave as an orifice of variable area, with larger opening at higher flows.[12–14] Hence, preoperative atrial fibrillation is an important consideration in deciding the choice of valve device. If patients in atrial fibrillation could be identified who are likely to maintain sinus rhythm after valve replacement, they might be as good candidates for a bioprosthetic valve implant as patients who present with preoperative sinus rhythm.

TABLE II Predictive values

	Positive*	Negative†
Preoperative atrial fibrillation <1 year	91%	8%
Left atrial size		
≤40 mm	85%	34%
≤45 mm	54%	32%
≤50 mm	48%	30%
≤55 mm	45%	29%
≤60 mm	43%	22%
Cardiothoracic ratio		
≤50%	57%	32%
≤55%	53%	25%
≤60%	43%	25%
Right atrial pressure		
≤7 mmHg	43%	30%
No prior mitral commissurotomy	53%	43%

* Positive: percent patients who return to sinus rhythm after surgery.
† Negative: percent patients who remain in atrial fibrillation after surgery.

Previous studies have defined a subset of patients with atrial fibrillation in whom the odds of maintaining sinus rhythm following cardioversion are low.[2,4,15–19] According to De Silva et al,[4] cardioversion may not succeed in patients with atrial fibrillation of prolonged duration or in patients who have mitral valve disease with markedly enlarged left atrium or in the setting of left ventricular failure. Conversely, Warris et al[16] found that the patient younger than 50 years of age who has a normal-sized heart and atrial fibrillation of short duration (less than 2 years) and who have treated hypertension or hyperthyroidism as the precipitating mechanism have the best chance of maintaining sinus rhythm after cardioversion.

Lown[20] has shown that the rationale for cardioversion is based on the concept that the *initiating mechanism* and the *sustaining mechanism* of atrial fibrillation are different. Thus, if the sustaining mechanism is interrupted, sinus rhythm will ensue. If the *initiating mechanism* is still present, atrial fibrillation will persist or recur. That probably explains why cardioversion is of limited application in the setting of "lone" atrial fibrillation.[4] Watson et al[17] have shown that myectomy in idiopathic hypertrophic subaortic stenosis leads to a significant reduction in left atrial size in young patients, a change associated with the abolition of atrial fibrillation. Therefore restoration of sinus rhythm following surgery may be expected in a number of patients provided that a near normal hemodynamic state can be achieved.

In the present study, the age of atrial fibrillation prior to surgery was shown to be a main determinant of maintenance of a normal sinus mechanism, since atrial fibrillation of less than 1 year was found in 86% of patients of group 1 and in only 5% of group 2 ($p < 0.001$). In addition, the probability of return to sinus rhythm was 91% for patients presenting with atrial fibrillation of less than a year and 8% for patients in whom atrial fibrillation was of longer duration. Our findings are similar to those of Upton and Honey,[18] who found chronic atrial fibrillation greater than 1 year to be associated with failure to maintain sinus rhythm following mitral valvotomy. In their series, patients fibrillating for more than a year failed to remain in sinus rhythm 1 year after defibrillation; none of the patients remained in sinus rhythm for more than 5 weeks when atrial fibrillation had been present for 5 years before operation. A small proportion of their patients in whom atrial fibrillation had been present for less than a year, or had newly appeared following operation, maintained sinus rhythm for 1–2 years or more. They concluded that the attempt to restore sinus rhythm is only worthwhile when atrial fibrillation has been present for less than 1 year. The duration of atrial fibrillation before surgery could not be precisely determined in our study, since clinical and/or electrocardiographic documentation of the onset of the arrhythmia was lacking in a number of patients. It remains true, however, that return to sinus rhythm is very unlikely in patients who developed atrial fibrillation more than 1 year before the time of surgery.

Our study also confirms the importance of left atrial size in determining the return and maintenance of a normal sinus mechanism following valvular replacement. When considering left atrial size as an independent variable, only the few patients presenting with a left atrial diameter of ≤40 mm were found to have a high probability (85%) of return to sinus rhythm. This is not surprising, since left atrial enlargement provides conditions for a sustained fractionation of reentrant excitability, particularly in the case of patients who have a giant left atrium secondary to chronic mitral regurgitation. Henry et al[19] have quantified the relationship between atrial fibrillation and left atrial size assessed by M mode echocardiography. They found that in patients who had isolated mitral valve disease, isolated aortic valve disease, or asymmetrical septal hypertrophy, atrial fibrillation was rare (3%) when the left atrial size was less than 40 mm and common (54%) when this dimension was greater than 40 mm. In their series, the patients who were cardioverted were unlikely to maintain sinus rhythm longer than 6 months if the left atrial diameter exceeded 45 mm. Our results are somewhat at variance with these data, since we found that 22% of patients whose left atrial size was greater than 60 mm returned to and maintained sinus rhythm. Differences between the present study and that of Henry et al's may well be explained by the improved hemodynamic conditions achieved by our patients following correction of the primary valvular lesion.

The left atrial pressure was not a predictor of the outcome of the arrhythmia following surgery. This can easily be understood if one considers that left atrial pressure might not be the *sustaining mechanism* of atrial fibrillation after surgery, since it rapidly becomes normal or near normal following valvular replacement. Fisher et al[21] found high left atrial pressure to be associated with failure to maintain sinus rhythm in patients undergoing cardioversion after mitral valve replacement; the patients, however, invariably had an increased left atrial size.

Our study also shows right atrial pressure, cardiothoracic ratio, and incidence of previous mitral commissurotomy to be different in patients who return to sinus rhythm. The independent predictive value of these preoperative variables are weakened somewhat by their correlation to the age of atrial fibrillation before surgery and to preoperative left atrial size.

Clinical Implications

The finding that as many as a third of patients presenting with atrial fibrillation could be restored to sinus rhythm following valvular replacement is of particular interest, since predictors of conversion can be identified from baseline preoperative variables. Age of atrial fibrillation and size of left atrium appear to be the main predictors of sustained sinus rhythm. A bioprosthesis may be indicated in patients presenting with atrial fibrillation of recent onset and a left atrial diameter less than 60 mm.

References

1. McCarthy C, Vargheje PS, Barritt, DW: Prognosis of atrial arrhythmias treated by electrical countershock therapy: A three year follow-up. Br Heart J 31:496, 1969.
2. Morris JJ, Peter RH, McIntosh HD: Electrical conversion of atrial fibrillation. Immediate and long-term results and selection of patients. Ann Intern Med 65:216, 1966.
3. Dram S, Davies JPM: Further experience of electrical conversion of atrial fibrillation to sinus rhythm. Analysis of 100 patients. Lancet 1:1294, 1964.
4. De Silva RA, Graboys TB, Podrid PJ, Lown B: Cardioversion and defibrillation. Am Heart J 100:881, 1980.
5. Jenzer H, Lown B: Cardioversion of atrial fibrillation after valve replacement. Am Heart J 84:840, 1972.
6. Carpentier A, Deloche A, Relland J, Fabiani JN, Forman J, Camilleri JP, Soyer R, Dubost C: Six year follow-up of glutaraldehyde-preserved heterografts. With particular reference to the treatment of congenital valve malformations. J Thorac Cardiovasc Surg 68:771, 1974.
7. Hetzer R, Hill JD, Kerth WJ, Ansbro J, Adappa MG, Rodvien R, Kamm B, Gerbode F: Thromboembolitic complications after mitral valve replacement with Hancock xenograft. J Thorac Cardiovasc Surg 75:651, 1978.
8. Stinson EB, Griepp RB, Shumway NE: Clinical experience with a porcine aortic valve xenograft for mitral valve replacement. Ann Thorac Surg 18:391, 1974.
9. Stinson EB, Griepp RB, Dyer PE, Shumway NE: Long-term experience with porcine aortic valve xenografts. J Thorac Cardiovasc Surg 73:54, 1977.
10. Wallace RB: Tissue valves. Am J Cardiol 35:866, 1975.

11. Angell WW, Angell JD, Sywaka Kosek JC: The tissue valve as a superior cardiac valve replacement. Surgery 82:875, 1977.
12. Chaitman BR, Bonan R, Lepage G, Tubau JF, David PR, Dyrda I, Grondin C: Hemodynamic evaluation of the Carpentier-Edwards porcine xenograft. Circulation 60:1170, 1979.
13. Pelletier C, Chaitman BR, Baillot R, Guiteras Val P, Bonan R, Dyrda I: Clinical and hemodynamic results with the Carpentier-Edwards porcine bioprostheses. Ann Thorac Surg 34:(Dec) 1982.
14. Ubago JL, Figuerda A, Colman T, Ochoteco A, Duran CG. Hemodynamic factors that affect calculated orifice areas in the mitral Hancock xenograft valve. Circulation 61:388, 1980.
15. Ewy GA, Ulfers L, Hager WD, Rosenfeld AR, Roeske WR, Goldman S: Response of atrial fibrillation to therapy: Role of etiology and left atrial diameter. J Electrocardiol 13:119, 1980.
16. Warris E, Kreus KE, Salokannel J: Factors influencing persistence of sinus rhythm after AC shock treatment of atrial fibrillation. Acta Med Scand 189:161, 1971.
17. Watson DC, Henry WL, Epstein JE, Morrow AG: Effects of operation on left atrial size and the occurrence of atrial fibrillation in patients with hypertrophic subaortic stenosis. Circulation 55:178, 1977.
18. Upton ARM, Honey M: Electroconversion of atrial fibrillation after mitral valvotomy. Am Heart J 81:732, 1971.
19. Henry WL, Morganroth J, Pearlman AS, Clark CE, Redwood DR, Iscoitz SB, Epstein SE: Relation between echocardiographically determined left atrial size and atrial fibrillation. Circulation 53:273, 1976.
20. Lown B: Electrical reversion of cardiac arrhythmias. Br Heart J 29:469, 1967.
21. Fisher RD, Mason DT, Morrow A: Restoration of sinus rhythm after mitral replacement. Circulation 37:173, 1968.

18

Porcine Bioprostheses Versus Mechanical Valvular Substitutes: A Retrospective Comparative Analysis

M. SCHÖNBECK, L. EGLOFF, J. KUGELMEIER, M. ROTHLIN, Å. SENNING, M. TURINA

Over the past 5 years, we have used porcine bioprostheses and mechanical valvular substitutes in equal numbers for aortic and mitral valve replacement. Repeated analyses of our clinical results have formed the basis of our present policy for the use of one or the other type of prosthetic device.[1,2] In this study we attempt to compare survival, valve-related complications, and quality of life after valve replacement with bioprostheses and mechanical substitutes implanted during the same time period.

Patients and Methods

From 1976–1980, 604 patients underwent either aortic or mitral valve replacement (AVR, MVR). Included in this series were patients with concomitant 1 or 2 vessel coronary artery disease, ascending aortic aneurysm, noncomplex congenital heart defects, functional tricuspid regurgitation, and with prior valve reconstruction or autologous fascia lata AVR. Bioprostheses of 3 different manufacturers were used: Carpentier-Edwards (194), Angell-Shiley (72), and Hancock (36). The mechanical prostheses employed were Björk-Shiley (256), St. Jude Medical (45), and Lillehei-Kaster (1). Indication for a bioprosthesis or a mechanical device depended largely on the patient's and surgeon's attitude toward the risk of long-term anticoagulation or possible future reoperation in case of prosthesis degeneration. Patients with mechanical prostheses were informed about the risk of long-term anticoagulants; those receiving a bioprosthesis were told of the uncertain durability of presently available biologic valves.

From the Surgical Clinic A, University Hospital, Zurich, Switzerland.

Preoperative data are summarized in Table I. Patients receiving a bioprosthesis generally were younger with less advanced cardiac disease, indicated by a lower functional class, a higher cardiac index, and, in the MVR group, a lower incidence of atrial fibrillation. The average size of bioprosthesis was 28.3 mm for AVR and 31.5 mm for MVR; for the mechanical devices it was 28.1 mm and 30.6 mm, respectively. Concomitant procedures are listed in Table II. There were no statistically significant differences between the 2 groups with regard to incidence or type of procedure.

The operation was performed under moderate hypothermia and cold potassium cardioplegia. The prostheses were inserted by means of interrupted pledgeted sutures. Rarely, a running monofilament was preferred. All patients with mechanical prostheses were kept on long-term anticoagulants, whereas in those with bioprostheses anticoagulation was discontinued after 3 months in the absence of other factors predisposing to thromboembolism.

TABLE I Preoperative data

	Bioprostheses	Mechanical prostheses	Total
AVR	201	188	389
Age	47.6 (5–74)*	53.6 (17–22)*	50.4 (5–74)
Functional class	2.2 ± 0.8*	2.5 ± 0.8*	2.3 ± 0.8
Cardiac index (mean)	3.0 ± 0.9*	2.7 ± 0.7*	2.9 ± 0.8
Lesion			
Predominant stenosis	40%	45%	42.5%
Predominant regurgitation	30%	31%	30.5%
Mixed lesion	30%	24%	27.0%
Prior heart surgery			
Commissurotomy or aortic valve replacement with fascia lata	12 (6%)	11 (6%)	23 (6%)
MVR	101	114	215
Age	47.6 (14–72)*	53.5 (1–69)*	50.6 (1–72)
Functional class	2.9 ± 0.6	3.0 ± 0.6	3.0 ± 0.6
Cardiac index (mean)	2.7 ± 0.7*	2.2 ± 0.6*	2.4 ± 0.6
Lesion			
Predominant stenosis	46%	43%	44.5%
Predominant regurgitation	39%	32%	35.5%
Mixed lesion	15%	25%	20.0%
Prior heart surgery			
Commissurotomy or reconstruction	8 (8%)	31 (27%)	39 (18%)
Electrocardiogram			
Sinus rhythm	54%	23%	34.5%
Atrial fibrillation	46%	77%	66.5%

* $p < 0.05$.

TABLE II Concomitant surgical procedures

	Bioprostheses	Mechanical prostheses	Total
AVR	201	188	389
Graft replacement of ascending aorta	12 (6%)	20 (10%)	32 (8%)
Coronary artery bypass grafting	10 (5%)	15 (8%)	25 (6%)
Resection of subvalvular stenosis	14 (7%)	3 (2%)	17 (4%)
Outflow patch	15 (7%)	7 (4%)	22 (6%)
Miscellaneous*	5 (2%)	3 (2%)	8 (2%)
MVR	101	114	215
Tricuspid anulorrhaphy	22 (22%)	30 (26%)	52 (24%)
Coronary artery bypass grafting	1 (1%)	1 (3%)	1 (2%)
Tricuspid anulorrhaphy and coronary artery bypass	1 (2%)	—	1 (0.5%)

* Closure of ventricular septal defect (2), resection of aortic coarctation (1), commissurotomy of the pulmonary valve (1), pericardiectomy (1), tricuspid anulorrhaphy (1), plication of a membraneous septal aneurysm (1), division of Kent's bundle (1).

Postoperatively, patients were seen at follow-up visits after 6 months and, thereafter, at yearly intervals. Patients living abroad or unable to attend arranged visits were followed by written questionnaires. Overall, 51 patients were lost during the follow-up period. Data were analyzed for early and late survival and valve-related complications. Thromboembolism, anticoagulant hemorrhage, prosthesis dysfunction, paravalvular leakage, and endocarditis were considered valve-related. Actuarial survival and complication-free survival rates were derived, using the method proposed by Kaplan and Meier[3] and Anderson et al.[4]

Results

Early Mortality

The 30-day mortality was very similar for patients undergoing AVR or MVR, independent of the type of prosthesis. It averaged 2%. None of the causes of death listed in Table III were prosthesis related.

Late Mortality

Late death rates of patients undergoing AVR or MVR have been the same, 1.4% and 1.6% per year, respectively (Table IV). There was no differ-

TABLE III Cause of early death

	Bioprostheses	Mechanical prostheses	Total
AVR	201	188	389
Low cardiac output		3	3
Sudden death		1	1
Dissection of ascending aorta		1	1
Myocardial infarction	1		1
Cerebrovascular insult	1		1
Tamponade		1	1
Total	2 (1%)	6 (3.2%)	8 (2.1%)
MVR	101	114	215
Posterior rupture of the left ventricle	1	1	2
Myocardial infarction		1	1
Sepsis		1	1
Total	1 (1%)	3 (2.6%)	4 (1.9%)

ence between patients receiving a bioprosthesis or a mechanical substitute. In 3 patients death was valve related: lethal cerebrovascular accidents occurred twice (once after AVR with a mechanical prosthesis and once after MVR with a bioprosthesis), and 1 patient died of an acute valve dehiscence 8 months after implantation of a bioprosthesis in the mitral position. Actuarial survival curves show 90–95% of patients alive 4 years after AVR or MVR with no significant differences between the 2 types of prosthesis (Figs. 1 and 2).

Late Valve-Related Complications

The incidence of valve-related complications, including valve-related deaths, varied after AVR from 2% per year for patients with bioprosthesis to 5.2% per year after replacement with a mechanical prosthesis (Table V). Reoperation rate, however, was almost identical (0.9 and 1.2% per year, respectively). After MVR with either type of prosthesis, valve-related complications and reoperations occurred with frequencies differing less than 1% per year. Thromboembolism and anticoagulant hemorrhages were the most frequent cause of complication for patients with bioprostheses and mechanical devices. They occurred after AVR at a rate of 1.37 and 6.5% per year, respectively; after MVR the risk of thromboembolism or anticoagulant hemorrhage was 1.6% per year for patients with bioprostheses and 3.18% per year for those with mechanical devices, although 100% of patients with the latter type of prosthesis were on anticoagulants, whereas after bioprosthetic valve replacement only 33% of AVR and 36% of MVR patients received this form of long-term thromboembolism prophylaxis. In

TABLE IV Cause of late death

	Bioprostheses	Mechanical prostheses	Total
AVR	201	188	389
Sudden death	3	3	6
Congestive heart failure	2	1	3
Myocardial infarction	1	1	2
Cerebrovascular insult		1	1
Dissection of ascending aorta	1	1	2
Other*		3	3
Total	7 (1.1% per year)	10 (1.7% per year)	17 (1.4% per year)
MVR	101	114	215
Sudden death	1	3	4
Congestive heart failure	1	2	3
Paravalvular leak (valve dehiscence)		1	1
Cardiomyopathy	1		1
Cerebrovascular insult	1		1
Other	1		1
Total	5 (1.6% per year)	6 (1.7% per year)	11 (1.6% per year)

* Renal failure, gastroenteritis, carcinoma of the esophagus.
† Accident.

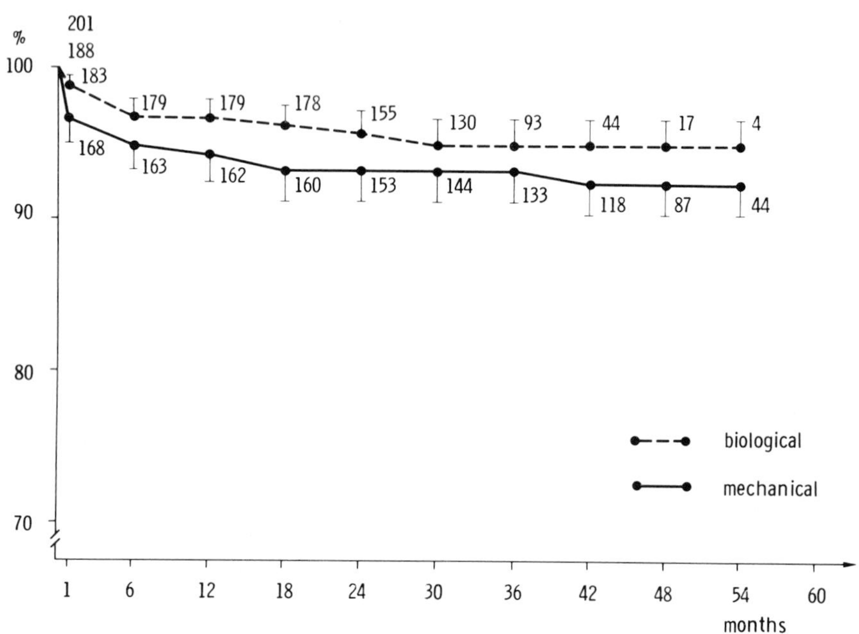

FIG. 1 Aortic valve replacement; actuarial survival curves.

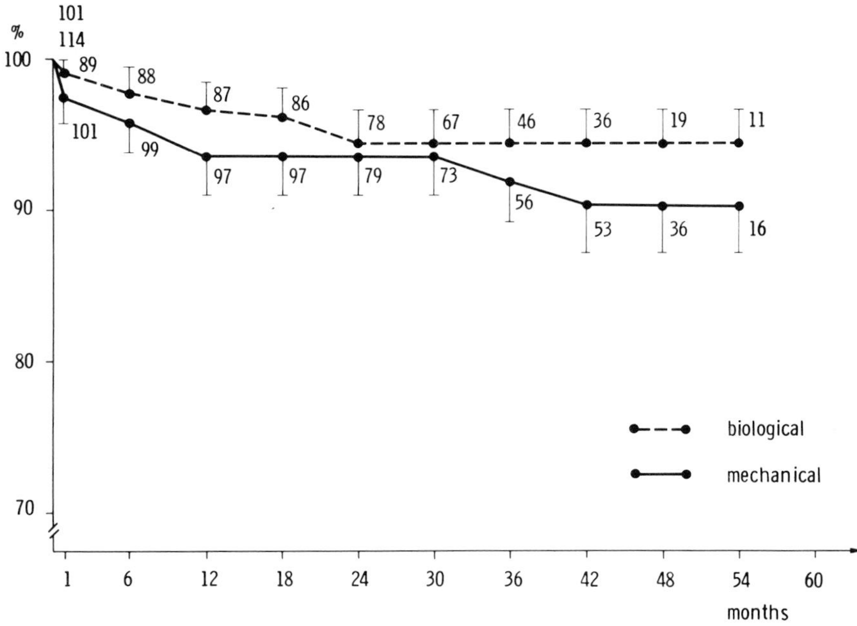

FIG. 2 Mitral valve replacement; actuarial survival curves.

3 patients the mitral prosthesis had to be replaced 3–7 months postoperatively because of dysfunction. The leaflets of 1 bioprosthesis became stiff soon after operation, causing again severe mitral stenosis. Two prostheses (1 biological, 1 mechanical) were acutely thrombosed and were successfully replaced. Actuarial valve-related complication-free survival curves show up to 36 months no difference between bioprostheses and mechanical prostheses after AVR or MVR; between 36 and 48 months the failure rate appears to be less for bioprostheses compared to mechanical prostheses after AVR and MVR (Figs. 3 and 4).

Comment

In this analysis we have attempted to compare 2 types of the most commonly used valvular substitutes for AVR and MVR: the tilting disc prosthesis versus the bioprosthesis. Although we are aware of the danger in comparing 2 groups of patients unequal with respect to age and preoperative status and whose prostheses were manufactured by different companies, an analysis of prosthesis-related complications may still be of some interest. Both groups were operated upon by the same team of surgeons and during the same time period. The same group of cardiologists and cardiac surgeons evaluated the indications for surgery and chose the valvular substitute to be

TABLE V Valve-related late complications

	Bioprostheses	Mechanical prostheses	Total
AVR	201	188	389
Thromboembolism	4	13 (1†)	17 (1*)
Anticoagulation hemorrhage	1	10	11
Endocarditis	3 (2*)	3 (1*)	6 (3*)
Paravalvular leak (excluding endocarditis)	4 (3*)	6 (6*)	10 (9*)
Total complications in % per year	2	5.2	3.6
Total reoperations in % per year	0.9	1.2	1.1
MVR	101	114	215
Thromboembolism	5 (1†)	6	11 (1†)
Anticoagulation hemorrhage	—	4	4
Endocarditis	2 (1*)	—	2 (1*)
Paravalvular leak (excluding endocarditis)	2 (2*)	4 (2*, 1†)	6 (4*, 1†)
Prosthesis dysfunction	2 (2*)	1 (1*)	3 (3*)
Total complications in % per year	3.1	3.9	3.5
Total reoperations in % per year	1.6	0.8	1.2

* Requiring reoperation.
† Resulting in death.

implanted. In general young and very old patients were more likely to receive a bioprosthesis and patients in their 50s and 60s, particularly those with impaired left ventricular function and atrial fibrillation, were more often candidates for the mechanical device. The patient's own feelings and preferences were respected. The criterion "valve-related complication" has been used to judge the overall performance of the 2 types of prostheses. Assuming that frequency of occurrence parallels seriousness of complications to a great extent, this parameter may be an acceptable standard for comparison.

Early Mortality

No valve-related complications were observed to cause early death in either group of patients. Both instances of posterior left ventricular rupture after MVR were related to circumflex coronary artery problems. The low total early mortality for AVR and MVR of 2% represents an improvement over the past decade observed at most institutions and related most likely to earlier indication for surgery (i.e., fewer candidates in preoperative functional class IV) and improved intraoperative myocardial protection.[5–9]

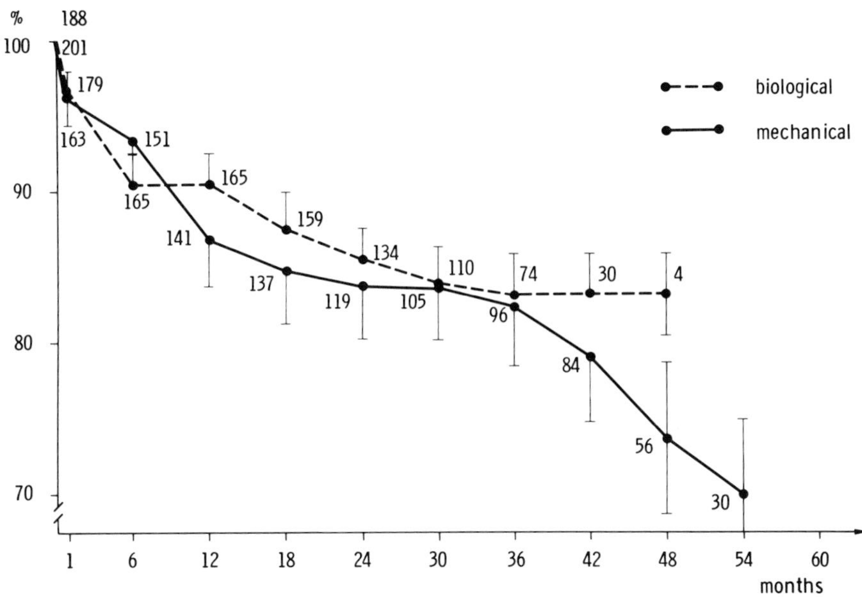

FIG. 3 Aortic valve replacement; complication-free survival curves.

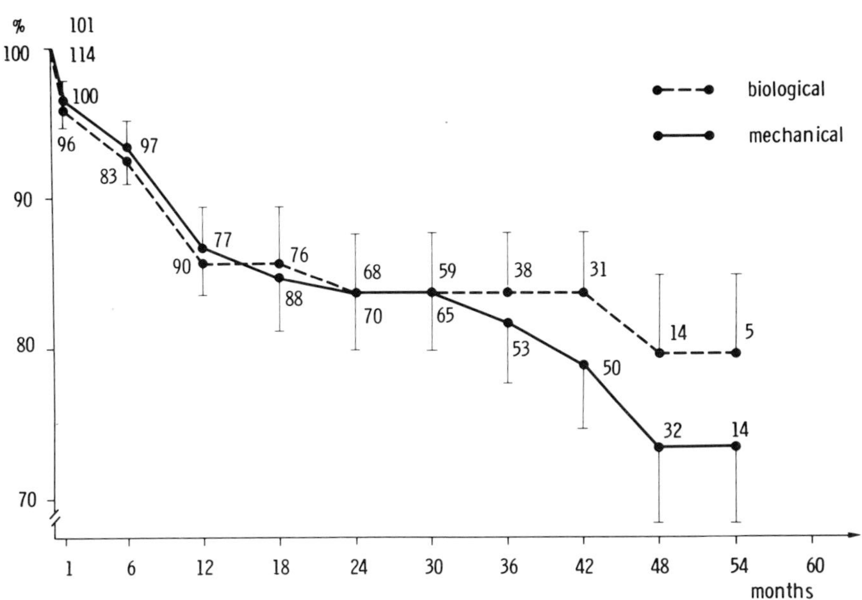

FIG. 4 Mitral valve replacement; complication-free survival curves.

Late Mortality

Sudden death has been the single most frequent cause of late death after AVR and MVR and was unrelated to the type of prosthesis. It occurred with almost equal frequency in both groups. Similarly, high incidences of sudden unexplained death are reported in other series.[10–12] Pre- and perioperative tachyarrhythmias may be an ominous sign in this regard. The minor differences in the actuarial survival rates between the mechanical and bioprosthetic group after 4 years of observation after AVR and MVR may be related to preoperative differences. Since they are statistically not significant, they are irrelevant.

Valve-Related Late Complications

No differences between the 2 groups can be observed after AVR or MVR up to 3 years (82% complication-free survival for both AVR and MVR). The slight differences between the third and fourth year favoring bioprostheses are difficult to explain. They are also statistically not significant because of too few patients in each group. The major interest focuses on thromboembolism and anticoagulant hemorrhage. For MVR patients, these complications have been similar for either type of valve (1.6 and 3.18% per year, respectively). After AVR, the thromboembolic rate has, with due reservations toward retrospective analysis, clearly been higher after replacement with a mechanical prosthesis, although only the latter patients were all on long-term anticoagulants (6.5 -vs- 1.3% per year). In the literature the rates of thromboembolism and anticoagulant hemorrhage are difficult to interpret and to compare. The diagnosis often is uncertain and the clinical manifestations vary from major findings to minor transient episodes. Recent reports indicate little differences after AVR and MVR between bioprostheses and Björk-Shiley valves if the latter patients are kept on anticoagulants. After AVR, the rate of thromboembolism in 4 series[13–15,17] averages 1.9% per year for bioprostheses and in 2 series,[6,8] 1.7% per year for Björk-Shiley valves. After MVR, the respective figures average 3.3% per year in 5 series[13–17] for bioprostheses and 3.3% per year in 3 series[6,18,19] for Björk-Shiley patients. Durability, besides thrombogenicity, is the second most important factor difference between the 2 types of valvular prostheses. The follow-up of 4 years in our series is not long enough to separate the 2 groups. In vitro studies[20,21] projecting a survival for Björk-Shiley valves 10 times as long as for a porcine bioprosthesis and clinical data[6,8,16,18,19,22,23] allow the conclusion that bioprostheses will fail earlier.

Conclusions

During a follow-up period of up to 4 years, the tilting disc prostheses and the porcine bioprostheses have performed remarkably similar after MVR and AVR. The disadvantage of the mechanical type of prosthesis is the absolute necessity for long-term anticoagulants. In bioprostheses they can soon be discontinued postoperatively if there are no other indications for their administration. The major drawback of biologic valves, however, remains their limited durability. At present, we continue to use both tilting disc prostheses and porcine bioprostheses for AVR and MVR. For AVR in young adults and good risk patients, we definitely prefer the bioprosthesis because of the low thromboembolic risk. Our previous experience with the autologous fascia lata valve supports the concept that a reoperation after several years is preferable to the continued risk of thromboembolism and anticoagulant hemorrhage.[24] At the other end of the age spectrum, durability is not a major issue and therefore the bioprosthesis is the device of choice for the elderly patient. The tilting disc prosthesis in aortic position is reserved for patients already on anticoagulants for other reasons and those definitely refusing a future operation. In the mitral position we have not been able to document significant differences between the 2 types except that all patients with mechanical prostheses had to take daily anticoagulants and had to control their prothrombin times at regular intervals. In the mitral position the bioprosthesis is therefore mainly indicated for patients difficult or impossible to anticoagulate (not a small group of patients), whereas for all other patients the tilting disc prosthesis still may be preferable.

References

1. Egloff L, Rothlin M, Krayenbühl C, Kugelmeier J, Senning Å, Turina M: Early valve related complications with porcine bioprostheses and a comparative analysis with the Björk-Shiley tilting disc valve. In: Bioprosthetic Cardiac Valves (F Sebening, WP Klövekorn, H Meisner, E Struck, Eds). Munich, Deutsches Herzzentrum, 1979, p 351.
2. Egloff L, Rothlin M, Turina M, Senning Å: Isolated aortic valve replacement with the Björk-Shiley tilting disc prosthesis and the porcine bioprosthesis. Eur Heart J 1:123, 1980.
3. Kaplan EL, Meier P: Nonparametric estimation from incomplete observations. J Am Stat Assoc 53:457, 1958.
4. Anderson RP, Bonchek LI, Grunkemeier GL, Lambert LE, Starr A: The analysis and presentation of surgical results by actuarial methods. J Surg Res 16:224, 1974.
5. Egloff L, Rothlin M, Turina M, Krayenbühl C, Kugelmeier J, Senning Å: Isolated mitral valve replacement with the Björk-Shiley tilting disc prosthesis. Thorac Cardiovasc Surg 27:223, 1979.
6. Björk VO, Henze A: Ten years' experience with the Björk-Shiley tilting disc valve. J Thorac Cardiovasc Surg 78:331, 1979.
7. Teply JF, Grunkemeier GL, Sutherland HD, Lambert LE, Johnson VA, Starr A: The ultimate prognosis after valve replacement: An assessment at twenty years. Ann Thor Surg 32:111, 1981.
8. Cheung D, Flemma RJ, Mullen DC, Lepley D Jr, Anderson AJ, Weirauch E: Ten-year follow-up in aortic valve replacement using the Björk-Shiley prosthesis. Ann Thor Surg 32:138, 1981.

9. Acar J, Ducimetiere P, Cadilhac M, Jallut H, Vahanian A: Prognosis of surgically treated chronic aortic valve disease. J Thorac Cardiovasc Surg 82:114, 1981.
10. Santinga JT, Kirsh MM, Flora JD, Brymer JF: Factors relating to late sudden death in patients having aortic valve replacement. Ann Thorac Surg 29:249, 1980.
11. Copeland JG, Griepp RB, Stinson EB, Shumway NE: Long-term follow-up after isolated aortic valve replacement. J Thorac Cardiovasc Surg 74:875, 1977.
12. Barnhorst DA, Oxman HA, Connolly DC, Pluth JR, Danielson GK, Wallace RB, McGoon DC: Isolated replacement of the mitral valve with the Starr-Edwards prosthesis. J Thorac Cardiovasc Surg 71:230, 1976.
13. Oyer PE, Stinson EB, Reitz BA, Miller DC, Rossiter SJ, Shumway NE: Long-term evaluation of the porcine xenograft bioprosthesis. J Thorac Cardiovasc Surg 78:343, 1979.
14. Rivera R, Infantes C, Delcan JL, Rico M: Clinical and hemodynamic assessment of the Angell-Shiley porcine xenograft. Ann Thorac Surg 30:455, 1980.
15. Davila JC, Magilligan DJ Jr, Lewis JW Jr: Is the Hancock porcine valve the best cardiac valve substitute today? Ann Thorac Surg 26:303, 1978.
16. Borkon AM, McIntosh CL, Von Rueden TJ, Morrow AG: Mitral valve replacement with the Hancock bioprosthesis: Five- to ten-year follow-up. Ann Thorac Surg 32:127, 1981.
17. Williams JB, Karp RB, Kirklin JW, Kouchoukos NT, Pacifico AD, Zorn GL Jr, Blackstone EH, Brown RN, Piantadosi S, Bradley EL: Considerations in selection and management of patients undergoing valve replacement with glutaraldehyde-fixed porcine bioprostheses. Ann Thorac Surg 30:247, 1980.
18. Lepley D Jr, Flemma RJ, Mullen DC, Motl M, Anderson AJ, Weirauch E: Long-term follow-up of the Björk-Shiley prosthetic valve used in the mitral position. Ann Thorac Surg 30:164, 1980.
19. Egloff L, Rothlin M, Turina M, Krayenbühl C, Kugelmeier J, Senning Å: Isolated mitral valve replacement with the Björk-Shiley tilting disc prosthesis. Thorac Cardiovasc Surg 27:223, 1979.
20. Clark RE, Swanson WM, Kardos JL, Hagen RW, Beauchamp RA: Durability of prosthetic heart valves. Ann Thorac Surg 26:323, 1978.
21. Clark RE, Swanson WM: In vitro durability of Hancock Model 242 porcine heart valve. J Thorac Cardiovasc Surg 78:277, 1979.
22. Oyer PE, Miller DC, Stinson EB, Reitz BA, Moreno-Cabral RJ, Shumway NE: Clinical durability of the Hancock porcine bioprosthetic valve. J Thorac Cardiovasc Surg 80:824, 1980.
23. Magilligan DJ Jr, Lewis JW Jr, Jara FM, Lee MW, Alam M, Riddle JM, Stein PD: Spontaneous degeneration of porcine bioprosthetic valves. Ann Thorac Surg 30:259, 1980.
24. Rothlin ME, Senning Å: 15 years experience with fascia-lata aortic valves and the outlook of modern bioprostheses. In: Bioprosthetic Cardiac Valves (F Sebening, WP Klövekorn, H Meisner, E Struck, Eds). Munich, Deutsches Herzzentrum, 1979, p 173.

SECTION IV

PEDIATRIC VALVE REPLACEMENT

19

Valved Conduits: A Panacea for Complex Congenital Heart Defects?

A. R. Castañeda, W. I. Norwood

Correction of congenital heart defects characterized by discontinuity between the systemic venous atrium and/or ventricle and the pulmonary artery is historically related to the development of a conduit to bridge the gap between the heart and the lungs. Experimental bypass of semilunar valves was first suggested by Carrell in 1910.[1] In 1949 Rodbard and Wagner[2] first bypassed in dogs the pulmonary valve by anastomosing the right atrial appendage to the main pulmonary artery. In 1964 Kirklin and associates[3] fashioned a (nonvalved) tubular conduit of pericardium to connect the right ventricle to the main pulmonary artery to treat a patient with a complex form of tetralogy of Fallot.

The first use of a valved conduit to bypass a pulmonary valve was reported by Donovan in 1950.[4] He used preserved femoral and jugular vein allografts to conduct blood from the right ventricle to a proximally ligated left pulmonary artery. The use of aortic allografts in clinical surgery was introduced by Gross in 1949 for the treatment of coarctation of the aorta. An ascending aortic allograft containing a functioning aortic valve was first used clinically by Ross and Somerville in 1966 to establish right ventricular pulmonary artery continuity in a patient with pulmonary atresia and ventricular septal defect. Such grafts were further popularized by Rastelli et al at the Mayo Clinic for the correction of truncus arteriosus communis[5] and transposition of the great arteries with ventricular septal defect and subpulmonary stenosis.[6] Finally, in the early 1970s, Dacron tube grafts containing either an allograft aortic valve or a preserved xenograft aortic valve were introduced and made commercially for the reconstruction of the pul-

---

From the Department of Cardiovascular Surgery, Children's Hospital Medical Center, Department of Surgery, Harvard Medical School, Boston, Massachusetts.

Dr. Castanẽda was an honor lecturer at the Second International Symposium on Cardiac Bioprostheses.

monary outflow tract.[7] The convenience of commercially available grafts has resulted in their widespread use and popularity in the last decade.

Much has been learned in the intervening years about the use of valved conduits and important advances have been made both in the understanding of complex congenital cardiac malformations and in surgical technique. Sufficient time has also elapsed to identify some of the early and late complications related to valved conduits used in the correction of these complex congenital heart defects.

Accordingly, in this presentation we review our experience at the Children's Hospital Medical Center, Boston, with Dacron conduits containing preserved xenograft valves positioned within the pulmonary circuit.

Clinical Material

Between October 1972 and December 1981, 189 patients had a valved conduit placed from the right side of the heart to the pulmonary circuit. The age of the patients at the time of repair ranged from 15 days to 35 years (mean, 9 years). Two operations were performed within the first months of life, and 11 patients were 6 years of age or younger. The primary diagnosis of these 189 patients and the surgical outcome are listed in Table I.

TABLE I Distribution of lesions repaired

Type of lesion*	Valved conduits, right sided			
	# pts		Mortality*	
			Hospital	Late
Tetralogy of Fallot	78		4 (5.1)	2 (2.5)
Pulmonary atresia		63	4	2
Single PA		11		
Anomalous ADC		3		
AV canal		1		
Tricuspid atresia	31		4 (12.9)	
Truncus arteriosus	20		7 (35.0)	
TGA {S,D,D}, VSD, PS	17		2 (11.7)	2 (11.7)
Double outlet RV	15		1 (6.6)	
Single V + other	14		8 (57.1)	
TGA {S,L,L}, VSD, PS	10			
Pulmonary atresia + IVS	4		1 (25.0)	
	189		27 (14.2)	4 (2.1)

* ADC: anterior descending coronary; AV: atrioventricular; PA: pulmonary artery; TGA: transposition of the great arteries; VSD: ventricular septal defect; PS: subpulmonary stenosis; RV: right ventricle; IVS: intact ventricular septum.

Seventy-eight patients had severe forms of tetralogy of Fallot, including 63 with infundibular or valvar atresia, 11 with congenital or acquired absence of 1 pulmonary valve, 3 with anomalous origin of the anterior descending coronary artery from the right coronary artery, and 1 patient had tetralogy of Fallot with complete atrioventricular canal and pulmonary atresia. Thirty-one patients with tricuspid atresia had a Fontan operation that included closure of the atrial communication and interposition of a valved conduit between the right atrium and either the right ventricle or the pulmonary artery. In none of these patients was a valve placed at the inferior vena cava to the right atrial junction. Twenty patients had truncus arteriosus communis. Seventeen had transposition of the great arteries with ventricular septal defect and subpulmonary stenosis. Fifteen had double outlet right ventricle with severe right ventricular outflow tract obstruction. A Fontan principle was applied to an additional 14 patients with single ventricle and other complex defects, such as single atrium and total anomalous pulmonary venous connection. Ten patients with corrected transposition of the great arteries, ventricular septal defect, and severe pulmonary outflow tract obstruction had a conduit placed from the anatomic left ventricle (functional right ventricle) to the main pulmonary artery. Valved conduits were also placed in 4 patients who had pulmonary atresia and an intact ventricular septum. These 4 patients had all previous palliative shunts and pulmonary valvotomies.

Generally, the clinical indications for operations were increasing cyanosis and decreasing exercise tolerance secondary to diminished pulmonary blood flow. In patients younger than 4 years of age, most of whom had truncus arteriosus communis, congestive heart failure and increased pulmonary artery pressure were the principal indications for operations. All operations were done on cardiopulmonary bypass with moderate hypothermia (30°C) except for infants who underwent repair by means of deep hypothermic circulatory arrest.

Since the total number of 189 patients includes such a heterogeneous group of lesions, we shall review in more detail the fate of the valved conduits in the cohort of 78 patients with complex forms of tetralogy of Fallot.

The age of patients with tetralogy of Fallot and pulmonary atresia ranged from 4 months to 35 years (median age, 12 years) (Table II). The ages and the number of patients with tetralogy of Fallot and other associated lesions are listed in Table III.

Routinely at the time of operation, left atrial, right atrial, and pulmonary artery catheters were placed to monitor blood pressure and ventricular filling pressures. An additional catheter was placed through the right ventricular free wall across the conduit and into the main pulmonary artery to

TABLE II Age and outcome of patients with tetralogy of Fallot and pulmonary atresia after valved conduit placement

Age (yr)	# pts	Mortality* Hospital	Mortality* Late	Reoperation*
0–1	2	0	0	0
1–3	4	0	0	0
3–6	5	1	0	1
6–10	16	0	1	2
10–15	21	1	0	2
15–35	15	2	1	0
Total	63	4 (6.3)	2 (3.1)	5† (7.9)

*( ): percent.
† Two were not conduit related.

identify residual left to right shunts and to measure pressure gradients across the conduit when the catheter is removed 24 to 48 hours postoperatively.

Cardiac catheterization was routinely recommended for all patients 1 year postoperatively. Hemodynamic data have been obtained so far on 94 patients 1 month to 5 years (mean, 1.5 years) after repair. However, only the postoperative data of 36 patients with tetralogy of Fallot will be presented.

Actuarial analyses were developed employing methods outlined by Anderson et al.[8]

Early Results

Hospital mortality of the entire group was 14.2% (27 of 189 patients). Four of the 78 patients (5%) with tetralogy of Fallot died shortly after operation. One 5 year old and one 14 year old died from uncontrolled hemorrhage during and 2 days after operation, respectively. The 5-year-old patient died early in our experience (1973) during dissection of a left Blalock-Taussig shunt. The other patient had a right Blalock-Taussig shunt and a Potts anastomosis. Because of continuing bleeding, he was returned to the operating room 2 days after the original procedure where he died during attempted control of bleeding from the left pulmonary hilum. An 18-year-old girl with stage IV pulmonary vascular obstructive disease secondary to long-standing bilateral Blalock-Taussig shunts had intermittent severe hemoptysis postoperatively and died from pulmonary complications. A 33-year-old man had undergone a Blalock-Taussig shunt in 1947 and had severe left ventricular failure and secondary renal insufficiency preoperatively. He remained in a low cardiac output state postoperatively and died of combined renal and cardiac insufficiency 2 weeks after the operation.

TABLE III Age and outcome of patients with tetralogy of Fallot and associated lesions after valved conduit placement

Age (Yr)	# pts	Mortality Hospital	Mortality Late	Reoperations
Tetralogy of Fallot and complete atrioventricular canal				
16	1	0	0	1
Tetralogy of Fallot and anterior descending coronary artery from the right coronary artery				
6–8	3	0	0	1
Tetralogy of Fallot and single pulmonary artery				
8–11	3	0	0	0
11–16	3	0	0	0
16–32	5	0	0	2
Total	15	0	0	4 (26.5%)

Six patients had early postoperative evidence of residual left to right shunts; 2 of these underwent reoperation during the first postoperative week for closure of a residual ventricular septal defect. Both survived reoperation and are well. The other 4 patients had smaller residual shunts (Qp/Qs $< 1.5:1$).

Late Results

There have been 4 (2.1%) late deaths in the total group of 189 patients. The survival rate of the 78 patients with tetralogy of Fallot is depicted in actuarial form in Fig. 1. Follow-up ranges from 1–8 years. Twenty patients are now being followed for more than 5 years postoperatively.

Almost all late complications were related to the valved conduits. For example, 1 patient treated with antibiotics alone for early postoperative Hancock conduit infection developed septicemia 1 year later and died during antibiotic therapy. Of the total group of 189 patients, 10 (5.3%) presented some conduit complication (Table IV). A relatively fresh thrombus was found 4 months after placement of an 18 mm Hancock conduit in a child with tetralogy of Fallot and complete atrioventricular canal. Obstructing internal peels and external conduit compression by the sternum was observed in 2 patients; 3 patients had obstructing internal peels combined with heavy calcification of the aortic xenograft valve 5.1–6.2 years after implantation. In 1 of these patients, a 5-year-old boy with tetralogy of Fallot and pulmonary atresia, a 20 mm Hancock conduit was replaced with a 20 mm Carpentier-Edwards valved conduit and at the same time, an insufficient aortic valve had to be replaced with a (27 mm Björk-Shiley) prosthetic valve. A 16-year-old patient with tricuspid atresia (type IB) had

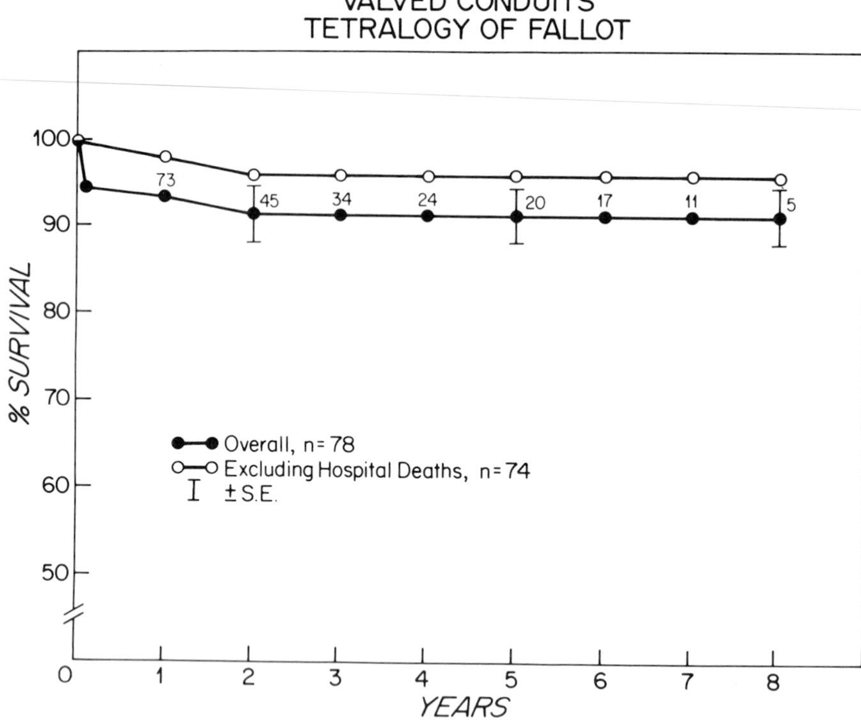

FIG. 1 Actuarial survival curves of patients after tetralogy of Fallot repair with valved conduit placement.

interposition of a 20 mm Hancock conduit between the right atrium and the pulmonary artery. He developed a 15 mm gradient across the conduit 4 years after the original operation. At reoperation, no trace of the xenograft valve could be found (vanished valve); the obstruction was caused by flattening of the distal conduit. This elongation of the graft seemed secondary to a significant growth spurt after the initial Fontan operation. The obstruction within the conduit was relieved by simply augmenting the distally narrowed conduit by a Dacron patch without repositioning of a valve. An isolated stenosis at the right ventricular conduit anastomosis site that had caused a 60 mm gradient was repaired by a patch-plasty of the proximal anastomosis.

Valved conduit-related reoperations in the patients with tetralogy of Fallot are outlined in Table V. Actuarial valved conduit durability is depicted in Fig. 2.

Three patients had reoperations not related to valved conduits. In 2, residual ventricular septal defects were closed approximately 1 year after

TABLE IV Reoperations for conduit complications

Lesion*	Conduit size (mm)	Δt reoperation	ΔP (mmHg)	Outcome*
Clotted valve				
TOF + AVC	18 H*	4 mo	80	NVC
Obstructing peel plus conduit compression				
TOF + PA	20 H	8.2 yr	50	RVOT patch
TGA + VSD + PS	20 H	4.5 yr	65	+
Obstructing peel plus Ca^{++}				
TOF + PA	20 H	5.1 yr	70	CE, 20 mm; BS, 27 mm
TGA + VSD + PS	18 H	6.0 yr	90	CE, 18 mm
TOF + PA	18 H	6.2 yr	80	NVC
Vanished valve plus graft elongation				
TA (RA-PA)	20 H	4.0 yr	15	Graft patch-plasty
Isolated anastomotic stenosis				
TOF + PA	20 H	3.0 yr	60	Patch-plasty
Sepsis				
TGA + VSD + PS	20 H	1.0 yr		+
TOF + PA	20 H	1.4 yr		+

* AVC: atrioventricular canal; BS: Björk-Shiley; CE: Carpentier-Edwards; H: Hancock; NVC: nonvalved conduit; PA: pulmonary artery; PS: subpulmonary stenosis; RA: right atrium; RVOT: right ventricular outflow tract; TGA: transposition of the great arteries; TOF: tetralogy of Fallot; VSD: ventricular septal defect.

TABLE V Reoperations for valved conduit complications after tetralogy of Fallot repair

Age 1st operation (yr)	Δt reoperation	Conduit size (mm) and type	Findings*	Operation*	Mortality
16	4 mo	18 H	Thrombosed valve	NVC	0
13	3.0 yr	20 H	ΔP Proximal anastomosis	Patch-plasty	0
8	5.1 yr	20 H	Ca^{++} + peel	CE, 20 mm; BS, 27 mm	0
14	6.0 yr	18 H	Ca^{++} + peel	NVC	0
19	8.2 yr	20 H	Peel	RVOT patch	0
7	1.1 yr	18 CE	VSD	VSD + NVC	0
17	1.2 yr	18 CE	ΔP LPA	LPA patch-plasty	0

* BS: Björk-Shiley; CE: Carpentier-Edwards; H: Hancock; LPA: left pulmonary artery; NVC: nonvalved conduit; RVOT: right ventricular outflow tract; VSD: ventricular septal defect.

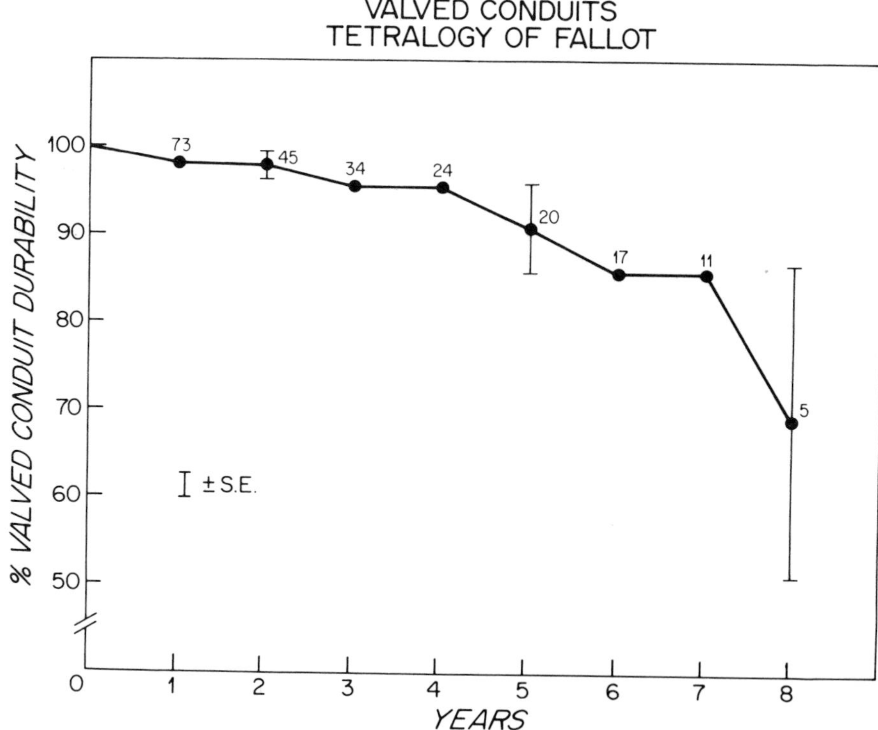

FIG. 2 Actuarial valved conduit durability curve in patients with tetralogy of Fallot repair and valved conduit placement.

the original surgery. The third patient had tricuspid atresia and required closure of a residual shunt at the atrial level. Concomitantly, the 16 mm Hancock conduit was replaced "electively" with a nonvalved conduit.

Follow-up hemodynamic data were obtained in 36 patients 1 month to 4 years (mean, 1.5 years) after repair of tetralogy of Fallot (Fig. 3). Ten patients had gradients greater than 40 mmHg. In 4, the gradient was localized at the right ventricular to conduit anastomosis and 1 at the xenograft valve level. In 5 patients, the gradients were measured across the area of the distal anastomosis. In the majority (26 of 36 patients), the gradient was less than 40 mmHg.

A significant residual shunt at the ventricular level (Qp/Qs > 2:1) was present in 2 of the 78 patients with tetralogy of Fallot.

Comment

In 1977 our initial experience with 56 valved conduits was reviewed.[9] At that time, we were interested in distinguishing those problems related to

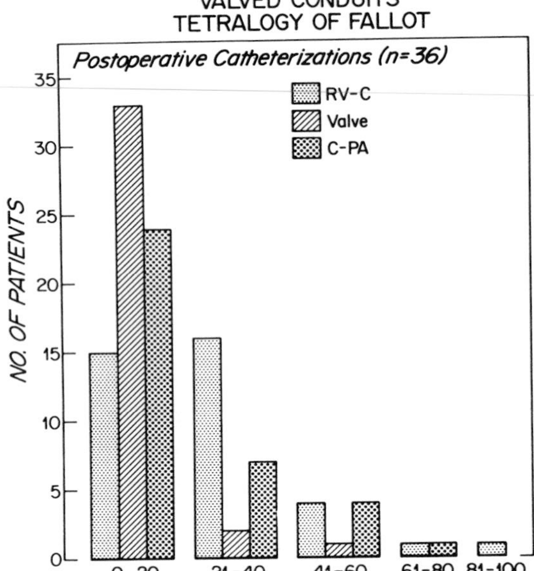

FIG. 3 Late postoperative pressure gradients across valved conduits in patients after tetralogy of Fallot repair. C: conduit.

technical details and therefore potentially subject to improvement from those inherent in the conduit itself. For example, in the initial review, it was recognized that progressive stenosis can occur from external compression by the sternum. By avoiding substernal positioning of conduits, only 2 of the patients in the present series had important external conduit compression causing gradients of 50 and 65 mmHg. Interestingly, both of these patients had an exuberant internal peel originating at the point of maximal conduit indentation by the sternum.

In addition to external compression, sites of potential obstruction within the conduit were identified. Although originally quite concerned about the high incidence of gradients across the distal anastomosis, subsequent experience has demonstrated that most of these gradients result from a narrowed or deformed main or branch pulmonary artery secondary to a previous systemic pulmonary artery shunt rather than the anastomosis itself. The primary cause of gradients at the proximal anastomosis has been appropriately identified to be related to the construction of the ventricular orifice. Since the use of a vertical ventriculotomy with little or no excision of ventricular muscle, no obstruction solely related to the proximal anastomosis has been identified in our patients.

Although during the first 26 months of follow-up we did not encounter any obstructive calcification of xenograft valves, 3 of the 162 long-term conduit valves became heavily calcified 5 to 6 years after implantation. This relatively low incidence of valve calcification (1.8%) contrasts markedly with a calcification rate of aortic or mitral xenograft valves placed in the pediatric age group.[10] In our experience with xenograft valves in the systemic circulation, valve failure began presenting approximately 30 months after implantation; in 16 patients followed 15 months or longer, 4 of the valves have required replacement. The reason for the significant difference in incidence of xenograft calcification between adults and children as well as between xenograft valves implanted within the left side of the circulation and those contained within Dacron conduits placed within the right side of the circulation remains unknown. Experimental and clinical studies to elucidate the possible role played by the vitamin K-dependent calcium-binding amino acid, γ-carboxyglutamic acid, continue but a causal relationship has yet to be established.[11]

Also, of recent concern is the appearance of proliferating and obstructing internal fibrous peels. It seems that the potential for the formation of internal peels, albeit not always obstructive, is inherent in all conduits. As suggested by Agarwal et al,[12] the lack of fibroblast and collagenous ingrowth to the graft fabric may set the stage for continuing dissection of luminal blood between the peel and conduit wall. In our experience, however, the incidence of obstructing internal peels has remained low.

These early and late results indicate that the use of valved conduits has greatly facilitated the management of complex congenital heart defects. Nevertheless, 10 patients in this series required reoperations for conduit-related complications (5.3%) and a continuing search for improved valved conduits is certainly warranted. In addition, the indications for valved conduits in the reconstruction of right atrial or ventricular to pulmonary artery continuity requires further clarification. At present, we have essentially abandoned the use of valved conduits for the Fontan repair, carrying out direct anastomosis between the right atrium and a pulmonary artery whenever possible. We are also experimenting with the use of nonvalved conduits in neonates or young infants with truncus arteriosus. Perhaps the use of valved conduits between the right ventricle and the pulmonary artery should be reserved primarily for patients with pulmonary hypertension or with a single pulmonary artery.[13] Clearly, the availability of valved conduits has greatly expanded the scope of corrective surgery for a large number of patients with complex congenital heart defects. Nevertheless, more long-term information is necessary to reach more definitive recommendations for their use.

References

1. Carrell A: On the experimental surgery of the thoracic aorta and the heart. Ann Surg 52:83, 1910.
2. Rodbard S, Wagner D: By-passing the right ventricle. Proc Soc Exp Biol Med 71:69, 1949.

3. Rastelli GC, Ongley PA, Davis GD, et al: Surgical repair for pulmonary valve atresia with coronary artery fistula: Report of a case. Mayo Clin Proc 40:521, 1965.
4. Donovan TJ: The experimental use of homologous vein grafts to circumvent the pulmonic valves. Surg Gynecol Obstet 90:204, 1950.
5. McGoon DC, Rastelli GC, Ongley PA: An operation for the correction of truncus arteriosus. JAMA 205:69, 1968.
6. Rastelli GC, McGoon DC, Wallace RB: Anatomic correction of transposition of the great arteries with ventricular septal defect and subpulmonic stenosis. J Thorac Cardiovasc Surg 58:545, 1969.
7. Bowman RO, Hancock WD, Malm JR: A valve containing Dacron prosthesis: Its use in restoring pulmonary artery-right ventricular continuity. Arch Surg 107:724, 1973.
8. Anderson RP, Bonchek LI, Grunkemeier GL, Lambert LE, Starr A: The analysis and presentation of surgical results by actuarial methods. J Surg Res 16:224, 1974.
9. Norwood WI, Freed MD, Rocchini AP, Bernhard WF, Castaneda AR: Experience with valved conduits for repair of congenital cardiac lesions. Ann Thorac Surg 24:223, 1977.
10. Sanders SP, Levy RJ, Freed MD, Norwood WI, Castaneda AR: Use of Hancock porcine xenografts in children and adolescents. Am J Cardiol 46:429, 1980.
11. Levy RJ, Zenker JA, Lian JB: Vitamin K-dependent calcium binding proteins in aortic valve calcification. J Clin Invest 65:563, 1980.
12. Agarwal KC, Edwards WD, Feldt RH, Danielson GK, Puga FJ, McGoon DC: Pathogenesis of non-obstructive fibrous peels in right-sided porcine-valved extracardiac conduits. J Thorac Cardiovasc Surg 83:584, 1982.
13. Mistrot J, Neal W, Lyons G, Moller J, Lucas R, Castaneda A, Varco R, Nicoloff D: Pulmonary valvulotomy under inflow stasis for isolated pulmonary stenosis. Ann Thorac Surg 21:30, 1976.

20

Factors Influencing Late Results of Extracardiac Conduit Repair for Congenital Cardiac Defects

D. C. McGoon, G. K. Danielson, H. V. Schaff, F. J. Puga, D. G. Ritter, D. D. Mair, D. M. Ilstrup, W. D. Edwards

Use of an extracardiac conduit between the right ventricle and the pulmonary artery has allowed repair of pulmonary atresia, persistent truncus arteriosus, transposition of the great arteries with pulmonary stenosis, and other complex forms of congenital heart disease. At this institution, a large experience with extracardiac conduit repair has accrued. Early results have been detailed by Ciaravella et al,[1] and analysis of late follow-up data has recently been reported.[2] This paper summarizes clinical experience with extracardiac conduit repair and focuses on those factors that might predict a good outcome.

Clinical Experience

From 1964 through June 1977, 468 patients received an extracardiac conduit for repair of congenital heart disease. As previously reported by Ciaravella et al,[1] there were 271 males (58%) and 197 females. Ages at the initial operation ranged from 14 days to 52 years (Table I). A summary of the diagnoses is presented in Table II. These 468 patients received a total of 474 conduits (6 patients also received conduits for left ventricular outflow reconstruction). Aortic homografts were used in 130 patients during the initial repair, and the Hancock (Hancock Laboratories, Anaheim, CA) conduit was used in 333 patients. In 4 patients a valveless Dacron tube graft was used, and a pericardial tube graft was constructed in 1 patient. In 244 patients a previous palliative operation had been performed, including 2

From the Mayo Clinic and Mayo Foundation, Rochester, Minnesota.

TABLE I Age distribution of patients at definitive operation

Age (yrs)	# pts	% total
0–1	28	6
2–4	75	16
5–9	174	37
10–19	146	31
20–52	45	10
Total	468	100

such procedures in 58 patients and 3 previous operations in 3 patients. At the time of surgical repair, 168 patients had closure of systemic pulmonary artery shunts. The details of operative repair were determined by the patient's particular anomaly. In general, an effort was made to provide the maximum diameter at the anastomoses of the conduit. By positioning of the valve as close as possible to the distal anastomosis, risk of compression by the sternum was minimized. The side of the aorta to which the conduit was

TABLE II Diagnoses*

	pts		
	#		%
Transposition of great arteries	121		26
With PS and VSD		94	
With VSD alone		9	
With VSD and previous banding		12	
With PS alone		6	
Truncus arteriosus	120		26
With previous banding		41	
Without banding		79	
Pulmonary atresia with VSD	113		24
Double-outlet right ventricle	30		6
With PS or banding		15	
With AV discordance, VSD, and PS		15	
Univentricular heart	28		6
Tetralogy of Fallot	23		5
AV discordance	15		3
Tricuspid atresia	9		2
Pulmonary and tricuspid atresia	3		<1
LV outflow tract obstruction	3		<1
Miscellaneous	3		<1
Total	468		100

*PS: pulmonary stenosis; VSD: ventricular septal defect; AV discordance: atrioventricular discordance (corrected transposition of great arteries); LV: left ventricular.

placed was determined by the relative position of the ascending aorta and the pulmonary artery. Right ventricular outflow reconstruction with conduit placement to the left of the aorta was possible in most patients with pulmonary atresia, truncus arteriosus, or tetralogy of Fallot (318 patients, 68%). When the ascending aorta was anterior or to the left, the conduit was generally placed on the right (141 patients, 30%).

Including all deaths within 30 days of operation, mortality was 25% (116 patients). Early mortality was similar within the diagnostic groups except that it was lower with pulmonary atresia and with tetralogy of Fallot and higher with univentricular heart. In general, the early mortality decreased during the years of the study. in spite of the fact that more complicated anomalies were undertaken for repair in the most recent period.

Late Follow-Up

Information supplied by return patient visits or reports supplied through correspondence or telephone contact were current to within 1 year of the study in 97.3% of patients. A clinical assessment (involving the patient or parent) was categorized as follows: good, in which the patient has no restrictions in activities and no known complications or illnesses; fair, in which the patient has one or more complications or illnesses or is restricted in activities; poor, in which the patient is restricted in activities and has not been improved by operation; and dead. Patients were further divided according to the principal congenital anomaly: truncus arteriosus, pulmonary atresia with ventricular septal defect, complete transposition of the great arteries with ventricular septal defect, pulmonary stenosis, or other. The final classification was by the type of conduit used: frozen, irradiated homograft aorta with valve, or Dacron tube with porcine valve (Hancock conduit). Patient survival was estimated by the Kaplan-Meier method, and the log rank test was used to test whether patient survival was associated with a discrete variable. The Cox regression method was used to assess associations between a continuous variable in patient survival and to measure the association with survival of more than 1 continuous or discrete variable in combination.

At the time of last follow-up, 296 (63%) of the 468 patients were living, and their mean length of follow-up was 65 months (±30, SD). One hundred sixteen patients had early deaths (within 30 days of operation) and 56 patients (12%) died late after repair. Clinical assessment could be defined in 349 patients and is presented in Table III. Of early survivors, 53% were classified in the good category and 28% were classified as fair; 16% have died late. Patients having pulmonary atresia showed a more favorable status by clinical assessment than did the remaining subgroups ($p < 0.001$, chi-square test). Of the 274 patients who were alive at the end of follow-up and

TABLE III Late status of operative survivors by clinical assessment

	#	%	Pulmonary atresia subgroup* (%)
Good	186	53	63
Fair	98	28	31
Poor	9	3	1
Dead	56	16	5
Total	349	100	100

* The pulmonary atresia subgroup had a better outcome (good plus fair) than the remaining subgroup ($p < 0.001$, chi-square test).

for whom information was available, 60% of the 25 who were not well and 23% of the 249 who considered themselves well were receiving cardiac medications, including digitalis or a diuretic, or both. The overall incidence of patients receiving medications was 26%.

Of the 352 patients who survived the first operation, 56 (16%) required reoperation. The major cause for reoperation was development of a gradient across the conduit (77% of reoperations). Residual septal defect was the cause for reoperation in almost all of the remainder of the patients. Five patients (9%) of the 56 patients who were reoperated on died of causes related to reoperation. Reoperation did not influence survival in comparison with all patients after the first operation. The probability of reoperation for the entire group who survived the initial conduit insertion was 3% at 1 year, 14% at 5 years, and 44% at 10 years. Patients who had complete transposition of the great arteries had a significantly higher incidence of reoperation than did patients with persistent truncus arteriosus or pulmonary atresia ($p < 0.005$) (Fig. 1). The incidence of reoperation according to the type of conduit used is shown in Fig. 2. At 5 years postoperatively, the likelihood of reoperation was 28% for patients having aortic homograft conduits and 6% for those with the Hancock conduit ($p = 0.001$). The likelihood of reoperation increased to 59% in 10 years for the homograft group. There was a higher incidence of reoperation in patients with conduits placed to the right of the aorta ($p = 0.08$).

For the entire group of 352 patients surviving initial operation, the estimated survival at 5 years is 85% and at 10 years, 73%. The decline averaged 2.7% per year. There was no significant difference in survival in patients with truncus arteriosus, transposition of the great arteries, or other groups. There was, however, a better survival for the group with pulmonary atresia with ventricular septal defect ($p < 0.006$). This improved rate of survival would have been further enhanced if the 23 patients with tetralogy of Fallot had been combined with the pulmonary atresia group. Survival curves for patients with a homograft conduit were similar to those for patients with the Hancock conduit.

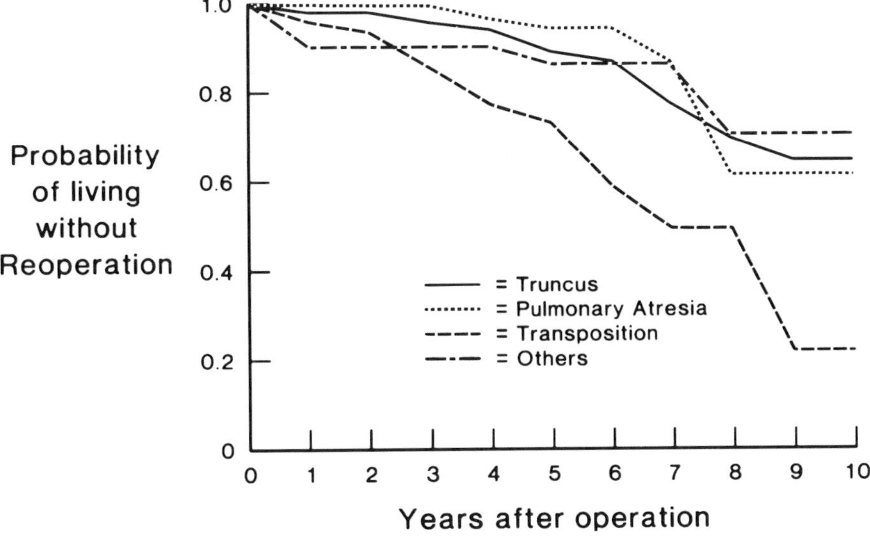

FIG. 1 Plots showing freedom from reoperation at various postoperative intervals among patients surviving initial operation, with respect to the type of congenital anomaly. The incidence of reoperation was higher for transposition of the great arteries ($p < 0.005$).

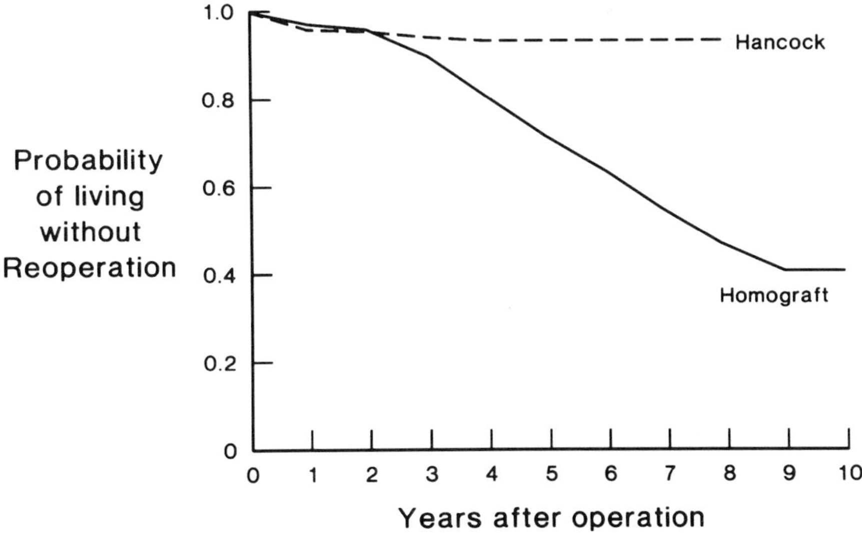

FIG. 2 Plots showing freedom from reoperation among patients surviving initial operation with respect to the type of extracardiac conduit which was placed. Reoperation was more common in the homograft group ($p = 0.001$).

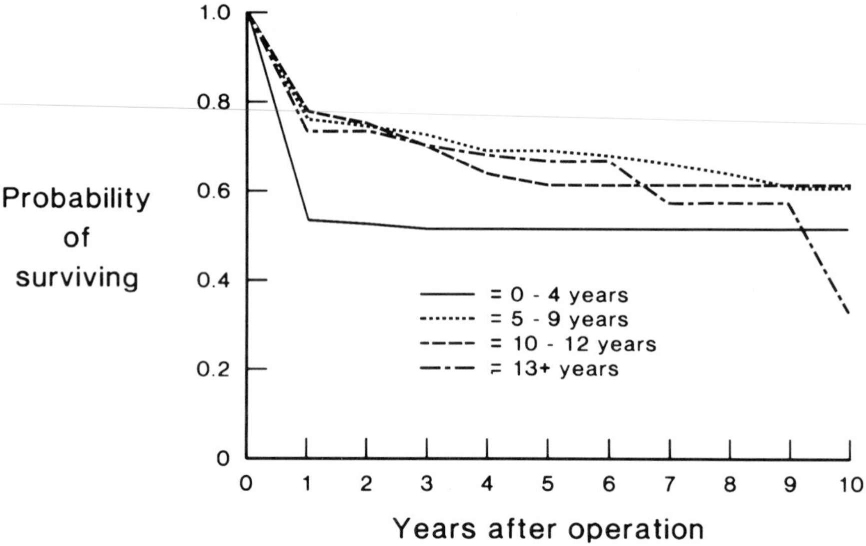

FIG. 3 Plots showing survival, including patients who died in the early postoperative period, with respect to age grouping. Overall survival was significantly less good ($p < 0.04$) for the youngest age group as a result of the high hospital mortality. Excluding the early operative deaths, this youngest age group had the lowest late mortality ($p < 0.03$).

Several variables were examined for their influence on late results of operation in patients who were early survivors. Because of the small number of patients operated on during infancy (12 patients were less than 1 year of age), this group was combined with that of children less than 5 years old. This youngest group had the highest operative mortality but also the lowest late mortality ($p < 0.03$). Late survival was not different among the other age groups. Actuarial survival for the age groupings, including perioperative death, is seen in Fig. 3.

Of the preoperative variables tested (Table IV), none had a bearing on risk of late death. Among the intraoperative variables, no influence on late death was found with respect to the side of the ascending aorta to which the conduit was placed or with respect to the postrepair transconduit gradient. The level of postrepair right ventricular to left ventricular peak pressure ratio and the postrepair pulmonary arterial peak systolic pressure did influence late survival (Table V).

Postoperative complications had an unfavorable effect on hospital mortality, as reported by Ciaravella et al[1] In addition, patients whose operative recovery was complicated, including those with arrhythmias, low cardiac output, congestive heart failure, or pulmonary failure, had a poorer long-term prognosis than patients with uncomplicated recoveries. The only complication for which this was not true was postoperative renal failure. There

TABLE IV Variables not influencing incidence of late death*

Variable*	Group	#	Late deaths (#)
Preoperative cardiothoracic ratio	≤0.6	273	42
	>0.6	79	14
Preoperative hemoglobin level	0–19 g	264	40
	>19 g	88	16
Preoperative pulmonary resistance	0–8 units·m^2	130	19
	>8 units·m^2	46	12
Prior cardiac operation	Yes	153	20
	No	199	36
Prior banding of pulmonary artery	Yes	19	2
	No	333	54
Side of aorta to which conduit was placed	Right	104	20
	Left	245	35
Intraoperative postrepair gradient across conduit	<15 mmHg	76	12
	15–30 mmHg	110	15
	>30 mmHg	69	10
Early postoperative renal dysfunction	Yes	7	1
	No	335	51

* $p > 0.05$.

TABLE V Variables influencing incidence of late death

Variable*	Group	#	Late death (#)	Probability of death (%) At 2 yrs	Probability of death (%) At 5 yrs	Significance†
Intraoperative postrepair P_{RV}/P_{LV}	<0.73	229	28	5	11	<0.02
	≥0.73	99	23	9	20	
Intraoperative postrepair P_p	<50 mmHg	204	25	3	11	<0.01
	≥50 mmHg	53	13	11	22	
Early postop complication	Yes	198	38	9	17	<0.05
	No	151	18	3	12	
Early postop rhythm disturbance	Yes	118	25	10	20	<0.05
	No	224	29	5	12	
Early postop low cardiac output	Yes	78	18	17	24	<0.02
	No	265	35	4	12	
Early postop congestive heart failure	Yes	42	13	14	33	<0.01
	No	300	40	6	12	
Early postop pulmonary failure	Yes	32	10	16	22	<0.05
	No	312	44	6	13	

* P_{RV}/P_{LV}: right ventricular over left ventricular peak systolic pressure ratio; P_p: pulmonary arterial peak systolic pressure.

† Log rank test for discrete variables and Cox regression model for continuous variables. Although the continuous variables were tested for significance as such, the data of the table are given in semiarbitrary groupings for comparison.

TABLE VI Causes of late death

Cause	Total #	
Congestive heart failure	22 (39%)	
Probable myocardial cause		13
Known hemodynamic burden*		9
Sudden death (probable arrhythmia)	18 (32%)	
Without } preceding congestive heart		13
With } failure or hemodynamic burden*		5
Associated with reoperation	5	
Persistent arrhythmia	2	
Dehiscence of aortic valve prosthesis	2	
Unrelated (noncardiovascular)	2	
Mediastinal hemorrhage (homograft)	1	
Renal failure	1	
Cerebral hemorrhage	1	
Bacterial endocarditis on conduit	1	
Unknown	1	
Total	56†	

* Intracardiac shunt, deficient pulmonary arterial "runoff," severe pulmonary vascular obstructive disease, aortic insufficiency, conduit stenosis, and so on.
† Total represents 16% of 352 early survivors.

was no relationship between late result and the side of the ascending aorta at which the conduit had been placed.

The primary causes of the 56 late deaths are listed in Table VI. Autopsies had been performed in 32 of the 56 patients. Progressive congestive heart failure, usually secondary to apparent myocardial failure, and sudden death, usually in the setting of stable active status, occurred most commonly, accounting for 39% and 32% of late deaths, respectively.

Surgical-Pathologic Findings

During the follow-up period, 11 patients with Hancock conduits required reoperation. In addition, 2 specimens were available in which the initial conduit operation was performed elsewhere but the obstructive conduits were replaced at our institution. The abnormalities of all 13 conduit specimens have been detailed.[3] Signs of conduit obstruction in these patients included increasing intensity of murmurs in 11 patients (85%), cyanosis in 2 patients (15%), and heart failure in 1. In only 6 of the 13 patients was the conduit stenosis correctly localized by angiography alone, but continuous pressure recordings during pullback of the catheter from the pulmonary arteries into the right ventricle provided reasonably accurate preoperative assessment of the site or sites of obstruction within the conduit.

The site of major obstruction was at the level of the valve in 9 patients (69%), and in 5 of these patients there was no other area of obstruction in the conduits. Calcification was present in the valvular stenosis in all 9 conduits (Fig. 4). It began as mineralization of the porcine aorta near the commissures and progressed until the leaflets were fixed in a semiclosed position. Valvular incompetence often coexisted with stenosis and was primarily due to cusp tears or to fusion of the cusps to either the porcine aorta or the distal conduit. A fibrous peel (neointima) was present within each conduit, but the thickness varied considerably. The fibrous peel re-

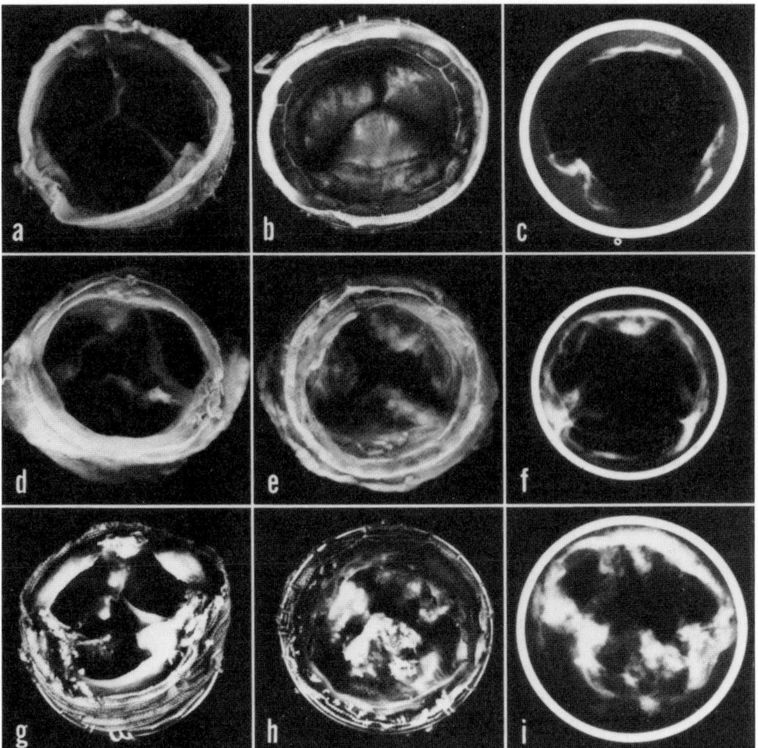

FIG. 4 Stenosis of porcine valves caused by progressive calcification and commissural fusion. Valves are viewed from above (*a, d,* and *g*) and from below, both grossly (*b, e,* and *h*) and roentgenographically (*c, f,* and *i*). Panels *a, b,* and *c* show early calcification of the porcine aorta and the aortic valve commissures, with mild stenosis resulting from muscular band in lower valve cusps. Panels *d, e,* and *f* demonstrate moderate calcification, resulting in rigid cusps and one fused commissure. In panels *g* through *i,* severe calcification of the porcine aorta and aortic valve cusps is seen with markedly deformed and rigid cusps and fusion of two commissures. Reproduced with permission of the C. V. Mosby Company from Agarwal et al.[3]

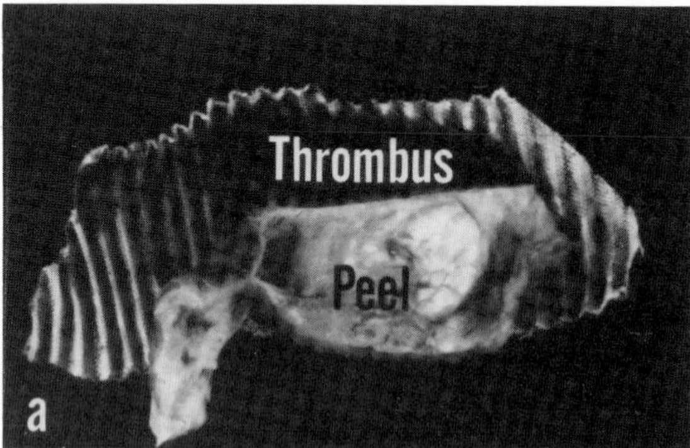

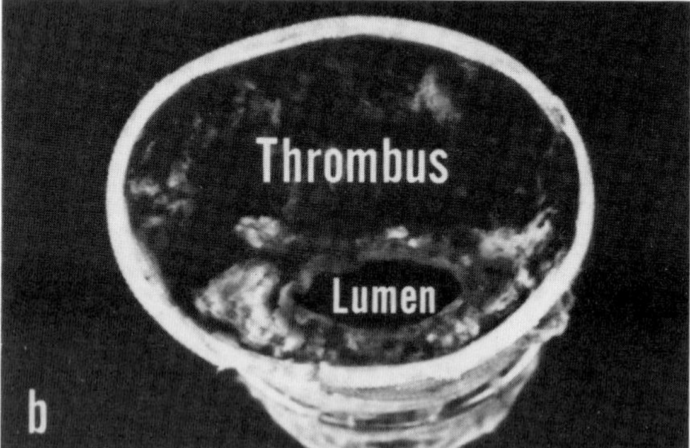

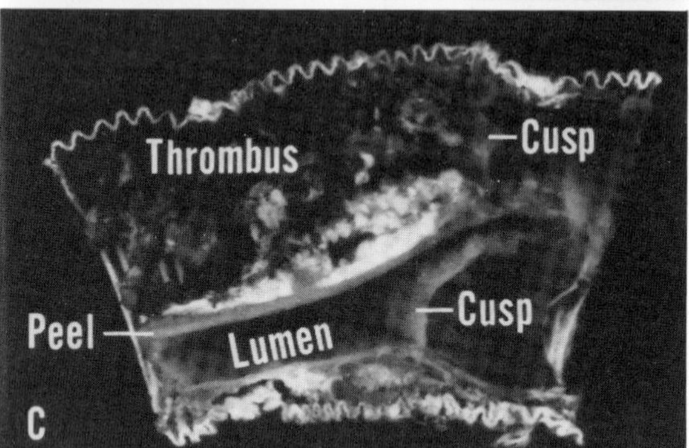

FIG. 5 Thrombus between peel and conduit. In panel *a* is seen a typical small thrombus. In panels *b* and *c* there is an unusually extensive thrombus, and marked conduit obstruction extends to the level of the porcine valve (*b:* cross section; *c:* longitudinal section). Reproduced with permission of the C. V. Mosby Company from Agarwal et al.[3]

sulted in major obstruction proximal to the porcine valve (proximal conduit) in 5 of the 13 cases (38%). In 6 patients, the peel produced obstruction beyond the valve in the distal conduit or side branches. In most cases, the peel was separated from the conduit by a layer of thrombus (Fig. 5). In 1 case, an extensive thrombus separated the peel from the conduit and caused severe obstruction similar to an aortic dissection. It appeared that the peel had become thickened by organization of thrombus between the conduit and the peel rather than by organization and progressive layering of mural thrombi.

Comment

In 1965, Rastelli and associates[4] described the use of an extracardiac conduit for correction of pulmonary atresia. One year later, Ross and Somerville[5] reported the repair of tetralogy of Fallot with pulmonary atresia with the use of an aortic homograft and an integral valve. The use of the aortic homograft with a valve was extended to the correction of truncus arteriosus and to complex transposition of the great vessels.[6,7] In 1973, Bowman and associates[8] first used clinically a glutaraldehyde-preserved porcine valve and a Dacron tube graft. Many variations in the use of the conduit to establish right ventricle to pulmonary artery continuity have been described and have permitted repair of a wide variety of complex congenital heart problems. Although several centers have reported satisfactory early results with the use of extracardiac conduits, long-term results of such operations are uncertain.[9–16] Although definitive hemodynamic data were not obtained regularly in patients in this study, clinical evaluation suggests that approximately three-fourths of patients who survived operation remain considerably improved in comparison with their preoperative status. In spite of the lack of comprehensive information regarding the natural history of these complex anomalies, it is probable that patients receiving extracardiac conduit repair had improved survival as a result of their "corrective" surgery.

In assessing factors that were predictive of a good result after extracardiac conduit repair, we found that patients with transposition of the great arteries required reoperation significantly more often than did patients having other anomalies. The causes for this are unclear, but perhaps the fact that the conduit was placed to the right of the ascending aorta most often in patients with transposition is a factor.

For the overall group, the probability of surviving beyond the first 10 postoperative years was 73%, and it was even more favorable for patients with pulmonary atresia and ventricular septal defect. This is consistent with the previous observation that late results of operation for patients having tetralogy of Fallott are excellent.[17] Conduit repair may provide dramatic improvement in clinical status, with elimination of cyanosis and considerable improvement in exercise tolerance. Late deaths were primarily due to progressive congestive heart failure or sudden death, probably as a consequence of arrhythmia. Inadequate technical repair was uncommonly implicated. Although these deaths might be attributable in part to inadequate myocardial protection during operation, it seems likely that long-standing myocardial hypertrophy and fibrosis that developed preoperatively and were aggravated by incisions, excisions, and suturing of the ventricular walls were important contributing factors. In this regard, it is interesting that patients who survived definitive repair during infancy or early childhood had strikingly reduced late mortality. If risk of perioperative mortality can be reduced, early operation is to be recommended.

It is our policy to advise complete repair promptly for patients who have truncus associated with heart failure and, in any case, before 2 years of age; for infants with truncus who have significant associated problems, such as pulmonary infection, bilateral proximal banding of the pulmonary arteries is often performed. Other patients with high pulmonary blood flow due to still more complex anomalies, such as univentricular heart, are palliated by banding the pulmonary artery if heart failure persists during infancy; and, in any case, their pulmonary vasculature should be protected by banding before age 2 years. For most patients who have pulmonary stenosis as part of a complex anomaly that, for repair, would probably require insertion of an extracardiac conduit, observation until age 5 is preferred unless pulmonary blood flow is severely reduced and disability is pronounced, in which case a systemic to pulmonary arterial shunt is constructive.

The other variable that was found to influence late survival was the post-repair ratio of peak systolic pressure in the right (pulmonary) ventricle divided by that in the left (systemic) ventricle (P_{RV}/P_{LV}). This ratio represents a composite of several determinants of right ventricular afterload, including 1) pulmonary vascular resistance, 2) adequacy of pulmonary arterial size, branching, and distribution, and 3) any obstruction between the pulmonary ventricle and the artery. When the patients are ranked according to groups of 10 percentiles from the lowest to the highest level of P_{RV}/P_{LV}, the point at which survival is affected is about the 70th percentile, which is at a P_{RV}/P_{LV} of 0.73. This is consistent with impressions from early experiences.

The durability of the conduit is of great importance in assessing late results. Previous reports from this clinic and from other institutions demonstrated a high incidence of aortic homograft calcification and obstruction.[1,9,18,19] It appears that calcification in the homografts is related to the method of preparation and sterilization. In this series, the homografts were frozen and sterilized with high-intensity radiation. Fresh homograft sterilized in antibiotic solution may have a much lower incidence of calcific obstruction than homografts prepared by physical-chemical means. Saravalli et al[15] observed that in 37 of 40 patients (92%) with congenital heart disease, calcification developed in the aortic homografts preserved by various techniques used for right ventricular outflow reconstruction. The degree of calcification, however, was mild to moderate in 35 patients and severe in only 2 patients. Of the 28 patients who had fresh homografts, none had exuberant proliferation of the calcium which caused obstruction.

In the present series, the risk of reoperation in patients with the Hancock conduit was 6% at 5 years.

As emphasized by Agarwal et al,[3] conduit stenosis was caused solely by degenerative changes in the porcine valve in about one-third of cases and by both valvular stenosis and peel formation in the conduit in another third of patients. This finding raises a question whether or not many patients with normal pulmonary vascular development and resistance might have a better long-term result if the conduit contained no valve at all, especially since patients who have had repair for tetralogy seem to tolerate absence of the functional pulmonary valve so well. This possibility is further supported by the failure in the present study to identify a single instance in which reoperation or a poor result could be attributed primarily to the presence of regurgitation through the degenerating valve conduit. However, the fact that Agarwal et al[3] found that conduit stenosis was a result only of peel formation inside the tubular portion of the conduit in one-third of cases, and was due to peel formation along with valvular degeneration in another third, suggests that the use of a valveless conduit of the same woven Dacron construction might reduce but would not eliminate the problem of progressive conduit stenosis. In addition, the woven Dacron is nonporous for reasons of hemostasis. This characteristic, however, hinders the formation of a fibrous anchor between the conduit wall and the neointima. Recurrent separation of the peel from the conduit may be the mechanism of the progressive fibrous thickening and in some patients may cause actual dissection of the fibrous peel and "acute" conduit obstruction.[3]

In summary, it appears that conduit reconstruction to establish right ventricle to pulmonary artery continuity has provided major improvement in quality of life and longevity for many patients with complex congenital heart disease. As emphasized in the present study, however, late conduit failure mandates a careful follow-up of these patients and suggests the need for exploration of new techniques and materials to obtain optimal long-term results.

References

1. Ciaravella JM Jr, McGoon DC, Danielson GK, Wallace RB, Mair DD, Ilstrup DM: Experience with the extracardiac conduit. J Thorac Cardiovasc Surg 78:920, 1979.
2. McGoon DC, Danielson GK, Puga FJ, Ritter DG, Mair DD, Ilstrup DM: Late results after extracardiac conduit repair for congenital cardiac defects. Am J Cardiol 49:1741, 1982.
3. Agarwal KC, Edwards WD, Feldt RH, Danielson GK, Puga FJ, McGoon DC: Clinicopathological correlates of obstructed right-sided porcine-valved extracardiac conduits. J Thorac Cardiovasc Surg 81:591, 1981.
4. Rastelli GC, Ongley PA, Davis GD, Kirklin JW: Surgical repair for pulmonary

valve atresia with coronary-pulmonary artery fistula: Report of case. Mayo Clin Proc 40:521, 1965.

5. Ross DN, Somerville J: Correction of pulmonary atresia with a homograft aortic valve. Lancet 2:1446, 1966.
6. McGoon DC, Rastelli GC, Ongley PA: An operation for the correction of truncus arteriosus. JAMA 205:69, 1968.
7. Rastelli GC: A new approach to "anatomic" repair of transposition of the great arteries. Mayo Clin Proc 44:1, 1969.
8. Bowman FO Jr, Hancock WD, Malm JR: A valve-containing Dacron prosthesis: Its use in restoring pulmonary artery-right ventricular continuity. Arch Surg 107:724, 1973.
9. Bailey WW, Kirklin JW, Bargeron LM Jr, Pacifico AD, Kouchoukos NT: Late results with synthetic valved external conduits from venous ventricle to pulmonary arteries. Circulation 56 (Suppl II):73, 1977.
10. Norwood WI, Freed MD, Rocchini AP, Bernhard WF, Castaneda AR: Experience with valved conduits for repair of congenital cardiac lesions. Ann Thorac Surg 24:223, 1977.
11. West PN, Hartmann AF Jr, Weldon CS: Long-term function of aortic homografts as the right ventricular outflow tract. Circulation 56 (Suppl II):66, 1977.
12. Heck HA Jr, Schieken RM, Lauer RM, Doty DB: Conduit repair for complex congenital heart disease: Late follow-up. J Thorac Cardiovasc Surg 75: 806, 1978.
13. Hazan E, Bex JP, Chétochine FL, Lecompte Y, Lemoine G, de Riberolles C, Neveux JY: Les tubes valvulés sur la voie pulmonaire: Résultats d'une série de 45 interventions. Arch Mal Coeur 72:470, 1979.
14. Shabbo FP, Wain WH, Ross DN: Right ventricular outflow reconstruction with aortic homograft conduit: Analysis of the long-term results. Thorac Cardiovasc Surg 28:21, 1980.
15. Saravalli OA, Somerville J, Jefferson KE: Calcification of aortic homografts used for reconstruction of the right ventricular outflow tract. J Thorac Cardiovasc Surg 80:909, 1980.
16. Bisset GS III, Schwartz DC, Benzing G III, Helmsworth J, Schreiber JT, Kaplan S: Late results of reconstruction of the right ventricular outflow tract with porcine xenografts in children. Ann Thorac Surg 31:437, 1981.
17. Fuster V, McGoon DC, Kennedy MA, Ritter DG, Kirklin JW: Long-term evaluation (12 to 22 years) of open heart surgery for tetralogy of Fallot. Am J Cardiol 46:635, 1980.
18. Moodie DS, Mair DD, Fulton RE, Wallace RB, Danielson GK, McGoon DC: Aortic homograft obstruction. J Thorac Cardiovasc Surg 72:553, 1976.
19. Park SC, Neches WH, Lenox CC, Zuberbuhler JR, Bahnson HT: Massive calcification and obstruction in a homograft after the Rastelli procedure for transposition of great arteries. Am J Cardiol 32:860, 1973.

21

Calcification of Porcine Bioprostheses in Children

J. A. ODELL

Valve replacement in children in undertaken with some reluctance. There is concern principally regarding the durability of the replaced valve in a population whose life expectancy following the valve replacement is far greater than that of adults. With the use of prosthetic valves without anticoagulants, there is concern regarding thromboembolism and valve clotting on the one hand and hemorrhage after trauma with the use of anticoagulants on the other hand. Because of difficulty in obtaining homograft valves and control of anticoagulation in children, the porcine bioprosthetic valve was implanted. This report documents the high incidence of valve dysfunction, principally calcification affecting mainly the mitral valve, in children.

Clinical Materials

During the period October 1975 to October 1980, 212 patients younger than 15 years received a porcine bioprosthetic heart valve. During the same period lonescu-Shiley and homograft valves were also used. Porcine valves were implanted in 701 patients older than 15 years during the same period.

The majority of the patients fell in the age group 11–15 years (Table I).

The mitral valve was replaced in 185 patients and the aortic valve in only 27 patients. Hancock and Carpentier-Edwards valves were used equally frequently in the mitral position but the Carpentier-Edwards valve was used more often in the aortic position (Table II).

The etiologic factors are listed in Table III. All patients were in functional class III or IV (NYHA classification). The majority of the patients demon-

From the Department of Thoracic Surgery, University of Natal, Durban, South Africa.

TABLE I Age and sex distribution of 212 children who underwent porcine valve replacement

	# cases		
Age (yrs)	Male	Female	Total
0–5	4	1	5
5–10	21	38	59
11–15	73	75	148
Total	98	114	212

TABLE II Distribution of replaced valves

	# children	
Site of replacement	Hancock	Carpentier-Edwards
Single		
Mitral	75	69
Aortic	4	23
Double		
Mitral and tricuspid		1
Mitral and aortic	13	27

TABLE III Etiologic factors

Aortic		
Congenital	6	
Rheumatic heart disease	19	(4 acute)
SBE	1	
Iatrogenic damage	1	
	27	
Mitral		
Congenital	3	
SBE	3	
Rheumatic heart disease	121	(16 acute)
Chordal rupture	3	
Cardiomyopathy	2	
Previous valve replacement (homograft)	11	
	143	
Multiple		
Rheumatic	42	(10 acute)
Total	212	

strated marked cardiomegaly radiographically. Four patients had atrial fibrillation.

Results

Mortality Rate

There were 16 deaths in the early postoperative period, giving an overall mortality rate of 7.6%. There were 9 deaths (6.3%) following mitral valve replacement, 2 deaths (7.4%) following aortic valve replacement, and 4 (10%) after mitral and aortic valve replacement. The 1 patient whose mitral and tricuspid valves were replaced died.

At follow-up, 29% were lost, leaving 138 patients available for follow-up. There were 18 known late deaths. In the mitral group there were 9 deaths. In 2 the cause was unknown, 4 patients had calcified valves, 1 died with clinical evidence of stenosis, 1 died following repeat cardiac surgery (she had 2 Hancock valves that had calcified and 2 St. Jude valves that clotted despite anticoagulation followed by insertion of a homograft); 1 patient died of subacute bacterial endocarditis (SBE). In the aortic group there were 4 deaths, 3 for unknown causes, 1 of SBE. In those having double valve replacement 5 died, 2 were proved to have calcified valves and 3 had clinical evidence of stenosis (1 died of pneumonia and 1 of SBE).

Reoperations

Further valve-related surgery was needed in 55 patients (Table IV). In the mitral valve replacement group 49 patients required further valve replacement; 46 (34.1% of survivors) had calcified valves, 1 had a disrupted valve replaced 8 months after implantation, and 2 patients had aortic valve replacements for continued rheumatic activity. Further valve replacements in this group were required in 7 patients: 4 had another tissue valve implanted that calcified; 2 patients had perivalvar leaks; 1 had SBE. One patient required 5 valve replacements, 2 for calcification and 2 for clotted St. Jude valves; 3 of these operations were emergencies. She died after the fifth operation.

One patient in the aortic valve replacement group required repeat replacement at 6 months for a disrupted valve. He unfortunately required further valve replacement for SBE. Moderate calcification was noted. Five patients in the combined mitral and aortic valve replacement group required further replacements. In 2, only the mitral valve was replaced. In the remainder there was only mild to moderate calcification of the aortic valve. Two of these 5 patients required further valve replacements.

The majority of patients with calcified valves presented at a late stage when there was severe valve obstruction, with acute symptoms of cardiac

TABLE IV Reoperations

Mitral valve replacement only	
Calcification	46*
Disruption	1
Continued rheumatic activity necessitating aortic valve replacement	2
	49
Aortic valve replacement only	
Valve disruption	1†
Mitral and aortic valve replacement	
Calcification	5‡
Total	55

* Five had concomitant aortic valve replaced for continued rheumatic activity, 2 had concomitant tricuspid valve replacement, 1 had a tricuspid anuloplasty; 7 patients had further valve replacements.
† Required further valve replacement for SBE. Calcification noted.
‡ Two patients had only the mitral valve replaced; 2 patients required further valve replacements.

decompensation in the presence of pulmonary hypertension and right heart failure. Episodic pulmonary edema is common, necessitating an emergency operation as was done on 14 of those reoperated on. Cardiac catheterization was done on 20 patients and confirmed severe pulmonary hypertension, severe gradients, and reduced valve areas. At present, echocardiography is used to diagnose this complication.

Pathologic Features of Calcified Valves

The pathologic findings are essentially similar. The leaflets were yellow, exhibiting a brittle calcific consistency similar to eggshell. The leaflets were held rigidly in the closed position. There were often calcific deposits deforming the valve surface. These granular deposits tended to be more common on the outflow portions of the valve and close to the commissures. In 1 patient who developed a hemiplegia there was a large piece of calcium attached to one of the cusps by a small piece of tissue, suggesting that calcific emboli may occur. In a number of patients there were tears and holes in the cusps. A hole was found frequently in the cusp lying in relation to the aortic valve. A few of these patients had some degree of aortic incompetence and the defect may represent a "wash back" lesion. It was, however, found in patients without aortic incompetence and may be related to this leaflet being exposed to the outflow portion of the left ventricle.

The calcified areas lay within the substance of the valves and suggested dystrophic calcification. Surface thrombus was occasionally seen and foci of calcification in the thrombus was noted in a few valves. Inflammatory cells

TABLE V Calcification of valves

	Requiring reoperation	Cause of late death
Mitral		
Hancock	26	3*
Carpentier-Edwards	20	1
Aortic		
Hancock	—	—
Carpentier-Edwards	—	—
Aortic plus mitral		
Hancock	1	1
Carpentier-Edwards	4 (in 2 mitral only replaced)	1
	51	6

* One patient died of a calcified second porcine valve.

were rarely seen. We have done electron microscopy on one of the calcified valves, which showed groups of collagen fibrils in amorphous material that presumably represent products of collagen degeneration.

Comment

This is one of the largest series of valve replacements in children and also one of the largest series with calcified valves. There has been evidence of severe calcification of valves, either requiring replacement or as a cause of known late death in 56 patients (28.6% of survivors) (Table V). Calcification affected mainly the mitral valve. In the double valve replacement group, replacement was primarily for calcified mitral valves in 2 patients; the other 3 patients had evidence of mild to moderate calcification of the aortic valve.

No patient having an aortic valve replaced only has developed calcification requiring replacement, nor has this condition been known to be a cause of late death. Hancock and Carpentier-Edwards valves are involved equally frequently. Patients requiring reoperation presented within 10–51 months (mean, 31 months). In our early experience, being unaware of the problem of porcine valve calcification in children, tissue valves were implanted at the second operation. Six had porcine valves implanted, 18 bovine pericardial valves, 1 had a homograft valve implanted. The remainder have all been replaced with St. Jude valves. Of the 6 who had porcine valves reimplanted, 3 developed further calcification (1 revealed at autopsy). One patient who had a St. Jude valve implanted developed a perivalvar leak and another heterograft was implanted in the large anulus; this valve calcified and required replacement. Previous studies[1–4] have confirmed that porcine valves implanted in children calcify.

In our patients older than 15 years only 5 valves have been removed because of calcification, the oldest patient being 22 years of age. The exact cause of the increased frequency of calcification in children is not known, but possible explanations are abnormalities of calcium metabolism, immune-mediated xenograft rejection, or excessive wear and tear leading to mechanical failure.

Growing children have a higher rate of calcium turnover than adults, so it is possible that this metabolic factor may be related to heterograft calcification in children. Soft tissue calcification with normal serum calcium levels has been noted in adults with chronic renal failure and Fishbein et al[5] and Lamberti et al[6] have reported calcification of porcine valves in patients maintained on chronic dialysis.

The role of immune-mediated xenograft rejection as a cause of calcification has been well documented by Rocchini et al.[7] Carpentier et al[8] and Zuhdi et al[9] concluded that histologic changes in the formalin-treated porcine xenograft were due to persistent immunogenetic factors in the porcine valve. In an attempt to make the porcine xenograft valves less immunogenetic Carpentier and associates[8] introduced glutaraldehyde as a better compound for preserving heterograft valves. Rocchini et al[7] found that the gross and histologic changes in the glutaraldehyde-preserved xenografts in their patients were qualitatively and quantitatively similar to those in the formalin-treated xenograft, so possibly the weakly immunogenic glutaraldehyde-preserved xenografts can induce a stronger immune response in children than it can in adults. Rocchini et al[7] had a high incidence of xenograft dysfunction only when intracardiac porcine valve replacement was performed and they believed this was due to the degree of host cell ingrowth.

If calcium homeostasis and/or an immunologic response are believed to be the cause of calcification, these effects should be operative to a similar degree in valves implanted in multiple sites. We have shown that calcification affects the mitral valve more severely when both the mitral and aortic valves have been replaced. We have also shown an implanted tricuspid valve with no calcification at postmortem, but the mitral valve was heavily calcified. Similar experience has been noted by others.[2,10]

The mitral valve, because of the higher pressure it is subjected to during systole, may be susceptible to an accelerated rate of mechanical damage. When the same porcine valve is implanted in the tricuspid position, where both level and rise of pressure are considerably lower, fatigue-induced lesions are likely to appear later. Similarly, implantation of a valve in the aortic position with a relatively small orifice size in children may result in these valves being subjected to a high degree of stress.

Rocchini et al[7] stressed that extracardiac porcine valves did not develop evidence of dysfunction and he believed this was due to an extracardiac Dacron conduit offering excellent mechanical protection against host cell ingrowth. However, most of these conduits were implanted on the right side of the heart and were subjected to lower pressures. Children have a resting heart rate and a level of activity much greater than that of adults and in fact their total number of cardiac cycles a day may approach twice that of adults. Calcification is found maximally in graft tissue and close to the commissures. This deposition may be the site of maximum stress, as determined by in vitro testing[11] of tissue valves. Thus, it is probable that all of these factors—calcium metabolism, immune-mediated xenograft rejection, and excessive wear and tear—are contributory to the problems of calcification of porcine valves in children. Stress-induced damage may cause release of immunogenic components of the porcine valve and permit the host to mount an immunologic response.

In developing countries, the choice of valve replacement is difficult to make. Follow-up and control of anticoagulation is poor. Calcification in children has been a disastrous complication and at present our policy is to use the St. Jude valve, if a homograft valve is not available, in those patients having repeat surgery for calcification and those younger than 20 years of age.

References

1. Geha AS, Laks H, Stansel HC, Cornhill JF, Kilman JW, Buckley MJ, Roberts WC: Late failure of porcine valve heterografts in children. J Thorac Cardiovasc Surg 78:351, 1979.
2. Curcio CA, Commerford PJ, Rose AG, Stevens JE, Barnard MS: Calcification of glutaraldehyde-preserved porcine xenografts in young patients. J Thorac Cardiovasc Surg 81:621, 1981.
3. Thandroyen FT, Whitton ID, Pirie D, Rogers MA, Mitha AS: Severe calcification of glutaraldehyde-preserved porcine xenografts in children. Am J Cardiol 45:690, 1980.
4. Silver MS, Pollock J, Silver MD, Williams WG, Trusler GA: Calcification in porcine xenograft valves in children. Am J Cardiol 45:685, 1980.
5. Fishbein MC, Gissen SA, Collins JJ, Barsamian EM, Cohn LH: Pathologic findings after cardiac valve replacement with glutaraldehyde-fixed porcine valves. Am J Cardiol 40:331, 1977.
6. Lamberti JJ, Wainer BH, Fisher KA, Kurunaraine HB, Al-Sadir J: Calcific stenosis of the porcine heterograft. Ann Thoracic Surg 28:28, 1979.
7. Rocchini AP, Weesner KM, Heidelberger K, Keren D, Behrendt D, Rosenthal A: Porcine xenograft valve failure in children: An immunologic response. Circulation 64 (Supp. II):162, 1981.
8. Carpentier A, Lemaigre G, Robert L, Carpentier S, Dubost C: Biological factors affecting long-term results of valvular heterografts. J Thorac Cardiovasc Surg 58:467, 1969.
9. Zuhdi N, Hawley W, Voehl V: Porcine aortic valves as replacement for human heart valves. Ann Thorac Surg 17:479, 1974.
10. Bortolotti U: Calcification of porcine heterografts implanted in children. Chest 80:117, 1981.
11. Clark RE, Swanson WM, Kardos JL, Hagan RW, Beauchamp RA: Durability of prosthetic heart valves. Ann Thorac Surg 26:323, 1978.

22

Valve Replacement in Children: Biologic Versus Mechanical Valves

D. F. SHORE, M. R. DE LEVAL, J. STARK

Many clinicians have discontinued the use of tissue valves in children because of the widely reported incidence of premature valve calcification resulting in valve malfunction and the need for reoperation. However, the survival of the patient and not of the valve is of paramount importance and the risks of reoperation for tissue valve failure may be less than those of the thromboembolic complications associated with mechanical prostheses. We have employed both mechanical and bioprosthetic valves for valve replacement in children and the aim of this largely retrospective study was to determine if the use of either prosthesis was associated with any advantage.

Clinical Material

Between January 1969 and June 1981, 51 patients underwent valve replacement at the Hospital for Sick Children, London. The mean age of the patients was 6 years, 6 months and the mean weight was 19.7 kg.

Five patients were younger than 1 year of age, 20 patients were between the ages of 1 and 5 years, and the remainder between the ages of 5 and 15.5 years.

Eight patients had replacement of the systemic ventriculoarterial valve and 6 patients, replacement of the pulmonary ventriculoarterial valve. The right atrioventricular valve was replaced in 1 patient and the left atrioventricular valve in 36 patients, including 11 with transposition or corrected transposition in whom the tricuspid valve was replaced.

Forty-nine patients had congenital heart disease. Two patients who had mitral valve replacement had rheumatic valve disease.

From the Thoracic Unit, Hospital for Sick Children, London, England.

In order to compare the pathology of those undergoing insertion of a mechanical valve with those undergoing insertion of a biologic valve, the patients were divided into 4 groups according to the following criteria (Table I): those with 1) isolated valve disease, 2) transposition complexes, 3) atrioventricular septal defects, and 4) other forms of complex congenital heart disease.

In 19 patients, a Björk-Shiley tilting disc valve was used, in 10 patients a Hancock valvular xenobioprosthesis was used and 22 patients received an Ionescu-Shiley pericardial xenobioprosthesis.

The expected area of each valve being replaced according to the patient's body surface area was calculated from regression equations based on the quantitative anatomy of the normal child's heart.[1] The mean value was taken and the effective orifice area of the prosthetic valve used was expressed as a percentage of this value in each case.

A second valve replacement was required in 8 patients. In 7 patients the valve used at the second operation was a Björk-Shiley. An Ionescu-Shiley valve was used in the remaining patient.

Results

The effective orifice area of the valve used expressed as a percentage of the calculated valve area for each valve replaced is represented in Fig. 1. A wide range of values was obtained for each of the prostheses used. It can be seen that some valves were severely stenotic even at the time of their insertion, whereas others in theory had the capacity to accommodate for the somatic growth of the patient. The difficulty of making valve match patient occurred in all age groups (Fig. 2).

Hospital Mortality

The overall hospital mortality was 24%. The hospital mortality after insertion of a mechanical valve was 36.8% and 15.6% after insertion of a biologic valve. This difference is statistically significant ($p < 0.05$).

TABLE I Comparison of mechanical and biologic valves in 4 groups of patients

	Mechanical valves		Biological valves	
	#	%	#	%
Isolated valve disease	10	53	7	22
Transposition complexes	1	5	10	31
Atrioventricular septal defects	4	21	1	3
Other complex congenital heart disease	4	21	14	74
Total	19		32	

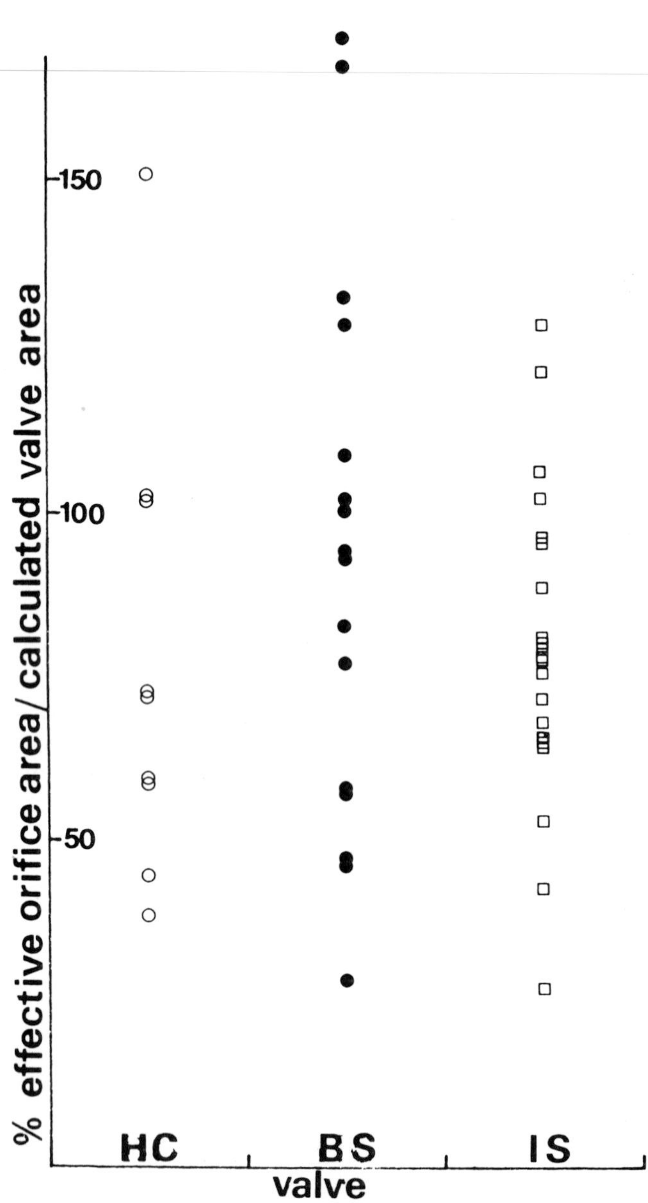

FIG. 1 The effective orifice area of the valve is expressed as a percentage of the calculated valve area in each patient and grouped according to the type of bioprosthesis.

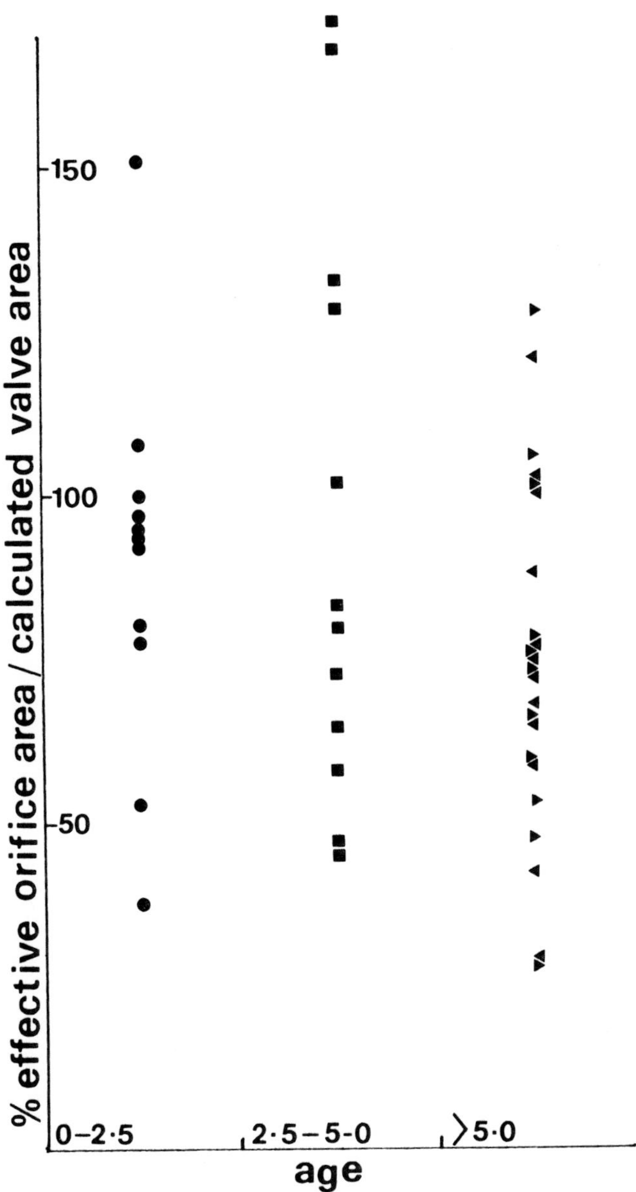

FIG. 2 The effective orifice area is expressed as a percentage of the calculated valve area according to the patient's age group.

Of the 7 patients who died following insertion of a mechanical valve, 5 had had previous heart operations; 4 of these patients had previously undergone repair of the mitral valve, 3 in association with correction of an atrioventricular septal defect and 1 had undergone a previous Mustard procedure and closure of a ventricular septal defect. Two patients died postoperatively as a result of prosthetic obstruction of the left ventricular outflow tract.

Five patients died after insertion of a biologic valve. Two of these patients had undergone a previous Mustard procedure for simple transposition, 2 patients had corrected transposition with incompetence of the left atrioventricular valve.

Late Survival

The 5-year survival calculated by actuarial methods was 53 ± 16% after insertion of a mechanical valve and 84 ± 8% after insertion of a biologic valve (Fig. 3). Four of the 6 late deaths that occurred after using a mechani-

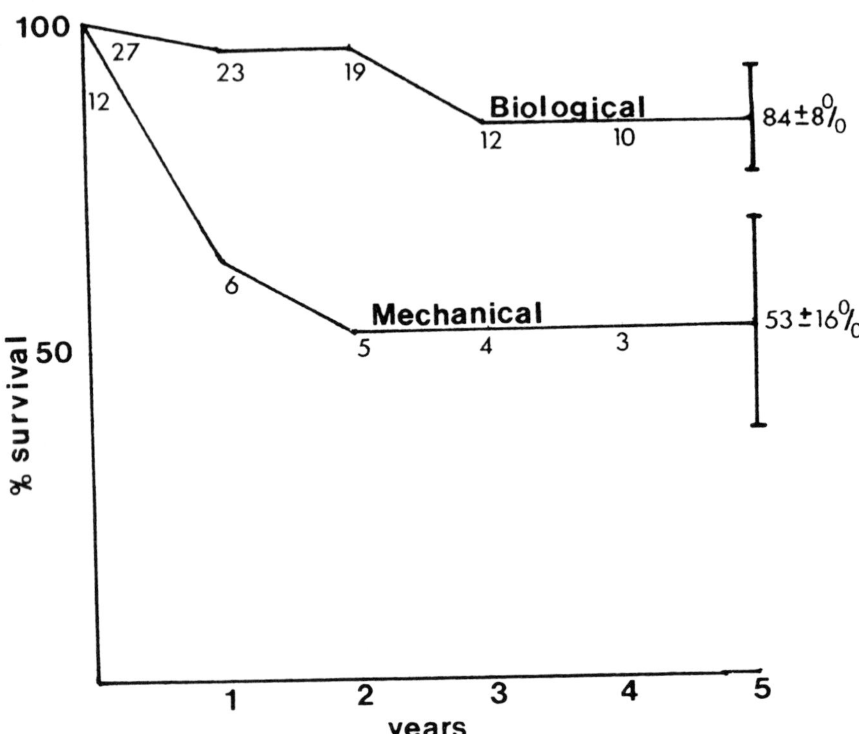

FIG. 3 The 5 year survival was calculated by actuarial methods.

cal valve were due to valve-related complications; 3 were due to valve thrombosis and malfunction and the fourth to staphylococcal endocarditis. The 2 remaining deaths were due to congestive cardiac failure, associated with pulmonary infection in one and a residual ventricular septal defect in the other.

In the group with biologic valves, 2 of the 3 late deaths were due to valve-related complications; one occurred as a result of a paraprosthetic leak and congestive cardiac failure and the other as a result of the severe stenosis from calcification of a valve in the aortic position.

Valve Degeneration

Calculated by actuarial methods, the probability that patients with tissue valves will not require a second valve replacement because of tissue valve calcification at 5 years is 27 ± 15%.

Seven valves have been replaced because of premature calcification. Six patients survived reoperation. Six of the 7 valves that required replacement were on the systemic side of the circulation. Only 1 valve required replacement because of calcification before 36 months; thereafter, there was a rapid increase in the number that required replacement (Fig. 4). There is evidence of tissue valve malfunction in 4 other patients, in 3 the valve is positioned on the pulmonary side of the circulation.

Thromboembolism

There were no incidences of thromboembolic complications in the late follow-up of patients with tissue valves. Eighty-one percent of patients with mechanical valves had an anticoagulant, warfarin, immediately after the insertion. Another patient received an anticoagulant after a cerebral embolus. One patient who did not receive an anticoagulant died as a result of prosthetic valve thrombosis, as did 2 other patients in whom anticoagulants were being administered. Calculated by actuarial methods, the chances of being free of a major thromboembolic episode 5 years after insertion of a mechanical valve was 59 ± 20% (Fig. 5).

Comment

Premature valve calcification in bioprostheses implanted in children has been widely reported.[2–6] This has resulted in many surgeons abandoning the use of bioprostheses in the pediatric and adolescent age groups. However, before accepting this view, we considered 2 points: 1) is the risk to the patient of the deteriorating function of the tissue valve and the eventual need for its replacement greater than the risks that accrue from the throm-

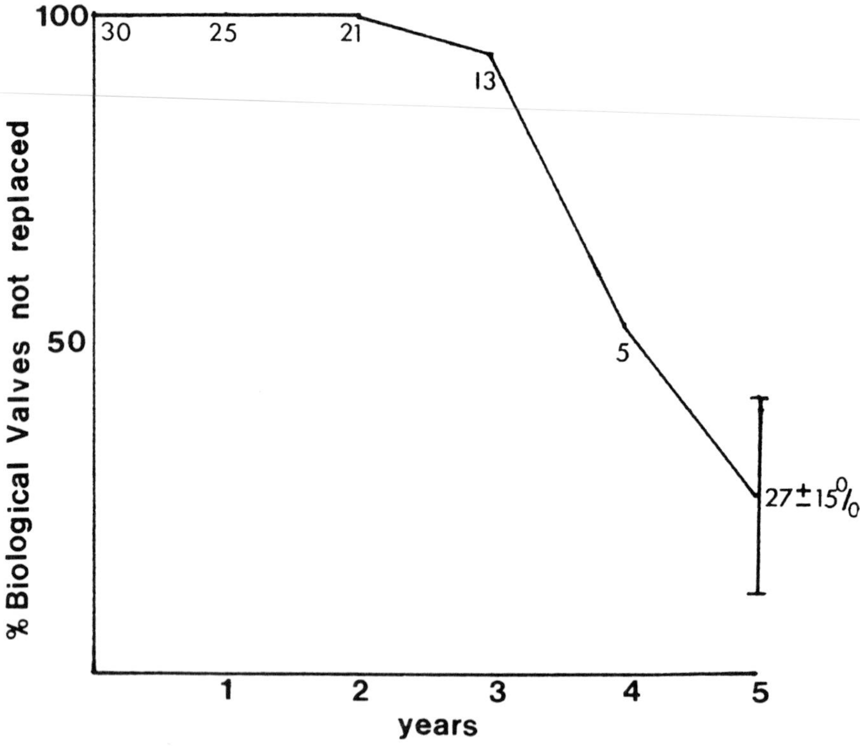

FIG. 4 The percentage of biologic valves inserted that will survive to 5 years is indicated.

boembolic complications of mechanical prostheses? 2) what is the likelihood of a second valve replacement being required because of the effect of somatic growth on prosthetic valve adequacy?

We have compared the early and late results after implantation of a Björk-Shiley tilting disc valve with those after insertion of a Hancock valvular xenobioprosthesis and an Ionescu-Shiley pericardial xenograft valve.

The overall hospital mortality of 24% in this series is high, when compared with other reported series[6–9] of between 4.3 and 12%. However, the patients in this series differ from the reported series in 2 important respects: 1) the mean age of our patients was 6.6 years and is considerably lower than that of 10–15 years in the other series; 2) the percentage of patients in our series with isolated valvular heart disease of 33% is considerably lower than the 59–100% in the other series.

The higher operative mortality in those patients undergoing valve replacement with a mechanical valve could not reliably be attributed to the prosthesis itself. Five of the 7 patients who died in this group had under-

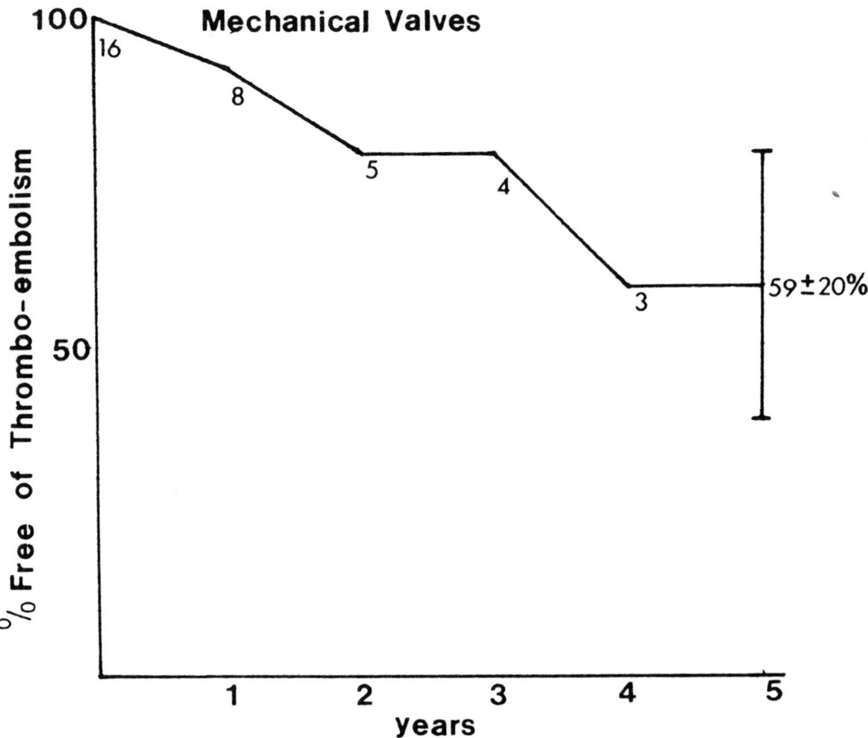

FIG. 5 The percentage of patients who will be free of thromboembolic complications at 5 years is calculated by actuarial methods.

gone a previous bypass procedure; 1 had undergone a previous Mustard procedure and 4 had undergone a previous repair of the mitral valve, in 3 of whom it was part of the correction of an atrioventricular septal defect. A high hospital mortality among patients requiring valve replacement who have previously undergone repair of an atrioventricular septal defect has been previously reported.[10] However, we performed a logistic analysis of probable short- and long-term risk factors that revealed that insertion of a mechanical valve significantly ($p < 0.05$) increased the risk of hospital death.

Our data strongly support the view that the risk to the patient of the thromboembolic complications of mechanical valves is greater than the risks of reoperation for tissue valve degeneration. It is difficult to compare the incidence of thromboembolism in our series with that of others.[7–10] The frequency of thromboembolic episodes is not presented in a standardized fashion and also the policy regarding anticoagulation varies greatly from one series to another. However, it would seem reasonable from published data to conclude that the incidence of thromboembolic complications following insertion of a mechanical prosthesis in our series is higher than that in other reported series in which the majority of patients received a Starr-Edwards valve. Indeed, the incidence of thromboembolic complications after insertion of a Starr-Edwards valve in the pediatric and adolescent age group is surprisingly low, considering that many of the patients had not been anticoagulated. In a recent report, Pass et al[12] reported no thromboembolic complications in 18 patients in the pediatric and adolescent age groups who received a St. Jude mechanical prosthesis and who were not maintained on anticoagulants.

One argument that can be applied in favor of tissue valves is that, since both tissue and mechanical valves will require replacement because of somatic growth, the problems of tissue valve degeneration and the consequent need for reoperation have been overemphasized.

However, this argument can only be generally applied if at the time of prosthetic insertion the valve and the patient are an ideal match. Reference to Figs. 1 and 2 show that this is not necessarily the case: whereas some valves are stenotic from the time of their insertion, other valves have the capacity to accomodate somatic growth. In our view a knowledge of the calculated valve area of the valve being replaced according to the patient's weight or body surface area, coupled with a knowledge of the effective orifice area of the prosthesis, is essential at the time of valve replacement. This will not only allow the surgeon to make the optimal choice of the valve in a particular case, but may also prevent insertion of an unnecessarily large valve and the production of left ventricular outflow tract obstruction, as occurred in 2 of our patients, which has previously been reported.[6]

In conclusion, there is no presently available satisfactory valvular prosthesis for use in children. Some of the early mortality following valve replacement in children may be attributed to the nature of the underlying congenital heart disease. But most of the long-term morbidity and mortality is related to complications of the prosthesis itself. The balance lies between the risks due to the thromboembolic complications of mechanical valves and the risks of reoperation, which becomes necessary because of tissue valve degeneration.

The problems of early calcification in tissue valves inserted in children is under investigation and recent reports on methods of delaying calcification are encouraging.[13] In addition, the antibiotic-sterilized or fresh aortic homograft valve inserted in the aortic position may have an extended life when compared with presently available commercial bioprostheses.[14] It is therefore possible that the homograft valve and the St. Jude mechanical valve will produce more satisfactory long-term results.

Addendum—We have recently heard of "thromboembolic" complications in patients with St. Jude's mechanical prostheses who were not anticoagulated, and we would like to clarify our present policy as follows:

All patients with mechanical prostheses are maintained on anticoagulants. Mechanical valves are used for the atrioventricular position, mechanical or fresh antibiotic preserved homografts for the aortic position, and fresh antibiotic preserved homografts for ventricular pulmonary conduits.

References

1. Rowlatt JF, Rimoldi HJA, Lev M: The quantitative anatomy of the normal child's heart. Pediatr Clin North Am 10:499, 1963.
2. Kutsche LM, Oyer P, Shumway N, Baum D: An important complication of Hancock mitral valve replacement in children. Circulation 60 (Suppl. I):98, 1979.
3. Geha AS, Laks H, Stansel HC, Cornhill F, Kilman JW, Buckley MJ, Roberts WC: Late failure of porcine valve heterografts in children. J Thorac Cardiovasc Surg 78:351, 1979.
4. Silver MM, Pollock J, Silver MD, Williams WG, Trusler GA: Calcification in porcine xenograft valves in children. Am J Cardiol 45:685, 1980.
5. Thandroyen FT, Whitton IN, Pirie D, Rogers MA, Mitha AS: Severe calcification of glutaraldehyde-preserved porcine xenografts in children. Am J Cardiol 45:690, 1980.
6. Sanders SP, Levy RJ, Freed, MD, Norwood WI, Casteneda AR: Use of Hancock porcine xenografts in children and adolescents. Am J Cardiol 46:429, 1980.
7. Horst RL, Roux BT, Rogers NMA, Gotsman MS: Mitral valve replacement in children; a report of 51 patients. Am Heart J 85:624, 1973.
8. Stansel HC, Nudel DB, Berman MA, Talner NS: Prosthetic valve replacement in children. Arch Surg 110:1397, 1975.
9. Chen S, Laks H, Fagan L, Terschluse D, Kaiser G, Barner H, Wellman VL: Valve replacement in children. Circulation 56 (Suppl II): 117, 1977.
10. Berry BE, Ritter DG, Wallace RB, McGoon DC, Danielson GK: Cardiac valve replacement in children. J Thorac Cardiovasc Surg 68:705, 1974.
11. Gardner TJ, Roland JA, Neill CA, Donahoo JS: Valve replacement in children; a fifteen year perspective. J Thorac Cardiovasc Surg 83:178, 1982.
12. Pass HI, Sade RM, Crawford FA, Donahoo J, Gardner T: St. Jude prosthesis without anticoagulation in children. Am J Cardiol 49:1035, 1982.
13. Carpentier A, Dubost C, Lane E, Nashef A, Carpentier S, Relland J, Deloche A, Fabiani JN, Chauvaud S, Perier P, Maxwell S: Continuing improvements in valvular bioprostheses. J Thorac Cardiovasc Surg 83:27, 1982.
14. Radley-Smith R, Fagan A, Yacoub M: An eleven year experience of fresh aortic homograft replacement in children. Am J Cardiol 49:1035, 1982.

23

Bioprosthetic Valve Replacement in Children

M. VILLANI, T. BIANCHI, V. VANINI, R. TIRABOSCHI, G. C. CRUPI, E. PEZZICA, L. PARENZAN

The main problems with cardiac valve replacement in children are related to: the expected somatic growth of the small patients, the unknown durability of the valve substitutes, the difficulty of achieving good anticoagulation, the long-term exposure to time-related complications, such as thromboembolism and sepsis, constraints in size, and the problems related to childbearing in the female patient.[1]

The introduction of porcine bioprosthetic valves in 1965 and the subsequent improvements in their manufacturing, preservation, and sterilization led to some enthusiasm that resulted in a more frequent use in children. However, it has become evident in the past few years that porcine xenograft deteriorate more rapidly in children than in adults.[2–8] These reports have prompted us to review our experience with pediatric valve replacement.

Patients and Methods

In the last 10 years (September 1971 to March 1982), 46 children had a porcine bioprosthetic valve replacement in the Department of Cardiac Surgery at our hospital. Valved conduits are excluded from this study. The age of the patients ranged from 1–15 years (mean, 7.5 years).

The types of substitutes and the age of patients are listed in Fig. 1. Fourteen patients (30%) were younger than 5 years of age. The majority of the children (42) had congenital heart disease, whereas only 4 had acquired valve disease.

From the Departments of Cardiac Surgery and Pathology, Ospedali Riuniti, Bergamo, Italy.

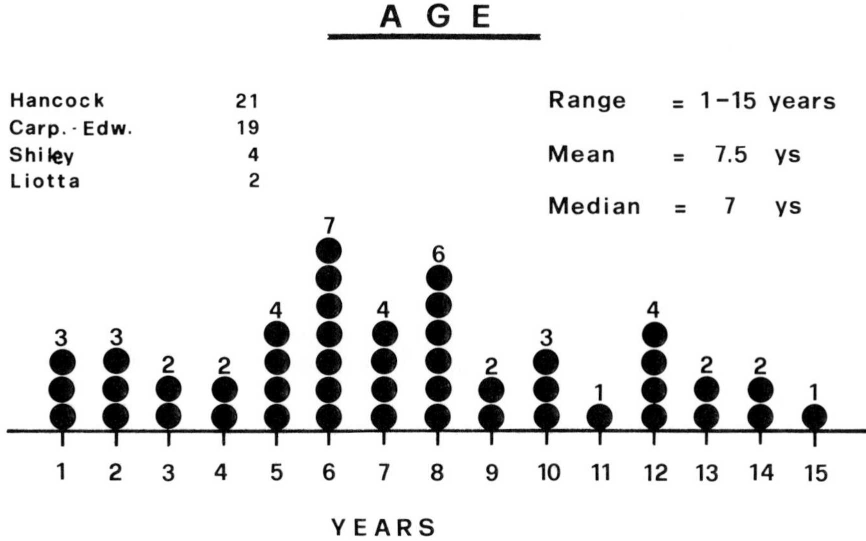

FIG. 1 Type of substitute and age of patients.

Tricuspid Valve

Four patients had Ebstein's anomaly of their tricuspid valve which required bioprosthetic valve replacement. One patient had a double outlet right ventricle (DORV) with pulmonary hypertension. Anomalous insertion of an important group of chordae tendinae on the anterior border of the ventricular septal defect (VSD) led to tricuspid excision, to allow the patch connection of the VSD to the aorta.

One 9-year-old girl with tricuspid atresia had received an uneventful Fontan type of repair by means of a Dacron conduit, between the right atrium (RA) and the good-sized right outlet chamber (RV). A few months later she developed inferior vena cava syndrome with a severe protein-losing enteropathy that was relieved by placing a porcine valve between the RA and the RV. Mean bioprosthetic size implanted in this group of 6 patients was 29.5 mm (range, 27–31). The mean age was 8.5 years and all patients survived the operation.

Pulmonary Valve

All 20 patients had a transanular patch reconstruction of their right ventricular outflow tract. Seven patients (6 tetralogy of Fallot and 1 pulmonary atresia plus VSD) had peripheral pulmonary stenosis that were considered not completely relievable by surgery. For fear of severe pulmonary stenosis and insufficiency, a free porcine valve was inserted at the valvular level. Five patients had residual VSD and/or stenosis after corrective repair of tetralogy of Fallot. At the time of reparative surgery, it was thought that unloading of the right ventricle from the volume due to the pulmonary insufficiency was indicated by bioprosthetic valve replacement.

Three patients had an absent left pulmonary artery. One of them died 15 days postoperatively because of a broncopneumonia in the right lung (the only functioning one). Two patients had a tetralogy of Fallot plus complete atrioventricular canal and 2 others had an absent pulmonary valve syndrome. One additional patient had a DORV. The mean bioprosthetic size was 21.4 mm (range, 16–27). The sizes most commonly used were 21 and 23 mm. Mean age of the group was 7.9 years. Only 1 patient died in the hospital (5%) (Table I).

Mitral Valve

Five children had mitral regurgitation: 2 had isolated rheumatic incompetence, and of the 3 congenital cases, 1 also had a large VSD and 1 an idiopathic hypertrophic subaortic stenosis, both of which were repaired at the time of valve replacement.

One 15-month-old child also had an aortic valve stenosis and endocardial fibroelastosis of the left ventricle which required additional surgery.

A 6-year-old girl with a parachute deformity of the mitral valve and aortic coarctation had received 4 years before a 1-stage repair of the valve and the aorta. Due to recurrent progressive valve dysfunction (stenosis and insufficiency), she had mitral replacement with a 21 mm Hancock valve.

A 2½-year-old boy had an attempted plastic repair of his double orifice mitral valve at time of surgery for partial atrioventricular (AV) canal in another institution. Because of severe heart failure due to the stenotic and

TABLE I Pulmonary valve

	# pts	Hospital mortality
Tetralogy of Fallot + peripheral stenosis	6	—
Tetralogy of Fallot (status postcorrection)	5	—
Tetralogy of Fallot + absent left pulmonary artery	3	1
Tetralogy of Fallot + complete atrioventricular canal	2	—
Tetralogy of Fallot + absent pulmonary artery	2	—
DORV + pulmonary stenosis	1	—
Pulmonary atresia + VSD + peripheral stenosis	1	—
	20	1

insufficient mitral valve, he received a 23 mm Liotta (low profile bioprosthetic valve).

Two patients with corrected transposition of the great arteries and left AV valve incompetence had valve replacement of their malformed valves. One patient also had a VSD. Even though the replaced valve is considered, anatomically, a tricuspid valve, from a clinical point of view, they are left-sided systemic AV valves and therefore are included in the mitral group. The mean bioprosthetic size was 26.2 mm (range, 21–31) and the mean age was 6.4 years. All 10 patients survived the operation.

Aortic Valve

Among the children with congenital aortic valve stenosis, 2 had received aortic valvotomy in the neonatal period. Both of them had an early recurrence of the stenosis that was associated with some degree of incompetence. At the time of the second operation, the dysplastic valve was not amenable to further commissurotomy and therefore an aortoventriculoplasty according to Konno was performed in both in order to insert an adequate-sized bioprosthetic (21 and 23 mm). One of the 2 died because of severe arrhythmias. Another patient in this group had endocarditis 2 years before and developed a fistula between the aorta and the right ventricle. Two of these 10 patients (mean age, 7.6 years) died early. Mean bioprosthetic size was 22.5 mm (range, 19–29), with the 21 and the 23 mm being the most commonly employed (Table II).

Late Results

Mortality

Nine patients died in a mean follow-up of 42 months (range, 2 months to 10.5 years). Two patients died 2 and 3 months postoperatively because of

TABLE II Aortic valve

	# pts	Hospital mortality
Aortic valve disease* (congenital)	4	1
Ventricular septal defect + aortic insufficiency	3	
Acute bacterial endocarditis	1	
Truncus arteriosus + transient ischemia	1	1
Aortic valve disease + myocardial infarct (rheumatic)	1	
	10	2† (20%)

* One patient had had acute bacterial endocarditis.
† Ages 2.5 and 4 years.

the congenital heart disease per se and therefore are considered nonvalve-related deaths. Six died because of endocarditis, documented in 5 with positive blood or valve culture (1 enterococcus, 2 *Pseudomonas aeruginosa,* 2 *Staphylococcus aureus*). Endocarditis appeared 2 months postoperatively in 2 patients and 7 months, 8 months, 2 years, and 4.5 years in the other children; endocarditis was present preoperatively in 2 of them.

The last patient, who died 3 years after surgery, had had in 1971 a 29 mm Carpentier-Edwards implanted at aortic level and a mitral Carpentier ring. At autopsy, the valve was severely calcified.

The other valve-related deaths occurred in patients with aortic (3), mitral (2), and tricuspid (1) replacements.

Re-replacement

Three patients had their bioprosthetic valve replaced because of endocarditis, which was associated with a suture dehiscence in one and a valve calcification in another. No patient survived reoperation. On the other hand, all 3 patients with a pure calcific malfunctioning valve survived reoperation 2, 3, and 4$^{1}/_{3}$ years after the first operation (Table III).

Valve Failures and Calcification

Six bioprostheses failed between 2 and 4.5 years postoperatively. Four valves degenerated from calcification 2–4 years postoperatively, 3 of which were successfully replaced (1 of them had also a third successful replacement).

The other 2 valve failures were both associated with endocarditis; in 1 of them severe calcification and valve tears were also present. In a mean follow-up period of 42 months, only 67% of the implanted bioprostheses were still in place (excluding 3 early and 9 late deaths and 3 successful reoperations). By 5 years, only 29% of aortic valves and 48% of mitral valves "at risk" were still in place and functioning. In the right side of the heart the situation was considerably better, since 62% of the tricuspid and

TABLE III Re-replacement

Position	Cause	Time postoperatively	Outcome
Aortic	endocarditis + dehiscence	8 mo	Death
Mitral	endocarditis	2 mo	Death
Mitral	endocarditis + malfunction	2 yr	Death
Tricuspid	malfunction	3 yr	OK
Mitral	malfunction	4 4/12 yr	OK
Aortic	malfunction	2 yr	OK

100% of the pulmonary devices were still in place. However, the numbers at 5 years were rather small (5 in each group).

Comment

During the past decade, the glutaraldehyde-preserved porcine xenograft has undergone extensive clinical use in adults because of the low incidence of acute complications, mainly thromboembolic episodes, and the possible avoidance of anticoagulation.[9–11] The enthusiasm created by the use of these valvular devices led to their use in children. However, during the last 5 years, several reports have indicated a more frequent occurrence of degeneration and calcification in young patients than in adults. Possible explanations for this early failure in children are: 1) mechanical fatigue due to the higher heart rate in children than adults, 2) the presence of transvalvular gradients in small valve sizes which create turbulence and predispose to thromboembolism and to mechanical damage, 3) calcium metabolism, such as the positive balance in children and the presence of vitamin K-dependent gamma-carboxyglutamic acid, which is a calcium-binding amino acid present in proteins involved in the process of all pathologic calcification,[12] 4) immunologic reaction,[6] and 5) increased host cell ingrowth.

We have had experience with 46 children who had valve replacement in the last decade for a variety of heart diseases, mostly congenital. The complexity of this very select group of patients is stressed by the fact that almost half had had previous heart surgery before the valve replacement (10 closed and 11 open heart procedures). In addition, 28 children (61%) had concomitant heart surgery at the time of bioprosthetic valve replacement.

Nevertheless, the hospital mortality in the last 6 years was only 2.8% (1 of 35 consecutive cases), the single death occurring in a 30 month old boy with congenital aortic stenosis who had an aortoventriculoplasty because of his very small aortic anulus. The youngest patient surviving operation and late follow-up (almost 5 years) was 15 months at time of valve replacement.

The sizes of valves used were rather large, since the majority of the children had valve incompetence with cardiomegaly. As a consequence of that, no child required re-replacement because of outgrowing the bioprosthesis, as determined in a mean follow-up of 42 months.

Anticoagulation, after the first 3 months' treatment, was not maintained in any child. Two episodes of thromboembolism occurred in this series: one 20 days postoperatively that resolved fully and very early and another that was a septic embolization in a patient with endocarditis who had already had endocarditis 2 years before the valve replacement.

The late mortality was rather high. The main cause of late death (6 patients) was bioprosthetic endocarditis, which is a highly lethal complication.[13] Two patients died because of the complexity of their congenital heart disease and it was coincidental that they had a bioprosthetic valve inserted a few months before. Another patient died because of a valve calcification 3 years after surgery, but we do not know how quickly the disease progressed. Interestingly enough, Dunn,[2] in a multicenter study on porcine valve durability in children, found that the porcine valve degeneration is not as slow as rheumatic valve degeneration and can occur within a few months. These data should encourage close follow-up of these patients even though they are in excellent clinical condition. The rather bad fate of the bioprosthesis in the left heart as compared with that of the same devices implanted in the right heart is rather significant and is in accordance with the multicenter study reported in 1981.[2] The cause of this is certainly not to be searched for in the calcium metabolism but probably in the less valve damage (which is the cause of stronger immunologic reaction and of faster calcium deposit) caused by the low pressure system of the right heart. To stress this consideration, of our 33 survivors of pulmonary conduit operations, only 2 had to be replaced after 2 and 5 years and both of them because of residual defects. Similar data were reported by Rocchini et al[6] who argued that the longevity of extracardiac porcine heterograft may be the direct result of retardation of host cell ingrowth given by the Dacron conduit. A different experience reported by Chen et al[14] noted 2 valve degenerations of 21 valved conduits (11.5%) within 3 years of implantation due to the fact that these conduits were left-sided (apicoaortic).

In conclusion, we believe that bioprosthetic valve replacement in children is a safe surgical procedure, but involves many late risks when performed on the systemic circulation. The risks are mainly endocarditis and valve failure (degeneration and calcification). For these reasons we feel that their use in the left heart in children should not be preferred to that of the prosthetic devices. The latter seem to be less thrombogenic in children than in adults[15] and in our experience of more than 20 mechanical devices implanted in children in the last years we have had, so far, no late valve failure and no late death.

References

1. Binet JP, Carpentier A: Implantation de valves heterologues dans le traitement des cardiopathies aortiques. CR Acad Sci 261:5733, 1965.
2. Dunn JM: Porcine valve durability in children. Ann Thorac Surg 32:357, 1981.
3. Curcio CA, Commerford PJ, Rose AG, Stevens JE, Barnard MS: Calcification of glutaraldehyde-preserved porcine xenografts in young patients. J Thorac Cardiovasc Surg 81:621, 1981.
4. Geha AS, Laks H, Stansel HC Jr, Cornhill JF, Kilman JW, Buckley MJ, Roberts WC: Late failure of porcine valve heterografts in children. J Thorac Cardiovasc Surg 78:351, 1979.
5. Kutsche LM, Oyer PE, Shumway N, Baum D: An important complication of

Hancock mitral valve replacement in children. Circulation 60 (Suppl I):98, 1978.

6. Rocchini AP, Weesner KM, Keidelberger K, Keren D, Behrendt D, Rosenthal A: Porcine xenograft valve failure in children: An immunologic response. Circulation 64 (Suppl II):162, 1981.
7. Silver MM, Pollock J, Silver MD, Williams WG, Trusler GA: Calcification in porcine xenograft valves in children. Am J Cardiol 45:685, 1980.
8. Thandroyen PT, Whitton IN, Pirie D, Roger MA, Mitha AS: Severe calcification of glutaraldehyde-preserved porcine xenografts in children. Am J Cardiol 45:690, 1980.
9. Carpentier A, Dubost C, Lane E, Nashef A, Carpentier S, Relland J, Deloche A, Fabiani JN, Chauvaud S, Perier P, Maxwell S: Continuing improvements in valvular bioprostheses. J Thorac Cardiovasc Surg 83:27, 1982.
10. Oyer PE, Stinson EB, Reitz BA, Miller DC, Rossiter SJ, Shumway NE: Long-term evaluation of the porcine xenografts bioprosthesis. J Thorac Cardiovasc Surg 78:343, 1979.
11. Cevese PG, Gallucci V, Morea M, Dalta Volta S, Fasoli G, Casarotto D: Heart valve replacement with the Hancock bioprostheses. Analysis of long-term results. Circulation 56 (Suppl III):221, 1976.
12. Sanders SP, Levy RJ, Freed MD, Norwood WI, Castaneda AR: Use of Hancock porcine xenografts in children and adolescents. Am J Cardiol 46:429, 1980.
13. Bortolotti U, Thiene G, Milano A, Panizzon G, Valente M, Gallucci V: Pathological study of infective endocarditis on Hancock porcine bioprostheses. J Thorac Cardiovasc Surg 81:934, 1981.
14. Chen R, Duncan JM, Nihile M, Cooley DA: Early degeneration of porcine xenograft valves in pediatric patients who have undergone apico-aortic bypass. Tex Heart Inst J 9:41, 1982.
15. Ebert PA: Discussion of the paper of Gardner TJ, Roland JMA, Neil CA and Donahoo JS: Valve replacement in children. J Thorac Cardiovasc Surg 83: 178, 1982.

24

Aortic Root Replacement

R. Gallotti, A. Bodnar, D. N. Ross

Our approach to the difficult aortic root in conventional and in most cases we apply a simple gusset within the aortotomy incision. This is usually a piece of autogenous pericardium and is facilitated by the fact that we use an oblique incision for our aortotomies. This is our standard incision in the aortic root.

In cases in which not only the aorta but the aortic ring itself is narrow and will not accommodate a large enough prosthetic or bioprosthetic valve, the problem can be overcome by using a free hand-sewn homograft that has no bulky sewing ring. Alternatively, we prolong our standard aortotomy incision down through the valve ring at the commissures between the left and noncoronary cusps and into the anterior cusp of the mitral valve. This incision can be extended for about half the length of the mitral valve. Since it extends into the junction of the left atrium and the posterior wall of the aorta, it may be necessary to dissect away the left atrial wall, or to repair it.

A piece of autogenous pericardium can now be sewn from the mitral valve leaflet, back up into the aortotomy, which has the effect of enlarging the ring considerably so that a much larger valve can be accommodated.

There is an additional group of difficult hypoplastic aortic outflow tract problems, appropriately named the "tunnel outflow tract obstruction." This generally consists of a hypoplastic valve ring, thickened stenotic valve, and often associated supravalvar and subvalvar obstructive lesions. The whole segment constitutes a tortuous track or tunnel-like obstruction.

In these circumstances, the surgical solution has been either to declare the situation inoperable or, as in our first 3 cases, virtually uncorrectable in terms of relief of obstruction.[1] Subsequently, surgeons have applied different solutions, one being the Kono type of operation[2] in which the right ventricle is first opened and then the left ventricular outflow tract is divided through the right ventricle by incising the septum and valve ring. Gussets of Dacron are then sewn in place.

From the Ospedale di Circolo, Varese, Italy, and the Cardio-Thoracic Institute, London, England.

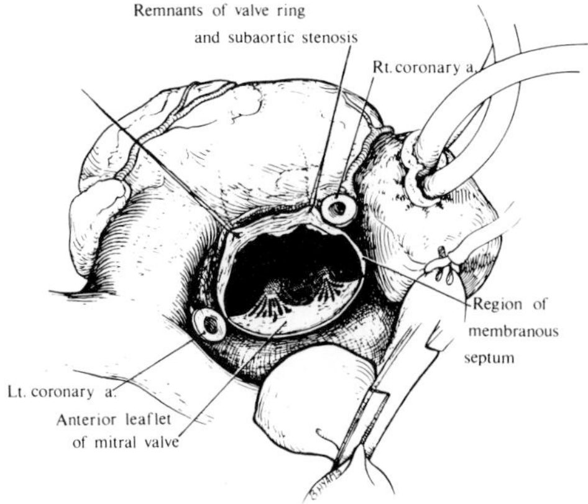

FIG. 1 Cross-section of operative field taken through the entire left ventricular outflow tract.

A second alternative has been offered by Denton Cooley, using the Sarnoff-type ventricular-aortic valved conduit procedure. This type of surgery has a widespread following, but in our view it is not a physiologic solution to the problem.

Our approach to these difficult tunnel-like obstructions has been to excise the entire aortic root, with its supravalvar component and to dissect out or enucleate the subvalvar thickening. The resulting orifice is wide and can then accommodate a full-sized adult aortic homograft, into which the child will grow as it gets older. The freeing of the root and the thickened tissues gives a markedly wide outflow, with the anterior cusp of the mitral valve occupying the posterior limit of the ring. The upper margin is formed by the membranous septum on the right and anteriorly by the ventricular septum. It is wise to leave remnants of ring tissue on the septum so as to give a good stitch attachment to the subsequent homograft replacement (Fig. 1.) Also one skirts the upper margin of the membranous septum to avoid the conducting tissue.

An adult sized homograft is now fixed in place in the outflow tract using multiple interrupted 4/0 Prolene sutures tied over a strip of Teflon felt.

An important consideration when excising the aortic root is to leave a good cuff of aortic wall, 2–3 mm wide, around each of the coronary orifices. Also it is particularly important that the left coronary artery is fully mobilized, since its subsequent anastomosis to the enlarged aortic root homograft would otherwise put it under undue tension. After completing the lower suture line of the homograft to the outflow tract, the left coronary artery is anastomosed with a running 6/0 suture to a corresponding hole in the back wall of the left coronary sinus of the homograft. The upper aorta is then sutured, anastomosing the homograft to the junction of the ascending aorta and the arch, using running 4/0 Prolene.

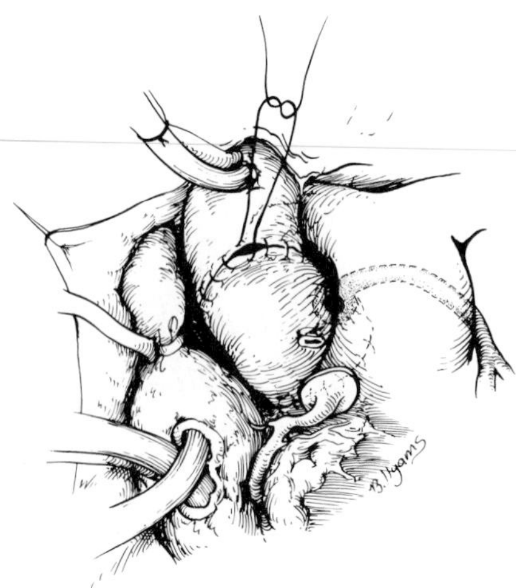

FIG. 2 Suture technique for implantation of homograft replacing patient's aortic valve, anulus, and ascending aorta.

It is now possible to open the aortic clamp and distend the homograft (Fig. 2.) This has the immediate effect of indicating precisely where the right coronary orifice should be attached to the homograft, and the aorta is again cross clamped, after which an appropriate incision is made in the front wall of the homograft and the right coronary artery is anastomosed.

The 1st of these procedures was carried out in a case of reoperation for calcified aortic valve stenosis. At the 2nd operation, the aortic root virtually disintegrated, and it was necessary to replace it with a homograft aortic root, with reanastomosis of the coronaries. This operation was carried out in 1973, and the patient has been fit and well since, with a perfectly competent aortic valve. Subsequent to this, 48 root replacement operations have been carried out in 219 cases of complex conditions. Of the root replacements, 30 have been for the hypoplastic root, and 18 were miscellaneous. A particularly suitable application for the technique, in our view, appears to be in advanced bacterial endocarditis, where the aortic root is virtually replaced by liquefying pus. Six of these patients have been operated upon with 2 deaths. Overall mortality has been 14% in the series and, in relation to the severity of the disease process, is probably acceptable.

References

1. Somerville J, Ross DN: Congenital aortic stenosis—an unusual form. Br Heart J 33:552, 1971.
2. Kono S, Ismai Y, Iida Y, Nakajima M, Tetsuno K: A new method for prosthetic valve replacement in congenital aortic stenosis associated with hypoplasia of the aortic valve ring. J Thorac Cardiovasc Surg 70:909, 1975.

25

Conduits Containing Antibiotic Preserved Homografts in the Treatment of Complex Congenital Heart Defects

D. DI CARLO, J. STARK, A. REVIGNAS, M. R. DE LEVAL

Extracardiac conduits opened a new era in the repair of some complex congenital heart defects. Following the pioneering work of Arai et al[1] and Ross and Somerville[2] with the aortic homograft, several large series of operations employing valved conduits have been reported.[3–11]

The early enthusiasm about the aortic homografts was dampened by the occurrence of late problems. The homografts sterilized by radiation and deep frozen showed a high incidence of calcification and subsequent conduit stenosis.[12–14] Additionally, the availability of homografts presented considerable difficulties; therefore efforts have been made to develop alternatives. Several valves were subsequently incorporated in the extracardiac conduits: these included porcine bioprosthetic valves,[15,16] pericardial valves, or even prosthetic valves.[17]

In our unit, we started to use conduits containing aortic homografts in 1971.[18] Since porcine valves became available, we have been using them frequently but the use of aortic homografts preserved in nutrient and antibiotic solution has always been our conduit of choice.[10,19]

The purpose of this presentation is to review our overall experience with homograft conduits.

Patients and Materials

Between 1971 and 1980, a total of 65 children received conduits containing fresh aortic homografts. There were 40 boys and 25 girls. The age at operation varied from 2 weeks to 15 years (mean, 6.8 years). Persistent

From the Thoracic Unit, the Hospital for Sick Children, London, England.

TABLE I Homograft conduits: hospital mortality

Diagnosis	Operation	# pts	Died	%
Persistent truncus arteriosus	Conduit repair	22	14	64
Transposition of the great arteries + ventricular septal defect + left ventricular outflow tract obstruction	Rastelli repair	20	3	15
Univentricular heart, including tricuspid atresia	Fontan-type repair	9	2	22
Pulmonary atresia + ventricular septal defect, plus complex tetralogy of Fallot	Ross repair	6	1	17
Miscellaneous*	Conduit repair	8	5	63
Total		65	25	38

* This included Taussig-Bing (2); double outlet right or left ventricle, ventricular septal defect, and subvalvar pulmonary stenosis (2); corrected transposition with ventricular septal defect and subpulmonary stenosis (4).

truncus arteriosus (PTA) and complex transposition were the most common diagnoses (Table I). Thirty-six children (55%) had undergone 48 previous operations. Thirty-five were performed to increase pulmonary blood flow, 4 to improve the mixing (Blalock-Hanlon operation), and 2 to reduce pulmonary blood flow by pulmonary artery constriction.

Operative Technique

The aortic homograft is prepared while the chest is being opened by trimming the excess muscle at the ventricular side and carefully oversewing the coronary ostia. The ventricular end of the homograft is usually extended with a segment of woven Dacron conduit of matching size. The aortic homograft valve is placed as close as possible to the pulmonary anastomosis to avoid compression and distortion under the sternum, leading to incompetence. Usually, the conduit is positioned to the left of the aorta to prevent compression between the heart and the sternum in the midline.

Results

The hospital mortality was high (25 patients, 38%). It was related to the type of lesion, as shown in Table I. The mortality for the repair of PTA was 64%: the main cause of death in this group of patients was poor preoperative condition in very young infants or pulmonary vascular obstructive disease (PVOD) in older children.

The most common cause of death was low cardiac output (19 patients). Three children died with severe residual right ventricular hypertension: 1 of these children, with pulmonary atresia and ventricular septal defect (VSD), was found at autopsy to have only very small peripheral pulmonary arteries. The other 2 patients were infants with PTA and histology showed grade III PVOD.

Factors Affecting Early Results

Age at surgery, diagnosis, and bypass time were found to affect significantly the early outcome.

Mean age at surgery was 8 years in early survivors and 4.6 years in those who died at operation ($p < 0.0027$).

Diagnosis influenced early results. PTA patients had higher hospital mortality than the entire remaining group (64% -vs- 25%, $p < 0.01$) and the transposition group separately (64% -vs- 15% $p < 0.01$). The difference from the other 2 groups was not significant due to the small number of patients.

Bypass time depended on the complexity of the repair. We found a significantly higher hospital mortality in patients with bypass time longer than 90 minutes (0% -vs- 43%, $p < 0.05$).

Hemodynamic Assessment

Twenty-one patients underwent postoperative cardiac catheterization. A routine postoperative study was performed 2 months to 6 years after surgery (mean, 2.2 years) in 13 children. The right ventricular (RV) pressure in these patients ranged from 18–100 mmHg. The gradients between the right ventricle and the pulmonary artery were 0–45 mmHg (mean, 14 mmHg). The RV to LV systolic pressure ratio was 0.2–0.8 (mean, 0.4). In 3 patients, hemodynamically insignificant residual VSD was diagnosed ($Qp/Qs \leq 1.2$). Two patients have elevated RV and pulmonary artery pressure without gradient across the valved conduit: a degree of PVOD is likely responsible for this hemodynamic abnormality. In one child, a 45 mmHg gradient across the conduit was found (20 mmHg at the valve level, 25 mmHg at the proximal anastomosis). She also has pulmonary artery pressure of 55 mmHg, suggesting the presence of PVOD; she is, however, asymptomatic.

Cardiac catheterization was required for recurrence of symptoms in 8 patients, 2 months to 6 years from surgery (mean 1.5 years). The RV pressure ranged from 30–130 mmHg (mean, 86 mmHg). The gradient across the conduit was 0–40 mmHg (mean, 10 mmHg). The RV to LV systolic pressure ratio was 0.4–0.95 (mean, 0.74). The most common problem with these patients was significant residual VSD. One of them also had conduit calcification and stenosis; severe PVOD was found in 1 case, without significant gradients across the conduit.

Two patients, among the 21 restudied, were found to have homograft valve incompetence: 1, already mentioned, also had residual VSD and conduit stenosis. The other, who has RV pressure of 60 mmHg and 25 mmHg gradient across the conduit, is currently asymptomatic. Further restudy is planned.

Our criteria for satisfactory performance of a homograft aortic valve are a peak systolic pressure gradient across the valve lower than 30 mmHg in RV to PA conduits and a mean systolic gradient lower than 5 mmHg in right atrium to PA conduits. These criteria were met by 18 of 21 restudied patients.

Conduit Calcification

Calcium deposits in the wall of the homografts were seen at chest xray in 56% of routinely examined patients. In most patients, this phenomenon became evident within 18 months of surgery. We found no evidence of increasing calcium deposits with time.

In 1 patient, heavy calcification of the homograft valve occurred, following an episode of endocarditis. This patient alone, in the whole series, required reoperation for this complication.

Reoperation

Five children were reoperated upon (Table II). In 1 case only was the reoperation necessary for stenosis of the homograft valve. A technical error (a conduit too long) was a contributory cause in 1 patient and endocarditis in 2. Four patients survived surgery, but 2 of them died 1.5 and 5.6 years later, the former of a second episode of endocarditis and the latter suddenly. One

TABLE II Homograft conduits: reoperations

# pts	Cause of reoperation	Early result	Late result
2	Residual VSD, suture line false aneurysm	Survived	1 well 1 died
1	Candida endocarditis	Survived	Died
1	Residual VSD, conduit calcification	Survived	Poor result
1	Residual VSD, tricuspid incompetence	Died	—

TABLE III Homograft conduits: causes of late deaths

	# pts
Sudden death	3
Mitral regurgitation, biventricular myocardial failure	1
Severe truncal valve regurgitation, biventricular myocardial failure	1
Endocarditis	1
Reoperation	1

patient had a poor result, due to irreversible biventricular failure proved at recatheterization.

Late Death

Late death occurred in 7 patients (Table III). Two had residual defects, leading to irreversible myocardial failure. Among the 3 patients who died suddenly, only 1 had had an uncomplicated course: he died 1 year after Rastelli operation for transposition, having been asymptomatic. Of the other 2, one required reoperation for residual VSD and false aneurysm of the suture line 5.6 years before death and was asymptomatic; the other was being treated for congestive heart failure due to truncal valve incompetence.

On a *clinical basis,* 40% of the long-term survivors had an excellent result, being asymptomatic without medication; 53% were improved by surgery and 7% were not improved.

Actuarial analysis of the long-term results shows 74% expected chance of homograft valve survival 9 years from implantation (Fig. 1). "Survival" indicated a long-term satisfactorily working homograft valve. All valve-related reoperations and deaths were accounted for as valve failures in this curve.

Comment

The technique of sterilization and preservation of aortic homografts have been reported by several authors.[20,21] It has been generally accepted that irradiated and deep-frozen homografts calcify and cause obstruction.[12–14] However, the hemodynamic performance and the long-term results with antibiotic-sterilized fresh homografts are excellent. We found no significant gradient across the valve in 18 out of 21 restudied cases. Similar results have been reported by others.[10,11,22]

In the past, late calcification of the aortic homografts has represented a considerable problem, leading to the discontinuation of their use. Antibi-

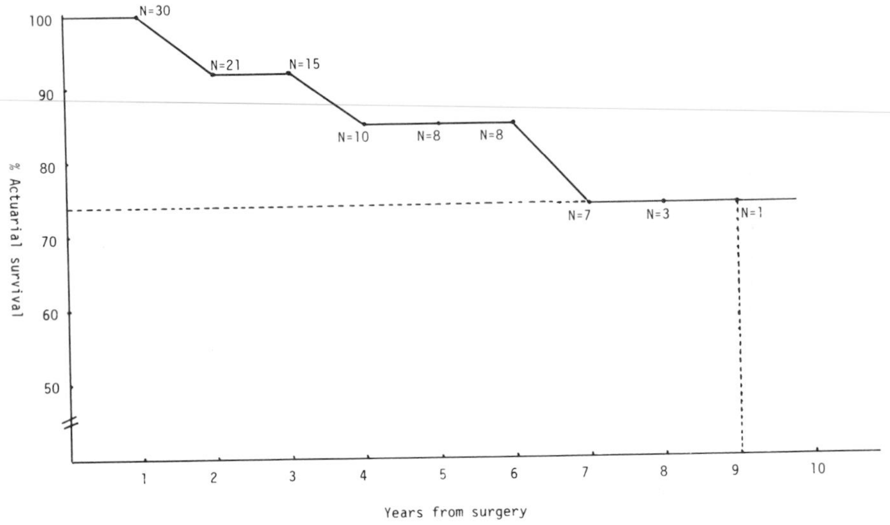

FIG. 1 Actuarial survival of homograft valve conduits 9 years after implantation.

otic sterilization proved useful in changing this course of events, as recently demonstrated by the extensive investigations of Saravalli et al.[23]

In our own experience, although calcium deposits in the wall of the homografts were commonly observed, only 1 patient required conduit replacement because of calcification of the valve leaflets and obstruction, secondary to a previous infective episode.

We conclude that fresh, antibiotic-preserved homografts perform well when used in extracardiac valved conduits. They are easier to insert and better hemostasis can be achieved. In our experience, degeneration of the valve leaflets was rare and development of homograft valve incompetence infrequent.

References

1. Arai R, Tsuyki Y, Nogi M, et al: Experimental study on bypass between the right ventricle and pulmonary artery, left ventricle and aorta by means of a homograft with valve. Bull Heart Inst Jpn 9:49, 1965.
2. Ross DN, Somerville J: Correction of pulmonary atresia with a homograft aortic valve. Lancet 2:1446, 1966.
3. Kouchoukos NT, Barcia A, Bargeron LM Jr, Kirklin JW: Surgical treatment of congenital pulmonary atresia with ventricular septal defect. J Thorac Cardiovasc Surg 61:70, 1971.
4. McGoon DC, Wallace RB, Danielson GK: Homografts in reconstruction of congenital cardiac anomalies. Mayo Clin Proc 47:101, 1972.
5. Moore CH, Martelli V, Ross DN: Reconstruction of right ventricular outflow

tract with a valved conduit in 75 cases of congenital heart disease. J Thorac Cardiovasc Surg 71:11, 1976.

6. Marcelletti C, Mair DD, McGoon DC, Wallace RB, Danielson GK: The Rastelli operation for transposition of the great arteries. Early and late results. J Thorac Cardiovasc Surg 72:427, 1976.
7. Bailey WW, Kirklin JW, Bargeron LM Jr, Pacifico AD, Kouchoukos NT: Late results of synthetic valved external conduits from venous ventricle to pulmonary arteries. Circulation (Suppl II) 56:73, 1977.
8. Norwood WI, Freed MD, Rocchini AP, Bernhard WF, Castaneda AR: Experience with valved conduits for repair of congenital cardiac lesions. Ann Thorac Surg 24:223, 1977.
9. Ciaravella JM, McGoon DC, Danielson GK, Wallace RB, Mair DD: Experience with the extracardiac conduit. J Thorac Cardiovasc Surg 78:920, 1979.
10. Moulton AL, de Leval MR, Macartney FJ, Taylor JFN, Stark J: Rastelli procedure for transposition of the great arteries ventricular septal defect and left ventricular outflow tract obstruction. Early and late results in 41 patients (1971 to 1978). Br Heart J 45:20, 1981.
11. Fontan F, Vosa C, Deville C, Scalia D, Choussat A, Doutremepuich C: Aortic valve homografts in the surgical treatment of complex cardiac malformations. Presented at the First Symposium on Cardiac Surgery, Naples, Italy, April, 1981.
12. Merin G, McGoon DC: Reoperation after insertion of an aoritc homograft as a right ventricular outflow tract. Ann Thorac Surg 16:122, 1973.
13. Park SC, Neches WH, Lenox CC, Zuberbuehler JR, Bahnson HT: Massive calcification and obstruction in a homograft after the Rastelli procedure for transposition of the great arteries. Am J Cardiol 32:860, 1973.
14. Moodie DS, Mair DD, Fulton RE, Wallace RB, Danielson GK, McGoon DC: Aortic homograft obstruction. J Thorac Cardiovasc Surg 72:553, 1976.
15. Bowman FO, Hancock WD, Malm JR: A valve-containing Dacron prosthesis. Arch Surg 107:724, 1973.
16. Carpentier A, Deloche A, Relland J, Fabiani JN, Forman J, Camilleri JP, Soyer R, Dubost C: Six-year follow-up of glutaraldehyde-preserved heterografts. J Thorac Cardiovasc Surg 68:771, 1974.
17. Cartmill TB, Celermajer JM, Stuckey DS, Bowdler JD, Johnson DC, Hawker RE: Use of the Björk-Shiley tilting disc prosthesis in valved conduits for right ventricular outflow reconstruction. Br Heart J 36:1106, 1974.
18. Breckenridge IM, Stark J, Oelert H, Waterston DJ: Transposition of the great arteries with ventricular septal defect and pulmonary stenosis treated by the Rastelli operation. Z Kinderchir 11:205, 1972.
19. Stark J, Gandhi D, de Leval MR, Macartney F, Taylor JFN: Surgical treatment of persistent truncus arteriosus in the first year of life. Br Heart J 40:1280, 1978.
20. Yacoub M, Kittle CF: Sterilization of valve homografts by antibiotic solutions. Circulation 41-42 (Suppl II):29, 1970.
21. Lockey E, Al-Janabi N, Gonzalez-Lavin L, Ross DN: A method of sterilizing and preserving fresh allograft heart valves. Thorax 27:398, 1972.
22. Shabbo FP, Wain WH, Ross DN: Right ventricular outflow reconstruction with aortic homograft conduit: Analysis of the long-term results. Thorac Cardiovasc Surg 28:26, 1980.
23. Saravalli OA, Somerville J, Jefferson KE: Calcification of aortic homografts used for reconstruction of the right ventricular outflow tract. J Thorac Cardiovasc Surg 80:909, 1980.

26

Dura Mater Bioprostheses in Young Patients

P. R. Brofman, R. G. Carvalho, E. J. Ribeiro, R. S. S. Almeida, A. Coelho, D. R. R. Loures

Despite the advance in cardiac valve surgery, it has been clearly shown that all valvular substitutions are palliative instead of long-lasting procedures.[1] If one compares the evolution of patients after valve replacement against the natural history of cardiac valve disease, one can be assured of a much better life, regarding quality and longevity.[2]

In 1971, Puig and Verginelli first implanted the dura mater bioprosthesis (DMB) preserved in 98% glycerol[3] and the use of the DMB was started in our hospital in 1972.[4] Despite the satisfactory clinical results in patients, the first complications (calcification, infectious endocarditis, and cusp rupture) were registered in 1975.[5] This report summarizes our experience with pediatric patients receiving the mitral DMB.

Patients

From January 1972 to November 1978, 38 pediatric patients had a mitral valve replaced by a DMB. In this group the following types of valvular dysfunction were observed: 25 patients (65.8%) with mixed mitral lesion and 13 patients (34.2%) with pure mitral insufficiency. The clinical history revealed that rheumatic fever was causative in 28 patients (73.7%).

The patients' ages varied from 5–15 years, with a mean of 12.8 years. Among the patients, 22 were females (57.8%). Six patients (15.8%) were functional class II (NYHA), 27 (71%) class III, and 5 (13.2%) class IV.

From the Section of Cardiac Surgery, Hospital Evangelico de Curitiba, Faculdade Evangelica de Medicina, Curitiba-Parana, Brasil.

Preparation of the DMB

Collection of the material. The dura mater was obtained at Instituto Medico Legal do Parana in Curitiba from persons who had suffered violent deaths. It was removed within 8 hours after the death. Any person with infectious, degenerative, or neoplastic disease was rejected. After the dura mater had been collected, it was washed in physiologic salt solution and preserved at room temperature in 98% glycerol for 12 days.

Preparation of the valve. the DMB was prepared on the basis of the fascia lata valve allograft.[6] The DMB has some characteristics of the rigid prosthesis; it is formed by 3 similar cusps, fixed to a rigid support of inox steel, covered by Dacron. Each cusp (Fig. 1) is obtained by sectioning a dura mater piece, obeying the shape and dimensions of the metalic blades that serve as a mold. The dura mater cusp was fixed and sutured to the Dacron of the rigid ring and molded with the acrylic molds.

Results

Five of 38 patients (13.2%) died in the early postoperative period (30 days). The causes of death were: low cardiac output in 2 patients, cerebrovascular accident in 2, and respiratory insufficiency in 1.

During an average follow-up period of 40 months (range, 7–81), 4 patients died (12.2%). Three of the deaths were due to bioprosthesis dys-

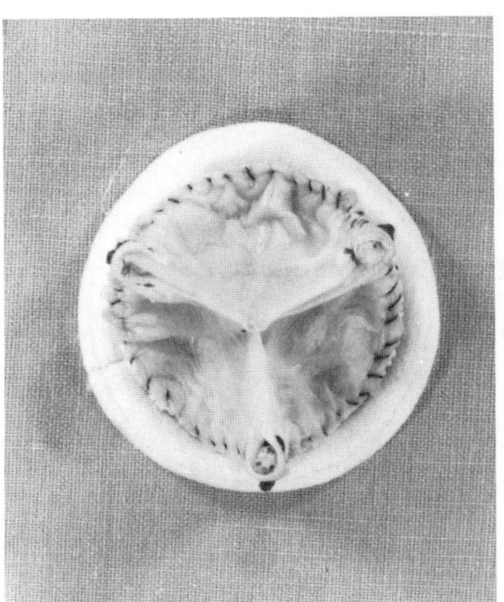

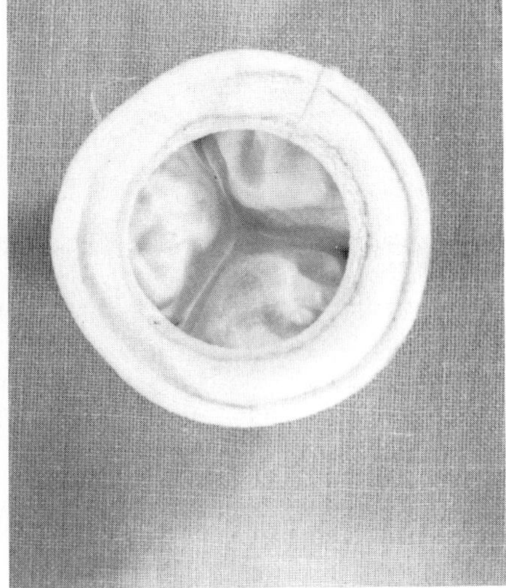

FIG. 1 The dura mater bioprosthesis.

function: 2 were calcified and 1 had infectious endocarditis. The other patient died from an unknown cause. After an average period of 41.8 months, 60.6% of the patients were graded as NYHA class I, 27.2% as class II, and 12.1% as class III.

Nine of 33 patients at risk (27.3%) were reoperated on due to bioprosthesis dysfunction and 1 of them was reoperated on for a 2nd time. The indications for reoperation were: 7, calcification; 2, infectious endocarditis, and 1, ruptured cusps. Calcification appeared between 22 and 59 months (mean, 36.8 months), infectious endocarditis between 9 and 17 months (mean, 13 months), and ruptured cusps at 26 months postoperatively. Of the 9 patients reoperated on due to bioprosthesis dysfunction, 5 (55.6%) died in the early postoperative period due to low cardiac output. Two patients (22%) died in late postoperative period due to bronchopneumonia leading to respiratory insufficiency in one and cardiac failure in the other. After a follow-up period of 7 years, actuarial analysis showed that only 38% of the bioprostheses were functioning acceptably. The durability of 73% was acceptable at 3 years but it was 40% at 7 years (Fig. 2).

Of the 13 DMB analyzed pathologically, 10 were from patients who were reoperated on and 3 from patients who died in the late postoperative period. Three bioprostheses were dysfunctional due to infectious endocarditis from

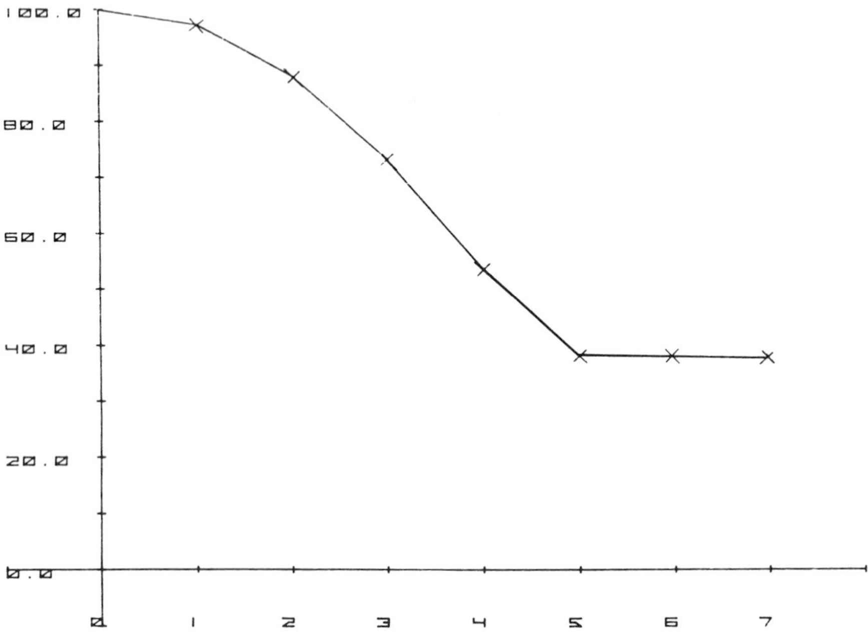

FIG. 2 Actuarial probability of an intact dura mater bioprosthesis at 7 years.

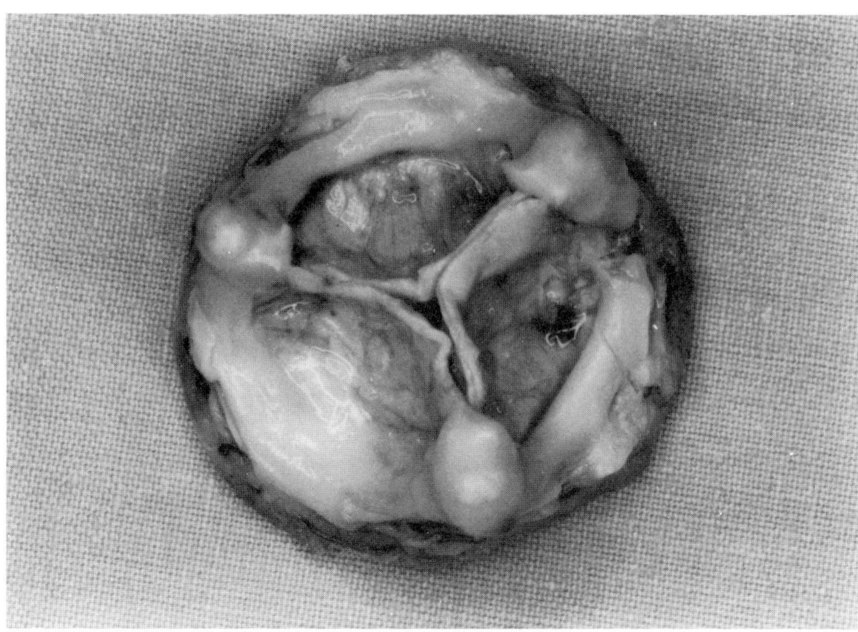

FIG. 3 (above) The dura mater bioprosthesis had a "porcelain" aspect with immobility and rigidity of one or more cusps. (below) The collagen with complete disorganization of bundles, altered by amorphous substances (calcium) in the thickness and surface of the tissue with the presence of fibroblasts (H&E ×150).

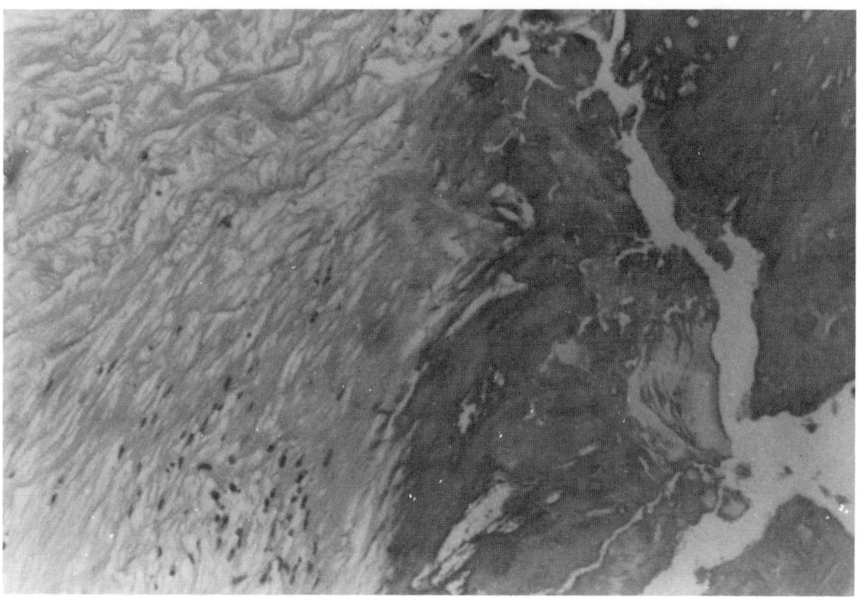

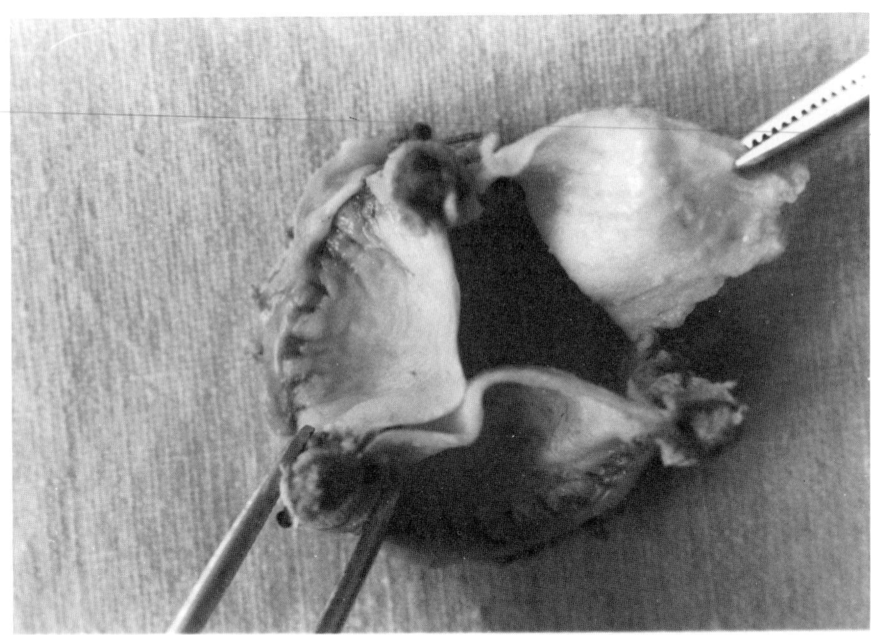

FIG. 4 (above) The dura mater bioprosthesis with cusp fenestrations next to the valvular struts. (below) The collagen with amorphous substances (calcium) more evident near the valvular struts with the disappearance of collagen bundles (H&E ×100).

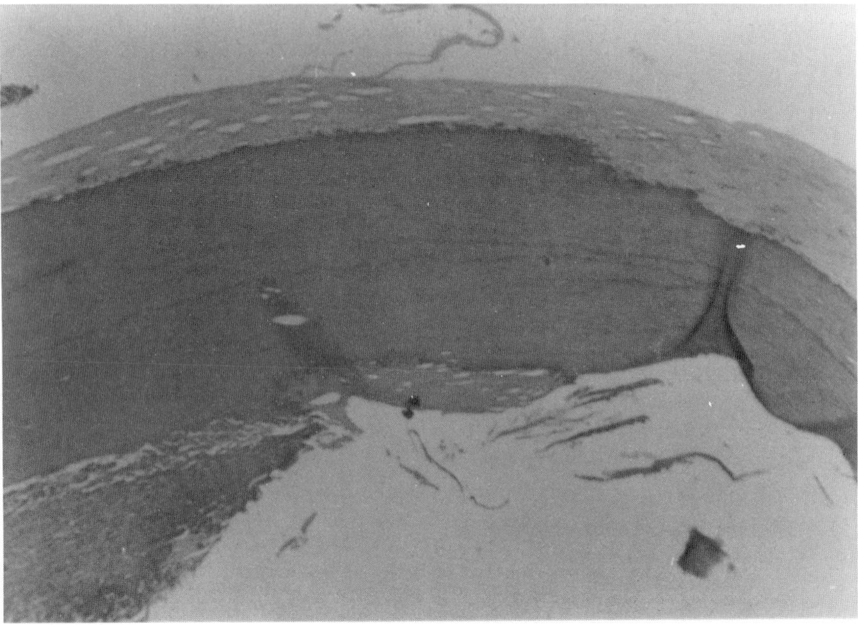

Escherichia coli (1), *Candida albicans* (1), and an unidentified organism in the third.

Nine bioprostheses exhibited leaflet calcification (Fig. 3, top). Macroscopically the dura mater had a "porcelain" aspect, with a yellowish color, with calcium pigments on the tissue's surface. This produced rigidity and immobility of 1 or more cusps. The light microscopic aspect showed an increased cellularity (with the presence of fibroblasts, histiocytes, macrophages, and lymphocytes), with a complete disorganization of the collagenous bundles, altered by amorphous substances (calcium) in the thickness and surface of the tissue (Fig. 3, bottom). One bioprosthesis had a ruptured cusp.

The macroscopic aspect showed cusp fenestrations next to the struts that sustain the valvular frame (Fig. 4, top). The light microscopic examination showed such areas to consist of a cellular collagenous matrix, areas with amorphous substance (calcium), and the disappearance of the collagenous bundle (Fig. 4, bottom).

Comment

Various reasons for early calcification in young patients with DMB have been suggested.[7,8] Bioprosthesis calcification occurs much more frequently in those implanted in young patients, probably because of increased calcium metabolism. An immunologic reaction is possible, although the preservation, such as with glycerol or glutaraldehyde, diminishes histologic antigenicity of the bioprosthesis. It is possible, however, that the collagenous fibers still provide a certain degree of antigenicity. This hypothesis is based on the presence of cells like histiocytes and lymphocytes.[9] In the present series, 25% of bioprostheses calcified in an average time of 37 months.

We conclude that DMB durability is a restrictive factor for its use in mitral replacement in young patients and should not be used in this clinical setting.

References

1. Rahimtoola SH, Ed: Symposium on the current status of valve replacement. Am J Cardiol 35:710, 1975.
2. Rapaport E: Natural history of aortic and mitral valve disease. Am J Cardiol 35:221, 1975.
3. Puig LB, Verginelli G, Zerbini EJ, Kawabe L: Valva cardíaca de dura-máter homóloga; método de preparação de valva. Rev Hosp Clin Fac Med São Paulo 29:85, 1974.
4. Brofman PR, Loures DR, Carvalho RG, Coelho A, Ribeiro EJ, Pereira MA, Oliveira PF, Carvalho RD: Experiência com o uso da valva de dura-máter homóloga. Arq Bras Cardiol 29 (Suppl 1):66, 1976.

5. Brofman PR, Loures DR, Carvalho RG, Coelho A, Ribeiro EJ, Pereira MA, Carvalho RD: Complica ções com o uso da prõtese de dura-máter homóloga. Rev Bras Med 33:66, 1976.
6. Ionescu MI, Ross DN: Heart-valve replacement with autologous fascia lata. Lancet 2:335, 1969.
7. Bachet J, Bical O, Guilmet D, Goudot B, Menn P, Richard T, Barbagelatta M: Early structural failure of porcine xenografts in young patients. In: Bioprosthetic Cardiac Valves (F Sebening et al, Ed). Munich, Deutsches Herzzentrum, 1979, p 341.
8. Christo MC, Fiqueroa CS, Gomes MU, Stortini MJ, Santana F GP, Salles CA, Figueiró FVU, Coutinho AO: Complicações tardias das próteses de dura-máter homóloga. Arq Bras Cardiol 34 (Suppl 1):30, 1980.
9. Abdulmassih CN, Souza LC, Paulista P, Falantier M, Oliveira FB, Soutell F AS; Lopes E, Jatene AD: Complicações das próteses de dura-mater. Rev Bras Cardiol 33:54, 1976.

SECTION V

EXPERIMENTAL PATHOLOGY

27

Experimental Evaluation of Bioprosthetic Valves Implanted in Sheep

M. JONES, G. R. BARNHART, A. M. CHAVEZ, G. K. JETT, D. M. ROSE, T. ISHIHARA, V. J. FERRANS

With the development of cardiopulmonary bypass and open heart operations, the replacement of cardiac valves became a practical therapeutic modality in early 1960s. Because of the need for anticoagulation in patients with mechanical cardiac valvular substitutes, investigators sought other forms of materials for the replacement of cardiac valves. During the late 1960s and early 1970s, valves made of biologic materials, including fascia lata, dura mater, and porcine aortic valves, became alternative cardiac valvular substitutes. Satisfactory hemodynamic function and the lack of the need for anticoagulation permitted bioprosthetic valves to become acceptable alternatives for mechanical cardiac prosthetic valves.

As long-term clinical experience developed, it became apparent that fascia lata valves were not acceptable because of their propensity to undergo early tissue failure.[1] Glutaraldehyde-preserved porcine aortic valvular bioprostheses, however, gave excellent early results[2-4] and became the prosthetic valves of choice in many centers. Unfortunately, as experience with the use of these valves has increased, their long-term durability is questionable. Clinical and pathologic studies have demonstrated that these glutaraldehyde-preserved porcine aortic bioprosthetic valves undergo degeneration and calcification.[5-12] Lipson et al[13] demonstrated that many bioprosthetic porcine aortic valves implanted in the mitral position for 5 or more years evidence hemodynamic deterioration. Degeneration and calcification of porcine bioprosthetic valves occur earlier following implantation in children and adolescents than in adults.[14-19] Recently, bovine pericardial bio-

---

From the Surgery and Pathology Branches, National Heart, Lung and Blood Institute, National Institutes of Health, Bethesda, Maryland.

prosthetic cardiac valves have become established clinically, but little is known of their long-term durability.

The reasons for degeneration and calcification of cardiac bioprosthetic valves are not clear. Research in human beings is limited to studies of valves recovered after death or reoperation; therefore detailed prospective studies investigating the mechanisms of valvular degeneration and calcification, and of the effects of modifications in valvular preparation and design, are not possible in the human. Thus, it is imperative that an in vivo investigational model be established for these studies.

We have developed an experimental animal model in juvenile domestic sheep (*Ovis aries*) to study the problems of degeneration and calcification of bioprosthetic cardiac valves. Presently, we have implanted 157 bioprosthetic cardiac valves in the sheep animal model. Of these 157 valves, 23 were explanted early (less than 1 month), 76 were explanted late (after 1 month; mean, 4.2 ± 1.7 months), and 58 remain implanted.

The purpose of this communication is to outline the techniques employed for implantation of bioprosthetic valves in sheep and their postoperative management; to summarize the clinical, hemodynamic, and morphologic results of the studies of the 99 sheep having valves explanted; and to present this experimental animal model for in vivo investigations of bioprosthetic cardiac valves. All 99 bioprosthetic valves were of clinical quality and consisted of 64 glutaraldehyde-preserved porcine aortic valves, 29 glutaraldehyde-preserved bovine pericardial valves, and 6 glycerol-treated human dura mater valves.

Technique of Valvular Implantation

Animal Preparation

A mixed breed of male and female Ramboulet and Dorset sheep with body weights of 20–25 kg, 2–4 months of age, were used for replacement of the tricuspid or mitral valves. The sheep were fasted overnight prior to the day of operation. Anesthesia was induced with sodium thiamylal (2.5%) or sodium thiopental (2.5%). A large bore catheter was positioned percutaneously in the external jugular vein for intravenous fluids and medications. The trachea was intubated per os and inhalation anesthesia maintained with halothane until cardiopulmonary bypass was instituted; thereafter, anesthesia was maintained by intravenous doses of barbiturates as necessary. The fleece of the animal's lateral thorax was sheared and the operative field was scrubbed with antiseptic soap. A sterile operative field was prepared.

Monitoring

Pressure measurements were obtained with the aid of Statham P23Db transducers (Statham Instruments, Oxnard, CA) at the time of implantation and terminal elective studies; signals were recorded on an 8 channel Gould Brush 480 recording system (Gould, Cleveland, OH). The electrocardiogram, systemic arterial blood pressure, and pulmonary arterial pressure were continuously monitored. A 20 gauge catheter was placed in the sartorius muscular branch of the femoral artery and advanced into the femoral artery for monitoring systemic arterial pressure. Through a groin incision on the contralateral side, a Swann-Ganz thermistor catheter was placed in the femoral vein and advanced to the pulmonary artery. To avoid postoperative impairment of ambulation, care was taken not to damage the femoral nerve during the groin dissection. A thermistor probe was positioned in the esophagus for monitoring body temperature.

Tricuspid Valve Implantation

A right thoracotomy incision was made through the fourth intercostal space (see Figs. 1–3). Snares were placed around the superior and inferior venae cavae outside the pericardium. Care was taken not to encircle the right phrenic nerve with the snares. Within the pericardium, purse-string sutures were placed in both venae cavae. Heparin, 300 units/kg body weight, was administered intravenously. A 12 gauge cannula was positioned in the femoral artery for systemic arterial perfusion during cardiopulmonary bypass, and 21 gauge cannulae were positioned in the venae cavae through incisions within each purse string for the return of systemic venous blood to the oxygenator. Cardiopulmonary bypass was instituted and the animal's body temperature cooled to 30°C. Replacement of the tricuspid valve was performed without cardiac arrest. Ventilation was discontinued with the airway maintained at a pressure of 5 cm of water. The left azygos vein, which drains into the coronary sinus in sheep and related animals, was ligated intrapericardially at its entry into the coronary sinus. The previously placed caval snares were secured to prevent caval blood from returning to the right atrium. An atriotomy was made extending from the right atrial appendage to the sulcus terminalis. The thermistor catheter in the pulmonary artery was retracted from the operative field. The tricuspid valve was excised, leaving a 2 to 3 mm remnant of valvular tissue. The papillary muscles were transected at their bases. Nonabsorbable interrupted horizontal mattress sutures buttressed with pledgets were passed through the atrial aspect of the anulus and the remaining valvular tissue. The sutures were placed superficially between the coronary sinus and the membranous

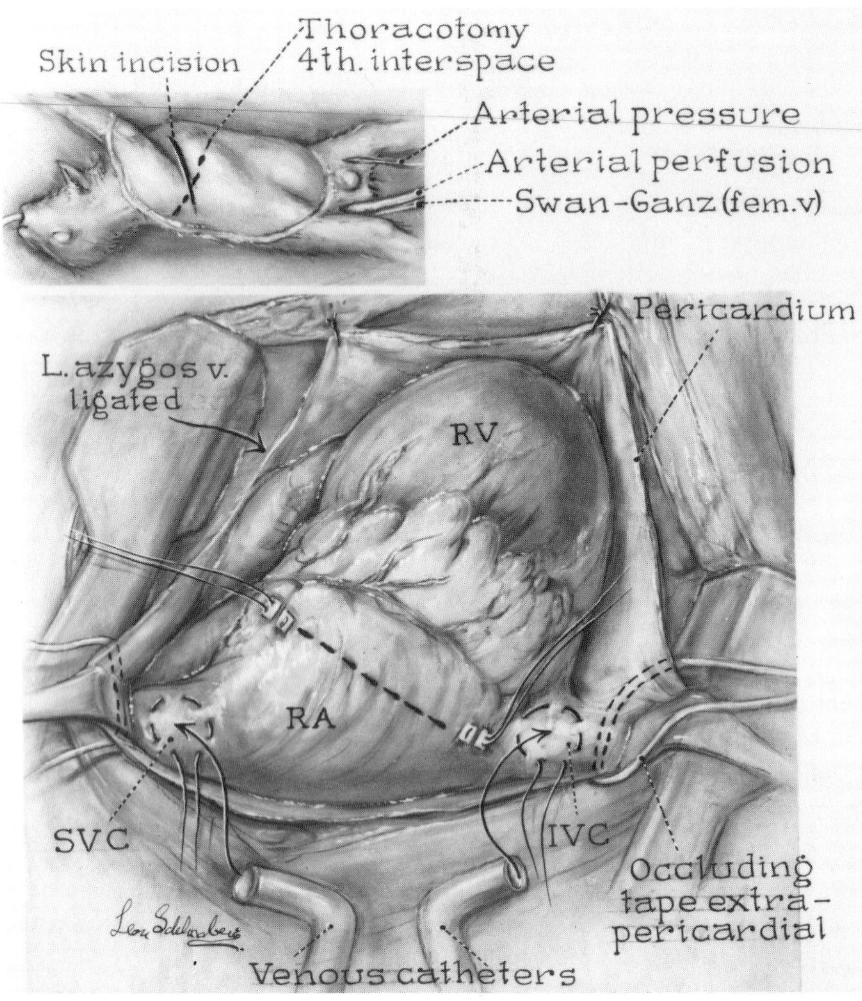

FIG. 1 Replacement of the tricuspid valve. The left of the figure is cephalad and the right of the figure is caudad in the sheep. The atriotomy extends from the atrial appendage to the sulcus terminalis. Cannulae are positioned in the venae cavae so that they remain outside of the operative field.

ventricular septal region of the tricuspid anulus to avoid injury to the conduction system. The sutures were passed through the sewing ring of the bioprosthesis, the valve was seated in the anulus, and the sutures were tied and cut. The valve was oriented so that the widest interstrut distance spanned the right ventricular outflow tract. The thermistor catheter was repositioned through the bioprosthesis into the pulmonary artery. Just prior to

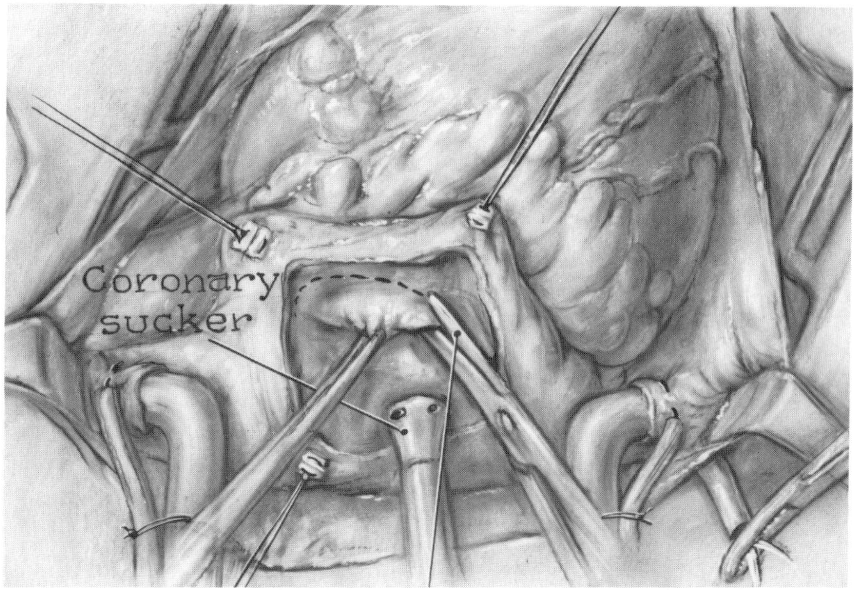

FIG. 2 Replacement of the tricuspid valve. The tricuspid valve is excised, leaving a 2–3 mm remnant of tricuspid valvular tissue and the papillary muscles are excised at their bases.

completion of atrial closure, the caval tapes were released. Air was evacuated from the right heart and the animal was rewarmed to 38°C. Ventilation was resumed and cardiopulmonary bypass was discontinued. The arterial and venous perfusion cannulae were removed; the femoral artery was ligated. Protamine sulfate, 3 mg/kg body weight, was given intravenously to counteract the heparin. A chest tube was placed through the sixth intercostal space and positioned anteriorly for dependent drainage. The ribs were approximated with nonabsorbable suture material and the chest wall muscles and skin were closed with absorbable sutures. Following the completion of the hemodynamic studies described later, the catheter in the pulmonary artery was removed and the femoral vein ligated. Both groin incisions were closed with absorbable sutures. Thereafter, the animal was placed in the position of sternal recumbency and was weaned from the ventilator and extubated.

Mitral Valve Implantation

After the animal was positioned in the right lateral decubitus position and the operative field was prepared as already described, a left thoracotomy

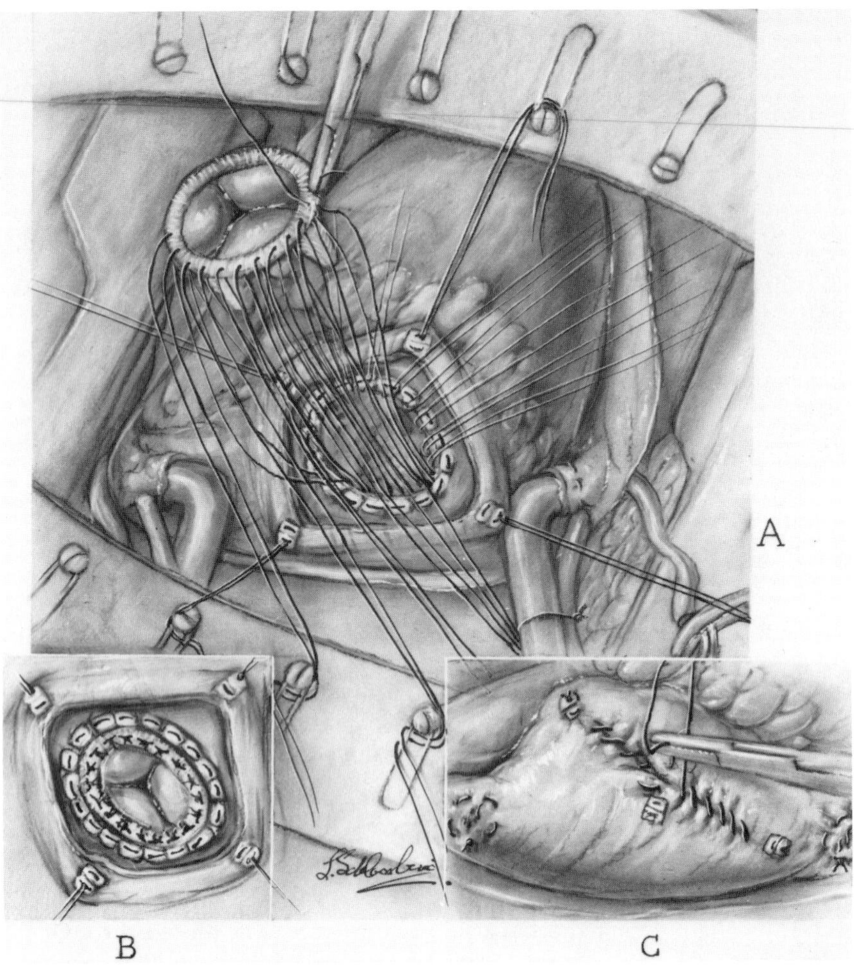

FIG. 3 Replacement of the tricuspid valve. Horizontal mattress sutures are placed along the tricuspid anulus. The sutures are passed through the sewing ring of the bioprosthetic valve, the valve is positioned in the tricuspid anulus, and the atriotomy is closed with a double row of simple continuous sutures. See text for details.

incision was made through the fourth intercostal space. (See Figs. 4–6). A snare was placed around the main pulmonary artery. A purse-string suture was placed in the main pulmonary artery for cannulation of the right ventricle. Heparin, 300 units/kg body weight, was administered intravenously and cannulation of the femoral artery and pulmonary artery was completed. Cardiopulmonary bypass was instituted and the animal's body temperture cooled to 25°C. The ascending aorta was cross clamped and cardioplegic solution consisting of 20 mEq potassium chloride, 5 mEq sodium bicarbo-

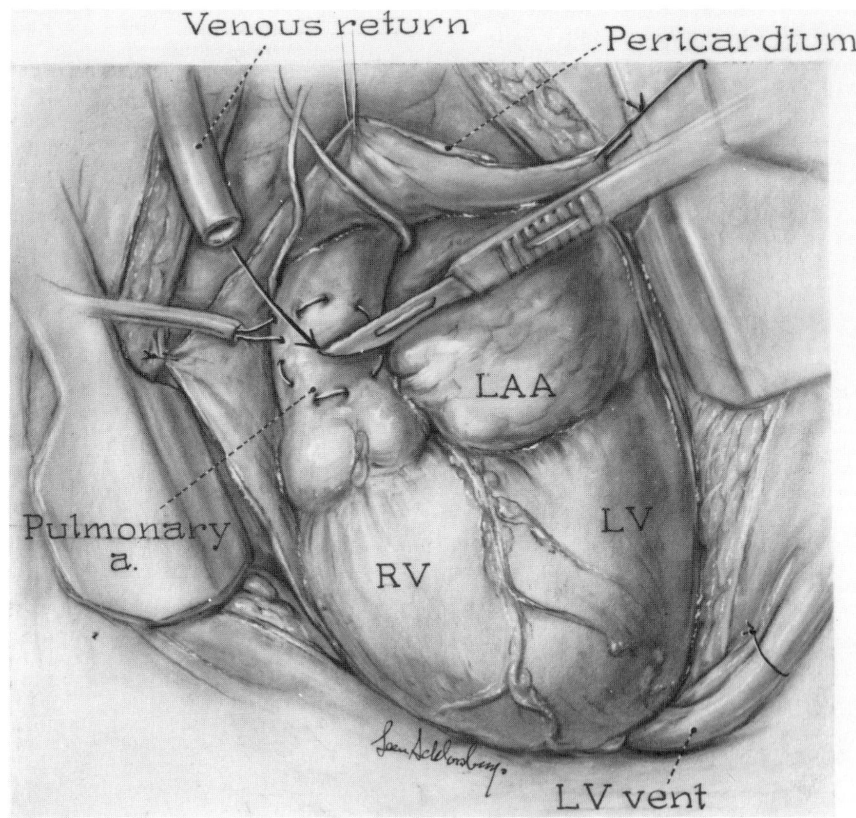

FIG. 4 Replacement of the mitral valve. Orientation is as in Fig. 1. Cannulation for return of systemic venous blood to the cardiopulmonary bypass circuit is performed by positioning a cannula via the pulmonary artery into the right ventricle. A left ventricular vent is placed in the left ventricular apex.

nate, 6.25 g mannitol in 1000 ml of 2.5% dextrose, and 0.44% sodium chloride (pH 7.60, 370 mOsm) at a dose of 10 ml/kg body weight was injected into the aortic root. It is important that the aortic cross clamp be applied so that blood flow to the brain through the brachiocephalic trunk, an anatomic variant in sheep and related animals, is not compromised. All the cranial arteries originate from this vessel. Once cardioplegic arrest had been achieved, an atriotomy was made extending from the left atrial appendage to the left inferior pulmonary vein. The mitral valve was excised and the papillary muscles were transected at their bases; a 2–3 mm remnant of valvular tissue was left in place. Nonabsorbable interrupted mattress sutures buttressed with pledgets were passed through the atrial aspect of the mitral anulus and remaining valvular tissue. The sutures were passed

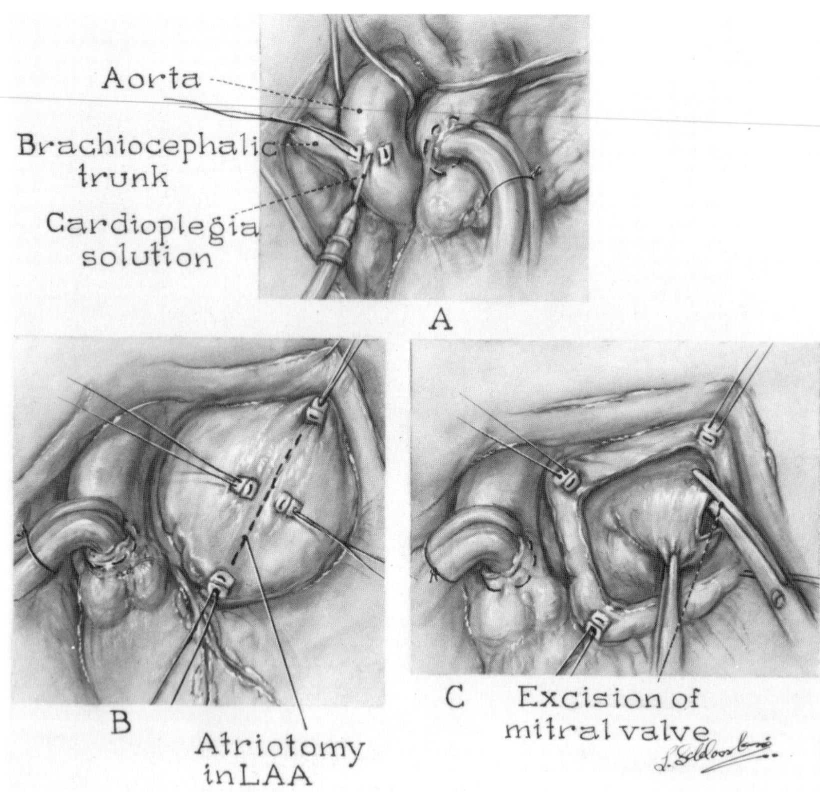

FIG. 5 Replacement of the mitral valve. The ascending aorta is cannulated for injection of cardioplegic solution; note the location of the brachiocephalic trunk from which all the cranial arteries arise. An atriotomy is made extending from the left atrial appendage to the left inferior pulmonary vein and the mitral valve and papillary muscles are excised.

through the sewing ring of the bioprosthesis; the bioprosthesis was oriented so that the widest interstrut distance spanned the left ventricular outflow tract. The valve was seated and the sutures tied and cut. The venous line was momentarily occluded to allow the right heart to fill, and a stab incision was made in the fossa ovalis of the atrial septum for acute left atrial decompression. A catheter was introduced via the left atriotomy and through the bioprosthetic valve to decompress the left ventricle and evacuate air during atrial closure. Before completion of the artiotomy closure, the pulmonary artery snare was released, the aortic cross clamp was removed, the aortic valve was made regurgitant by distorting the aortic root and the lungs were expanded to insure that all air was removed from the left heart structures. The left ventricular vent was removed and closure of the atriotomy com-

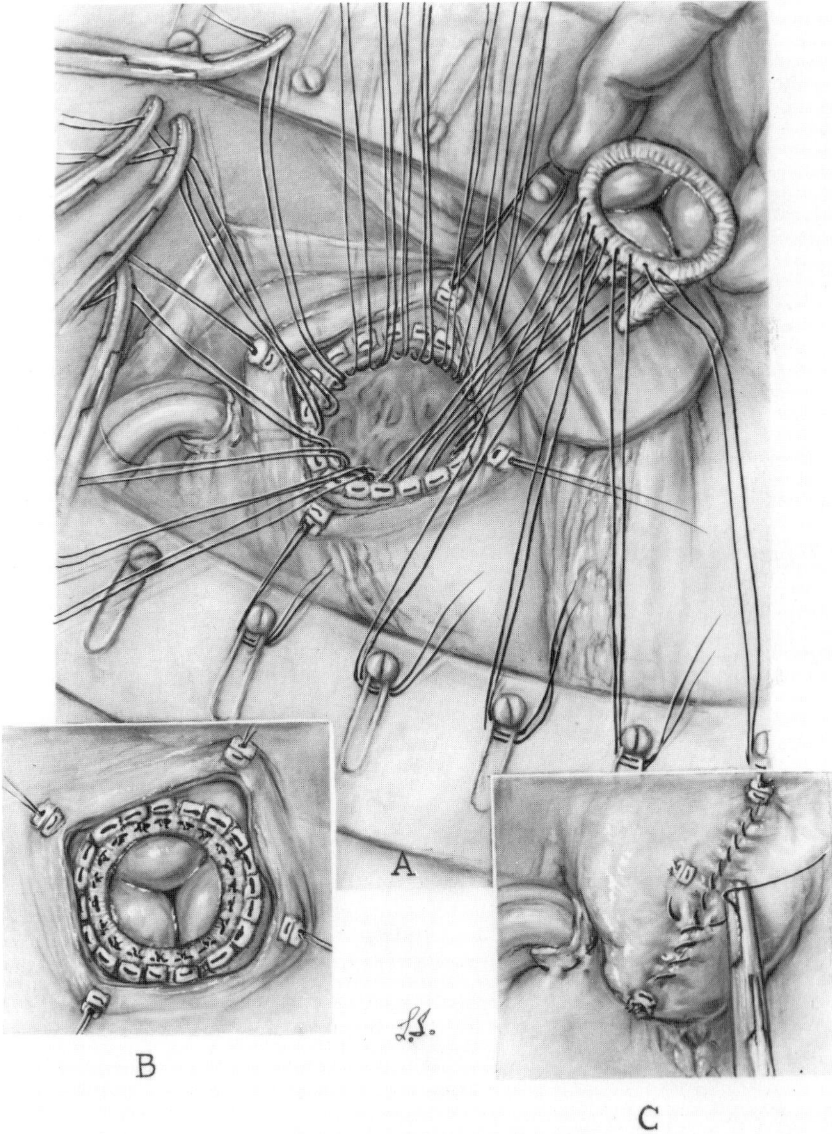

FIG. 6 Replacement of the mitral valve. Horizontal, pledgeted reinforced mattress sutures are placed along the mitral anulus. The bioprosthetic valve is positioned in the mitral anulus and the atriotomy is closed. See text for details.

pleted. The animal's body temperature was rewarmed to 38°C and cardiopulmonary bypass was discontinued. The perfusion cannulae were removed and the remainder of the procedure completed as described for replacement of the tricuspid valve.

Hemodynamic Studies

Following termination of cardiopulmonary bypass and stabilization of the cardiopulmonary status, cardiac outputs were determined by thermodilution technique (See Table I). In the animals that had undergone replacement of the tricuspid valve, right ventricular and right atrial pressure measurements were obtained by pullback of the catheter from the pulmonary artery to determine tricuspid transvalvular mean and end diastolic pressure gradients. In animals that had undergone replacement of the mitral valve, simultaneous left atrial and left ventricular pressure measurments were obtained with small catheters introduced by transmural punctures of these cardiac chambers. Mitral transvalvular mean and end diastolic pressure gradients were determined. Cardiac outputs/kg of body weight, valve orifice areas, and valve areas /kg of body weight were calculated.

Postoperative Care

Following removal of the endotracheal tube, the animal was placed in a warm (70–75°F), humidified (70%), oxygenated (40%) compartment for 24 hours. We emphasize that the position of sternal recumbency must be maintained until the animal is fully conscious. This position is the only one in which sheep can expel the gases that collect in the rumen as a consequence of fermentation. Unless this position is maintained, serious and often fatal respiratory or cardiovascular embarrassment may occur due to distension of the rumen leading to decreased diaphragmatic excursion and due to compression of the inferior vena cava. The chest tube is aspirated at

TABLE I Pathologic findings in 76 bioprosthetic valves implanted for one or more months

Implantation site	#	Duration of implantation (months)	Calcific deposits	Fibrous sheaths	Infection	Intracuspal* hematomas
Tricuspid	41	4.7 ± 1.7	41 (100%)	39 (95%)	5 (12%)	3 (7%)
Mitral	35	3.7 ± 1.4	33 (91%)	32 (91%)	7 (20%)	2 (6%)
Total	76		74 (97%)	71 (93%)	12 (16%)	5 (7%)

* Excludes an additional 2 tricuspid and 6 mitral valves with intracuspal hematomas implanted for less than 1 month.

30 minutes, and at 1, 2, and 8 hours on the day of operation. Usually, chest tubes were removed within the first 48 hours following operation. Antibiotics (penicillin and streptomycin) were given intramuscularly twice a day for the first 5 postoperative days. After 2 weeks, the animals were transferred to our larger facility (National Institutes of Health Animal Center, Poolesville, MD) and maintained using conventional husbandry techniques until elective hemodynamic terminal studies were performed. Monthly physical examinations were performed by staff veterinarians and laboratory studies were performed when indicated.

Terminal Elective Studies

At 3–6 months following implantation, the sheep underwent terminal, elective hemodynamic studies. The studies were performed with the sheep anticoagulated with heparin to prevent the development of postmortem microthrombi on the valves. Thermodilution cardiac outputs and transvalvular mean and end diastolic pressure gradients were obtained. Cardiac outputs/kg body weight, valve orifice areas, and valve orifice areas/kg body weight were calculated. The hemodynamic studies were performed for comparison with the values obtained immediately after implantation of the bioprosthetic valves (See Table I). The animals were then terminated by the injection of potassium chloride. Necropsy examinations were performed. The bioprosthetic valve was photographed and radiographed. Sections of each leaflet were submitted for quantitative analyses of calcium and phosphorus, and for histologic and ultrastructural (scanning and transmission electron microscopic) evaluations.

Results

Tricuspid Valve Implantation

Forty-one (93%) of the 44 sheep that underwent tricuspid valvular implantation survived 1–6 (mean, 4.7) months. Ten sheep died prior to terminal, elective hemodynamic studies: one died of respiratory failure and another of complete heart block within the first 24 hours after operation; the other 8 sheep died of infection of the bioprosthetic valves (4 sheep), cold exposure (2 sheep), and failure of the bioprosthetic valves (2 sheep) from 1–5 months after operation. One animal developed hind limb paralysis due to injury of the femoral nerve; this injury led to an open wound infection, pyarthrosis, bioprosthetic valvular infection, sepsis, and death. No animals developed complications caused by ligation of the femoral artery and vein. Thirty sheep had elective hemodynamic studies performed at an average of 4.9 ± 1.7 months after operation. These results are summarized in Table I.

Mitral Valvular Implantation

Of the 55 sheep that had undergone implantation of bioprosthetic valves in the mitral position, 35 (64%) survived from 1–6 (mean, 3.7 ± 1.4) months. Twenty sheep died within 4 days after operation from: cardiopulmonary failure (17 sheep), coronary arterial air emboli (1 sheep), respiratory failure (1 sheep), and hemorrhage (1 sheep). Eighteen sheep died 1–5 (mean, 2.8) months from cardiopulmonary problems related to bioprosthetic valvular failure (11 sheep), infection of the bioprosthetic valves (7 sheep), and late pericardial tamponade (1 sheep). Fifteen sheep had elective hemodynamic studies performed at an average of 4.6 ± 0.7 months after operation. These results are also summarized in Table I. None of the sheep with mitral bioprostheses developed wound infections, hind limb paralyses, or complications due to ligation of the femoral artery and vein.

Pathologic Observations

Pathologic (including clinical, hemodynamic, and morphologic) observations were limted to those 76 sheep surviving 1 or more (mean, 4.2 ± 1.7) months. Clinical, hemodynamic, and/or morphologic deterioration occurred in all 76 of these valves. Clinical deterioration, as determined by the staff veterinarians, was followed by prompt hemodynamic evaluation. Technically satisfactory early and late hemodynamic evaluations were performed upon 45 of the 76 sheep. Each of the 30 sheep having bioprosthetic valves implanted in the tricuspid position had decreased cardiac outputs/kg body weight, increased mean transvalvular gradients and end diastolic gradients, and/or decreased valve areas. Similar abnormalities were found in each of the 15 sheep studied hemodynamically with bioprosthetic valves implanted in the mitral position. Calcific deposits were documented by quantitative, radiographic, and/or histologic analyses in 74 of the 76 valves. By quantitative analyses, in the explanted tricuspid valves (n = 34) calcium averaged 196 ± 44.4 mg/g of tissue dry weight and in the explanted mitral valves (n = 26) it averaged 96.4 ± 13.6 mg/g of tissue dry weight. In comparison, calcium content averaged 1.2 ± 0.2 mg/g tissue dry weight in nonimplanted valves (n = 27). Morphologic abnormalities, including calcific deposits within the cuspal connective tissue, the muscle shelves, and/or microthrombi, fibrous sheathing of the leaflet tissue, intracuspal hematomas, and/or infection, were observed in all 76 valves. These morphologic findings are itemized in Table II and illustrated in Fig. 7.

Comment

The present study demonstrates that sheep constitute a satisfactory animal model for the evaluation and testing of bioprosthetic cardiac valves. We

TABLE II Hemodynamic alterations of 51 bioprosthetic valves implanted for one or more months

Implantation site	#	Duration of implantation (months)	Decreased CO/kg	Increased end-diastolic gradient	Increased mean gradient	Decreased valve area
Tricuspid	34	4.9 ± 1.7	28 (82%)	12 (32%)	15 (44%)	21 (62%)
Mitral	17	4.6 ± 0.7	12 (71%)	3 (18%)	7 (41%)	8 (47%)
Total	51		40 (78%)	15 (29%)	22 (43%)	29 (57%)

CO/kg = cardiac output per kg body weight.
Hemodynamic values compare those values obtained immediately after implantation of the bioprosthetic valves to those obtained at the time of elective, hemodynamic terminal studies.

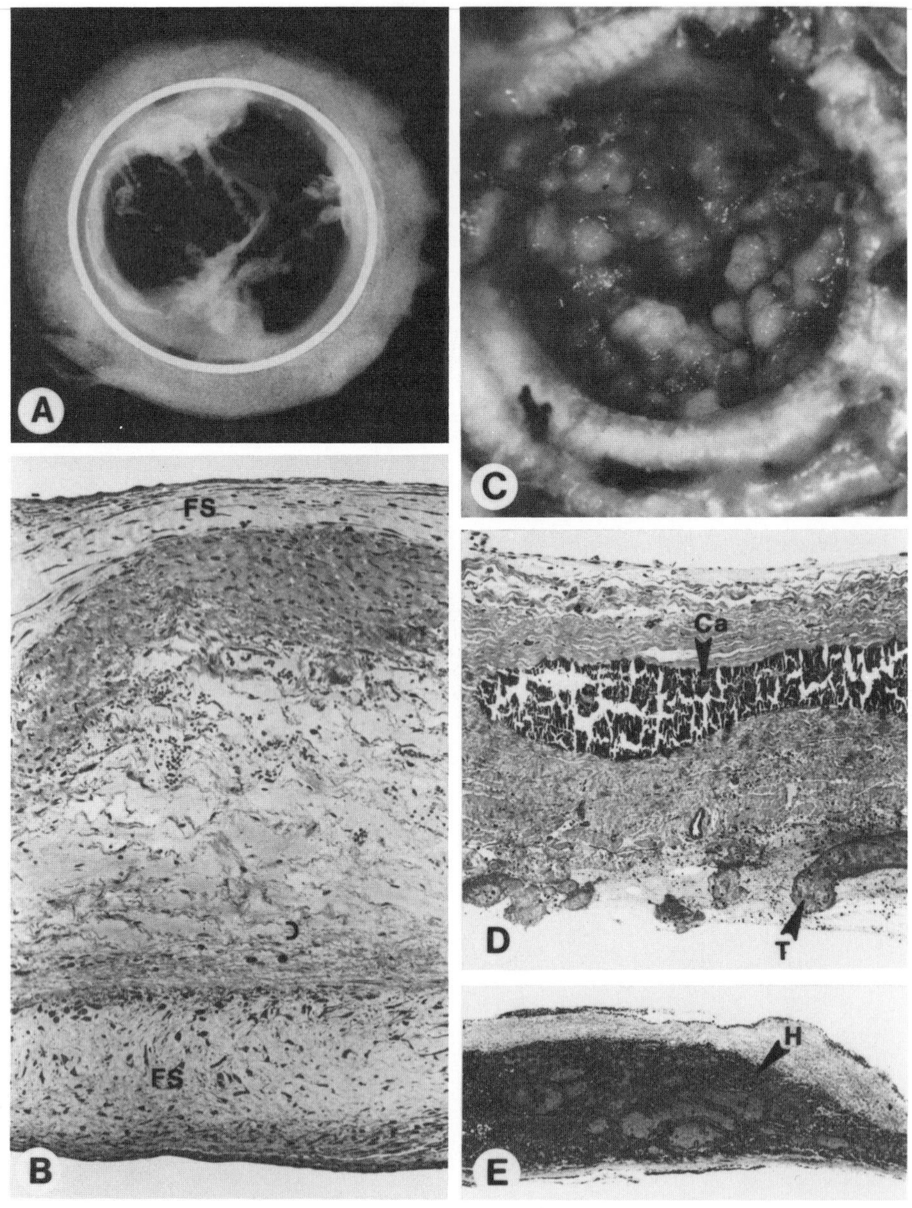
A
B
C
D
E
FS
FS
Ca
T
H

also describe the techniques employed by our laboratory in this experimental animal model. Little experience is available with bioprosthetic valvular implantation in sheep.[19] Other animal species that have been used as experimental models for the evaluation of biologic materials used as cardiac valvular substitutes include calves and dogs. Yarbrough et al[20] reported the occurrence of structural alterations in valvular bioprostheses constructed from fresh autogenous pericardium, fresh autogenous or glutaraldehyde-preserved human fascia lata, and formalin-preserved porcine valvular bioprostheses implanted in human beings and calves. This study concluded that cardiac valvular substitutes constructed from these biologic materials were unacceptable; in contrast, glutaraldehyde-preserved porcine valvular bioprostheses were found acceptable as substitutes for cardiac valves. Harasaki et al[21] noted bioprosthetic valvular degeneration and calcification in bovine aortic and human dura mater valvular bioprostheses in artificial hearts implanted in calves. The rapid rate of growth and weight gain of calves within their first year of life make them undesirable as models for long-term bioprosthetic valvular testing. The placement of bioprosthetic valves within artificial hearts for the purposes of testing seems much less practical than intracardiac implantation.

Dogs have also been used for the experimental evaluation of bioprosthetic valves. Geroulanos et al[22] reported a study in dogs demonstrating the scanning electron microscopic changes of bioprosthetic valvular surfaces. No reports are available of changes in bioprosthetic valves that have been implanted in dogs for long periods of time. The small tricuspid and mitral anular sizes of dogs during their juvenile period of life make the intracardiac implantation of clinically available valvular bioprostheses technically difficult in this species.

Sheep are an excellent laboratory animal model for the study of bio-

---

Fig. 7 Morphologic alterations in explanted bioprosthetic valves. A. Roentgenogram showing calcific deposits, particularly in regions of commissures, in porcine aortic valvular bioprosthesis implanted for 5 months in mitral position. B. Well-developed fibrous sheaths (FS) are present on inflow (bottom) and the outflow (top) surfaces of porcine valvular bioprosthesis implanted for 6 months in tricuspid position. Large, clear spaces are seen in the spongiosa (center). (One micron-thick plastic embedded section, H & E, × 120.) C. Numerous vegetations are present on inflow surface of bovine pericardial bioprosthesis recovered at necropsy 4 months after implantation in tricuspid position. D. Calcific deposits (Ca) form a large nodule in the central 3rd of bovine pericardial bioprosthesis implanted for 6 months in the tricuspid position. Microthrombi (T) developed on the inflow surface (bottom). (One micron-thick plastic section, alkaline toluidine blue stain, ×100.) E. Intracuspal hematoma (H) forms a wide zone separating fibrosa (top) and ventricularis (bottom) of porcine aortic valvular bioprosthesis that had been implanted for 12 hours in mitral position. (H & E, ×20.)

prosthetic valvular degeneration and calcification for several reasons. Standard cardiopulmonary bypass techniques with modifications may be used in juvenile sheep without difficulty, and the hearts of juvenile sheep are of a size suitable for the implantation of clinically available valvular bioprostheses. Sheep hearts do not grow so rapidly as to produce relative stenosis of the bioprosthetic orifices. The degenerative alterations and calcification in valves removed from sheep appear morphologically similar to those found in the same types of valves removed from the human. These pathologic alterations occur over several months (rather than over several years, as is the case in humans), allowing expeditious study of the valves. Sheep also offer a model in which valves can be implanted in juvenile animals and harvested at the animals' maturity for evaluation. The rate of growth and absolute size increase of sheep from approximately 3 months of age to maturity at 10 to 12 months of age impose no restrictions for valvular implantation. Implantation in juvenile sheep also allows for the study of these pathologic alterations in young, growing animals; this situation is analogous to that found in children and adolescents, in whom bioprosthetic valvular degeneration and calcification is known to occur much sooner following implantation than in the adult human.[14–19] In our experience, the serum calcium levels in young sheep, like those in the young human, are in the high normal range; their serum phosphorus and alkaline phosphatase levels are elevated as compared to those of adults. These alterations, which appear to be related to bone growth, are thought to be of importance in the pathogenesis of calcific deposits in bioprostheses.[14]

Conclusions

Valvular bioprostheses have become established as the cardiac valvular substitutes of choice in many centers. Bioprosthetic valvular degeneration and calcification occur at variable times following implantation, and the occurrence of these pathologic processes increases with the passage of time after implantation. It is clear that bioprosthetic valves potentially offer advantages over mechanical valves; however, it is imperative that the problems of degeneration and calcification be better understood before further improvements can be made in the technology of bioprosthetic valvular development. Thus, we offer the ovine in vivo experimental animal model as a system for the study of the problems of bioprosthetic valvular degeneration and calcification.

References

1. Buch WS, Kosek JC, Angell WW: Deterioration of formalin-treated aortic valve heterografts. J Thorac Cardiovasc Surg 60:673, 1970.

2. Carpentier A, Deloche A, Relland J, Fabiani JN, Forman J, Camilleri JP, Soyer R, Dubost C: Six-year follow-up of glutaraldehyde-preserved heterografts. J Thorac Cardiovasc Surg 68:771, 1974.
3. Oyer PE, Stinson EB, Griepp RB, Shumway NE: Valve replacement with the Starr-Edwards and Hancock prosthesis: Comparative analysis of late morbidity and mortality. Ann Surg 186:301, 1977.
4. Pipkin RD, Buch WS, Fogarty TJ: Evaluation of aortic valve replacement with a porcine xenograft without long-term anticoagulation. J Thorac Cardiovasc Surg 71:179, 1976.
5. Ferrans VJ, Boyce SW, Billingham ME, Jones M, Ishihara T, Roberts WC: Calcific deposits in porcine bioprostheses: Structure and pathogenesis. Am J Cardiol 46:721, 1980.
6. Ferrans VJ, Spray TL, Billingham ME, Roberts WC: Structural changes in glutaraldehyde-treated porcine heterografts used as substitute cardiac valves. Am J Cardiol 41:1159, 1978.
7. Fishbein MC, Gissen SA, Collins JJ, Barsamian EM, Cohn LH: Pathologic findings after cardiac valve replacement with glutaraldehyde-fixed porcine valves. Am J Cardiol 40:331, 1977.
8. Riddle JM, Magilligan DJ Jr, Stein PD: Surface morphology of degenerated porcine bioprosthetic valves four to seven years following implantation. J Thorac Cardiovasc Surg 81:279, 1981.
9. Magilligan DJ, Jr, Lewis JW, Jr, Jara FM, Lee MW, Alam M, Riddle JM, Stein PD: Spontaneous degeneration of porcine bioprosthetic valves. Ann Thorac Surg 30:259, 1980.
10. Hetzer, R, Hill JD, Kerth WJ, Wilson AJ, Adappa MG, Gerbode F: Thrombosis and degeneration of Hancock valves: Clinical and pathological findings. Ann Thorac Surg 26:317, 1978.
11. Gordon MH, Walters MB, Allen P, Burton JD: Calcific stenosis of a glutaraldehyde-treated porcine bioprosthesis in the aortic position. J Thorac Cardiovasc Surg 80:788, 1980.
12. Bloch WN, Karcioglu Z, Felner JM, Miller JS, Symbas PN, Schlant RC: Idiopathic perforation of a porcine aortic bioprosthesis in the aortic position. Chest 74:579, 1978.
13. Lipson LC, Kent KM, Rosing DR, Bonow RO, McIntosh CL, Condit J, Epstein SE, Morrow AG: Long-term hemodynamic assessment of the porcine heterograft in the mitral position. Late development of valvular stenosis. Circulation 64:397, 1981.
14. Sanders SP, Levy RJ, Freed MD, Norwood WI, Castaneda AR: Use of Hancock porcine xenografts in children and adolescents. Am J Cardiol 46:429, 1980.
15. Kutsche LM, Oyer P, Shumway N, Baum D: An important complication of Hancock mitral valve replacement in children. Circulation 60 (Suppl I):98, 1979.
16. Geha AS, Laks H, Stansel HC, Cornhill JF, Kilman JN, Buckley MJ, Roberts WC: Late failure of porcine valve heterografts in children. J Thorac Cardiovasc Surg 78:351, 1979.
17. Bortolotti U, Milano A, Mazzucco A, Gallucci V, Valenti M, Del Maschio A, Valfre C, Thiene G: Alterazioni strutturali delle bioprotesi di Hancock applicate in età pediatrica. G Ital Cardiol 10:1520, 1980.
18. Williams WG, Pollock JC, Geiss DM, Trussler GA, Fowler RS: Experience with aortic and mitral valve replacement in children. J Thorac Cardiovasc Surg 81:326, 1981.
19. Reis RL, Hancock WD, Yarbrough JW, Glancy DL, Morrow AG: The flexible

stent. A new concept in the fabrication of tissue heart valve prostheses. J Thorac Cardiovasc Surg 62:683, 1971.

20. Yarbrough JW, Roberts WC, Reis RL: Structural alterations in tissue cardiac valves implanted in patients and in calves. J Thorac Cardiovasc Surg 65:364, 1973.
21. Harasaki H, Kiraly RJ, Jacobs GB, Snow JL, Nosé V: Bovine aortic and human dura mater valves. A comparative study in artifical hearts in calves. J Thorac Cardiovasc Surg 79:125, 1980.
22. Geroulanos S, Gossler W, Walpoth B, Turina M, Senning A: Frühe rasterelektronenoptische Oberflächenveränderungen nach orthotoper Pulmonalklappen-Xenotransplantation durch glutaraldehyd-konditionierte Schweineklappen. Helv Chir Acta 46:91, 1979.

28

Role of Mechanical Stress in Calcification of Bioprostheses

J. D. Deck, M. J. Thubrikar, S. P. Nolan, J. Aouad

Bioprosthetic valves have been used with increasing frequency as successful replacements for diseased human valves for more than 10 years.[1] Commonly employed bioprosthetic valves now include porcine aortic valves and trileaflet prostheses constructed from pericardial tissue.[2] In recent years calcific deterioration of these valves has increasingly proved to be a problem: in children after brief implantations[3] and in adult patients 3–8 years after implantation.[4] By the time that calcification has been sufficiently advanced in these valves to require replacement, the sites of initial calcification and their causes have been substantially obscured. Calcium deposits, however, have been most consistently described in association with sites of collagen disorganization or disintegration.[4,5] It is reasonable to suspect that the breakdown of collagen is caused by excessive wear from functional movements of the implanted valves.

How to investigate these movements of implanted valves during actual in situ operation was already apparent from our earlier studies of natural valve function in vivo.[6,7] In these studies we had exposed the valves by aortotomy and attached radiopaque markers to leaflets at selected places to permit the postrecovery fluoroscopic recording of tagged leaflet movements on videotape. Analysis of these movements demonstrated where and how much leaflets flexed as they opened and closed. This provided the basis for calculating their elasticity in vivo and the stresses they sustained. A combination of differences in elastic properties between open and closed leaflets[8] and renewability of their tissues[9] appears to confer durability on the natural

---

From the Departments of Anatomy, Surgery and Comparative Medicine, University of Virginia, Charlottesville, Virginia.
Supported by U.S. National Institutes of Health Research Grants HL-16935 and HL-17969.

valve.[10] In the preserved tissues of the bioprosthetic valves, on the other hand, it seemed reasonable to suppose elasticity would differ from the natural valves and, of course, tissue renewal would be foreclosed. Tracing the movements of implanted bioprosthetic leaflets by the same marker techniques was expected to demonstrate the regions of maximal bending and the stresses associated with them.

We chose to implant the tagged bioprosthetic valves in young calves, because of their similarity to the human in size of aorta and postoperative function of valves.[11–13] Early in the experiments we discovered that the implanted valves began to calcify within a few weeks. Realizing that this event occurred in calves precociously with respect to most human cases, we undertook to study the location of calcium deposits in implanted valves (subsequently recovered from the calves) in an effort to understand the steps of calcification.

Materials and Methods

Observations were made on 4 Carpentier-Edwards, 5 Hancock porcine valves, and 7 Ionescu-Shiley pericardial valves, all of 23 mm mounting diameter. These valves were implanted in the aortic position in calves 4–6 weeks old by means of aortotomy and cardiopulmonary bypass and were observed over a period of 4–11 weeks. Most implanted valves had platinum markers 1 mm long placed variously on the leaflets and walls to permit fluoroscopic tracing of valve movements, but at least 2 valves of each kind were without markers, removing any influence the markers might have on subsequent developments. Valve movements were studied within a week and once again 4–11 weeks postoperatively and recorded on videotape at 60 fields/s. Field by field analysis of the tapes with respect to marker positions and distance between markers made it possible to reconstruct leaflet geometry in the fully open and closed positions and demonstrated the degree of leaflet flexion that occurred. Bending stresses associated with this flexion deformation could then be calculated by using the modulus of elasticity for bioprosthetic tissue. This elasticity was determined initially in vitro and secondarily related to the in vivo situation by data from the marker studies. Along with the studies of valve movements, diastolic pressure gradients across leaflets of at least 2 bioprostheses of each kind were measured to permit the calculation of associated membrane stresses. Systolic pressure gradients measured to be less than 10 mmHg.[12,13] Total stresses on the functioning valves consisted of the summation of membrane and bending stresses.

Calves were killed 4–11 weeks after valve implantation. Valves were excised and visually examined for evidence of calcification. Surface deposits, including thrombi and vegetations, were then removed from the valves, with care not to disturb the tissue, and radiographs of whole valves and detached leaflets were made to locate sites of calcification. Finally, leaflets were embedded in paraffin or plastic for histologic or ultrastructural examination. Representative sections were cut in both the radial and the circumferential directions. Paraffin sections were stained by the calcium identification method of Dahl.[14] Thick plastic sections were stained with hematoxylin and eosin for optical microscopy. Thin sections were stained for electron microscopy with uranyl acetate and lead citrate. Prior to embedding, valves excised from the calves were kept in their original commercial fixative containing glutaraldehyde, which effectively fixed any calf-derived material in the tissues.

Results

Functional wear as a suspected cause of collagen disintegration in calcifying bioprosthetic valves is necessarily a reflection of stresses in the valves. We obtained stress/strain curves in vitro for strips of tissue from bioprosthetic leaflets, using an Instron tensile testing machine. We were then able to calculate in vivo stresses in the leaflets from our marker studies.

Total stresses in the leaflets consisted of membrane and bending stresses. Membrane stresses result from pressure gradients across the leaflets and changes in leaflet curvature, but pressure gradients produce the most significant effect. Pressure gradients were measured directly at 2 different times from transducers above and below the implanted valves. As in natural valves, the diastolic gradient was high (80–100 mmHg) with concomitant high stresses, and the systolic gradient was low (5–10 mmHg). Membrane stress was high in closed leaflets because of the pressure differential across the leaflet and low in open leaflets as the gradient dropped. Membrane stresses represent the total stresses in diastole, since bending stresses are not present during this portion of the cycle.

Bending stresses are the other component of total leaflet stress in systole. Bending stresses occur at the leaflet attachments as well as within the body of the leaflets as a result of change in the configuration of the leaflet. These stresses are a function of angular displacement of tissue, length of the bending zone, thickness of the tissue, and change in the curvature of the leaflet. Angular displacement, length of the bending zone, and change in the curvature of the leaflet were determined from the marker studies in vivo, which quickly demonstrated the principal bending zones and their approximate breadth in the several kinds of leaflets (Fig. 1). The most acute bending of leaflets occurred at their mural attachments as they opened, although in porcine valves significant stressful bending also took place in the centers of the leaflets. After bending zones had been identified in vivo, tissue thickness was measured directly from the leaflets themselves follow-

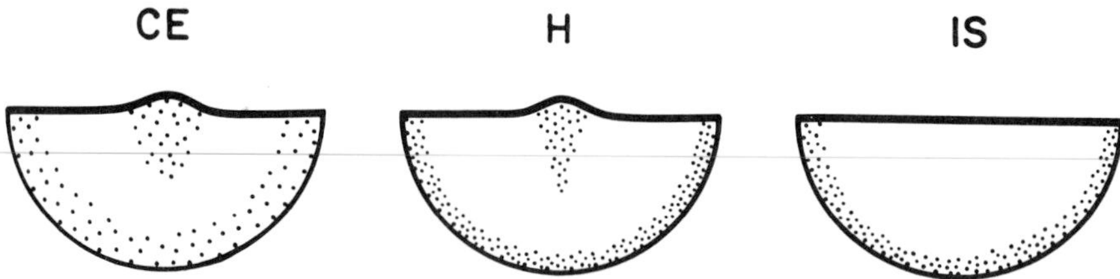

FIG. 1 Drawings of aortic valve leaflets stippled to show where each type of valve flexed as it opened and closed. The Carpentier-Edwards (CE) leaflet had the broadest zone of sharp bending, both along its attachment and in the center. In the Hancock (H) leaflet acute bending was concentrated more intensely in narrower zones. The Ionescu-Shiley (IS) leaflet underwent sharp bending only around its attachment margin.

ing valve excision. From these data, bending stresses were calculated over the whole leaflet. Bending stresses were then added to the membrane stresses to determine the total stresses in systole. The total stresses were highest at the leaflet attachment, being maximum at the upper point of attachment and decreasing toward the base. Furthermore, the stresses were compressive on the aortic surface and tensile on the ventricular surface. In the middle of the leaflet, small compressive stresses occurred on the ventricular side. At about 3 mm away from the leaflet attachment, small compressive stresses occurred on the aortic surface. The details of stress distribution are reported elsewhere.[12,13] Stress/strain curves from the bioprosthetic tissues indicate that the tissues are well adapted for tensile stresses but are unable to sustain compressive stresses. As a consequence, localized tissue buckling accompanied by internal cavitation is likely to take place where compressive bending stresses are high, leading ultimately to tissue disintegration (see Fig. 2).

Clues from histologic studies, which are described later, raised the question whether the flexion of opening and closing in pericardial valve leaflets produced shearing. It was possible to resolve the question very simply by directly observing the behavior of pericardial leaflets during bending. Two vertical lines were drawn across flattened leaflets to simulate sharp edges; microscopic examination of the direction taken by these lines as the leaflets were flexed then demonstrated the nature of stresses produced. If bending resulted only in tensile and compressive stresses, extensions of both lines would pass through the center of the circle of curvature (Fig. 2). One of the lines instead passed outside the center, indicating that internal shearing had caused slippage between layers and created an angular edge.[15]

By these combinations of observation and calculation, it has been possible to discover what kinds of stresses occur in bioprosthetic leaflets and where they are most intense. To consider whether such stresses play a role in tissue calcification, presumably by way of disintegration and cavitation

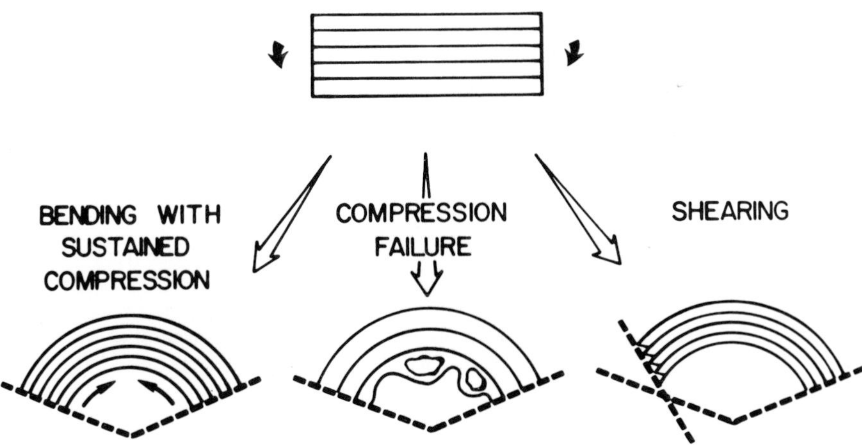

FIG. 2 How bending stresses can affect a laminated structure like the valve leaflet. If the structure, the ends of which are cut perpendicular to its surface (upper sketch), is flexed downward at the ends (solid arrows), it will respond by true bending, by buckling, or by shearing. In true bending (sketch at lower left) the upper surface stretches and the lower surface is compressed (arrows) so that lines drawn across the cut ends pass through the center of bending curvature. If the structure tolerates compression poorly (sketch in lower center), its compressed surface tends to buckle and holes may be formed within it. If the laminated structure shears between its layers as it bends (sketch at lower right), a line drawn across its cut ends will pass outside the center of bending curvature. Thus, response to stress can be assayed by looking at the ends and the concave surface.

within the tissues, it was necessary to determine where the earliest calcifications occurred. Valves were excised from calves between 4 and 11 weeks postoperatively and examined grossly for signs of calcification. Whitish, mineralized deposits were evident in all porcine valves implanted as long as 7 weeks and in all pericardial valves after 4 weeks. In porcine valves the mineralized deposits appeared within the tissue as parallel streaks originating in zones of leaflet attachment and tapering into the leaflets themselves. Deposits occurred first in commissural and later in basal regions of leaflets and were more prominent toward the aortic surfaces than toward the ventricular surfaces. In one porcine valve of each type, mineralized material ultimately was deposited toward the center of the leaflet as well. In pericardial valves, mineralized material also appeared in regions of leaflet attachment, but as clusters of nodular deposits (rather than localized streaks) both within tissues and superficially. Deposits increased with time but continued to be confined mainly to the attachment zones.

Radiographs were taken of all leaflets after removal of surface thrombi, vegetations, and encrustations. Mineralized materials appeared as opacities in the radiographs (Figs. 3 and 4). In porcine valves, radiography revealed

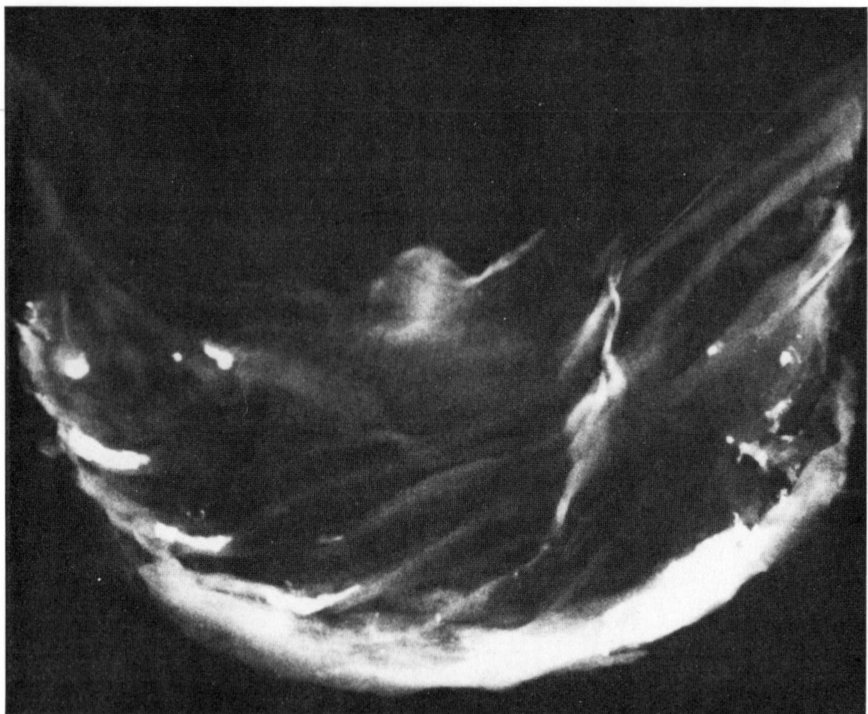

FIG. 3 Radiogram of a porcine leaflet showing early deposits of calcium as 3 radiopaque (very white) streaks on the left edge and 1 on the right edge along collagenous cords. Less intensely white areas in the radiograph represent tissue folds and edges. Note that no calcification occurred in the center of the free edge, where a leaflet marker had been attached.

calcification as early as 4 weeks after implantation, even though it was not apparent visually until several weeks later. As in the visual examinations, leaflet radiography demonstrated mineralization as parallel streaks passing into the leaflets from their areas of wall attachment, first in the commissural regions and later at the bases of leaflets (Fig. 3). Mineralization was also evident in the aortic wall of the porcine tissue. Radiography similarly confirmed the visual examinations of pericardial valves, displaying calcifications as opaque clusters of material around the margins of leaflet attachment (Fig. 4). In any particular valve, all 3 leaflets contained radiographic opacities, without influence from valve orientation in the animal. It is important to note that placement of markers on leaflets, which may have crushed or punctured the tissue, was not accompanied by calcification (Fig. 3). To reiterate both visual and radiographic observations, calcification in all types of valves began near the leaflet attachments, which were shown by marker

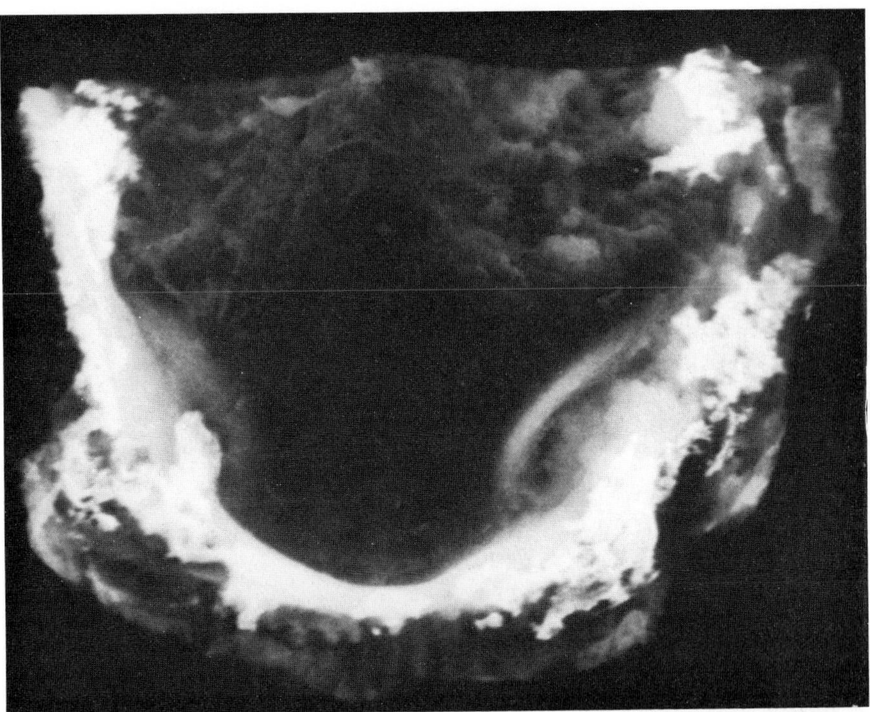

FIG. 4 Radiogram of a pericardial leaflet showing clustered deposits of calcium at the upper and lower right and left and at the middle right, all along the margin of leaflet attachment. The U-shaped tissue opacity that follows the same margin and partially obscures the calcified areas resulted from curvature of the leaflet that increased its depth and its radiodensity.

studies to be the areas of most acute flexion, and increased in amount with length of implantation.

Three valves of each type were studied histologically to confirm the identification of calcific deposits and to relate them to structural features of the leaflets. Dahl's stain for calcium revealed calcific deposits as reddish-purple granulations in otherwise unstained tissues. Hematoxylin-eosin staining also produced a sharp staining of the same features of leaflets (Figs. 5 and 6) and hence was utilized for most of the verification studies. It was readily apparent from these histologic sections that calcification occurred not only within the leaflets of porcine valves, but on the surface as well as within the leaflets of pericardial valves. In porcine leaflets, calcific material was deposited in early stages, mainly within tendinous cords of the lamina fibrosa, which are especially marked in these valves (Fig. 5). In one Carpentier-Edwards leaflet the only accumulation of calcium was found at

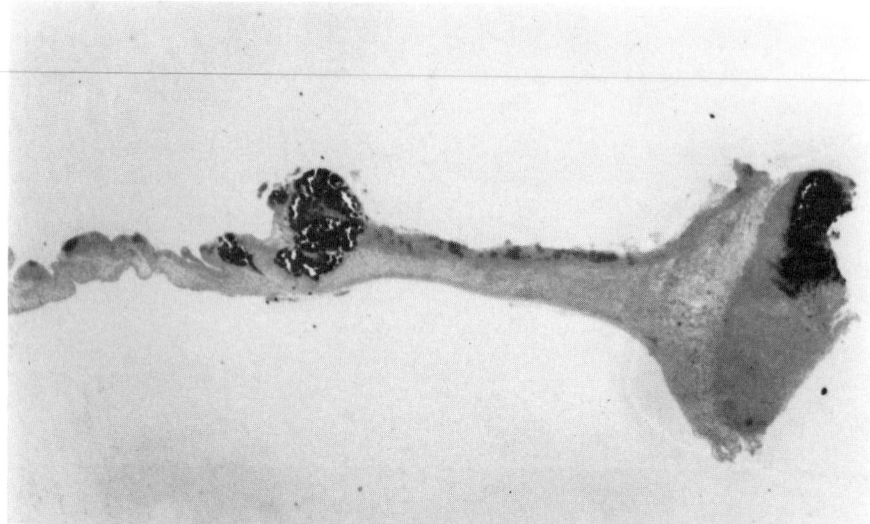

FIG. 5 Histologic section from a porcine leaflet cut in the radial direction. Dense calcified masses can be seen in the aortic wall (at right) and in an enlarged and protruding collagenous cord of the leaflet just beneath its aortic surface. At least one other transected cord contains a smaller amount of calcified material. The free edge of the leaflet is out of the figure to the left. (×18.)

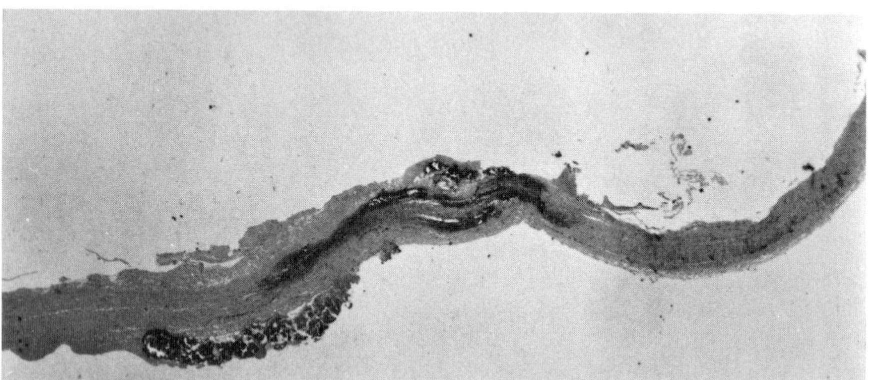

FIG. 6 Histologic section from a pericardial leaflet cut in the radial direction. Several layers of dense collagenous tissue make up the leaflet. Darly stained calcified material occurs along and between these layers, which appear to have been separated by shearing. Note that calcification is not limited to one part of the leaflet tissues but occurs through its entire thickness. (×18.)

the place in these collagenous cords where they would have been most severely compressed by opening of the valve. Leaflet appearance and function were not altered in these valves, which subsequently were found histologically to contain early stages of calcification, indicating that apparent normalcy is not a reliable indicator of the absence of calcification. Longer implantations of the porcine valves produced calcification at bases of leaflets within the lamina spongiosa as well as within the collagenous cords of the fibrosa. Within the aortic wall of the porcine valves, calcification occurred along the parallel planes of musculoelastic tissue, coinciding thus with the dominant architectural lamination and differing markedly from the pattern found in the leaflets.

Histologic sections of leaflets made from pericardial tissue reveal a structure markedly different from the porcine bioprostheses. Instead of the porcine *fibrosa* with its tendinous cords and *spongiosa* backed up by an elastic layer, pericardial leaflets consist of a number of essentially identical layers of dense collagenous sheets parallel to the surface. In spite of these differences, calcification occurred in the same zones of each kind of leaflet. In pericardial leaflets, however, it was indicated histologically that the calcium deposits were laid down more diffusely in all layers of the bending zone, both within and especially between the sheets of collagenous fibers (Fig. 6). It was the discovery of this pattern of interlaminar calcification that first called our attention to the possible damage to continually flexed leaflets from shearing stresses. It is worth noting that the laminar pattern of calcification which we saw in the walls of porcine valves is essentially similar to that which occurred in pericardial leaflets.

Ultrastructural studies of calcification in these bioprosthetic valves are still incomplete but nevertheless have provided some recurrent observations. In leaflet tissues from zones of bending, we find calcified material most often associated with collagenous fibrils (Fig. 7). Enlargement of an area of calcification shows it to be composed of needle-shaped crystals in dense masses (Fig. 8). The calcium content of the crystals and masses has been verified by x-ray elemental analysis. Crystals can be found surrounding or even within the collagenous fibrils. Other visible structural features of the tissue besides collagen are not regularly seen as foci for the masses of crystals. We have not yet recognized consistent evidence of collagenous fibrillar disintegration where low and presumably initial concentrations of crystals are found, nor does obvious breakdown of collagen characterize areas of high calcium density. Therefore our expectation that continued stress would be manifested in the disruption of collagen accompanied by calcification has not yet been substantiated by our observations. We have not explored the role of extracellular matrix materials other than collagen in calcification of leaflet tissues.

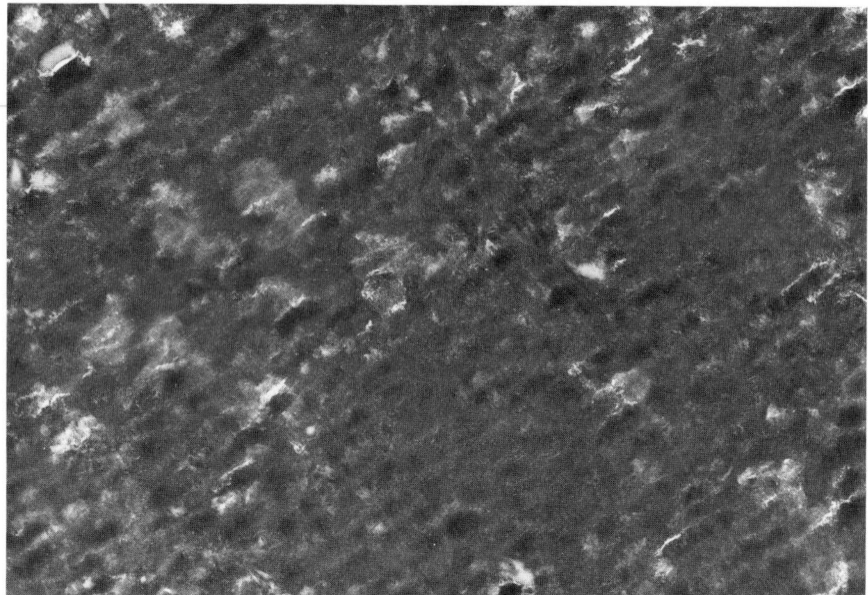

FIG. 7 Low power electron micrograph of collagenous fibrils in the dense tissue of a pericardial leaflet darkened throughout by the presence of electron-dense calcified material. The calcification has occurred unevenly but follows the course of the fibrils from lower left to upper right. Cross banding of the fibrils is hardly visible at this magnification but has not been totally obscured by the calcification. (×15,600.)

Comment

Many observations[1,3,5,16–21] have now reported calcification within cardiac valve bioprostheses. Several causes of calcification have been proposed, including the presence of infection,[16,22] the disintegration of collagenous tissues,[5] and the insudation of calcium-binding proteins.[23] We believe, however, that none of these several possibilities is sufficient by itself to explain the focal nature of calcification observed in our study.

The calcifications that we observed most likely represented initial stages of calcification because they occurred in valves implanted for a relatively brief time and caused no clinically significant changes in transvalvular gradients of systolic pressure. In the absence of any evidence of infection, the initial stages of calcification occurred as a similar pattern in all types of valves, coincident with sites of high mechanical stress in the zones of leaflet flexion. Our calculations show that large compressive and tensile stresses are found in these zones of all the valves. In porcine valves, calcification occurred first in the commissural region where the stresses are highest and

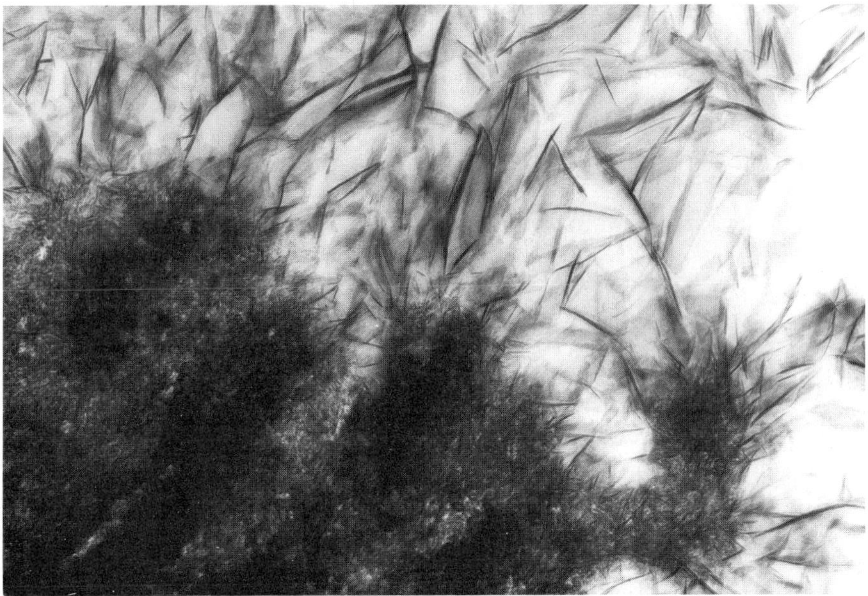

FIG. 8 High power electron micrograph demonstrating massed crystals of calcified material associated with collagenous fibrils out of the figure at the lower left. Individual needle-shaped structures resembling hydroxyapatite crystals are easily seen at the edge of the dense masses but are mostly indistinguishable when packed tightly together. (×96,500.)

somewhat later in the basal region. Longer implantation of these valves also produced calcification in leaflet centers, where reversal of curvature in systole tends to cause elevated mechanical stresses. Pericardial valve leaflets exhibited a somewhat different degree of bending both at the attachments and centrally, perhaps related to a difference in how the tissue was mounted on the valve frame, and calcification in them was limited to the leaflet bending zones.

Mechanical stresses can affect the leaflet in several ways. Primarily they cause deformations that produce structural and other changes within the tissues.[11,12] The 2 simple modes of deformation are pure bending and internal shearing. If a flexed material undergoes pure bending and has little or no tolerance to compressive stress, it will buckle on the compressed face and form voids internally as its substance deteriorates. This appears to describe what we have observed in the collagenous cords of porcine leaflets exposed to large compressive stresses in the zones of bending as these leaflets open. These cords are relatively homogeneous structures that pass obliquely or perpendicularly across the line of bending. Like the leaflet as a whole, they are unable to withstand compressive stresses and may respond by cavitating internally and depositing calcium, in the fashion suggested by our histologic sections. We must acknowledge, of course, that calcification in these cords is not entirely limited to the bending zone but with time spreads for a variable distance along the cords. It may be that compressive stresses are propagated along these cords as well as in the plane of bending itself in response to the beginning of calcification.

The second mode of deformation is by internal shearing. It is most likely to occur in a structure obviously composed of a number of similarly constituted layers, a condition that pericardial leaflets readily meet. In such leaflets, if the various layers are forced to shear or slide over each other, the bonds between layers are progressively broken and clefts between layers can result. From observing pericardial tissue as it is bent, we have concluded that shearing does indeed occur. Shearing may be restrained initially by interlaminar bonds, but if they fail the continued shearing would produce splits between layers. The calcification of pericardial leaflets within and between the layers seems to have delineated just such splits. The lamination of calcified material in the walls of porcine valves may well have resulted from similar shearing stresses.

The actual conditions of bioprosthetic valve function may produce stresses considerably more complex than these simplified versions depict. Nevertheless, our representation offers an initial approximation to the forces that may be generated by valve operation and has the virtue of exposing a pattern of stresses that correlates well with the sites of early calcification seen in the diverse types of valves. Actually, not only the location but also the degree and kind of stress that occur correlate well with calcification. We therefore conclude that mechanical stresses initiate calcification by means that still remain to be clarified. Although tissue destruction appears to be a likely factor, we have not yet identified the ultrastructural features of this condition. The loss of tissue components during valve manufacture and the insudation of extrinsic materials from the host circulation are other possible factors that we have not yet examined, although they seem to offer less obvious ways to explain the patterns we have observed.

References

1. Cohn LH, Koster JK, Mee RBB, Collins JJ: Long-term follow-up of the Hancock bioprosthetic heart valve. Circulation 60 (Suppl 1):87, 1979.
2. Ionescu MI, Tandon AP, Mary DAS, Abid A: Heart valve replacement with the Ionescu-Shiley pericardial xenograft. J Thorac Cardiovasc Surg 73:31, 1977.
3. Geha AS, Laks H, Stansel HC, Cornhill JF, Kilman JW, Buckley MJ, Roberts WC: Late failure of porcine heterografts in children. J Thorac Cardiovasc Surg 78:351, 1979.
4. Ferrans VJ, Boyce SW, Billingham ME, Jones M, Ishihara T, Roberts WC:

Calcific deposits in porcine bioprostheses: Structure and pathogenesis. Am J Cardiol 46:721, 1980.

5. Ferrans VJ, Spray TL, Billingham ME, Roberts WC: Structural changes in glutaraldehyde-treated porcine heterografts used as substitute cardiac valves. Am J Cardiol 41:1159, 1978.
6. Thubrikar M, Harry R, Nolan SP: Normal aortic valve function in dogs. Am J Cardiol 40:563, 1977.
7. Thubrikar M, Bosher LP, Nolan SP: The mechanism of opening of the aortic valve. J Thorac Cardiovasc Surg 77:863, 1979.
8. Thubrikar M, Piepgrass WC, Bosher LP, Nolan SP: The elastic modules of canine aortic valve leaflets *in-vivo* and *in vitro*. Circ Res 47:792, 1980.
9. Schneider PJ, Deck JD: Tissue and cell renewal in the natural aortic valve of rats: An autoradiographic study. Cardiovasc. Res 15:181, 1981.
10. Deck JD, Thubrikar M, Schneider PJ, Nolan SP: Structure, Stress and Tissue Repair in Aortic Valve Leaflets, Proc Annu Conf Engin Med Biol 21:169, 1979.
11. Thubrikar M, Skinner JR, Aouad J, Nolan SP: Geometry and performance of aortic bioprostheses *in vivo*. Surg Forum 31:341, 1980.
12. Thubrikar M, Skinner JR, Eppink RT, Nolan SP: Stress analysis of porcine bioprosthetic heart valves *in vivo*. J Biomed Mater Res 1982. In press.
13. Thubrikar MJ, Skinner JR, Nolan SP: Design and stress analysis of bioprosthetic valves *in vitro*. International Symposium on Cardiac Bioprostheses, 1982. In press.
14. Dahl LK: A simple and sensitive histochemical method for calcium. Proc Soc Exp Biol 80:474, 1952.
15. Thubrikar M, Eppink RT: Analysis of bending and shearing deformations in biological tissue. J Biomech, 1982. In press.
16. Fishbein MC, Gissen SA, Collins JJ Jr, Barsamian EM, Cohn LH: Pathologic findings after cardiac valve replacement with glutaraldehyde-fixed porcine valves. Am J Cardiol 40:331, 1977.
17. Hetzer R, Hill JD, Kerth WJ, Wilson AJ, Adappa MG, Gerbode F: Thrombosis and degeneration of Hancock valves: Clinical and pathological findings. Ann Thorac Surg 26:317, 1978.
18. Rose AG, Forman R, Bowen RM: Calcification of glutaraldehyde-fixed porcine xenograft. Thorax 33:111, 1978.
19. Lamberti JJ, Wainer BH, Fisher KA, Karunaratne HB, Al-Sadir J: Calcific stenosis of the porcine heterograft. Ann Thorac Surg 28:28, 1979.
20. Sanders SP, Levy RJ, Freed MD, Norwood WI, Casteneda AR: Use of Hancock porcine xenografts in children and adolescents. Am J Cardiol 46:429, 1980.
21. Silver MM, Pollock J, Silver MD, Williams WG, Trusler GA: Calcification in porcine xenograft valves in children. Am J Cardiol 45:685, 1980.
22. Ferrans VJ, Boyce SW, Billingham ME, Spray TL, Roberts WC: Infection of glutaraldehyde-preserved porcine valve heterograft. Am J Cardiol 43:1123, 1979.
23. Levy RJ, Zenker JA, Lian JB: Vitamin K-dependent calcium binding proteins in aortic valve calcification. J Clin Invest 65:563, 1980.

29

Inhibition of Mineralization of Glutaraldehyde-Fixed Hancock Bioprosthetic Heart Valves

D. J. Lentz, E. M. Pollock, D. B. Olsen, E. J. Andrews, J. Murashita, W. L. Hastings

Since the introduction of glutaraldehyde-fixed bioprosthetic heart valves in the late 1960s, numerous reports have attested to their efficacy and durability. These valves have good hemodynamic properties and in addition have low rates of thromboembolism in patients without anticoagulation.[1–7] However, with the increased clinical use and the availability of information on long-term implants, it has also been shown that the tissue valve is subject to mineralization in certain individuals. Considering the low incidence of primary tissue failure reported,[8–10] mineralization may be a major factor in the long-term failure of these valves.[11–18] Tissue valve mineralization has become an increasingly important issue in pediatric applications, where the lack of anticoagulation and the long-term durability of the bioprosthesis would be distinct advantages. Clinical evidence, however, suggests that the onset of mineralization is more rapid and the incidence more common in children, presumably as a result of their dynamic calcium metabolism during growth.[7,19–23] Mineralization has therefore emerged as a significant drawback to the extended durability of the tissue valve, and also to its desired use in pediatrics.

The solution to the problem of bioprosthetic mineralization has been hindered by a lack of understanding of the pathogenesis of ectopic mineralization. Both the highly structured collagen of tissue valves and their amorphous ground substance matrix have been implicated as possible causes of mineralization.

From Hancock/Extracorporeal, Inc., Anaheim, California, and The University of Utah, Salt Lake City, Utah.

In vitro experiments on the pathogenesis of ectopic mineralization have concentrated on the metastable solution approach of calcium and phosphate being present physiologically and, in the presence of an appropriate "nucleator," calcium phosphate salts precipitating and transforming into the mineral form of hydroxyapatite. Collagen, in the form of tendon or demineralized bone, has been shown to be a very effective nucleator in this type of system.[24–28]

Experiments in vitro with modified collagen have shown that blockage of ϵ-NH_2 side chains on lysine, hydroxylysine, or of phenolic hydroxyls on tyrosine could inhibit mineralization, presumably as a secondary consequence of steric hindrance or conformational change.[29–32]

The involvement of collagen in mineralization has been suggested by detailed morphologic studies of tissue where early calcification has been described in degenerating fibrils of collagen.[33–36] The collagen may simply act as a passive nucleator, or the calcium of the matrix vesicles may be an active initiating factor in the mineralization process.

These concepts of mineralization suggest the presence of an in vivo regulatory mechanism to prevent a generalized mineralization of the ubiquitous calcium and phosphate into hydroxyapatite. Pyrophosphates have been implicated as regulators, in that diphosphonates can prevent mineralization in both in vivo and in vitro systems.[37–43]

More recent studies on in vivo aspects of mineralization have concentrated on the search for compounds unique to mineralized tissue and therefore possibly involved in its pathogenesis. A class of proteins (GLA proteins) rich in the calcium-binding residues, γ-carboxyglutamic acid, has been described.[44–46] Although the precise role of these GLA proteins is unknown, they have been identified in a wide range of natural and pathologic calcified tissue, and an association, whether causative or not, seems clear.[47–51]

Utilizing the experience of previous workers, we systematically analyzed a large series of chemicals and processes having the potential of preventing or altering the onset of ectopic mineralization of bioprostheses in vivo.

The following studies detail our efforts with particular emphasis on one process designated as T6. This process involves the use of a water-soluble C-12 alkyl sulfate (U.S. Patent #4,323,358).

Materials and Methods

Rat Model

Previous studies in this laboratory had demonstrated that glutaraldehyde-fixed tissue, either porcine cusp or bovine pericardium, would calcify within 8 weeks when implanted intramuscularly in the abdominal wall of rats, an animal well established in calcification research.[29,45,52,53] We therefore used the rat model as a standard screening system for in vivo mineralization and employed 3 independent measures of the presence or degree of mineralization.

Small pieces, each 20–30 mg wet weight, were prepared from glutaraldehyde-fixed tissue (either Hancock porcine valve cusp or bovine pericardium). The tissue pieces were appropriately processed for the particular experiment, rinsed in balanced electrolyte solution, sterilized by standard valve processing procedures, and stored at room temperature in stabilized glutaraldehyde solution. Immediately prior to implantation, tissues were rinsed 3 times in sterile physiologic saline.

The tissue pieces were aseptically implanted in the abdominal wall muscles of anesthetized male Sprague-Dawley rats, weighing 180–200 g. Six tissue replicates were placed in each animal and 5 animals were used for each group, i.e., 30 samples per experiment.

The animals were housed in groups of 5, provided tap water and laboratory chow *ad libitum,* and maintained in appropriate environmental conditions for the species. After specified time intervals, the animals were sacrificed, and the entire abdominal wall was removed with the intramuscular implants in situ.

The abdominal wall was radiographed, using a Hewlett-Packard Faxitron with Kodak Industrex M film. Two implant samples, with surrounding muscle, were then removed, fixed in a solution of 10% nonbuffered formalin, and routinely processed for histologic examination. The remaining 4 implant samples from each animal were dissected free of surrounding host tissue and extracted in 5 ml of 6N hydrochloric acid at 78°C for 96 h. Calcium was measured in the acid extract by atomic absorption spectrophotometry. Control extracts were prepared from unimplanted glutaraldehyde-fixed xenograft tissue, which had been appropriately processed. Rat abdominal muscles, remote from the sites of implant, were also used for control extracts.

Calf Model

Further studies were done to study the potential effects of the experimental anticalcification processes on functional valves in the vascular system.

The calf was chosen as the experimental model, because of its known propensity for accelerated mineralization of glutaraldehyde-fixed materials, such as porcine xenograft valves.[54–57] Porcine bioprosthetic valves, size 30 mm, were evaluated in conduits, implanted from the apex of the left ventricle to the aorta, with a partial ligation of the proximal aorta. This design ensured suitable flow through the valved conduit, adequate coronary perfusion, and continued survival and growth of the animal, regardless of the state of the valved conduit.

Control valved conduits were prepared according to the standard Hancock manufacturing process. Test valves were similarly prepared except for the introduction of the T6 process during fabrication. The valved conduits were then implanted in castrated male Holstein calves, weighing 70–90 kg. Five control and 8 test valves were implanted. Animals were sacrificed at predetermined intervals: controls after 4 months, and test animals after 4, 8, or 12 months. At necropsy, a gross examination of all organs was performed, with appropriate samples taken for microscopic examination, particularly from the kidneys, to evaluate thromboembolic phenomena. The valved conduits were removed, radiographed, photographed, and examined both grossly and microscopically.

In Vitro Studies

A number of in vitro tests were done on T6-processed materials, either as tissue samples or as whole valves, to determine the strength and durability of the processed tissue, the integrity of the valve collagen cross-linking, and the funtionality of whole valves.

1. Accelerated durability testing was carried out under controlled conditions on high speed testers. Eight clinical quality valves, size 27 mm or 25 mm, were prepared for fatigue testing, photographed, and evaluated. Four of the valves, two of each size, were then processed in T6, while the control valves were held in 0.2% stabilized glutaraldehyde. All valves were rinsed 3 times, placed in fresh 0.2% glutaraldehyde, reevaluated, photographed, and placed on the fatigue test rigs. The fatigue tests were carried out in balanced electrolyte solution at 37°C, and a back-closing pressure of 85 mmHg. The valves were evaluated at appropriate intervals, to more than 10^8 cycles. Valve function was evaluated by standard flow testing procedures.

2. Standard Hancock porcine valves were prepared for in vitro testing in a pulse duplicator. The valves were tested at room temperature in balanced electrolyte solution; differential pressure across the valve, regurgitation in comparison to a check valve, and leaflet function as shown by opening sequence and peak pulsatile flow were determined. The valves were then processed by T6, rinsed, and immediately reevaluated.

3. The stability of the collagen cross-links from the glutaraldehyde fixation was determined by the measurement of the tensile strength, the resistance to collagenase digestion, and the shrink temperature, before and after T6 processing of the tissue.[58]

Collagen tape or bovine pericardium samples were prepared for tensile testing, fixed in 0.2% glutaraldehyde, tested on an Instron tensiometer, processed in T6, and subsequently retested. These samples were then held in 0.2% glutaraldehyde, and retested at prescribed intervals.

The integrity of the glutaraldehyde cross-linking of collagen was also measured by resistance to collagenase digestion. Pieces of glutaraldehyde-fixed porcine cusp and bovine pericardium were treated at ambient temperature in either 0.2% glutaraldehyde or T6. The samples were then held for appropriate times in 0.2% glutaraldehyde. Prior to assay, the individual samples were weighed and washed 3 times in balanced electrolyte solution. Ten samples from each group were assayed at any one point, and fresh, unfixed tissue was included as a control. In the assay, samples were incubated at 37°C for 96 hours in a collagenase solution. After incubation, the solution was assayed for free amino acids by a ninhydrin method.

Shrink temperature was measured on samples of porcine cusp and bovine pericardium, treated as in the enzyme digestion experiment, and assayed after the appropriate holding time.

Results

Rat Model. This system was used initially to screen a number of different processes for their anticalcification potential for porcine cusp. The results of these studies are summarized in Table I. As shown in the table, two processes, designated T5 and T6, resulted in a delay in the onset of mineralization, as measured in this system. More detailed experiments were then carried out, and it was determined that the anticalcification efficacy of T5 waned rapidly after 12 weeks. Accordingly, all further experiments addressed variations of the T6 process, including different implant times, and the efficacy of the T6 process on bovine pericardium in addition to porcine cusp. These data are summarized in Table II for porcine cusp and in Table III for bovine pericardium.

The data clearly indicate that the T6-processed materials do not mineralize over extended time periods (up to 5 months for porcine cusp and 3 months for bovine pericardium). Histologic sections of implants both confirmed the absence of mineralization and showed that the material was well tolerated by the host, there being very little host reaction in terms of inflammation. The results of extractable calcium measurements were significantly different between standard and T6 processed material.

Calf model. As a consequence of these results in the rat model, experiments were done to determine the efficacy of the T6 process in porcine xenograft valves in the vascular system of calves, an accepted model for accelerated mineralization. A number of T5 processed valves also were included in this study.

The results of the calf studies are given in Table IV. The control valves were all removed after 4 months. At this time intrinsic mineralization could be identified within the spongiosa of the leaflet, except in cases where the mineralization was so extensive as to obliterate the normal leaflet architecture (Fig. 1). In such cases, a distinction between intrinsic versus extrinsic mineralization could not be made. The valves processed in T5 were re-

TABLE I Effect of various compounds on mineralization of porcine cusp after 8 weeks implantation in rat muscle

Treatment	Radiography	Histology	Extractable calcium
Trinitrobenzenesulfonic acid	+*	+†	44.32 ± 21.16‡
Carbodiimide	+	+	25.00 ± 21.41
Hyaluronidase	+	+	55.54 ± 24.39
Neuraminidase	+	+	17.84 ± 17.54
N-ethylmaleimide	+	+	26.24 ± 16.61
Alkyl sulfate (T6)	−	−	0.005 ± 0.018
Tetrasodium ethylenediaminetetraacetic acid	+	+	29.65 ± 19.84
Leuco toluidine blue (T5)	−	−	2.46 ± 3.39

* + Mineralized implants clearly visible on radiograph.
† + Positive von Kossa stain for calcium.
‡ μg calcium/mg tissue, $\bar{X}$ ± SD.

TABLE II Effect of T6 processing on mineralization of porcine cusp implanted in rat muscle

	Radiography	Histology	Extractable calcium
Standard			
8 wk	5/5 positive	5/5 positive	7.2 ± 3.2*
T6 Processed			
8 wk	5/5 negative	5/5 negative	0.001 ± 0.001
16 wk	5/5 negative	5/5 negative	0.1 ± 0.05
20 wk	5/5 negative	5/5 negative	0.00 ± 0.00
Control			
Rat abdominal muscle	Negative	Negative	0.48 ± 0.85
Unimplanted cusp			0.10 ± 0.05

* μg calcium/mg sample, $\bar{X}$ ± SD.

TABLE III Effect of T6 processing on mineralization of bovine pericardium implanted in rat muscle

	Radiography	Histology	Extractable calcium
Standard			
8 wk	5/5 positive	5/5 positive	50.0 ± 46*
T6 Processed			
8 wk	5/5 negative	5/5 negative	0.03 ± 0.01
12 wk	5/5 negative	5/5 negative	0.00 ± 0.00

* μg calcium/mg, $\bar{X}$ ± SD.

TABLE IV Mineralization of explanted porcine valves in the calf

	# explanted valves	Time of implant (mo)	Result
Control	6	4	Mineralized
T5 Processed	2	4	Mineralized
	2	8	Mineralized
T6 Processed	4	4	No intrinsic mineralization
	2	8	No intrinsic mineralization

moved, 2 after 4 months, 2 after 8 months, and all showed extensive intrinsic mineralization of the valve leaflets.

In contrast, the T6 processed valves removed after 4 and 8 months showed no intrinsic mineralization (Figs. 1 and 2), and even in the presence of vegetative endocarditis in some animals in the series. Vegetations were also found in some control animals early in the series. The use of systemic antibiotics was instituted and prevented further cases of endocarditis.

At necropsy, special attention was given to the gross and microscopic examination of the kidneys to determine if there were any significant thromboembolic phenomena. Although kidneys from animals with both standard and T6 processed valves showed evidence of thromboembolic events, there were no significant differences between the 2 groups.

In vitro testing. Of the 8 valves subjected to accelerated fatigue testing, 3 T6-processed and 4 control valves were fatigued to more than 10^8 cycles. The 4th T6-processed valve was removed at 8×10^7 cycles because of excessive wear due to leaflet abrasion from the bias, an artifact of this in vitro system.[59] There were no significant differences between the processed and the control valves.

The results of the leaflet function testing are summarized in Table V. Again, there were no significant changes as a result of the T6 process.

Tables VI and VII summarize the data from the enzyme digestion and shrink temperature experiments on porcine valve cusp. Statistically, there is no difference between the control and the T6-processed material, indicating that the T6 process has no effect on the integrity of the glutaraldehyde-introduced cross-links. This is further demonstrated in Fig. 3, which depicts the stress-strain curves for collagen tape and bovine pericardium before and after T6 processing.

Comment

The results presented here clearly show that the T6 process inhibits the onset of intrinsic mineralization in glutaraldehyde-fixed xenograft tissues.

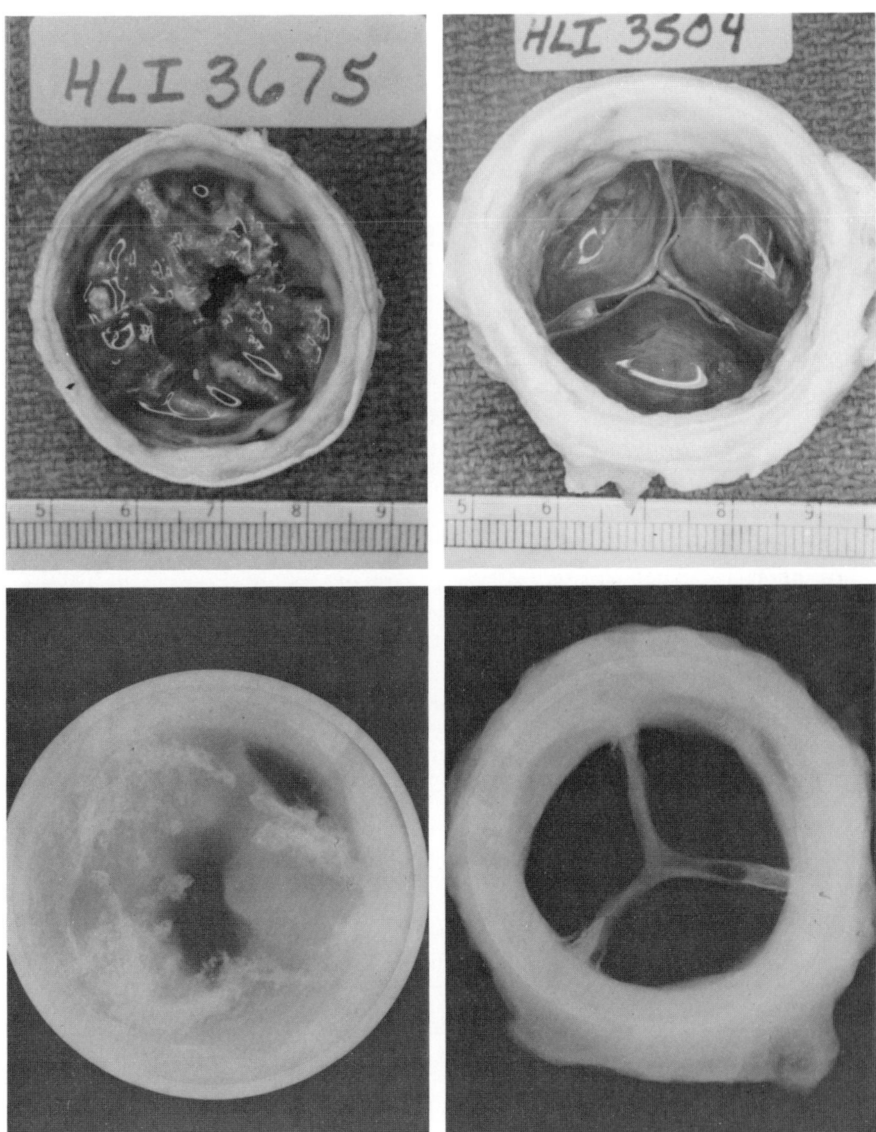

FIG. 1 Radiographs and gross appearance of porcine valves explanted from calves after 4 months. Standard valve (left) and T6-processed valve (right). Note extensive mineralization and distortion of leaflets in standard valve.

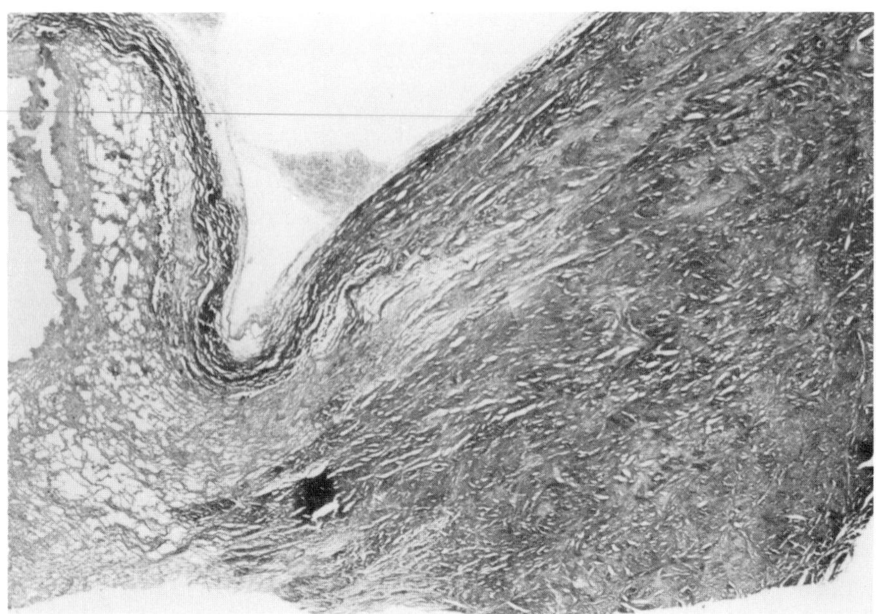

FIG. 2 Histologic appearance of T6-processed valve after 8 months implant in calf. This section through the commissure shows no mineralization in aortic wall (right) or cusp leaflet (left). (Von Kossa stain, ×60).

TABLE V Effect of T6-processing on leaflet function of porcine valves

Parameter	# valves	Mean change after process
Regurgitation	17	0.7 ± 1.1%
Effective orifice area	17	2.0 ± 3.0%
Opening characteristics	14	No change

TABLE VI The effect of T6 on glutaraldehyde-induced collagen cross-linking in porcine valve cusp: collagenase susceptibility

Time*	Control†	T6 processed
0	98.4	98.6
1 wk	98.2	99.0
1 mo	95.5	98.4
2 mo	85.9	90.1
3 mo	86.7	92.2
4 mo	80.9	96.1
5 mo	95.7	98.6

* Time after T6 processing.

† Calculated percent of fixation of cross-links based on detectable amino acid residues.

TABLE VII The effect of T6 on glutaraldehyde-induced collagen cross-linking in porcine valve cusp: shrink temperature

Time*	Control†	T6 processed
0	83.3 ± 1.2	81.2 ± 0.5
1 wk	83.1 ± 0.8	84.0 ± 0.6
1 mo	84.3 ± 0.5	84.8 ± 0.3
2 mo	84.5 ± 0.4	84.5 ± 0.6
3 mo	83.7 ± 0.3	84.7 ± 0.3
4 mo	83.8 ± 0.3	84.1 ± 0.7
5 mo	83.3 ± 0.3	83.2 ± 0.3

* Time after T6 processing.
† Temperature, °C, $\bar{X}$ ± SD.

In the rat model, the T6-processed material was not mineralized, even after 5 months for porcine cusp. In the control unprocessed material, the loose spongiosa of the cusp tissue was almost obliterated by mineralization after only 8 weeks.

Other experimental treatments, as shown in Table I, failed to affect the onset of mineralization, although several of these should have blocked reactive groups in collagen in a manner similar to that reported by Urist[29] in in vitro systems.

Those processes that should remove mucopolysaccharides (hyaluronidase, neuraminidase) also failed to influence the course of mineralization. Since these matrix materials can be presumed to be replaced rapidly in vivo, no significance can be placed on the efficacy of such compounds from these experiments.

The mechanism of action of the T6 process is not understood, but it may affect membrane surface charge, ground substance, or the collagen fibrils. Further studies using the T6 process may not only provide clarification of its mechanism but also assist in the understanding of the pathogenesis of mineralization of bioprosthetic material.

The results of the calf study indicated that the T6 process was as efficacious in a physiologic (blood-contact) system as in the intramuscular rat screening model. The valves remained free of intrinsic mineralization, and extensive thromboembolic complications were not observed, except in the presence of vegetative endocarditis, a condition independent of the valve (control or processed). The extended period free of mineralization is highly significant in the calf, for this species has been reported to mineralize not only bioprosthetic valves (in fewer than 150 days) but also synthetic polymers.[55–57]

In conclusion, the in vivo studies presented in this communication were designed to determine the effect of the T6 process on the strength, durability, and functionality of the porcine valve. The results show that the dura-

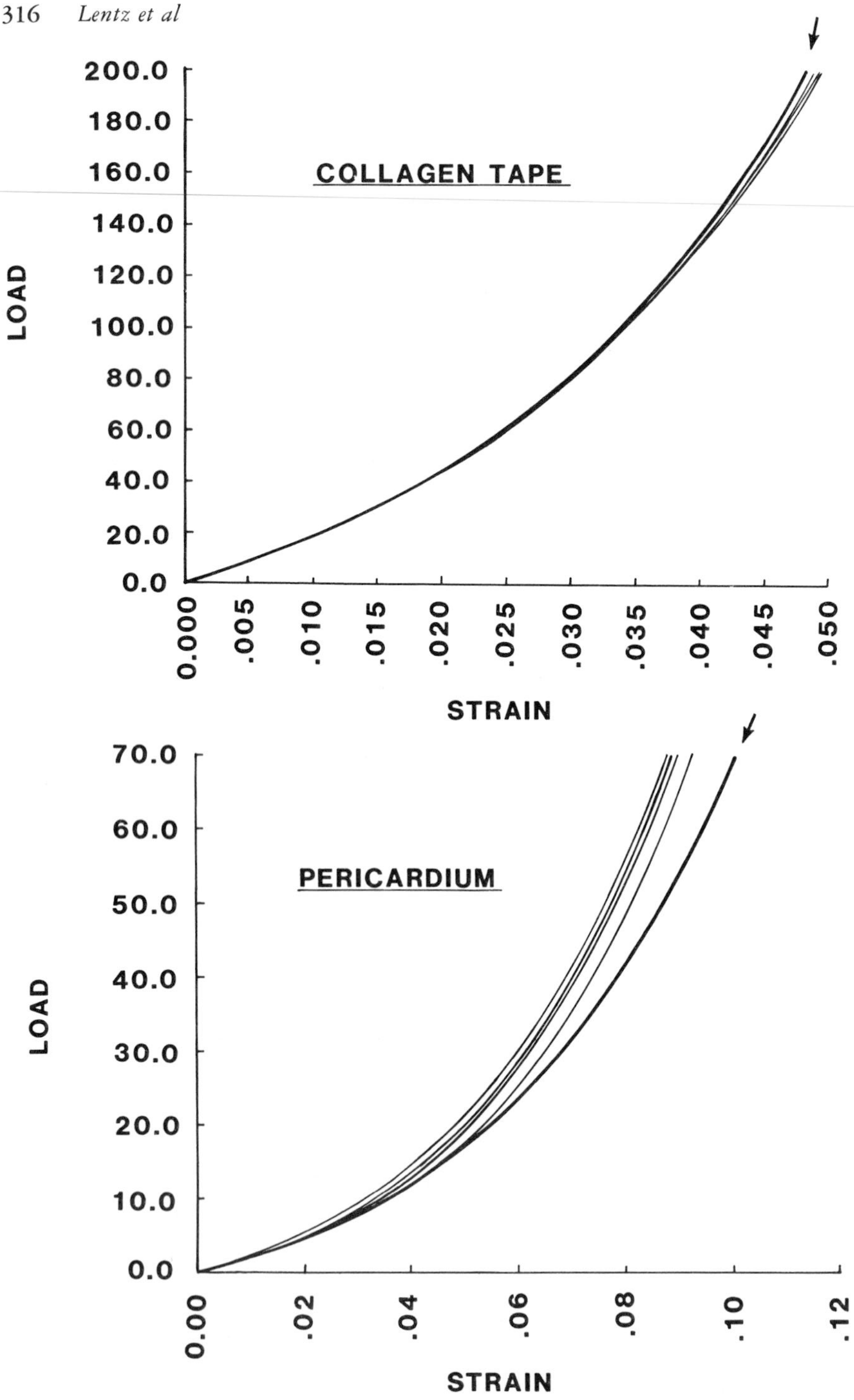

COLLAGEN TAPE

PERICARDIUM

FIG. 3 Effect of T6 process on tensile strength of collagen tape and bovine pericardium. In both graphs the arrow indicates the curve prior to treatment; the other lines represent stress-strain curves 1, 4, 8, 12 weeks after T6 processing.

bility, hemodynamics and strength of the valve, and the integrity of the tissue fixation were unaffected by the process. The development of the T6 process represents a significant advance in the inhibition of mineralization of bioprosthetic heart valves in experimental animals, without sacrificing any of the other advantages of tissue heart valves.

References

1. Horowitz MS, Goodman DJ, Fogarty TJ, Harrison DC: Mitral valve replacement with the glutaraldehyde-preserved porcine heterograft. J Thorac Cardiovasc Surg 67:885, 1974.
2. Baxley WA, Soto B: Hemodynamic evaluation of patients with combined mitral and aortic prostheses. Am J Cardiol 45:42, 1980.
3. Williams JB, Karp RB, Kirklin JW, Kouchoukos NJ, Pacifico AD, Zorn GL, Blackstone EH, Brown RN, Painnados IS, Bradley EL: Considerations in selection and managements of patients undergoing valve replacement with glutaraldehyde-fixed porcine bioprostheses. Ann Thorac Surg 30:247, 1980.
4. Cohn LH, Mudge GH, Pratter F, Collins JJ: Five to eight-year follow-up of patients undergoing porcine heart valve replacement. N Engl J Med 304:258, 1981.
5. Geha AS, Hammond GL, Laks H, Stansel HC, Glenn WWL: Factors affecting performance and thromboembolism after porcine xenograft cardiac valve replacement. J Thorac Cardiovasc Surg 83:377, 1982.
6. Missirlis YF, Chong M: Aortic valve mechanics—Part I: Material properties of natural porcine aortic valves. J Bioeng 2:287, 1978.
7. Rossiter SJ, Stinson EB, Oyer PE, Miller DC, Shapira JN, Martin RP, Shumway NE: Prosthetic valve endocarditis. J Thorac Cardiovasc Surg 76:795, 1978.
8. Oyer PE, Stinson EB, Reitz BA, Miller DC, Rossiter SJ, Shumway NE: Long-term evaluation of the porcine xenograft bioprosthesis. J Thorac Cardiovasc Surg 78:343, 1979.
9. Oyer PE, Miller DC, Stinson EB, Reitz BA, Moreno-Cabral RJ, Shumway NE: Clinical durability of the Hancock porcine bioprosthetic valve. J Thorac Cardiovasc Surg 80:824, 1980.
10. Durability Assessment of the Hancock Porcine Bioprosthesis. Hancock Laboratories, April, 1980.
11. Fishbein MC, Gissen SA, Collins JJ, Barsamian EM, Cohn LH: Pathologic findings after cardiac valve replacement with glutaraldyhyde-fixed porcine valves. Am J Cardiol 40:331, 1977.
12. Spray TL, Roberts WC: Structural changes in porcine xenografts used as substitute cardiac valves. Am J Cardiol 40:319, 1977.
13. Sade RM, Greene W, Kurtz SM: Structural changes in a porcine xenograft after implantation for 105 months. Am J Cardiol 44:761, 1979.
14. Dale J, Levang O, Enge I: Long-term results after aortic valve replacement with four different prostheses. Am Heart J 99:155, 1980.
15. Lewis BS, Bakst A, Rod JL, Rein A, Gorsman MS, Appelbaum A: Early calcification and obstruction of a mitral porcine bioprosthesis. Ann Thorac Surg 30:592, 1980.
16. Magilligan DJ, Lewis JW, Jara FM, Lee MW, Alam M, Riddle JM, Stein PD: Spontaneous degeneration of porcine bioprosthetic valves. Ann Thorac Surg 30:259, 1980.

17. Platt MR, Mills LJ, Estrera AS, Hillis LD, Buja LM, Willerson JT: Marked thrombosis and calcification of porcine heterograft valves. Circulation 62:862, 1980.
18. Thiene G, Bortolotti U, Panizzon G, Milano A, Gallucci V: Pathological substrates of thrombus formation after heart valve replacement with the Hancock bioprosthesis. J Thorac Cardiovasc Surg 80:414, 1980.
19. Rose AG, Forman R, Bowen RM: Calcification of glutaraldehyde-fixed porcine xenograft. Thorax 33:111, 1978.
20. Geha AS, Laks H, Stansel HC, Cornhill JF, Kilman JW, Buckley MJ, Roberts WC: Late failure of porcine valve heterografts in children. J Thorac Cardiovasc Surg 78:351, 1979.
21. Silver MM, Pollock J, Silver MD, Williams WG, Trusler GA: Calcification in porcine xenograft valves in children. Am J Cardiol 45:685, 1980.
22. Thandroyen FJ, Whitton IN, Pirie D, Rogers MA, Mitha AS: Severe calcification of glutaraldehyde preserved porcine xenografts in children. Am J Cardiol 45:690, 1980.
23. Weesner KM, Rocchini AP, Rosenthal A, Behrendt D: Intravascular hemolysis associated with porcine mitral valve calcification in children. Am J Cardiol 47:1286, 1981.
24. Sobel AE, Burger M: Calcification XIV: Investigation of the role of chondroitin sulfate in the calcifying mechanism. Proc Soc Exp Biol Med 87:7, 1954.
25. Strates B, Neuman WF: On the mechanisms of calcification. Proc Soc Exp Biol Med 97:688, 1958.
26. Robertson WG: Factors affecting the precipitation of calcium phosphate *in vitro*. Calcif Tissue Res 11:311, 1973.
27. Eanes ED: The interaction of supersaturated calcium phosphate solutions with apatitic substrates. Calcif Tissue Res 22:75, 1976.
28. Boskey AL, Posner AS: The role of synthetic and bone extracted Ca-phospholipid-PO_4 complexes in hydroxyapatite formation. Calcif Tissue Res 23:251, 1977.
29. Urist MR, Adams JM: Effects of various blocking agents upon local mechanism of calcification. Arch Pathol 81:325, 1966.
30. Schubert G, Pras M: Ground substance proteinpolysaccharides and the precipitation of calcium phosphate. Clin Orthop 60:235, 1968.
31. Glimcher MJ, Andrikides A, Kossiva D: Studies of the mechanism of calcification. In: Structure and Function of Connective and Skeletal Tissues. Proceedings of an advanced Study Institute organized under the auspices of NATO. London, Butterworths. 1965, pp 342.
32. Wadkins CL, Luben R, Thomas M, Hunphreys R: Physical biochemistry of calcification. Clin Orthop 99:246, 1974.
33. Ashraf M, Bloor CM: Structural alteration of the porcine heterograft after various durations of implantation. Am J Cardiol 41:1185, 1978.
34. Ferrans VJ, Spray TL, Billingham ME, Roberts WC: Structural changes in glutaraldehyde-treated heterografts used as substitute cardiac valves. Am J Cardiol 41:1159, 1978.
35. Ishihara T, Ferrans VJ, Jones M, Cabin HS, Roberts WC: Calcific deposits developing in a bovine pericardial bioprosthetic valve 3 days after implantation. Circulation 63:718, 1981.
36. Barnhart GR, Jones M, Ishihara J, Rose DM, Chavez AM, Ferrans VJ: Degeneration and calcification of bioprosthetic cardiac valves. Am J Pathol 106:136, 1982.
37. Jung A, Bisaz S, Fleisch H: The binding of pyrophosphate and two diphosphonates by hydroxyapatite crystals. Calcif Tissue Res 11:269, 1973.

38. Larsson FV: The metabolic heterogeneity of glycosaminoglycans of the different zones of the epiphyseal growth plate and the effect of ethane-1-hydroxy-1, 1-diphosphonate (ENDP) upon glycosaminoglycan synthesis *in vivo.* Calcif Tissue Res 21:67, 1976.
39. Francis MD, Slough CL, Briner WW, Oertel RP: An *in vitro* and *in vivo* investigation of mellitate and ethane-1-hydroxy 1, 1-diphosphate in calcium phosphate systems. Calcif Tissue Res 23:53, 1977.
40. Meyer JL, Lee KE, Bergert JH: The inhibition of calcium oxalate crystal growth by multidentate organic phosphonates. Calcif Tissue Res 23:83, 1977.
41. Barone JP, Nancollas GH: The growth of calcium phosphates on hydroxyapatite crystals. The effect of fluoride and phosphonate. J Dent Res 57:735, 1978.
42. Pojokar M, Schnidt-Dunker M: The inhibitory effect of new diphosphonic acids on aortic and kidney calcification *in vivo.* Atherosclerosis 30:313, 1978.
43. McClure J: A comparison of the inhibitory effects of disodium pyrophosphate and disodium ethane-hydroxy-1, 1-diphosphonate on simple calcergy. J Pathol 129:149, 1979.
44. Hauschka PV, Lian JB, Gallop PM: Direct identification of the calcium-binding aminoacid, γ-carboxyglutamate, in mineralized tissue. Proc Natl Acad Sci USA 72:3925, 1975.
45. Christakos S, Norman AW: Vitamin D_3-induced calcium binding protein in bone tissue. Science 202:70, 1978.
46. Lian JB, Hauschka PV, Gallop PM: Properties and biosynthesis of a vitamin K-dependent calcium binding protein in bone. Fed Proc 37:2615, 1978.
47. Reddi AH, Hascall VC, Hascall GK: Changes in proteoglycan types during matrix-induced cartilage and bone development. J Biol Chem 253:2429, 1978.
48. Wagner WD, Salisbury BG: Aortic total glycosaminoglycan and dermatansulphate changes in atherosclerotic rhesus monkeys. Lab Invest 39:322, 1978.
49. Levy RJ, Lian JB: γ-Carboxyglutamate excretion and warfarin therapy. Clin Pharmacol Ther 25:562, 1979.
50. Levy RJ, Zenker JA, Lian JB: Vitamin K-dependent calcium binding proteins in aortic valve calcification. J Clin Invest 65:563, 1980.
51. Gabbiani G, Tuchweber B: Studies of the mechanism of calcergy. Clin Orthop 69:66, 1970.
52. Johnson WC, Alker DS: Histopathology and histochemistry of cutaneous calciphylaxis. Clin Orthop 69:75, 1970.
53. Kato Y, Ogura H: Mineral phase in experimental ectopic calcification induced by lead acetate in the rat. Calcif Tissue Res 25:69, 1978.
54. Yarbrough JW, Roberts WC, Reis RL: Structural alterations in tissue cardiac valves implanted in patients and in calves. J Thorac Cardiovasc Surg 65:364, 1973.
55. Harasaki H, Gerrity R, Kiraly R, Jacobs G, Nose Y: Calcification in blood pumps. Trans Am Soc Artif Intern Org 25:305, 1979.
56. Pierce WS, Donachy JH, Rosenberg G, Baier RE: Calcification inside artificial hearts: Inhibition by warfarin-sodium. Science 208:601, 1980.
57. Coleman DL, Lim D, Kessler T, Andrews JD: Calcification of nontextured implantable blood pumps. Trans Am Soc Artif Intern Organs 27:97, 1981.
58. Bluel KE, Saul TA, Lentz DJ, Woo SLY: Evaluation of reconstituted collagen tape as a model for chemically modified soft tissues. Biomater Med Devices Artif Organs 9:37, 1981.
59. Saul T, Myers DJ, Gibbs ML, Wright JTM: Problems associated with high speed durability of tissue heart valve studies. Proceedings of the AAMI 16th Annual Meeting. In press.

30

Prevention of Tissue Valve Calcification by Chemical Techniques

A. Carpentier, A. Nashref, S. Carpentier, N. Goussef, J. Relland, R. J. Levy, M. C. Fishbein, B. El Asmar, M. Benomar, S. El Sayed, P. G. Donzeau-Gouge

Tissue calcification is a major concern in bioprosthetic valve replacement, whether porcine valves or bovine pericardial valves are used.[1,2] According to various reports, the incidence of valve failure due to calcification averages 10% at 10 years in the adult and 50% at 5 years in children.

This stimulated extensive investigation in our Laboratory in Paris in order to determine, and if possible influence, the various factors involved in the process of bioprosthetic tissue calcification. These factors are either patient related or valve related. Among the latter, preservation techniques are of primary importance and form the basis of this paper.

Rationale

The mechanism of calcification is not totally elucidated yet. It is possible, however, to summarize what is known in a diagrammatic representation (Fig. 1). As one can see on this diagram, calcium phosphate and blood metabolites, such as phospholipids, are important determinants, for they act as initiators of the process of calcification. Our approach was to influence these initiators by various chemical techniques used in addition to glutaraldehyde fixation. Among these techniques, the following proved to be the most efficient: HEPES buffer, magnesium chloride, surfactant, and polymer incorporation.

From Laboratoire d'Etude des Prothèses Cardiaques, C.N.R.S. and Association Claude-Bernard, Hôpital Broussais, Paris, France, and Edwards Laboratories, Santa Ana, California, the Department of Cardiology, Children's Hospital and Medical Center, Boston, Massachusetts, and the Department of Pathology, Cedars-Sinai Medical Center, Los Angeles, California.

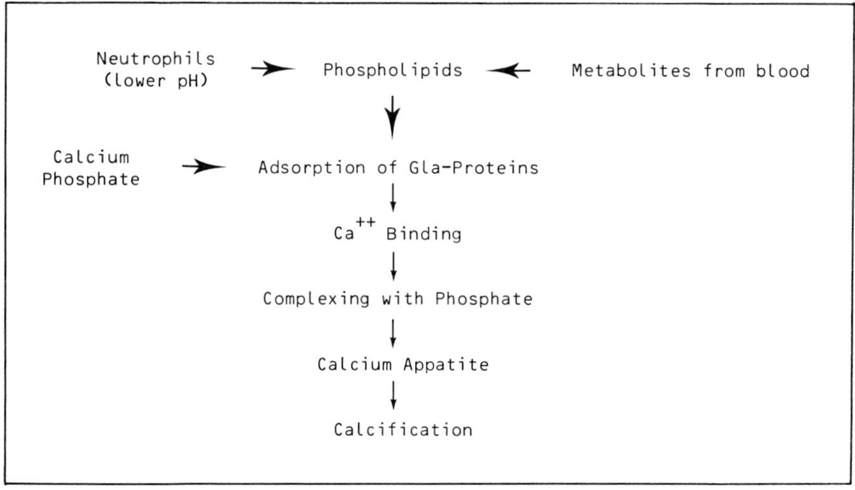

FIG. 1 Proposed mechanism for intrinsic calcification of tissue valves.

Techniques

The efficacy of these methods was studied in an animal model we proposed and described in previous publications.[1,3,4] Control and treated tissues were subcutaneously implanted in the growing rabbit and subsequently explanted at 1, 2, 3, and 4 weeks. The degree of calcification was determined on a scale of 0, 1, 2, and 3 using von Kossa-stained tissue sections. The validity of this model was established by histologic and chemical similarities found between explants from the animal model and valves explanted from the human: same location of calcium in the spongiosa, similar calcium to phosphate radio and similar calcium to carboxyglutamic acid-containing protein ratio.[4,5] The validity of this model was further supported by implanting control tissues and treated tissues in the same animal, thus allowing accurate comparison. The efficacy of the various techniques was also assessed by physical and chemical tests, i.e., heat shrinkage temperature, moisture content, lysin to glutamic acid ratio, amino group analysis, enzymatic digestion, radioisotope labeling, histologic studies, and flow testing.

Results

HEPES Buffer plus Magnesium Chloride

The aim of this technique was to decrease phosphate in the tissue, and hence the phosphate to calcium ratio, and to block calcium-binding sites with

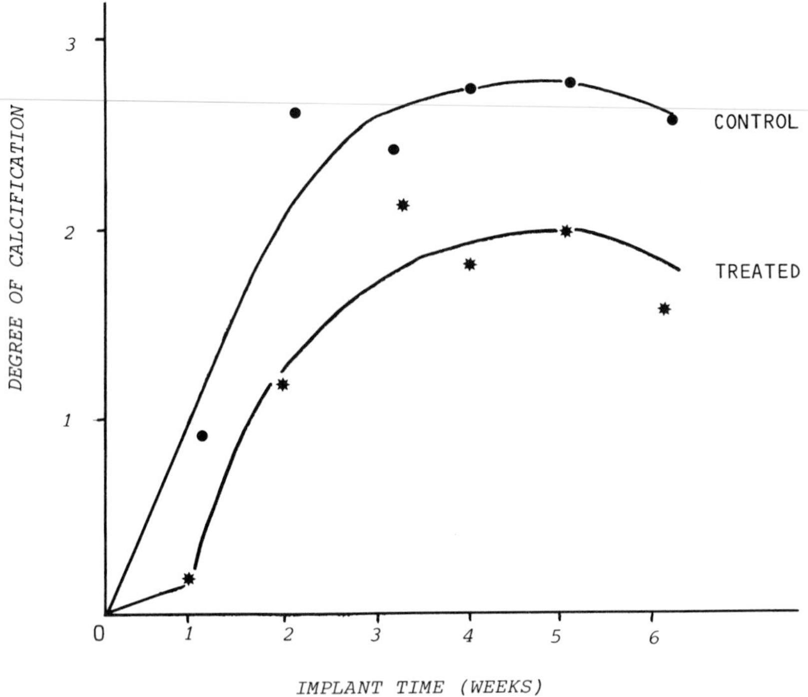

FIG. 2 Calcification curve of subcutaneously implanted valves treated by HEPES and magnesium chloride.

magnesium, a divalent cation like calcium. Fragments of valvular tissue were treated in a solution containing glutaraldehyde, 0.625%, HEPES, 0.02*M*, and magnesium chloride, 0.26% in saline for 8 days. The solution was isotonic (285 ± 15 mOsm) with a final pH 7.3 ± 0.2.

Results in the rabbit model are summarized in Fig. 2 (average value from 60 implants). They do show a significant reduction in calcification in the treated tissue. Stability tests showed no statistically significant difference between control and treated tissues, demonstrating the absence of deleterious effects of the treatment, in particular no impairment of the physicochemical stability of the tissue (heat shrinkage temperature tests and moisture content), nor any changes in its ultrastructure (Table I).

Surfactant

The demonstration that surfactant could decrease the risk of calcification in tissues resulted from systematic studies conducted to enhance the efficacy of cold sterilization. Among the numerous agents investigated, surfac-

TABLE I Control tests of valves treated by HEPES plus magnesium chloride

Test	Control	Treated
Shrinkage temperature (°C)	83.97	84.94
Moisture content (%)	93.91	93.19
Lysine to glutamic acid ratio	0.054	0.051
Amino group analysis	2.08	1.82
Scanning electron microscopy	No difference	
Transmission electron microscopy	No difference	
Histologic evaluation	No difference	
Flow testing	No difference	

tant was used to increase the permeability of the spore membrane to sterilizing agents. Control tests showed, in addition to improved sterilization, a reduced incidence of calcification, an observation that interestingly enough was also made by others following the same approach at the same time.

A surfactant is comprised of 2 parts: one hydrophobic and one hydrophilic. Most probably the hydrophilic portion inhibits lipids and phos-

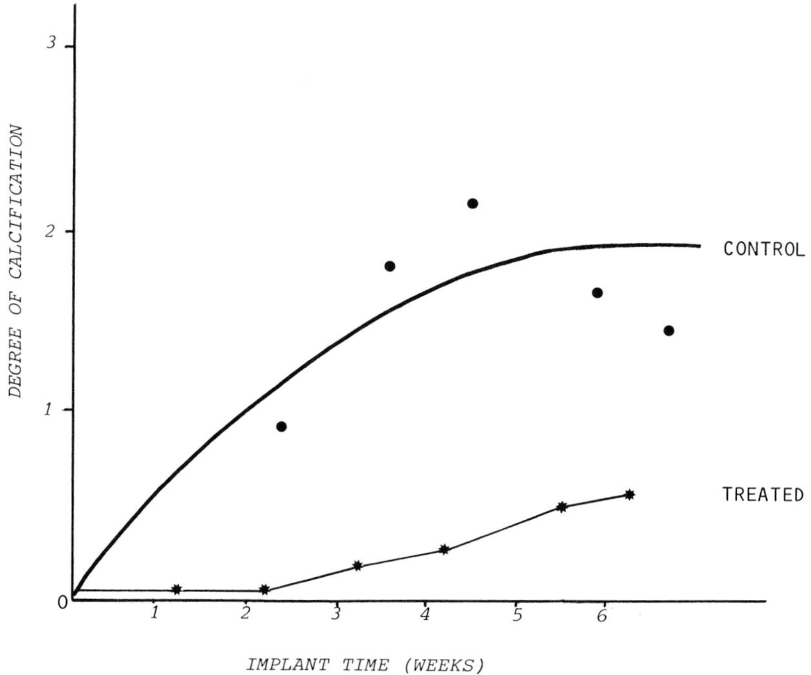

FIG. 3 Calcification curve of subcutaneously implanted valves treated by surfactant.

TABLE II Control tests of valves treated by surfactant

Tests	Control	Treated
Shrinkage temperature (°C)	82.6	83.0
Moisture content (%)	94.02	94.64
Lysine to glutamic acid	0.04	0.04
Amino group analysis	1.2	1.1
Enzymatic digestion	2.9	3.2
Radioisotope labeling	Negligible*	
Histologic evaluation	No different	
Flow testing	No different	

* <0.1 mole/mole collagen.

pholipid penetration into the tissue, thus acting on the phospholipid pathways.

The technique consists of first fixing the tissue in a phosphate buffered glutaraldehyde solution (0.62%) for 8 days followed by treatment with the surfactant in an aqueous solution for 8 days. The valve is then rinsed in saline and stored in a glutaraldehyde solution. Figure 3 summarizes the results obtained in the animal model, showing a reduced incidence of calcification in the treated series (average values from 22 implants). The stability tests (Table II) showed no significant differences between the treated group and the control group, demonstrating the absence of deleterious effect following treatment by surfactant. Radioisotope labeling of surfactant showed minimal incorporation of the surfactant within the tissue.

HEPES, Magnesium Chloride plus Surfactant

Combination of the 2 previous techniques was achieved with the aim of acting on 2 pathways of the process of calcification: phosphate/calcium and phospholipids. Reduction of calcification was further improved as seen in Fig. 4.

Polymer Incorporation

This technique consisted of incorporating acrylic acid coupled to carboxyl via diamine within the tissue, with subsequent polymerization in acrylamide. Hydrogel incorporation prevents phospholipid penetration and binding of phosphate and calcium to collagen, thus acting on 2 initiators of the process of calcification: phospholipids and calcium/phosphate.

Results in the animal model are summarized in Fig. 5. They do show a significant reduction in calcification. Stability tests did not show any delete-

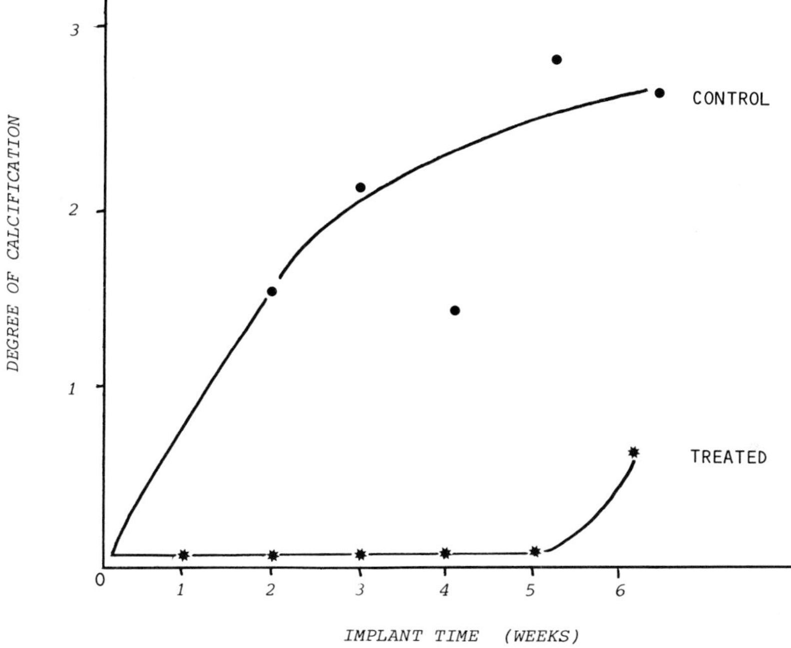

FIG. 4 Calcification curve of subcutaneously implanted valves treated by HEPES, magnesium chloride, and surfactant.

rious effect on physical stability of the tissue, nor did they show any impairment of its ultrastructure (Table III). Further investigations are being carried out to evaluate the stability of the polymer incorporation and absence of adverse secondary reactions.

Conclusions

Numerous factors either patient related or valve related may play a role in the process of bioprosthetic valve calcification. In previous publications, we stressed the importance of avoiding dehydration of the valve during implantation and excess calcium intake through intravenous calcium or high calcium diet after the operation.[3,6] Reduction of turbulence and stress by improving valve design and stent flexibility was also an important consideration.[7] In this paper, we have studied the possibility of influencing calcification of bioprosthetic valves by various chemical treatments in addition to glutaraldehyde fixation of the tissue. Among the numerous techniques

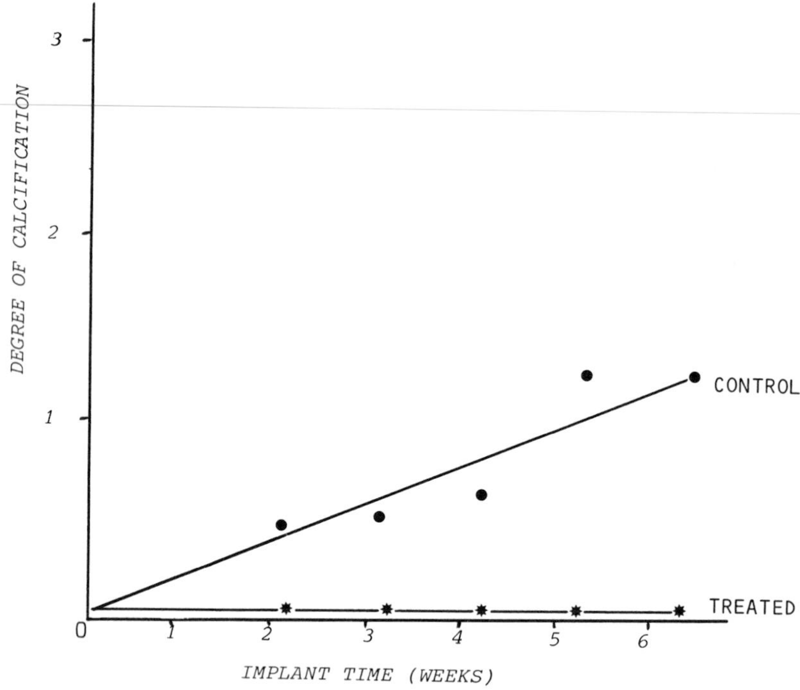

FIG. 5 Calcification curve of subcutaneously implanted valves treated by polymer incorporation.

investigated, HEPES buffer, magnesium chloride, surfactant and hydrogel incorporation used either alone or in association appear to be promising. Further investigation in particular implantation of treated valves in the mitral position in the calf are being carried out to evaluate the possibility of using these techniques clinically.

TABLE III Control tests of valves treated by polymer incorporation

Test	Control	Treated
Shrinkage temperature (°C)	83.0	84.7
Moisture content (%)	90.05	88.03
Amino group analysis	0.03	0.39
Resistance to enzymatic digestion	1.43	0.95
Histology	No significant difference	
Flow testing	No significant difference	

References

1. Carpentier A, Lemaigre G, Robert L, Carpentier S, Dubost C: Biological factors affecting long-term results of valvular heterografts. J Thorac Cardiovasc Surg 58:467, 1969.
2. Carpentier A, Deloche A, Relland J, Fabiani JN, Forman J, Camilleri JP, Soyer R, Dubost C: Six-year follow-up of glutaraldehyde-preserved heterografts. J Thorac Cardiovasc Surg 68:771, 1974.
3. Carpentier A, Carpentier S, Nashef A, Levy RJ, Fishbein MC, Goussef N: Prevention of calcification in implanted glutaraldehyde treated biological tissue. Proceedings of the 8th Meeting of the European Society for Artificial Organs, 1981, p 96.
4. Fishbein MC, Levy RJ, Ferrans VJ, Dearden LC, Nashef A, Goodman AP, Carpentier A: Calcification of cardiac valve bioprostheses. Biochemical, histologic and ultrastructural observations in a subcutaneous implantation model system. J Thorac Cardiovasc Surg 83:602, 1982.
5. Levy RJ, Lian JB, Gallop PM: Atherocalcin, a gamma-carboxyglutamic acid containing protein from atherosclerotic plaque. Biochem Biophys Res Commun 91:41, 1979.
6. Carpentier A, Carpentier S, Goussef N, Paillet C, Fishbein MC, Levy RJ, Nashef A: Calcium intake as a factor affecting calcification in glutaraldehyde-treated biological tissue. Proceedings of the 3rd Meeting of the International Society for Artificial Organs, Suppl Vol. 5: Artificial Organs, 1982.
7. Carpentier A, Dubost C, Lane E, Nashef A, Carpentier S, Relland J, Deloche A, Fabiani JN, Chauvaud S, Perier P, Maxwell S: Continuing improvements in valvular bioprostheses. J Thorac Cardiovasc Surg 83:27, 1982.

SECTION VI

EXPLANT PATHOLOGY

31

Complications of Replacement of Either the Mitral or Aortic Valve or Both by Either Mechanical or Bioprosthetic Valves

W. C. Roberts, V. J. Ferrans

It has been more than 21 years since successful replacement of 1 or more cardiac valves became a reality, and many thousands of patients with severely symptomatic valvular heart disease have had valve replacement with complete loss or sharp decrease in their symptoms of cardiac dysfunction. Although the chance of successful valve replacement in most patients is very high, occasional, often predictable, complications occur both early and late in some patients. Since 1960, we have examined at necropsy more than 600 hearts, submitted from around the United States, containing 1 or more prosthetic valves, and certain complications of cardiac valve replacement observed in them will be summarized in this chapter.

Complications Common to any Valve Site and to Most or All Presently Available Mechanical or Bioprosthetic Valves

Prosthetic Size Disproportion

The normal cardiac valves, of course, consist of thin, very pliable leaflet-like structures that allow central flow of blood and occupy very little space within the ventricles or great arteries in which they reside. Mechanical valves and even tissue valves attached to rigid or semirigid stents and rings, in contrast, are rigid except for movement of the occluder or cusps; they

---

From the Pathology Branch, National Heart, Lung and Blood Institute, National Institutes of Health, Bethesda, Maryland.

Dr. Roberts was the G. B. Morgagni Lecturer at the Second International Symposium on Cardiac Bioprostheses.

often prevent central flow and they occupy noncompressible space. Early in the history of cardiac valve replacement, there appeared to be a tendency to insert as large a prosthesis as possible because of their tendency to be less inherently obstructive than the smaller-sized prostheses. Experience taught, however, that if a mechanical prosthesis was too large for the ventricle or ascending aorta into which it was to reside then the movement of the occluder could be limited, with the potential for varying degrees of obstruction to flow.[1–15] At one time, a common view was that this disproportion problem was mainly produced by caged ball prostheses because they were larger than most subsequently utilized mechanical prostheses. This view, however, is incorrect. No mechanical valve and no tissue valve attached to a frame is immune to the problem of prosthetic disproportion.

The usual consequence in the mitral position is interference to left atrial emptying (or to left ventricular filling) and, rarely, in our experience, despite beliefs to the contrary, interference with left ventricular emptying (left ventricular outflow obstruction)[1] (Fig. 1). The usual consequence in the

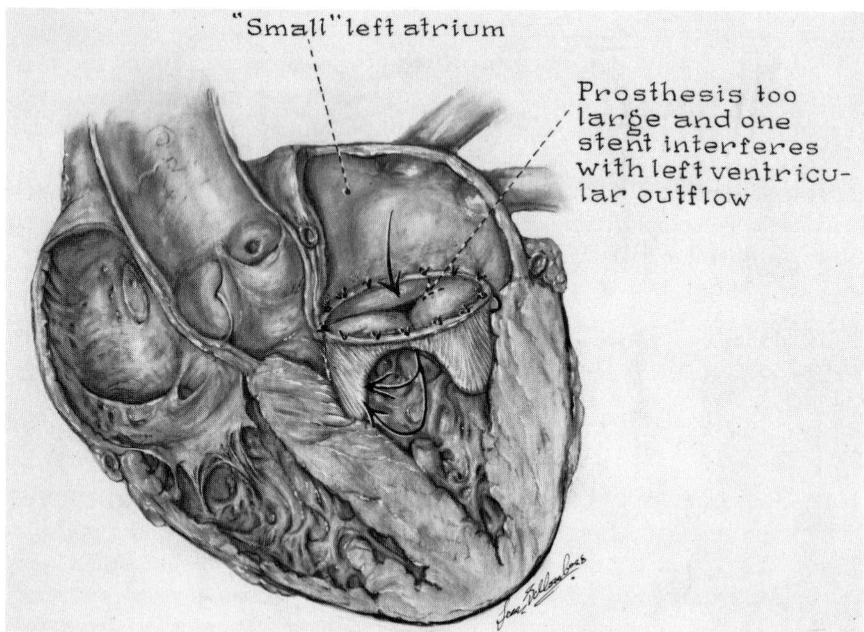

FIG. 1 Obstruction to LV outflow by stent of mitral prosthesis. Porcine bioprosthesis (33 mm) appears to be too large for the left ventricle in this woman with severe acute mitral regurgitation from sudden rupture of several chordae tendineae. Despite volume lesion, left ventricle had not had adequate time to dilate, and the large prosthesis was oriented so that one of its large stents partially obstructed LV outflow (and, additionally, contacted ventricular septum).

aortic position, of course, is interference to left ventricular emptying. Prosthetic disproportion is most likely to occur in the mitral position when valve replacement is carried out for pure mitral stenosis (or in combined mitral and aortic valve stenosis) and in the aortic position when the aorta is small because of aortic stenosis associated with mitral valve disease or because of acute aortic regurgitation when the aorta has not had adequate time to dilate. Large-sized prostheses, whether caged ball (Starr-Edwards), tilting disc (Björk-Shiley or St. Jude), or nontilting disc (Kay-Shiley) must be avoided in small-sized patients with purely stenotic valvular lesions. Determining proper prosthetic size only in the operating room without consideration of the hemodynamic lesion and the lean weight of the patient can lead to prosthetic disproportion, a major problem in the early years of valve replacement, but, even today, an occasional problem.[15]

Prosthetic Thrombosis

It took years to convince physicians dealing with patients who had mechanical prosthetic valves that anticoagulation (warfain sodium) was essential. After that principle was established, mechanical valve thrombosis became less of a problem. Nevertheless, prosthetic thrombus occurs in some patients with mechanical valves, who are well anticoagulated, and, occasionally, it does *not* occur in patients who have never received anticoagulants. Thrombus is often observed in porcine bioprostheses that have been in place for more than 2 months, but usually the thrombi are so small that function of the prosthesis is not altered.[15–17]

Paraanular Prosthetic Ring Discontinuity (Peribasilar Leak)

Parabasilar communications appear to result from placement of an inadequate number of sutures in the sewing ring (because of anular calcific deposits for example) or the pulling loose of one or more sutures, primarily after replacement of anatomically normal (as in papillary muscle dysfunction) or floppy mitral valves or in aortic regurgitation secondary to a disease of the wall of the aorta (as in Marfan's syndrome) rather than of aortic valve cusp or in infection (prosthetic endocarditis) at the site of attachment of a prosthesis.[4]

Prosthetic Degeneration or Wear

Almost all of the initial models of presently utilized mechanical prostheses had evidence of wear or variance of 1 or more parts. The silicone rubber poppet utilized in the initial models of the caged ball prosthesis took in lipids that resulted in their swelling (with impaction in the cage) or in large cracks that allowed some of them to dislodge from the cage.[4,8,12,18–20]

Hopefully, the change (about 1966) in the processing of the silicone rubber has alleviated this problem. The utilization of cloth around the struts of the cage led to "cloth wear" and the disastrous introduction by the manufacturer of the "close-clearance" cage that led to sticking of the poppet in the mid-portion of the cage and often sudden death. In the latest model Starr-Edwards valve, wear of the metallic studs on the inner lining of the ring has led to contact of the metallic poppet with the cloth of the ring with subsequent disruption of the cloth (Fig. 2). Fracture of the strut or occluder (Delrin) also occurred in a few of the earlier models of the tilting and nontilting discs.

Much evidence has accumulated to indicate that the cusps of the porcine bioprosthesis will eventually degenerate[15–17,21–24] and the same fate may be in store for the bovine parietal pericardial bioprosthesis. Numerous reports have described heavy calcification and cuspal disruption of the porcine bioprosthesis after the first 5 year period, enough evidence to convince us that this prosthesis should not be the prosthesis of choice for persons who can tolerate antiocoagulants and are older than age 20 and younger than age 60 or 65 years.

Suture Overhang of Prosthetic Orifice

If a suture or knots overhang the metallic ring of a caged disc or tilting disc prosthesis, the consequence might be prosthetic regurgitation.[25] Such was the case in 3 patients reported earlier from this laboratory: fatal aortic regurgitation was the consequence in 2, and the aortic regurgitation in the third was relieved simply by cutting one overhanging suture. More recently, the same mechanism caused mitral regurgitation after replacement with a tilting disc prosthesis. This mechanism is less likely to occur with caged ball prostheses because the margin of error is simply greater than with the more delicate tilting disc type prostheses.

Prosthetic Endocarditis

With mechanical prostheses, the infection is always beneath the site of attachment of the prosthesis, i.e., ring abscess is inevitable[26–31](Fig. 3). With tissue valves mounted on frames, the infection may be limited to the cusps. Thus, if one has a substitute cardiac valve that is infected, it is better that the infection involve a bioprosthesis rather than a mechanical valve. If endocarditis occurs in a patient in whom more than 1 mechanical or bioprosthetic valve is in place, the infection nearly always involves only the most downstream prosthetic valve.

Entanglement of Sutures Beneath the Occluder

Suture entanglement beneath the occluder during insertion of a mitral prosthesis may prevent descent of the occluder during ventricular dias-

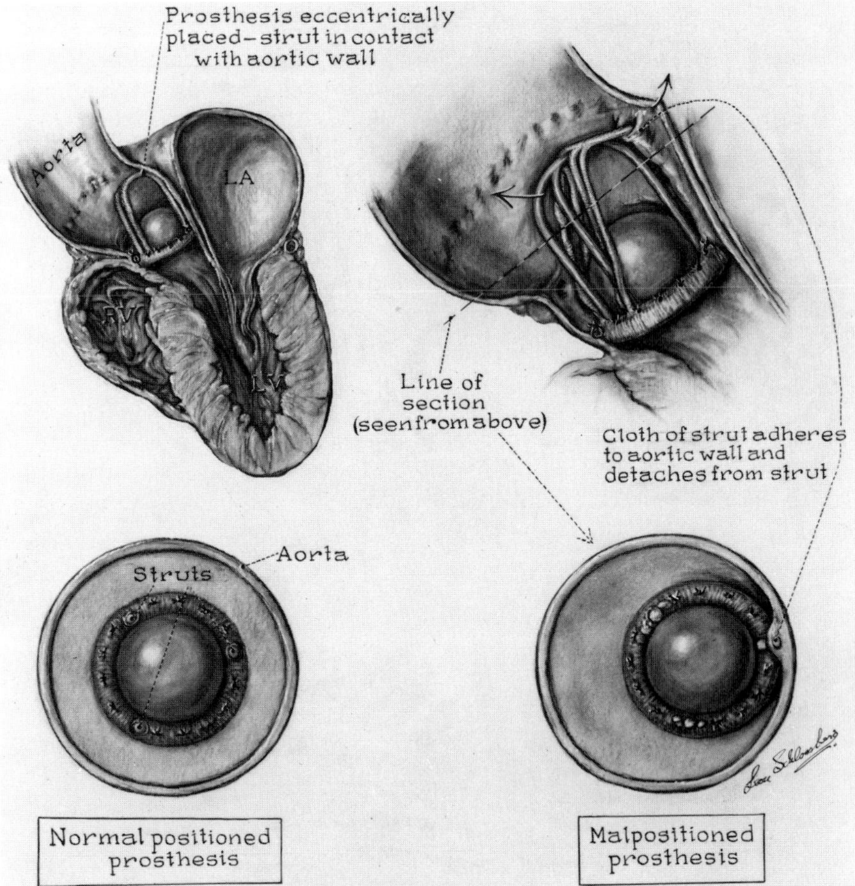

FIG. 2 Cloth wear on stents of a caged ball prosthesis in 76-year-old man who died of carcinoma many years after aortic valve replacement and asymptomatic postoperative course. At necropsy, 1 of the 3 stents contacted intimal lining of aorta and eventually aortic wall completely encircled 1 stent and cloth became detached from other 2 stents. Although a rather striking finding at necropsy, cloth degeneration and aortic wall overgrowth did not cause symptoms during life.

tole.[32] Simply making certain by manual manipulation that the mitral occluder descends freely before closing the left atriotomy incision might prevent this technical problem from being fatal.

Incomplete Removal of Native Valve or Its Calcific Deposits

If calcific deposits involve the attachment of a valve leaflet to its "anulus," complete debridement of the calcium may not be possible. If a rather sizable calcific nodule remains after valvular excision, the residual calcific debris, on rare occasion, may interfere with complete closure of the occluder.[3]

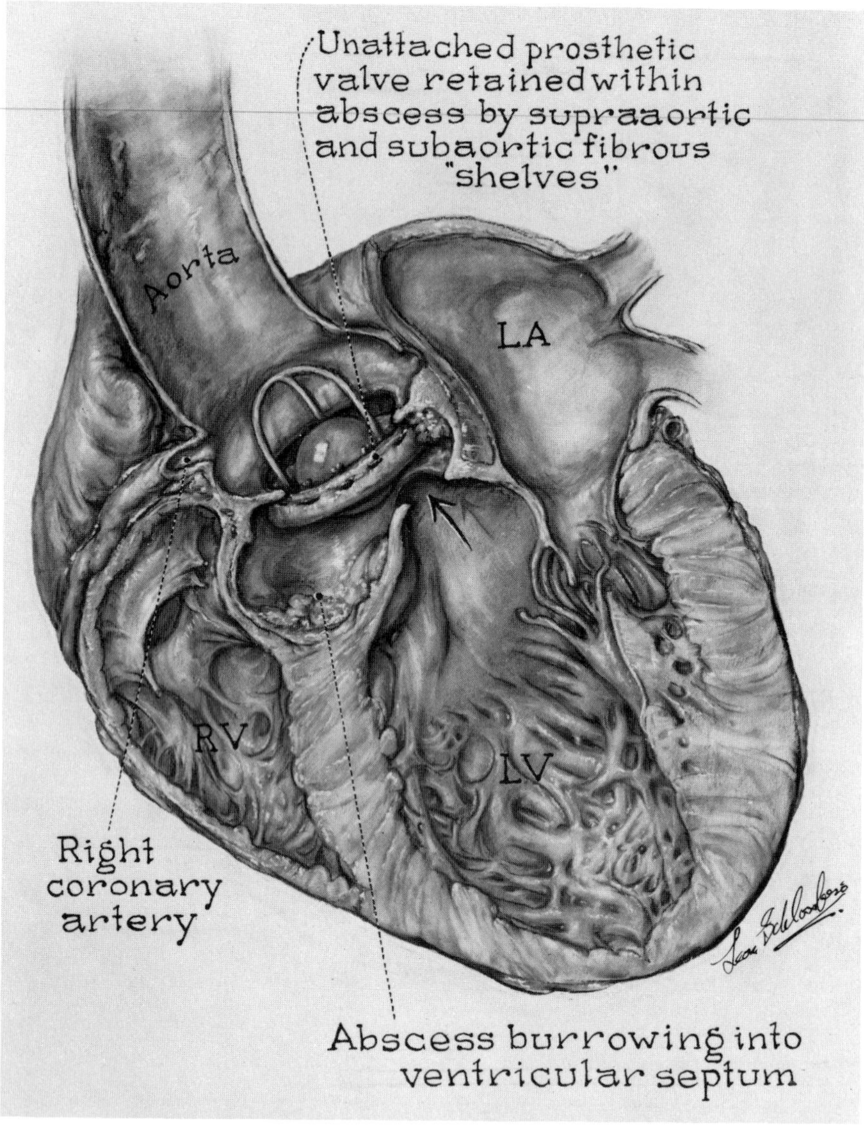

FIG. 3 Prosthetic valve endocarditis. Heart of a 39-year-old woman who underwent aortic valve replacement 8 years earlier because of severe aortic regurgitation secondary to intravenous heroin-induced infective endocarditis. She was asymptomatic thereafter, however, except for occasional ventricular arrhythmias, until 26 hours before death when she suddenly became unconscious and was found to have an intracerebral hemorrhage. At necropsy, the caged ball prosthesis was completely detached due to infection beneath the prosthetic ring. The prosthesis was prevented from dislodging by a "constricting" fibrous ring just cephalad to the prosthetic anulus. During her last 8 years of life, there was never clinical evidence of infective endocarditis.

Dislodgement of a Portion of Native Cardiac Valve During Its Excision

It is preferable to remove a calcified cardiac valve intact rather than in multiple fragments to prevent the possibility of embolism.[33]

Development of Calcific Deposits Beneath Site of Attachment of a Prosthetic Valve Ring

During both phases of the cardiac cycle, a rigid-framed prosthesis moves. This back and forth "rocking" motion over many years may stimulate the development of calcific deposits beneath the prosthetic anulus.[34] As long as the deposits are small, significant functional consequences are unlikely, but larger ones theoretically could disrupt a suture that holds the prosthetic ring in place. This "anular calcium" is most likely to develop more than 5 years after mitral replacement with a "heavy" prosthesis (caged ball) but to date we are aware of no functional consequences of its development.

Hemolysis of Blood Elements

Most mechanical cardiac valves decrease the half-life of erythrocytes, leukocytes, and even platelets, but in all but a few patients the bone marrow accelerates production and anemia or leukopenia or thrombocytopenia is rarely a consequence. On occasion, however, hemolysis is a problem, most frequently in patients with caged ball prostheses (particularly with the fully cloth-covered models), in patients with aortic valve prostheses as opposed to other replaced valves, and in patients with parabasilar leaks as opposed to patients with intact parabasilar regions.[35]

Complications Limited to a Particular Valve Site Irrespective of Type of Prosthesis

Mitral Valve Position

Disruption of connection between left atrium and left ventricle at mitral anulus with extravasation of blood into the atrioventricular sulcus. When calcific deposits are located in the mitral anular region in addition to their being located in the mitral leaflets, excision of the mitral valve, including one or more anular calcific deposits, may lead to loss of continuity between the walls of left atrium and left ventricle with extravasation of blood into the left atrioventricular sulcus with or without fatal bleeding into the pericardial sac.[3]

Excision of a portion of left ventricular free wall beneath papillary muscle during excision of papillary muscle with resulting rupture or aneurysmal formation If during mitral valve excision a left ventricular papillary muscle, grasped with a clamp, is pulled toward the left atrium before the papillary muscle incision is made, a portion of the left ventricular free wall in addition to papillary muscle may be excised.[3] Depending on how much left ventricular free wall is excised, the result may be through-and-through rupture of aneurysmal formation.[4]

Incision of left ventricular free wall midway between mitral anulus and stump of left ventricular papillary muscle during mitral valve excision. A number of reports have described rupture of the left ventricular wall after mitral valve replacement and most often the rupture was attributed to a stent of either a mechanical or a porcine valve's burrowing through the free wall.[36] Its mechanism was never been precisely determined, in our view, but the rupture or aneurysm site in the left ventricular free wall is midway between the mitral anulus and stump of the papillary muscle. This complication unfortunately is not rare. At 1 major medical center this complication was reported in 1980 to be the most common cause of early death after mitral valve replacement.[36] We believe its cause is inadvertent incision of the left ventricular free wall during the incision of the chordae tendineae, for the "tear" into left ventricular free wall is linear and often involves the entire free wall of the left ventricular[37] (Fig. 4). Furthermore, it may be a considerable distance from a prosthetic stent. I have seen this complication in about 10 patients at necropsy. All have had relatively small hearts with normal-sized left atrial and left ventricular cavities. The mitral hemodynamic lesion in each was either chronic mitral stenosis or acute mitral regurgitation. The atrium was entered in all but 1 by an interatrial groove incision and this incision was relatively short in length due to the small size of the heart. The distance from the interatrial groove incision to the inadvertent left ventricular circular incision was about 8–9 cm, exposure of the mital valve was poor, visualization of the tips of the incising or excising mitral valve scissors had to be poor or inadequate, and during either the opening or closing maneuver or both the scissor tips incised a portion of left ventricular free wall while the mitral valve was being excised.

Damage to the left circumflex coronary artery or coronary sinus during insertion of a mitral prosthesis or during suture obliteration of the entrance into the left atrial appendage. Although we have not seen this complication personally, damage to the left circumflex coronary artery or coronary sinus or both during mitral replacement has been observed by others. Both of these vessels, of course, are located in the left atrioventricular sulcus, which is less than 1 cm from where sutures are placed into the most basal portion of mitral leaflet during insertion of the prosthesis. Occlusion of the left circumflex coronary artery by a suture may result in a ventricular arrhythmia or acute myocardial infarction or both, whereas occlusion of the coronary sinus usually does not produce a clinically recognized functional conse-

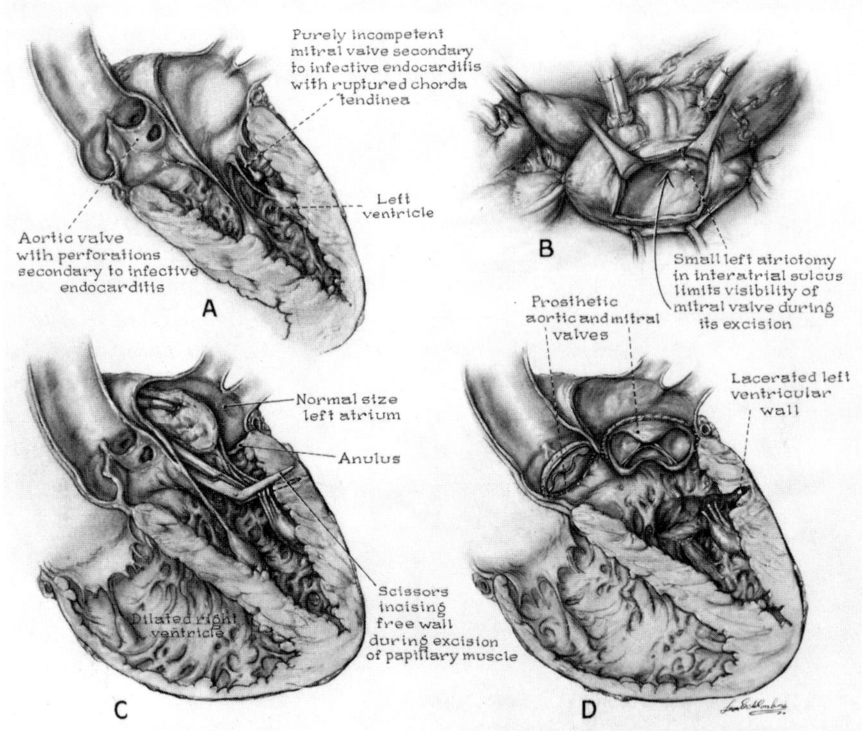

FIG. 4 Mechanism of LV rupture in a 44-year-old man who had rupture of the LV free wall 4 days after mitral valve replacement.

quence. During suture obliteration of the mouth of a left atrial appendage, complete obliteration by a suture of the lumen of the left circumflex coronary artery that courses just beneath the entrance into the appendage may occur (Fig. 5).

Contact of cage or stent of mitral prosthesis with ventricular septum or left ventricular free wall producing a ventricular arrhythmia. Contact of the cage or stent of a mitral or tricuspid valve prosthesis with the ventricular septum or even left ventricular free wall not only may result in left ventricular inflow or outflow obstruction, but the "tickling" of the myocardium by the prosthesis may produce a ventricular arrhythmia that may be fatal (Fig. 6). This mechanism has been documented by echocardiography during life and indentations of the ventricular septum, particularly by the cage of a caged ball prosthesis or by a stent of a porcine bioprosthesis, may be observed at necropsy. This situation, of course, is most liable to occur when relatively large prostheses are employed in relatively small-sized ventricules.

Diffuse or extensive left ventricular fibrosis. Whenever the left ventricular

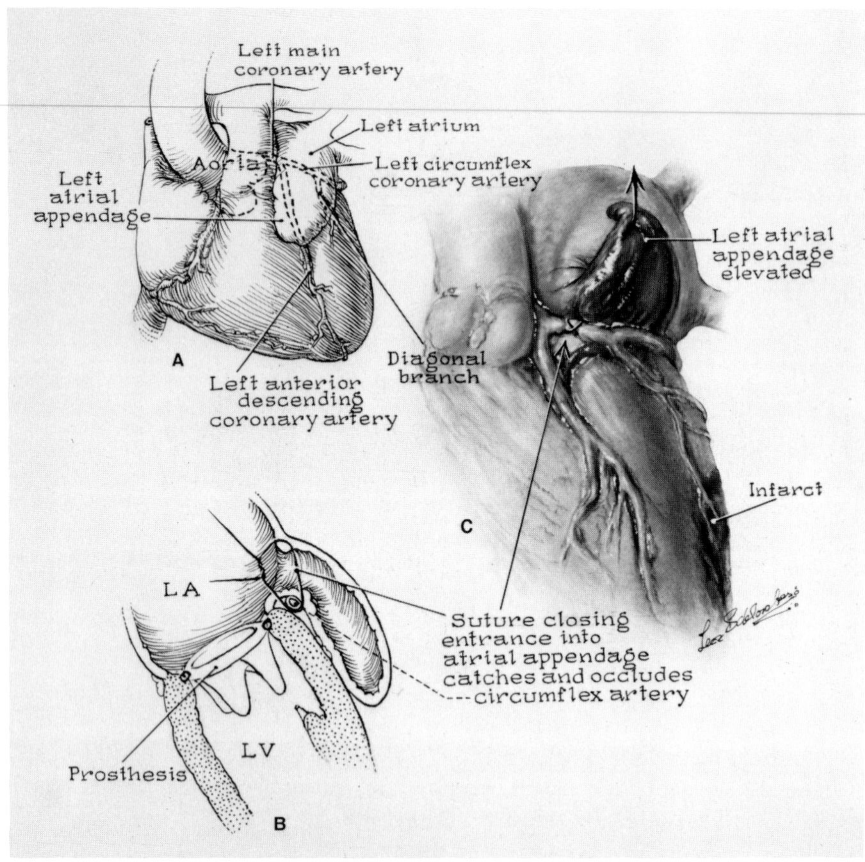

FIG. 5 Occlusion of left circumflex coronary artery by sutures utilized to close mouth of left atrial appendage in 62-year-old man who died with lateral wall LV acute infarct 5 days after mitral valve replacement.

papillary muscles are excised, their "raw" stumps are eventually covered by dense fibrous tissue. Thus, mural endocardial fibrosis over the stumps of the papillary muscles is an expected late finding after mitral valve replacement. On rare occasion, not only is the endocardial covering over the papillary muscles thickened by fibrous tissue but the same process may involve most of the remaining portion of left ventricle.[38] The mechanism of this diffuse or extensive endocardial fibrosis is unclear. Initially, the concept was presented that the ball in a cage prosthesis "stirred up" the blood in the left ventricular cavity and the anatomic consequence of the "churning" up and down movement was intimal thickening. Another view has been that the entensive endocardial thickening was the consequence of poor myocardial protection at the time of valve replacement, but the endocardial thick-

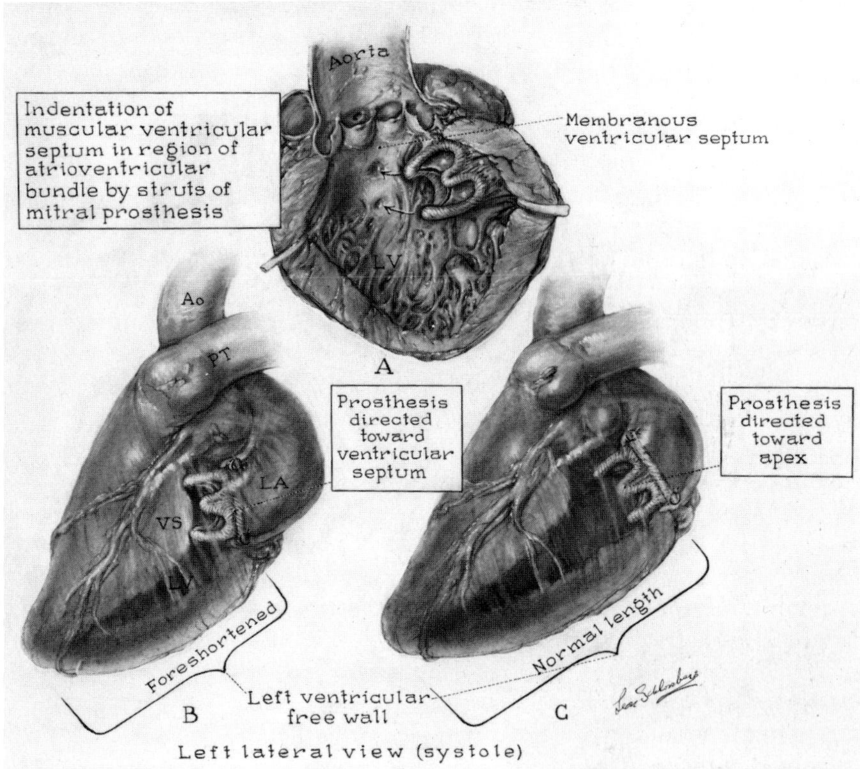

FIG. 6 Contact of stents of porcine bioprosthesis in mitral position with ventricular septum, probably during ventricular systole only. This 71-year-old woman underwent mitral replacement 38 days before death because of severe mitral regurgitation associated with idiopathic dilated cardiomyopathy. Although no difinite consequence of this contact between prosthesis and ventricular septum was apparent, this type contact has been recognized as producing arrhythmias and possibly even sudden death.

ening, to our knowledge, has been observed only after mitral valve replacement and not after aortic valve replacement.

Aortic Valve Position

Obstruction of a coronary ostium by a prosthetic ring or stent. This complication, of course, is rare but it may result in fatal acute myocardial infarction or a ventricular arrhythmia. Utilization of a porcine valve, which has relatively large stents, in a small aorta with improper positioning of the stents is the most likely situation in which this complication may occur today.

Intimal thickening in the aortic root. Whenever the intimal surface of the aorta is touched, the endothetial cells are immediately removed and the underlying media is exposed. Usually healing occurs simply by proliferation of new endothelial cells but occasionally collagen is deposited in excess in these "exposed" areas. In addition to some expected focal intimal thickening in the aortic root after aortic valve replacement by the mechanism already mentioned, turbulent flow through particularly a peripheral flow type prosthesis may lead to severe intimal thickening in the aortic root. If the aortic root intimal thickening involves the aorta in the area of the coronary ostia, the latter may be narrowed and this may lead to myocardial ischemia.[2] This complication, however, has proved to be uncommon but, nevertheless, it is well documented after aortic valve replacement. In patients with clinical evidence of red blood cell hemolysis, the aortic root intimal thickening can be predicted to be particularly severe because its origin is primarily turbulence produced by flow through the prosthesis, the same mechanism that shortens the half-life of the red blood cells.[8]

Dissection of aorta. Aortic dissection is a well-known occurrence in certain patients with aortic valve disease, but its occurrence *after* aortic valve replacement is not widely appreciated. Fortunately, this complication is infrequent after aortic valve replacement (described in only 0.07% of such patients postoperatively[39]). Dissection, however, also may occur after aortotomy for any purpose, such as cannulation site, aortocoronary conduit anastomosis, and therefore its occurrence after aortic valve replacement may be more related to the aortotomy than to inherent disease of the aorta associated with aortic valve stenosis or regurgitation.

Complications Following Combined Mitral and Aortic Valve Replacement

Contact of Aortic Valve Poppet with Stent or Ring of Mitral Prosthesis Causing Aortic Regurgitation

The basal attachment of the anterior mitral leaflet is about 1 cm caudal to the bases of the aortic valve cusps, and after replacement of both valves the fixation rings of the 2 prostheses are in close proximity. Ordinarily, of course, this juxtaposition produces no hemodynamic disturbance, but if the mitral prosthesis is particularly large, one of its stents or even its ring may lie directly beneath the orifice of the aortic prosthesis and during ventricular diastole the poppet of the aortic prosthesis may contact the stent or ring of the mitral prosthesis, the aortic poppet may be prevented from seating, and aortic regurgitation, which may be fatal, may result.[40] This complication has been observed only when the mitral valve has been replaced with a very large prosthesis.

Compression of Anomalous Left Circumflex Coronary Artery by Mitral and Aortic Prosthetic Fixation Rings

The most common important coronary anomaly is origin of the left circumflex coronary artery from the right coronary artery with subsequent coursing behind the aorta on its way to the left atrioventricular sulcus. Although potentially this anomalous artery could be damaged during isolated mitral or aortic valve replacement, such has not been reported. Damage to this artery, however, is a distinct danger if both mitral and aortic valves are replaced because the anomalous coronary artery courses between the fixation rings of these 2 prosthesis and thus it may be compressed by them.[41] Fortunately, because this coronary anomaly occurs about once in 300 human hearts and combined replacement of both mitral and aortic valves is even less frequent, this complication of valve replacement is extremely rare.[41]

References

1. Roberts WC, Morrow AG: Mechanisms of acute left atrial thrombosis after mitral valve replacement. Pathologic findings indicating obstruction to left atrial emptying. Am J Cardiol 18:497, 1966.
2. Roberts WC, Morrow AG: Late postoperative pathologic findings after cardiac valve replacement. Circulation 36 (Suppl I):48, 1967.
3. Roberts WC, Morrow AG: Causes of early postoperative death following cardiac valve replacement. Clinico-pathologic correlations in 64 patients studied at necropsy. J Thorac Cardiovasc Surg 54:422, 1967.
4. Roberts WC, Morrow AG: Anatomic studies of hearts containing caged-ball prosthetic valves. Johns Hopkins Med J 121:271, 1967.
5. Roberts WC, Morrow AG: Causes of death and other anatomic observations after cardiac valve replacement. Adv Cardiol 7:226, 1972.
6. Winter TQ, Reis RL, Glancy DL, Roberts WC, Epstein SE, Morrow AG: Current status of Starr-Edwards cloth-covered prosthetic cardiac valves. Circulation 45, 46 (Suppl I):14, 1972.
7. Shepard RL, Glancy DL, Stinson EB, Roberts WC: Hemodynamic confirmation of obstruction to left ventricular inflow by a caged-ball prosthetic mitral valve. Case report. J Thorac Cardiovasc Surg 65:252, 1973.
8. Roberts WC, Bulkley BH, Morrow AG: Pathologic anatomy of cardiac valve replacement: A study of 224 necropsy patients. Prog Cardiovas Dis 15:539, 1973.
9. Roberts WC: Operative treatment of hypertrophic obstructive cardiomyopathy. The case against mitral valve replacement. Am J Cardiol 32:377, 1973.
10. Seningen RP, Bulkley BH, Roberts WC: Prosthetic aortic stenosis. A method to prevent its occurrence by measurement of aortic size from preoperative aortogram. Circulation 49:921, 1974.
11. Fishbein MC, Roberts WC, Golden A, Hufnagel CA: Cardiac pathology after aortic valve replacement using Hufnagel trifleaflet prostheses: A study of 20 necropsy patients. Am Heart J 89:443, 1975.
12. Roberts WC, Fishbein MC, Golden A: Cardiac pathology after valve replace-

ment by disc prosthesis. A study of 61 mecropsy patients. Am J Cardiol 35:740, 1975.
13. Roberts WC, Hammer WJ: Cardiac pathology after valve replacement with a tilting disc prosthesis (Björk-Shiley type). A study of 46 necropsy patients and 49 Björk-Shiley prostheses. Am J Cardiol 37:1024, 1976.
14. Roberts WC: Choosing a substitute cardiac valve: Type, size, surgeon. Am J Cardiol 38:633, 1976.
15. Spray TL, Roberts WC: Structural changes in porcine xenografts used as substitute cardiac valves. Gross and histologic observations in 51 glutaraldehyde-preserved Hancock valves in 41 patients. Am J Cardiol 40:319, 1977.
16. Ferrans FJ, Spray TL, Billingham ME, Roberts WC: Structural changes in glutaraldehyde-treated procine heterografts used as substitute cardiac valves. Transmission and scanning electron microscopic observations in 12 patients. Am J Cardiol 41:1159, 1978.
17. Ferrans VJ, Boyce SW, Billingham ME, Jones M, Ishihara T, Roberts WC: Calcific deposits in porcine bioprosthesis: Structure and pathogensis. Am J Cardiol 46:721, 1980.
18. Roberts WC, Morrow AG: Fatal degeneration of the silicone rubber ball of the Starr-Edwards prosthetic aortic valve. Am J Cardiol 22:614, 1968.
19. Roberts WC, Levinson GE, Morrow AG: Lethal ball variance in the Starr-Edwards prosthetic mitral valve. Arch Intern Med 126:517, 1970.
20. Fishbein MC, Roberts WC: Late postoperative anatomic observations after insertion of Hufnagel caged-ball prostheses in descending thoracic aorta. Chest 68:6, 1975.
21. Yarbrough JW, Roberts WC, Reis RL: Structural alterations in tissue cardiac valves implanted in patients and in calves. J Thorac Cardiovasc Surg 65:364, 1973.
22. Geha AS, Laks H, Stansel HC Jr., Cornhill JF, Kilman JW, Buckley MJ, Roberts WC: Late failure of porcine valve heterografts in children. J Thorac Cardiovasc Surg 78:351, 1979.
23. Ishihara T, Ferrans VJ, Jones M, Cabin HS, Roberts WC: Calcific deposits developing in a bovine pericardial bioprosthetic valve 3 days after implantation. Circulation 63:718, 1981.
24. Ishihara T, Ferrans VJ, Jones M, Boyce SW, Roberts WC: Structure of bovine parietal pericardium and of unimplanted Ionescu-Shiley pericardial valvular bioprostheses. J Thorac Cardiovas Surg 81:747, 1981.
25. Waller BF, Jones M, Roberts WC: Postoperative aortic regurgitation from incomplete seating of tilting-disc occluders due to overhanding knots or long sutures. Chest 78:565, 1980.
26. Cohn LH, Roberts WC, Rockoff SD, Morrow AG: Bacterial endocarditis following aortic valve replacement. Clinical and pathologic correlations. Circulation 33:209, 1966.
27. Archard HO, Roberts WC: Bacterial endocarditis after dental procedures in patients with aortic valve prostheses. J Am Dent Assoc 72:648, 1966.
28. Roberts WC, Morrow AG: Bacterial endocarditis involving prosthetic mitral valves. Clinical and pathologic observations. Arch Pathol 82:164, 1966.
29. Arnett EA, Roberts WC: Prosthetic valve endocarditis. Clinicio-pathologic analysis of 22 mecropsy patients with comparison of observations in 74 necropsy patients with active infective endocarditis involving natural left-sided cardiac valves. Am J Cardiol 38:281, 1976.
30. Arnett EN, Kastl DG, Garvin AJ, Roberts WC: A conversation on prosthetic valve endocarditis. Am Heart J 93:510, 1977.

31. Ferrans VJ, Boyce SW, Billingham ME, Spray TL, Roberts WC: Infection of glutaraldehyde-preserved porcine valve heterografts. Am J Cardiol 43:1123, 1979.
32. Jones AA, Otis JB, Fletcher GF, Roberts WC: A hitherto undescribed cause of prosthetic mitral valve obstruction. J Thorac Cardiovasc Surg 74:116, 1977.
33. Roberts WC, Morrow AG: Cardiac valves and the surgical pathologist. Arch Pathol 82:309, 1966.
34. Bulkley BH, Morrow AG, Roberts WC: Calcification of prosthetic valve anuli: A late complication of cardiac valve replacement. Am Heart J 87:129, 1974.
35. Roberts WC, Morrow AG: Renal hemosiderosis in patients with prosthetic aortic valves. Circulation 33:390, 1966.
36. Cobbs BW Jr, Hatcher CR Jr, Craver JM, Jones EL, Sewell CW: Transverse midventricular disruption after mitral valve replacement. Am Heart J 99:33, 1980.
37. Roberts WC, Mason DT, Engle MA, Cohn LH: Cardiology 1981. New York, Yorke Medical Books, 1981.
38. Roberts WC, Morrow AG: Secondary left ventricular endocardial fibroelastosis following mitral valve replacement. Cause of cardiac failure in the late post-operative period. Circulation 37, 38 (Suppl II):101, 1968.
39. Muna WF, Spray TL, Morrow AG, Roberts WC: Aortic dissection after aortic valve replacement in patients with valvular aortic stenosis. J Thorac Cardiovasc Surg 74:65, 1977.
40. Roberts WC, Lambird PA, Gott VL, Morrow AG: Fatal aortic regurgitation following replacement of the mitral and aortic valves. A mechanical complication of double valve replacement. J Thorac Cardiovasc Surg 52:189, 1966.
41. Roberts WC, Morrow AG: Compression of anomalous left circumflex coronary arteries by prosthetic valve fixation rings. J Thorac Cardiovasc Surg 57:834, 1969.

32

Pathogenesis and Stages of Bioprosthetic Infection

V. J. Ferrans, T. Ishihara, M. Jones, G. R. Barnhart, S. W. Boyce, A. B. Kravitz, W. C. Roberts

Although the clinical manifestations of infection of bioprosthetic cardiac valves have been described previously,[1-10] only limited information is available on the morphologic features of infected bioprostheses.[11-13] The pathogenesis of bioprosthetic infection has not been fully clarified, although it has been suggested that bacteria first attach to thrombotic material on the cuspal surfaces and subsequently invade the cuspal collagen.[11] It also has been pointed out that infection in bioprostheses tends to remain localized in the cusps, with little tendency to form ring abscesses, such as occurs with infection involving mechanical valve prostheses.[14] This report provides a detailed analysis of morphologic findings in 30 infected bioprosthetic valves: 15 of these (group I) had been implanted in patients; the other 15 (group II) had been implanted in sheep as part of a program of experimental evaluation of the processes of calcification and degeneration of bioprostheses in animals.[15,16]

Materials and Methods

Group I bioprostheses. The 15 bioprostheses in group I (13 porcine aortic valvular bioprostheses, and two bovine pericardial bioprostheses) had been implanted in 11 patients, 10 men and 1 woman, aged 28–68 years (mean, 46; Table I). The bioprostheses had been in place from 6 days to 42 months (mean, 19 months) before removal at reoperation (7) or necropsy (8). Six bioprostheses had been in the mitral position; 7, in the aortic position; and 2

From the Pathology and Surgery Branches, National Heart, Lung, and Blood Institute, National Institutes of Health, Bethesda, Maryland.

in the tricuspid position. Twelve bioprostheses had been infected by Gram positive cocci; the others, by a variety of other organisms.

Group II bioprostheses. Fifteen bioprostheses (7 porcine aortic valvular bioprostheses and 8 bovine pericardial bioprostheses) became infected after having been implanted in 25 young sheep, which were 4–6 months of age at operation (Table II). Eight bioprostheses had been implanted in the tricuspid position, and 7 in the mitral position. These 15 bioprostheses represent 10% of the 148 bioprostheses that we have implanted in sheep. The bioprostheses were recovered at necropsy in 14 animals, which died suddenly 4 days to 5 months after operation, and at terminal elective study, 1 month after operation, in the remaining animal. Twelve bioprostheses had been infected by Gram positive cocci, 2 by Gram negative rods, and 1 by a fungus.

The bioprostheses were photographed and radiographed immediately after removal. Tissue blocks were then obtained and processed for histologic study and transmission and scanning electron microscopic examination according to methods described elsewhere.[17]

Results

Gross Anatomic Observations

Group I bioprostheses. Vegetations were evident grossly in 12 of 15 bioprostheses. They were nodular, friable, and varied from whitish-yellow to brownish-red. They were limited to the cusps and were more extensive on the outflow surfaces than on the inflow surfaces. Of the other 3 bioprostheses, 1 had been in place for only 6 days and contained only a few colonies of bacteria associated with fibrin on the cuspal surfaces;[11] the other 2 had abundant thrombi that contained microorganisms.

Ring abscesses occurred in 2 patients, who had staphylococcal infection of porcine aortic valvular bioprostheses that had been implanted in the mitral position. Calcific deposits were detected by gross inspection and roentgenogram or microscopic study in 12 of the 15 bioprostheses. In the porcine aortic valvular bioprostheses, the calcific deposits were multinodular, whereas in the pericardial bioprostheses they involved the cusps much more diffusely.

Valvular regurgitation due to cuspal damage occurred in 5 bioprostheses, all of which were porcine aortic valvular bioprostheses. The tears or perforations involved only 1 cusp in 2 bioprostheses, 2 cusps in another, and each of the 3 cusps in the remaining 2 bioprostheses. Large, centrally located perforations (type III according to the classification of Ishihara et al[18]) were present in 4 of these 5 bioprostheses. Each of the 4 bioprostheses had been implanted in the mitral position and had been infected by Gram positive

TABLE I Morphologic findings in 15 bioprosthetic cardiac valves that became infected after implantation in patients*

BP #	Pt. #	Age	Sex	BP implanted: Type	BP implanted: Position	BP implanted: Time (mo)	Reason for BP removal	Infecting organism	Stage of infection	Surface thrombi	Ca++ deposits	Fibrous sheaths	Perforation
1	1	66	F	H	A	0.2	N	My	I	0	0	0	0
2	2	68	M	H	A	5	N(S)	C, rods(−)	I	+	0	0	0
3	3	61	M	H	A	14	S,R	C	IV	+	0	0	+
4	4	35	M	CE	A	27	S,R	C	IV	+	+	0	+
5	5	40	M	CE	A	33	S,R	Staph	IV	+	+	0	+
6	6	55	M	H	A	40	N(R)	Str	IV	+	+	0	+
7	7	45	M	IS	A	4	N(S)	Staph	III	+	+	0	0
Total					7		S = 5 R = 4		I = 2, III = 1, IV = 4	6	4	0	4
8	8	28	M	H	M	4.5	S	Staph	II	+	+	0	0
9	9	29	M	H	M	8	N	Staph	I	+	+	0	0
10	10	42	M	H	M	28	S	Rods(+)	II	+	+	0	0
11	5	40	M	CE	M	33	S	Staph	III	+	+	+	+†
12	11	36	M	H	M	42	S	Staph	III	+	+	+	0
13	7	45	M	IS	M	4	N(S)	C	II	+	+	0	0
Total					6		S = 5		I = 1, II = 3 III = 2	6	6	2	1
14	9	29	M	H	T	8	N	Staph	I	+	+	0	0
15	6	55	M	H	T	40	N	Str	II	+	+	+	0
Total				2					I = 1, II = 1	2	2	1	0
Overall Total		46.5 (avg)			A = 7 M = 6 T = 2	19.4 (avg)	S = 10 R = 4		I = 4, II = 4 III = 3 IV = 4	14	12	3	5

* A: aortic; BP: bioprosthesis; C: Gram positive cocci; CE: Carpentier-Edwards porcine aortic valvular bioprosthesis; F: female; H: Hancock porcine aortic valvular bioprosthesis; IS: Ionescu-Shiley bovine pericardial bioprosthesis; M: mitral, male; My: *Mycobacterium chelonei;* N: necropsy; R: regurgitation; Rod (−); Gram negative rods; Rod (+): Gram positive rods; S: stenosis; Staph: staphylococci; Str: streptococci; T: tricuspid.

TABLE II Morphologic findings in infected cardiac valvular bioprostheses in 15 sheep*

Sheep	BP implanted			Infecting	Stage of	Surface	Ca++	Fibrous	Bacteria	
#	Type	Position	Time	organism	infection	thrombi	deposits	sheaths	in FS	Perforation
1	H	T	4 days	C	†	0	0	0	0	0
2	CE	T	1 mo	C	III	+	+	0	0	0
3	CE	T	2.5 mo	C	III	+	+	0	0	0
4	CE	T	3 mo	C	III	+	+	+	0	0
5	H	T	5 mo	R	III	+	+	+	0	0
6	H	M	2 mo	F	III	+	0	+	0	0
7	H	M	2.5 mo	C	II	+	+	+	0	0
8	IS	T	3 mo	C	III	+	+	+	0	0
9	IS	T	5 mo	C	II	+	+	+	+	0
10	IS	T	6 mo	C	III	+	+	+	0	0
11	IS	M	1 mo	R	III	+	0	0	0	0
12	IS	M	1.5 mo	C	II	+	0	0	0	0
13	IS	M	2.5 mo	C	II	+	+	+	0	0
14	IS	M	3 mo	C	II	+	+	+	0	0
15	IS	M	3 mo	C	II	+	+	+	+	0
Totals	H = 4 CE = 3 IS = 8	T = 8 M = 7	2.75 mo (avg)	C = 12 R = 2 F = 1	II = 6 III = 8	14	11	10	2	0

* BP: bioprosthesis; C: gram-positive cocci; CE: Carpentier-Edwards porcine aortic valvular bioprosthesis; F: fungus; FS: fibrous sheath; H: Hancock porcine aortic valvular bioprosthesis; IS: Ionescu-Shiley bovine pericardial bioprosthesis; M: mitral; R: gram-negative rods; T: tricuspid; +: present; 0: absent.

† Infection limited to the muscle shelf of the right coronary cusp.

cocci. Two of the 4 bioprostheses also had tears (type I lesions) involving the free edges of the cusps; in each of these 2 bioprostheses, 2 cusps were affected by the tears and the remaining cusp was the site of a large (type III) perforation. The fifth perforated bioprosthesis had been implanted in the mitral position and contained multiple, minute perforations (type IV), which were associated with calcific deposits but not with destruction of tissue by bacteria. At the time of removal, 10 bioprostheses were judged to have been stenotic due to vegetations and calcified, poorly mobile cusps.

Group II bioprostheses. Vegetations and thrombi causing stenosis were found in 14 of the 15 infected group II bioprostheses. Ring abscesses and cuspal tears and perforations were absent. In 5 of the porcine aortic valvular bioprostheses, the vegetations were more prominent on the outflow surfaces than on the inflow surfaces. In contrast, the vegetations in 5 of the 8 pericardial bioprostheses were more prominent on the inflow surfaces than on the outflow surfaces. The only bioprosthesis in which vegetations were not grossly evident had been implanted for only 4 days. This porcine aortic valvular bioprosthesis was anatomically normal except for the presence of bacteria in the muscle shelf of the right coronary cusp. Calcific deposits were present in 11 bioprostheses, including 5 porcine aortic valvular bioprostheses and 6 pericardial bioprostheses.

Histologic and Ultrastructural Observations

Based on the topographic localization of the infecting organisms and the tissue alterations in the bioprostheses, we have formulated a system for evaluating the degree of involvement of bioprosthetic tissue and host tissue. Infection in bioprosthetic cardiac valves is classified into 4 stages (Fig. 1): *stage I* is characterized by localization of organisms only on thrombotic material adherent to the surfaces of the bioprosthetic cusps; *stage II,* by the presence of organisms on thrombotic material as well as on immediately subjacent cuspal collagen; *stage III,* by penetration of the organisms into centrally located areas of cuspal tissue (i.e., the spongiosa in porcine aortic valvular bioprostheses and the middle third of the pericardial fibrosa in pericardial bioprostheses); and *stage IV,* by cuspal perforation.

Group I bioprostheses. Four bioprostheses implanted in patients were judged to have stage I infection (Fig. 2). One bioprosthesis had been implanted in the aortic position in a patient who had Ehlers-Danlos syndrome and died of an aortic dissection 6 days after operation; another bioprosthesis had been in the mitral position in a patient who died of coronary embolus 5 months after operation. The other 2 bioprostheses had been implanted for 8 months, in the mitral and in the tricuspid positions, in a patient who developed signs and symptoms of infection only 2 days before dying of staphylococcal sepsis. Only 2 of the 4 bioprostheses with stage I infection had a calcific deposit. A fibrous sheath was not present on any of these 4

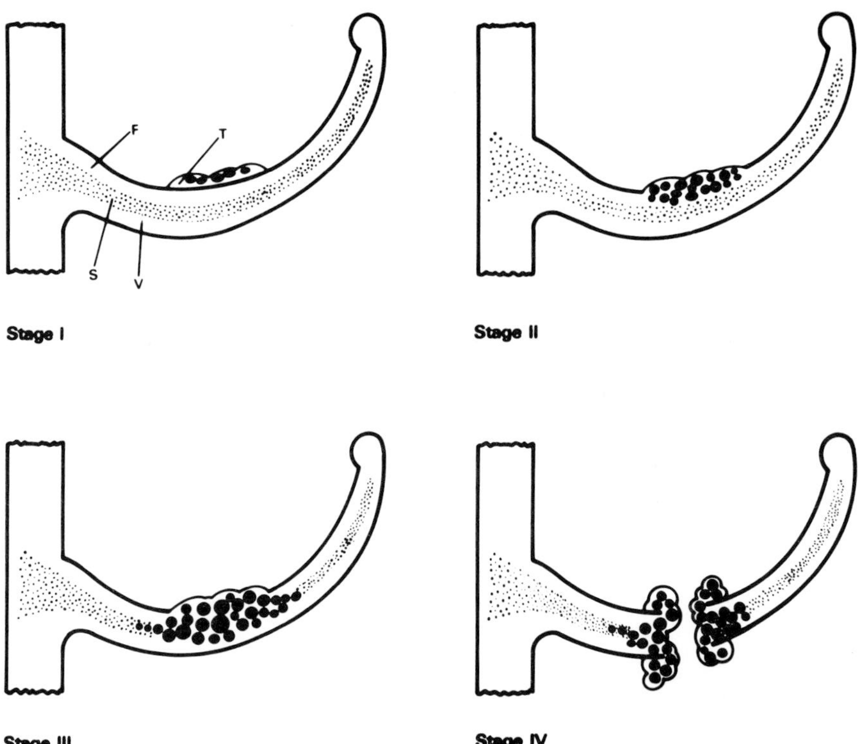

FIG. 1 The 4 stages of infection of bioprosthetic cardiac valves.

bioprostheses, and bacteria in these bioprostheses did not extend into the basal portions of the cusps.

Four other group I bioprostheses were classified as having stage II infection (Fig. 3). Each of these 4 bioprostheses contained calcific deposits. In 1 porcine aortic valvular bioprosthesis, these were localized only to healing vegetations; in 2 others they involved cuspal connective tissue, and in a pericardial bioprosthesis they involved both cuspal connective tissue and vegetations. Numerous neutrophils and macrophages were found in thrombi and in superficial regions of cuspal connective tissue in each of the 4 bioprostheses.

Three bioprostheses had stage III infection, including 2 porcine aortic valvular bioprostheses in which the bacteria had accumulated in empty spaces in the spongiosa (Fig. 4). These bacteria were not associated with inflammatory cells, which were mostly confined to thrombotic material on the surfaces of the cusps. In 1 pericardial bioprosthesis with stage III infection[13] (Fig. 5) the bacteria involved deeply located spaces between bundles of collagen in the pericardial fibrosa. These bacteria were associated with

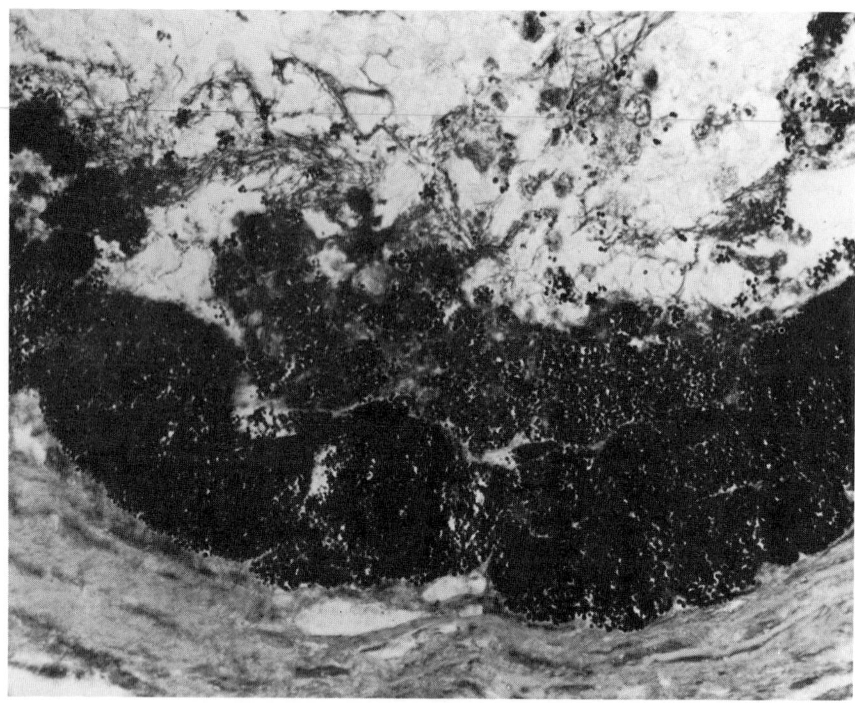

FIG. 2 Stage I infection, limited to thrombotic material overlying cusps, is shown in this section of porcine aortic valvular bioprosthesis that became infected with staphylococci. A dense layer of organisms, shown here in black, covers surface of cusp. Plastic section, alkaline toluidine blue, ×750.

only small numbers of inflammatory cells; a few bacteria and many macrophages were present in thrombotic material in the surface. Each of the bioprostheses with stage III infection contained calcific deposits. In the pericardial bioprosthesis the deposits were localized both in thrombi and in the cusps; in the other 2 bioprostheses, they were localized in the cusps only.

Four bioprostheses were found to have stage IV infection (Fig. 6). Each of these bioprostheses was a porcine aortic valvular bioprosthesis, had been implanted in the aortic position, had been infected with Gram positive cocci, and had bacteria and macrophages both in thrombi and in cuspal tissue, including the spongiosa. In each instance, the perforations were due to disruption of cuspal collagen, a process that appeared to terminate in the formation of a very finely granular material of moderate electron density. Strands of fibrin and lipid droplets often were interspersed with this material. Three of the bioprostheses had calcific deposits in cuspal connective

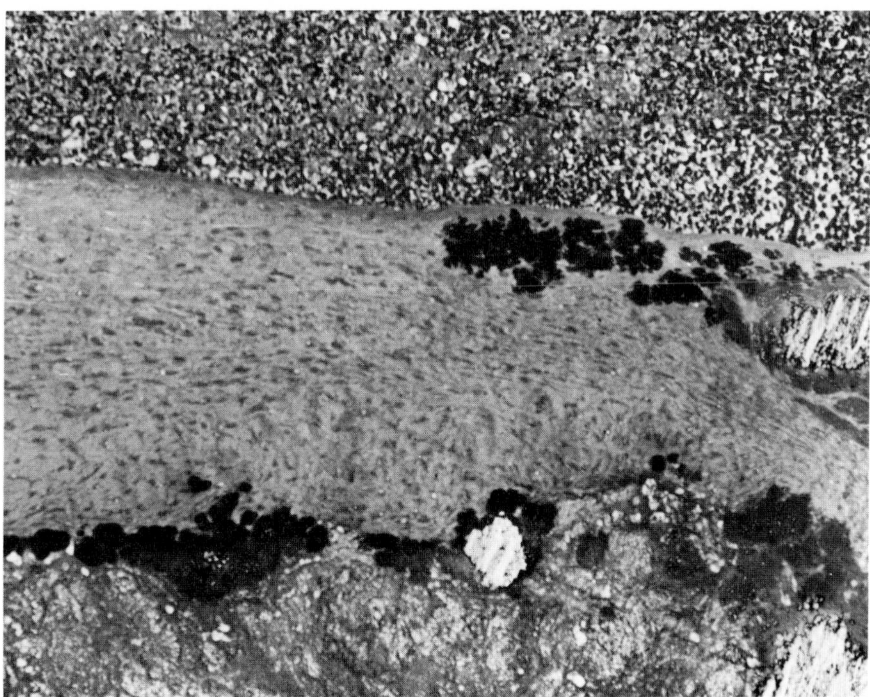

FIG. 3 Stage II infection, involving superficial layers of fibrous connective tissue in pericardial bioprosthesis, is associated with calcific deposits and with large thrombi on both surfaces. Plastic section, alkaline toluidine blue, ×250.

tissue; however, the calcific deposits were judged not to have been responsible for the large perforations.

Calcified bacteria were identified by transmission electron microscopic study in 9 bioprostheses (2 with stage I infection, 1 with stage II, 3 with stage III, and 3 with stage IV). In histologic sections stained with hematoxylin-eosin, calcified bacteria could not be distinguished clearly from minute calcific deposits unrelated to bacterial infection. Macrophages containing abundant phagocytosed bacteria were found in 3 bioprostheses, 1 with a stage II infection, the other 2 with stage IV infection.

Group II bioprostheses. Of the 7 infected porcine aortic valvular bioprostheses in this group, 1 (which had been implanted for only 4 days) had clusters of bacteria localized only to the area of the cardiac muscle shelf of the right coronary cusp. These bacteria were not associated with thrombi or with inflammatory cells. Therefore it is unclear whether the organisms were indicative of postimplantation infection or of preimplantation contamination. Of the other 6 porcine aortic valvular bioprostheses, 1 had stage II infection

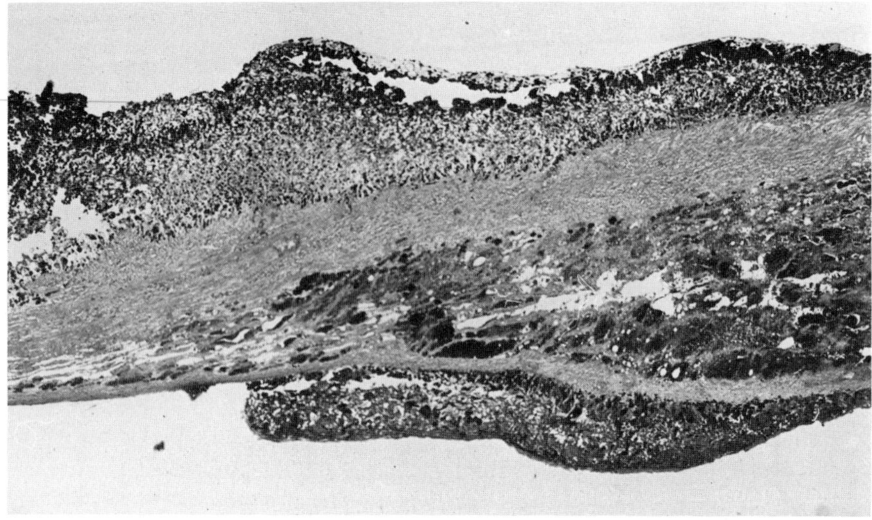

FIG. 4 Stage III infection, with invasion of spongiosa by organisms, is shown in this section of a porcine aortic valvular bioprosthesis. Both surfaces are covered by infected thrombi. The spongiosa on right side is widened considerably and filled with infecting organisms; on left side, it is much narrower and less severely affected. Plastic section, alkaline toluidine blue, ×150.

and 5 had stage III, with organisms invading all layers of the cuspal tissue, including the spongiosa, as well as surface vegetations.

Calcific deposits were present in thrombi, cusps, or muscle shelves in 5 porcine aortic valvular bioprostheses. In addition, calcific deposits within bacteria were identified by electron microscopic study in 4 bioprostheses. Fibrous sheaths were observed on 4 bioprostheses, and in none of these was the sheath invaded by bacteria. Five of the 7 porcine aortic valvular bioprostheses were infected by Gram positive cocci, 1 by Gram negative rods, and 1 by a fungus (Fig. 7).

Of the 8 infected pericardial bioprostheses, 7 had been infected by Gram positive cocci and 1 by Gram negative rods. The infection was stage II in 5 bioprostheses and stage III in the other 3. In each bioprosthesis the bacteria were more numerous in the thrombi than in the cusps, and in each the bacteria in cuspal tissue were localized in the spaces between adjacent bundles of collagen in the pericardial fibrosa. Fibrous sheaths[19] were present in 6 of the 8 pericardial bioprostheses, and only in 2 (which had severe infection) of these were they invaded by bacteria. Calcific deposits were present in 6 bioprostheses. In 1, they were located in the cusp; in the other 5, in thrombi and cuspal tissue. Calcified bacteria were observed in 5 pericardial bioprostheses. In infected pericardial bioprostheses, the inflammatory cells were essentially confined to the thrombi and cuspal surfaces.

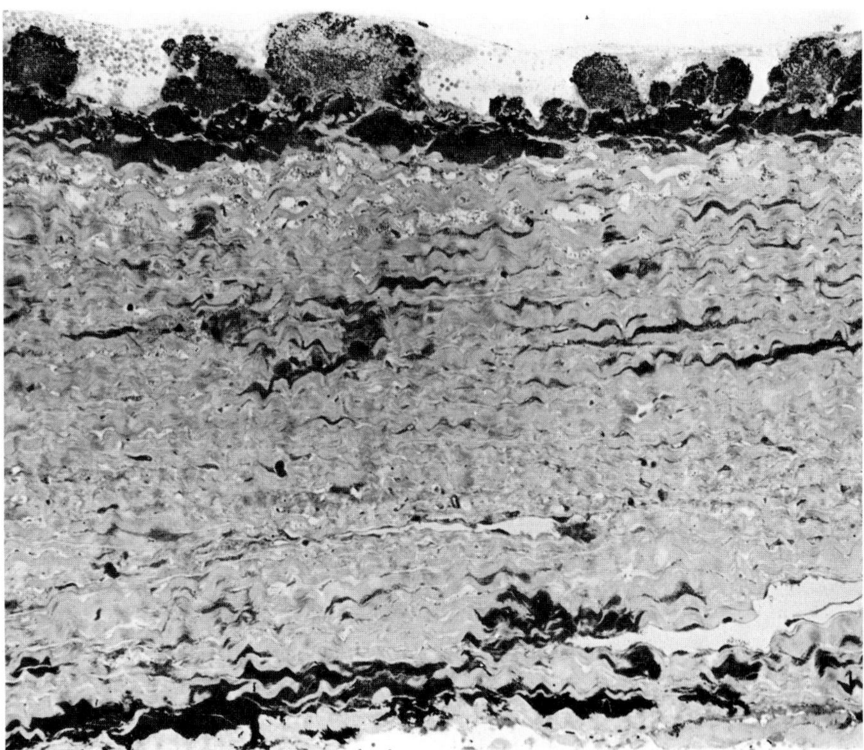

FIG. 5 Stage III infection in bovine pericardial bioprosthesis, showing bacterial colonies not only in superficial areas but also in deeper regions of pericardial fibrosa. Plastic section, alkaline toluidine blue, ×200.

Comment

Our observations serve as the basis for formulating a staging system to evaluate the structural damage produced by infection and to compare the anatomic changes in infected porcine aortic valvular bioprostheses and pericardial bioprostheses.

Stage of Bioprosthetic Infection

The stages of bioprosthetic infection were found to be related to 2 important factors: 1) the time elapsed between the onset of clinical manifestations of infection and the removal of the infected bioprosthesis either at reoperation or at necropsy, and 2) the position in which the bioprosthesis had been implanted. Stage I infection, with organisms confined to thrombi on the cuspal surfaces, was found only in the 4 bioprostheses from the 3 patients (#1, 2, 9) who had had signs and symptoms of infection for less

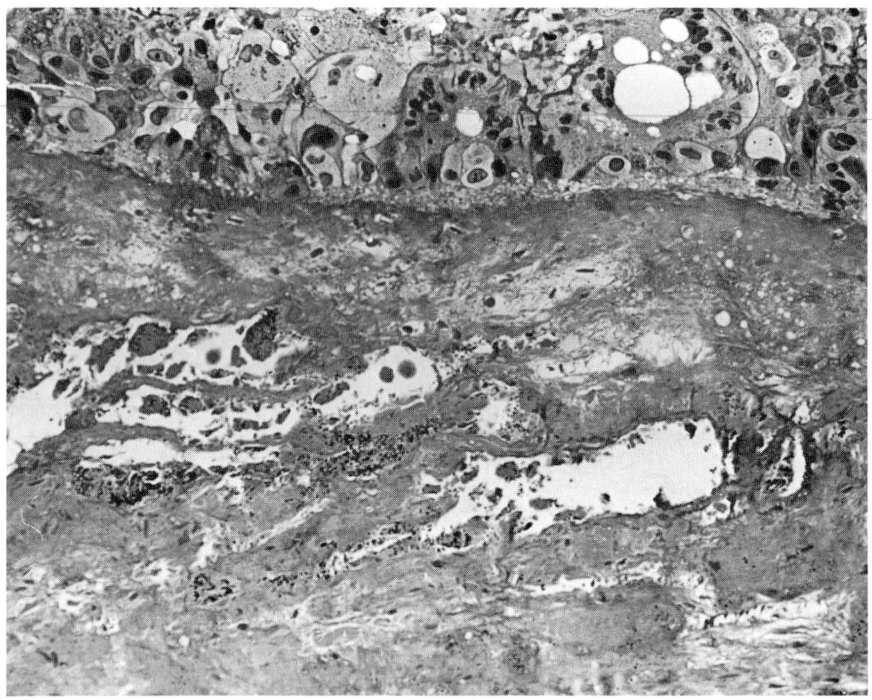

FIG. 6 Stage IV infection in porcine aortic valvular bioprosthesis. Surface of fibrosa (top) is covered by layer of histiocytes. Bacterial colonies are present in spongiosa, which also shows several zones of complete loss of connective tissue. Plastic section, alkaline toluidine blue, ×450.

than 1 month before removal of the bioprosthesis. Of 10 bioprostheses that were recovered from 7 patients (#3–8, 11) who had signs and symptoms of infection for longer than 1 month, 3 had stage II, 3 had stage III, and 4 had stage IV infection. The remaining patient (#10) did not have definite signs and symptoms of infection; this patient, who had stage III infection, underwent reoperation because of bioprosthetic stenosis, and infection was diagnosed only on morphologic examination of the bioprosthesis. A correlation between duration of symptoms and staging of infection could not be established in sheep, since the presenting symptom in most of the animals with infected bioprostheses was sudden death.

The stage of infection of a bioprosthetic heart valve was not necessarily related to patient mortality. Stage I infection was lethal in 2 patients who died of coronary embolus and staphylococcal sepsis. Late stages of infection also can be fatal because of sepsis, embolic phenomena, or prosthetic dysfunction. The latter complication can present in 2 ways: as bioprosthetic stenosis, caused by vegetations, and as bioprosthetic regurgitation, caused

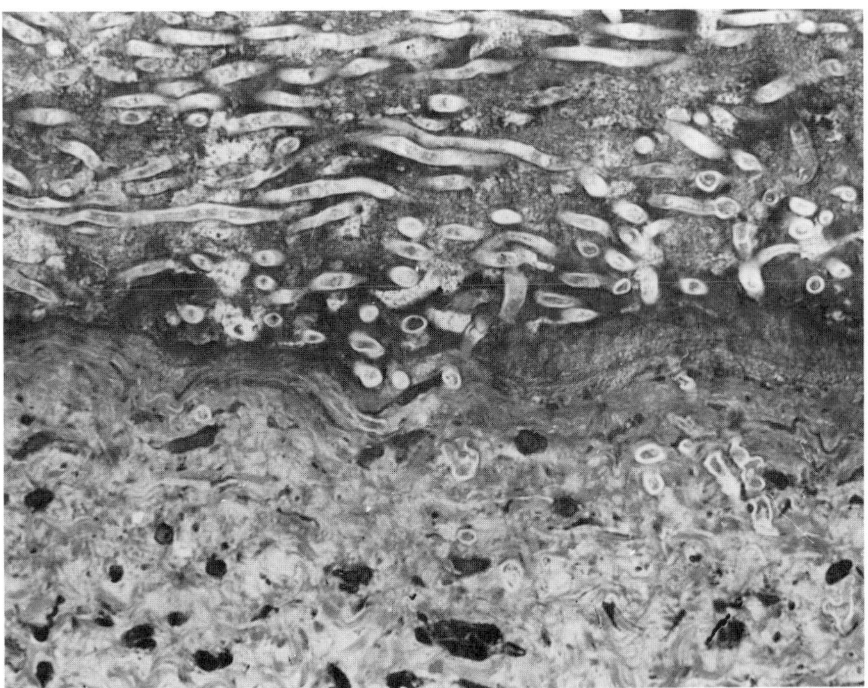

FIG. 7 Stage II infection, caused by a fungus, involves bovine pericardial bioprosthesis implanted in a sheep. Fungal hyphae are mostly localized on valvular surface and show only minimal penetration into cuspal tissue. Plastic section, alkaline toluidine blue, ×750.

by cuspal perforations (stage IV infection). Large, centrally located cuspal perforations (type III perforations) are a consequence of infection-related, extensive breakdown of cuspal connective tissue.[18] It is presumed that such a breakdown is caused by the release of proteolytic enzymes by the bacteria and/or the inflammatory cells. Mechanical factors also appear to be of importance in the pathogenesis of perforations related to infection, as shown by the fact that in our study such perforations were found to occur only in bioprostheses that had been implanted in the aortic position, in which the hemodynamic forces exerted on the cusps are of greater magnitude than in the atrioventricular position. Eight of the 30 bioprostheses in the present study had been implanted in the aortic position, and type III perforations occurred in 4 of these. In contrast, no type III perforations occurred in any of the 22 bioprostheses that had been implanted (7 in patients and 15 in sheep) in the mitral or tricuspid position. One of these bioprostheses had type IV perforations, which were judged to be related to calcific deposits rather than to infection. Two of the perforated aortic bioprostheses also had tears involving the free edge of each of the 2 cusps not affected by the perforation related to infection. These tears were caused by mechanical fragmentation of collagen near the free edge of the cusp and not by bacterial invasion of the tissue.

Spread of Infection in Bioprosthetic Cusps

Invasion of the spongiosa of porcine aortic valvular bioprostheses by bacteria is important as a mechanism of tissue destruction in deeper regions of the cusps and as route of spread of infection toward the basilar portions of the cusps and the sewing ring. The empty spaces left in the spongiosa by the loss of proteoglycan material during commercial processing of the bioprostheses[17] serve as sites through which bacteria grow and spread throughout the cusp. This spread may be facilitated in bioprostheses that have been implanted for a long time and also have undergone degenerative changes and delamination (i.e., separation of layers) in cuspal connective tissue. The spongiosa widens in the basilar regions of the cusps, thus providing a pathway by which the infection can spread from the cusps to the sewing ring. No evidence was found to indicate that infection tends to spread along the surfaces of the cusps to the sewing ring. The tissue-sewing ring interface in bioprostheses becomes covered by a fibrous sheath of host origin, which extends to a variable extent into the basal portions of the cusps. This fibrous sheath develops gradually, as a function of time elapsed after implantation, in bioprostheses implanted in the atrioventricular position, and tends to become lined by endothelial cells.[19] However, fibrous sheaths have very little tendency to cover bioprostheses implanted in the aortic position.[19]

Fibrous sheaths have two contrasting effects: 1) a favorable effect in reinforcing the structure of the cusps and protecting the cuspal surfaces against thrombosis and infection, and 2) a deleterious effect related to mechanical stiffening of the cusps when the formation of fibrous tissue becomes excessive. In the present study, a protective effect against infection was noted in the bioprostheses implanted in sheep, in which fibrous sheaths were more extensive and frequent than in bioprostheses implanted in human beings. This host tisssue appears to be more resistant to infection than is the bioprosthetic tissue itself. Thus, it appears that 2 anatomic paths can be followed by infection of a prosthetic heart valve to cause a ring abscess. The first is through a large thrombus that covers the sewing ring (as can be found in mechanical valves). The second, found in bioprostheses, is from surface thrombus to superficial regions of the cusp, to spongiosa, to regions of the spongiosa in the most basilar portion of the cusp, and to the sewing ring. Such bacterial spread appears to constitute a late, uncommon phenomenon in infected bioprostheses, particularly in comparison with mechanical prostheses.[11,12] Ring abscesses are not encountered more frequently in association with infected bioprostheses because considerable destruction of cuspal tissue and clinical manifestations of severe bioprosthetic dysfunction are likely to occur well before infection spreads along the spongiosa into the sewing ring area. Bacterial invasion of the spongiosa indicates that the bioprosthesis probably cannot be salvaged by antibiotic therapy and eventually will be destroyed by the infection. Unfortunately, there is no way of determining before removal of the bioprosthesis whether or not the spongiosa has been invaded by organisms. The majority (7 of 10) of the bioprostheses that had been infected for longer than 1 month had stage III or IV infection.

Comparison of Morphological Features of Infection in Porcine Aortic Valvular Bioprostheses and Pericardial Bioprostheses

Our observations provide the first detailed comparison of morphologic alterations caused by infection in infected bovine pericardial bioprostheses and porcine aortic valvular bioprostheses. From the gross anatomic standpoint, the 2 types of infected bioprostheses differed in that vegetations were more prominent on the inflow surfaces than on the outflow surfaces of pericardial bioprostheses; the reverse was true in porcine aortic valvular bioprostheses. This difference may have been due to the texture of the inflow surfaces of pericardial bioprostheses being much rougher than that of their outflow surfaces.[20] This rough texture may favor the development of thrombi, which are the sites of initial infection, on the inflow surfaces. In contrast, the inflow and outflow surfaces of porcine aortic valvular bioprostheses are similar in texture and are smoother than the surfaces of pericardial bioprostheses.[20]

From the microscopic standpoint, the 2 types of bioprostheses differ in their layered arrangement[17,20] and in their tendency to become covered by fibrous sheaths.[15,16] Pericardial bioprostheses are composed of a single major layer, the pericardial fibrosa, which consists mainly of densely packed collagen. This layer would seem to present more resistance than does the spongiosa of porcine aortic valvular bioprostheses to the spread of infection both locally and in the direction of the sewing ring. Histologic observations in the present study showed that bacteria were less numerous in deeper portions of infected pericardial bioprostheses than in the spongiosa of infected porcine aortic valvular bioprostheses. These observations also were reflected in the finding that stage III infection (invasion of deeper layers of the bioprosthetic cusps by bacteria) was more common in porcine aortic valvular bioprostheses (5 of 7 bioprostheses) than in pericardial bioprostheses (3 of 8 bioprostheses). It is not known whether these differences, and the greater tendency to become covered by fibrous sheaths, would result in a more favorable response of pericardial bioprostheses to treatment of infection with antibiotics or in a lesser tendency to form ring abscesses.

References

1. Magilligan DJ, Quinn EL, Davila JC: Bacteremia, endocarditis and the Hancock valve. Ann Thorac Surg 24:508, 1977.
2. Lakier JB, Khaja F, Magilligan DJ, Goldstein S: Porcine xenograft valves. Long-term (60–89 month) follow-up. Circulation 62:313, 1980.
3. Oyer PE, Stinson EB, Reitz BA, Miller DC, Rossiter SJ, Shumway N: Long-term evaluation of the porcine xenograft bioprosthesis. J Thorac Cardiovasc Surg 78:343, 1979.
4. Rossiter SJ, Stinson EB, Oyer PE, Miller DC, Schapira JN, Martin RP, Shumway N: Prosthetic valve endocarditis. Comparison of heterograft tissue valves and mechanical valves. J Thorac Cardiovasc Surg 76:795, 1978.
5. Wilson WR, Nichols DR, Thompson RL, Giuliani ER, Geraci JE: Infective endocarditis: Therapeutic considerations. Am Heart J 100:689, 1980.
6. Gallo JI, Ruiz B, Carrion MF, Gutierrez JA, Vega JL, Duran CMG: Heart valve replacement with the Hancock bioprosthesis: A 6-year review. Ann Thorac Surg 31:444, 1981.
7. Angell WW, Angell JD: Porcine valves. Prog Cardiovasc Dis 23:141, 1980.
8. Le Clerc JL, Deuvaert FE, Wellens F, Goffin Y, Primo G: A four year experience of bioprosthetic cardiac valve replacement. Early and late results. In: Bioprosthetic Cardiac Valves (F Sebening, WP Klövekorn, H Meisner, E Struck, Eds). Munich, Deutsches Herzzentrum, 1979, p 27.
9. Myerowitz PD, Lamberti JJ, Replogle RL, Schwarz D, Anagnostopoulos E: Delayed complications following heterograft valve replacement. In: Bioprosthetic Cardiac Valves (F Sebening, WP Klövekorn, H Meisner, E Struck, Eds). Munich, Deutsches Herzzentrum, 1979, p 335.
10. Jamieson WRE, Janusz MT, Munro AI, Miyagishima RT, Tutassura H, Gerein AN, Burr LH, Allen P: Early clinical experience with the Carpentier-Edwards porcine heterograft cardiac valve. Can J Surg 23:132, 1980.
11. Ferrans VJ, Boyce SW, Billingham ME, Spray TL, Roberts WC: Infection of glutaraldehyde-preserved porcine valve heterografts. Am J Cardiol 43:1123, 1979.
12. Bortolotti U, Thiene G, Milano A, Panizzon G, Valente M, Gallucci V: Pathological study of infective endocarditis in Hancock porcine bioprostheses. J Thorac Cardiovasc Surg 81:934, 1981.
13. Williams EH, Conti VR, Nishimura A, Stout LC, Ferrans VJ: Early calcific stenosis of aortic and mitral Ionescu-Shiley valves in a patient with bioprosthetic infection. J Thorac Cardiovasc Surg 41:391, 1981.
14. Arnett EN, Roberts WC: Prosthetic valve endocarditis. Clinicopathologic analysis of 22 necropsy patients with comparison of observations in 74 necropsy patients with active infective endocarditis involving natural left-sided valves. Am J Cardiol 38:281, 1976.
15. Barnhart GR, Jones M, Ishihara T, Chavez AM, Rose DM, Ferrans VJ: Bioprosthetic valvular failure: Clinical and pathological observations in an experimental animal model. J Thorac Cardiovasc Surg 83:618, 1982.
16. Barnhart GR, Jones M, Ishihara T, Rose DM, Chavez AM, Ferrans VJ: Degeneration and calcification of bioprosthetic cardiac valves. Animal model: Bioprosthetic tricuspid valve implantation in sheep. Am J Pathol 106:136, 1982.
17. Ferrans VJ, Spray TL, Billingham ME, Roberts WC: Structural changes in glutaraldehyde-treated porcine heterografts used as substitute cardiac valves. Transmission and scanning electron microscopic observations in 12 patients. Am J Cardiol 41:1159, 1978.

18. Ishihara T, Ferrans VJ, Boyce SW, Jones M, Roberts WC. Structure and classification of cuspal tears and perforations in porcine bioprosthetic cardiac valves implanted in patients. Am J Cardiol 48:665, 1981.
19. Ishihara T, Ferrans VJ, Jones M, Boyce SW, Roberts WC: Occurrence and significance of endothelial cells in implanted porcine bioprosthetic valves. Am J Cardiol 48:443, 1981.
20. Ishihara T, Ferrans VJ, Jones M, Boyce SW, Roberts WC: Structure of bovine pericardium and unimplanted Ionescu-Shiley pericardial valvular prostheses. J Thoarac Cardiovasc Surg 81:747, 1981.

33

Structure and Classification of Cuspal Tears and Perforations in Porcine Bioprosthetic Cardiac Valves Implanted in Patients

T. ISHIHARA, V. J. FERRANS, S. W. BOYCE, M. JONES, W. C. ROBERTS

Detailed studies have been made of morphologic changes related to infection, calcific deposits, and degeneration of collagen in implanted porcine aortic valvular bioprosthesis.[1-7] However, cuspal disruption, characterized by tears and perforations, has been the subject of only brief descriptions.[1-31] The patterns of anatomic distribution of these lesions in the different cusps of the bioprostheses have not been studied systematically. This communication presents detailed morphologic observations in 16 porcine valve bioprostheses that were found to have cuspal tears or perforations when recovered after implantation.

Patients and Methods

The 16 bioprostheses in the study were recovered from 14 patients (9 male, 5 female), who ranged in age from 2–65 years. Clinical findings on these patients and morphologic observations on their bioprostheses are summarized in Table I. Eleven bioprostheses had been in place in the mitral position for 30–123 months, 4 others had been in the aortic position for 15–40 months, and 1 had been in a valved pulmonary conduit for 96 months. Twelve bioprostheses were recovered at operation and 4 at necropsy. Four bioprostheses had clinical and morphologic evidence of bacterial infection.

From the Pathology and Surgery Branches, National Heart, Lung, and Blood Institute, National Institutes of Health, Bethesda, Maryland.

Immediately after removal, each bioprosthesis was fixed with cold 3% glutaraldehyde in phosphate buffer. Roentgenograms and gross photographs were then taken of the inflow and outflow surfaces. Selected portions of the cusps were taken for histologic study and for scanning and transmission electron microscopic examination.[1,3]

Detailed observations were made of the incidence and characteristics of the tears and perforations in each of the 3 cusps (anatomic left, right, and noncoronary) of each bioprosthesis. These lesions were classified into 4 types, according to the diagrams shown in Fig. 1. Type I lesions (Fig. 2) were defined as tears, which involved the free edges of the cusps. Type II, III, and IV lesions were perforations, which did not involve the free edges of the cusps. Type II lesions consisted of linear perforations that extended along the basal regions of the cusps forming an arc parallel to the sewing ring. Type III (Fig. 3) lesions were large, round, or oval perforations that occupied the central regions of the cusps, often in association with extensive destruction of cuspal tissue. Type IV lesions (Fig. 4) were small, pinholelike perforations; they usually were multiple and localized in central regions of the cusps, often in association with multiple calcific deposits.

Results

Gross Anatomic Observations

Overall incidence of the 4 types of lesions. A total of 30 tears and perforations were identified in the 48 cusps of the 16 bioprostheses (Table I). Of the 4 types of cuspal lesions, type I lesions accounted for more than 50% of the total number. Type II lesions occurred only once. Type III lesions also were uncommon, accounting for 4 perforations, 3 of which were associated with infection. Type IV lesions involved a total of 9 cusps and always were multiple.

Two-thirds of the total number of perforations, including 10 of type I, 1 of type II, 1 of type III, and 9 of type IV, occurred in the 11 bioprostheses that had been in the mitral position. Eight perforations, 5 of type I and 3 of type III, were found in the 4 bioprostheses that had been in the aortic position. The bioprosthesis that had been in a valved pulmonary conduit had a type I tear in the right coronary cusp.

Relation of lesion types to position in which the bioprostheses had been implanted. Type I lesions were equally frequent in bioprostheses implanted in the mitral and in the aortic position. The only type II lesion was found in a mitral bioprosthesis. Type III lesions were more frequently found in bioprostheses implanted in the aortic (3 of 8 lesions) than in the mitral (1 of 21 lesions) position; this difference was statistically significant ($p = 0.03$) according to the 2-tailed Student's t test. However, 3 of the 4 bioprostheses

TABLE I Clinical and morphologic observations on 16 perforated bioprostheses in 14 patients*

Patient #	Age/Sex	Time BP in place (mo)	Reason for BP removal	Ca++ in BP	Ca++ associated with perforation	Infected BP	Fibrous sheath	Type and location of perforation			Total # perforations
								RC	LC	NC	
Mitral valve											
1	5/F	30	S	+	+	0	0	IV	—	IV	
2	—M	33	IE	+	0	+	0	—	—	IV	
3	8/F	35	R	+	+	0	0	III	IV	—	
4	57/M	36	S	+	+	0	0	I	IV	I, IV	
5	55/M	40	N	+	0	0	0	I	I	I	
6	2/M	50	S, R	+	+	0	+	—	IV	IV	
7	65/F	63	R	+	+	0	+	—	II	—	
8	55/F	76	N	+	+	0	0	I	I	—	
9	65/M	94	N	+	+	0	0	I	I	—	
10	50/F	107	S	+	+	0	+	—	IV	—	
11	53/M	123	R	+	+	0	0	I	—	—	
Subtotals	41 (avg)	62 (avg)	S = 3	11	9	1	3	7	8	6	21
	M = 6		R = 3					I = 5	I = 3	I = 2	10
	F = 5		S, R = 1					II = 0	II = 1	II = 0	1
			N = 3					III = 1	III = 0	III = 0	1
			IE = 1					IV = 1	IV = 4	IV = 4	9

TABLE I—Continued

Aortic valve												
12	30	M	15	R	0	0	0	0	—	I	—	
13	35	M	27	IE	+	0	+	0	I	III	I	
2	—	M	33	IE	+	0	+	0	III	—	—	
5	55	M	40	N	+	0	+	0	I	III	I	
Subtotals	40 (avg)		29 (avg)	R = 1	3	0	3	0	3	3	2	8
	M = 4			N = 1					I = 2	I = 1	I = 2	5
				IE = 2					II = 0	II = 0	II = 0	0
									III = 1	III = 2	III = 0	3
									IV = 0	IV = 0	IV = 0	0
Pulmonic valve												
14	6	M	96	S	+	+	0	0	I = 1	—	—	1
Totals	37 (avg)		56 (avg)	S = 4	15	10	4	3	11	11	8	30
	M = 9			R = 4					I = 8	I = 4	I = 4	16
	F = 5			S, R = 1					II = 0	II = 1	II = 0	1
				N = 4					III = 2	III = 2	III = 0	4
				IE = 3					IV = 1	IV = 4	IV = 4	9

* BP: bioprosthesis; Ca++: calcific deposits; F: female; IE: infective endocarditis; LC: left coronary cusp; M: male; N: necropsy; NC: noncoronary cusp; R: regurgitation; RC: right coronary cusp; S: stenosis; +: present; 0: absent.

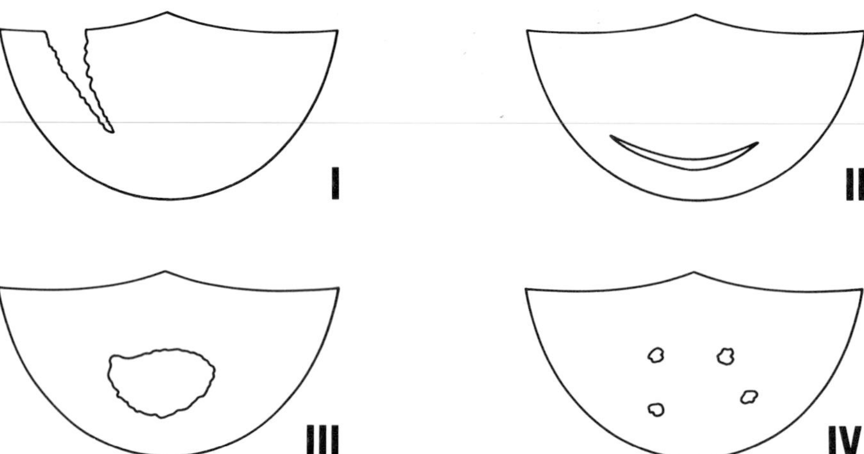

FIG. 1 Diagram of 4 types of cuspal tears (type I) and perforations (type II, III and IV) found in implanted cardiac valvular bioprostheses.

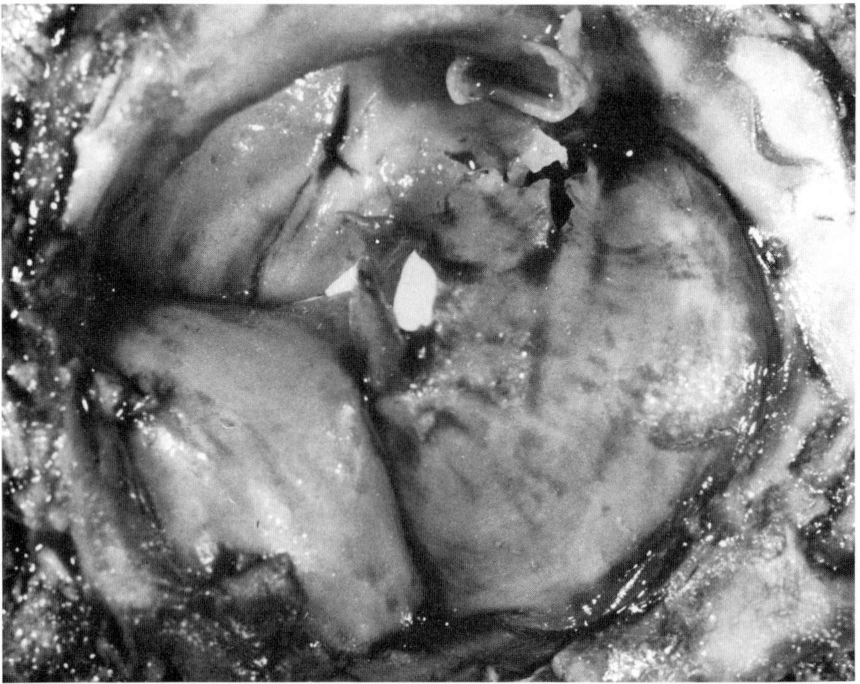

FIG. 2 Type I lesions, involving free edge, developed in 2 of the cusps of porcine aortic valvular bioprosthesis that was removed because of regurgitation 76 months after implantation in mitral position.

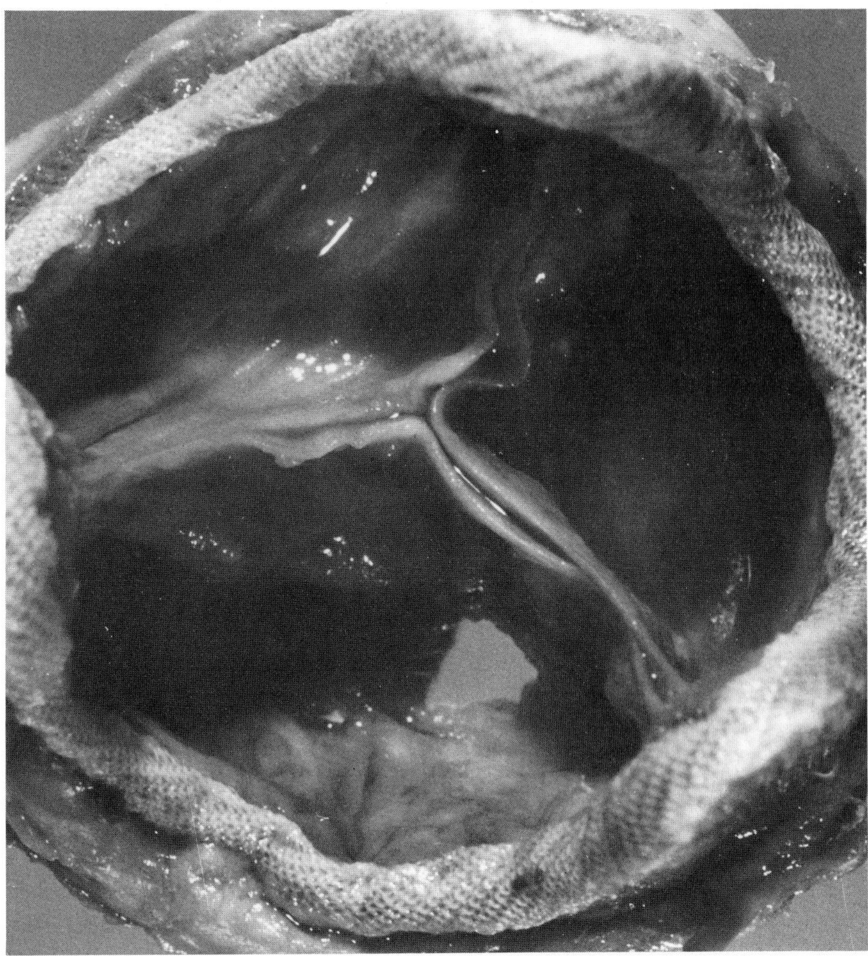

FIG. 3 Large, centrally located, type III perforation in infected porcine aortic valvular bioprosthesis.

that had been implanted in the aortic position were infected at the time of removal, and it was found to be more likely ($p = 0.02$, according to the 2-tailed Student's *t* test) that a type III perforation would occur in an infected than in a noninfected bioprosthesis. Nevertheless, a type III lesion did not occur in the only mitral bioprosthesis that was infected. Type IV perforations, which accounted for nearly half of all the lesions observed in the bioprostheses in the mitral position, occurred much more frequently ($p = 0.02$, according to the 2-tailed Student's *t* test) in mitral than in aortic bioprostheses.

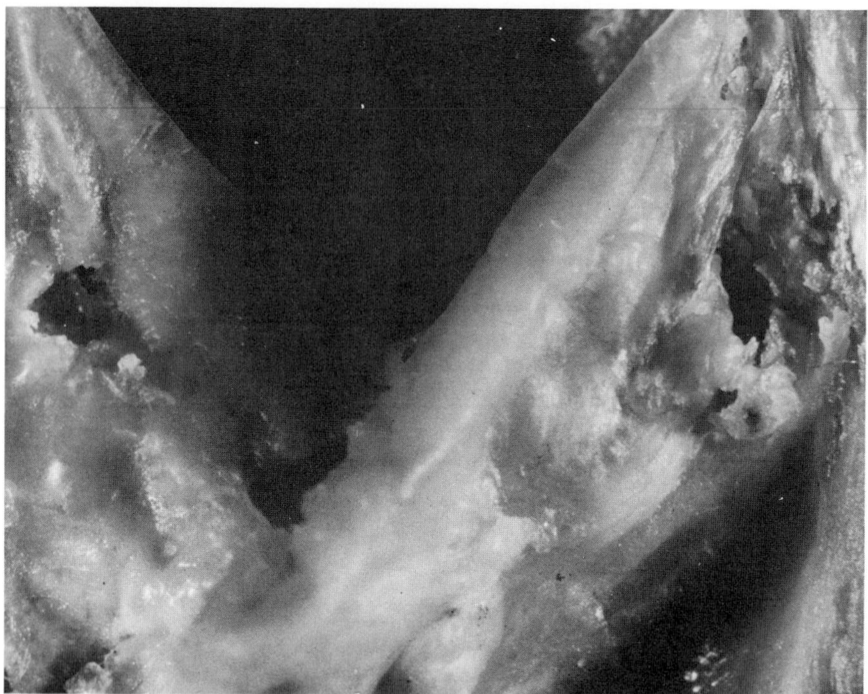

FIG. 4 View of part of cusp of porcine aortic valvular bioprosthesis removed from child 42 months after implantation in mitral position. This cusp was heavily calcified and was site of several type IV perforations, 2 of which are shown in this view.

Incidence of lesions in the three cusps of the bioprostheses. The total number of tears and of perforations were distributed with near equality in the right coronary, left coronary, and noncoronary cusps of the 16 bioprostheses. However, the frequency of occurrence of the different types of lesions varied in each cusp. In the right coronary cusp, type I tears occurred more frequently ($p < 0.05$, according to the chi-square test) than did type II, III, or IV perforations, regardless of the position of valve implantation. Type IV perforations were very uncommon in the right coronary cusp. In contrast, the left coronary cusp and the noncoronary cusp demonstrated an equal incidence of type I and type IV lesions, with type II and type III lesions being uncommon.

Other correlations between types of perforations and clinical and anatomic changes. Fifteen bioprostheses had been implanted for longer than 2 years; 1 noninfected aortic bioprosthesis developed a type I tear 15 months after implantation. The average time in place for the 16 bioprostheses was 56 months. The 4 perforated bioprostheses that had been in the aortic position had been in place for less than half of the time of those that had been in the mitral position (mean, 29 -vs- 62 months). However, because 3 of the 4 aortic bioprostheses were infected, a definite correlation could not be established between position of implantation and average time in place before removal for malfunction. Similarly, there was no relation between the patients' ages at the time of implantation and the type of cuspal lesions that developed subsequently.

Calcific deposits were present in 15 of the 16 bioprostheses. In 10 of these, the calcific deposits were immediately adjacent to the areas of perforation. Of the remaining 6 perforated bioprostheses, 4 were infected and the other 2 had only type I tears, which were not associated with infection.

Histologic Observations

The 4 types of cuspal lesions were consistently characterized by fragmentation or loss of cuspal connective tissue components. Type I lesions were associated with fragmentation of collagen. The affected areas of collagen appeared less intensely birefringent and less intensely stained with toluidine blue and with eosin than was normal collagen. Similar changes were evident in the type II lesion examined. The type III lesions associated with infection had considerable amounts of disorganized necrotic collagen along their edges, together with fibrin deposits, platelets, inflammatory cells, and infecting organisms. The noninfected type III lesion had extensive calcific deposits around its edges; thus, it resembled a large type IV lesion.

The edges of type IV lesions consisted of various combinations of damaged, fragmented collagen and large, nodular calcific deposits. The calcific deposits in areas of perforations occupied parts of the spongiosa, from which zone they extended toward surfaces, most often projecting into the cuspal pockets. The overall thickness of the cusps was appreciably increased in regions of calcification. The layers of cuspal connective tissue immediately overlying the calcific deposits often had been almost completely eroded.

Scanning Electron Microscopic Observations

Type I lesions (Fig. 5) extended irregularly from the free edges toward central regions of the cusps. The edges of these lesions were irregular, with fragmentation, separation, and breakage of connective tissue components, and marked thinning and erosion of the cuspal tissue. The latter changes progressed toward the lesion edges, in which successive layers of connective tissue showed increasing degrees of damage.

The type II lesion (Fig. 6) showed considerable separation of bundles of collagen that were oriented parallel to the free edges of the cusps. This lesion type was reproduced in bioprostheses subjected to accelerated fatigue testing in vitro.

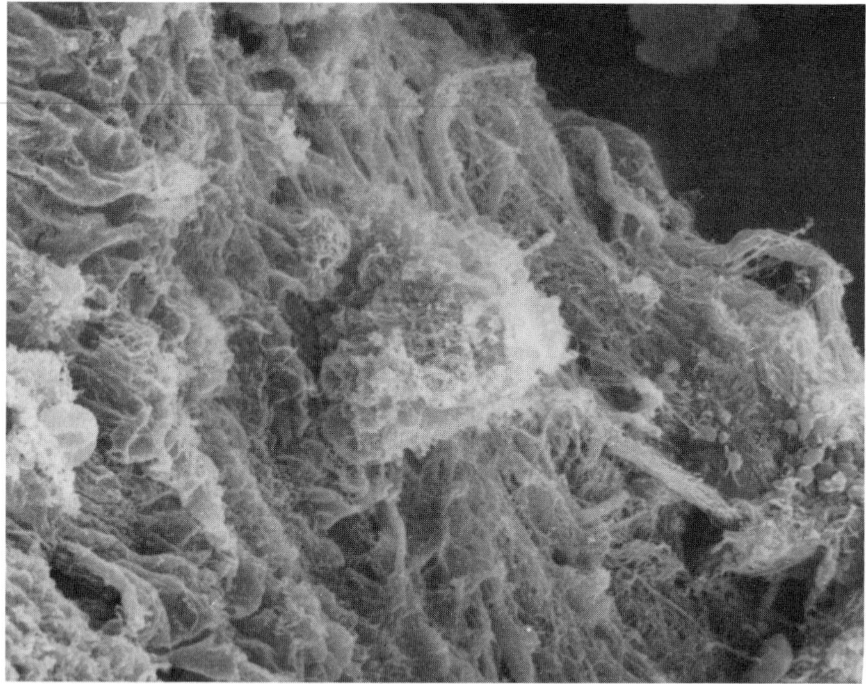

FIG. 5 Scanning electron micrograph showing edge of type I lesion similar to that illustrated in Fig 2. The collagen bundles along this edge have fractured. Space at upper right represents site of tear. ×1,700.

The edges of type III lesions appeared very irregular and had strands of fibrin and necrotic collagen that projected into the lumen of the perforation. In infected type III lesions, inflammatory cells were abundant and microorganisms were identified along the edges.

Type IV lesions (Fig. 7) often were associated with nodular calcific deposits. Some of these had raised but smooth surfaces composed of collagen and fibrin, whereas others had irregular surfaces composed of partially eroded calcific deposits and damaged collagen. Platelets were frequently adherent to collagen in these areas.

Transmission Electron Microscopic Observations

Connective tissue changes along the edges of perforations not associated with infection consisted of the following: 1) fragmentation of collagen fibrils; 2) marked decrease in the numbers of collagen fibrils; 3) large amounts of amorphous to finely granular material between the remaining collagen fibrils; 4) irregular stainability of the collagen; 5) infiltration by numerous

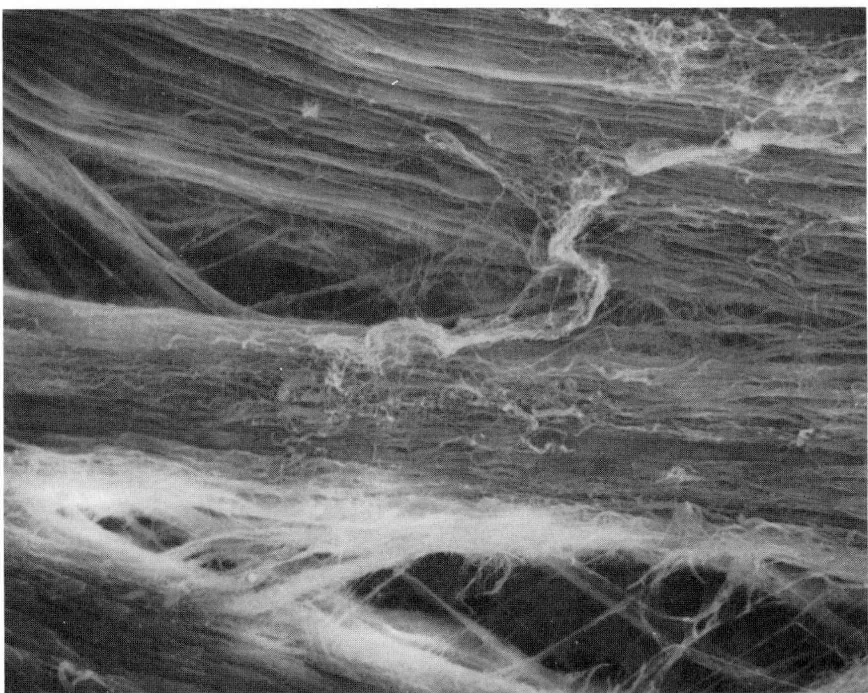

FIG. 6 Scanning electron micrograph of basilar region of porcine aortic valvular bioprosthesis that had been subjected to accelerated fatigue testing for 235 million cycles, showing 2 type II tears which developed in a direction parallel to the course of the collagen bundles. ×1,400.

lipid droplets that measured up to 1 μ in diameter and often were associated with the amorphous material described previously; 6) evidence of clacification of collagen fibrils;[3] and 7) few or no alterations involving elastic tissue. In addition to these alterations, areas of infection had marked necrotic changes and contained bacteria.

Comment

The observations in this study show that cuspal tears and perforations develop in bioprostheses as the final consequences of connective tissue failure. This failure appears to develop in areas in which mechanical forces are exerted in a highly localized manner either because of the patterns of opening and closure of the bioprosthetic cusps or because of the presence of calcific deposits. The 3 main connective tissue components of porcine bioprostheses are elastic fibers, proteoglycans, and collagen fibrils.

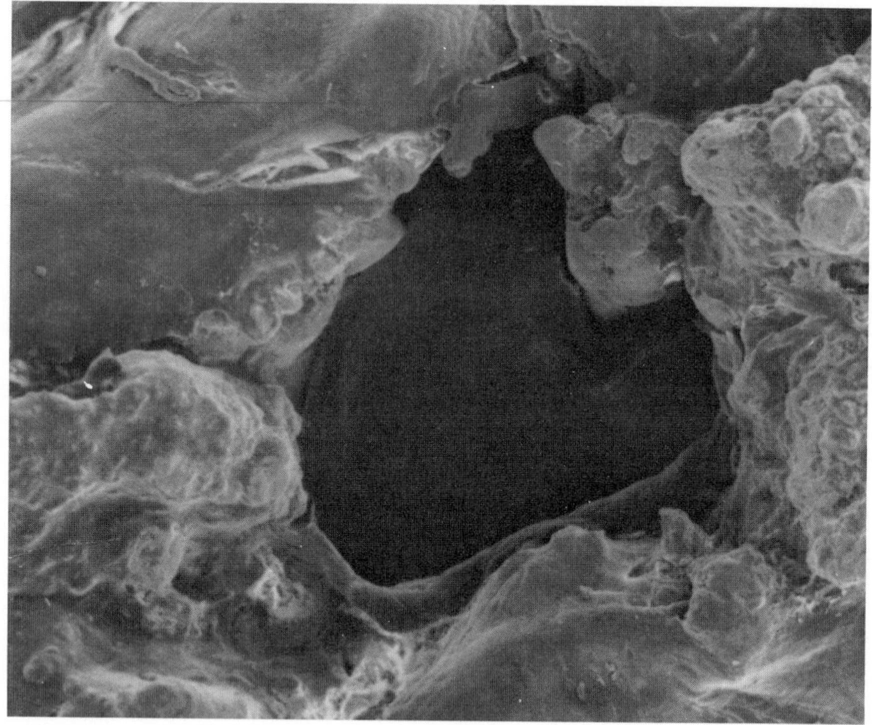

FIG. 7 Scanning electron micrograph of type IV perforation, similar to those shown in Fig. 4. This perforation is small, generally rounded, and its borders are closely associated with raised, nodular calcific deposits. ×250.

Elastic fibers in implanted bioprostheses are small in size, relatively few in number, mainly localized in the ventricularis layer, and show few structural alterations. Their role in maintaining the integrity of glutaraldehyde-treated bioprostheses is uncertain. In contrast, the proteoglycan material and the collagen fibrils play important but different roles with respect to the durability of bioprostheses.

Proteoglycans are major components of the spongiosa, from which they are largely extracted during preimplantation processing and soon after implantation.[1] Their loss from the spongiosa causes a marked change in the mechanical properties of this zone. Proteoglycans form a gel that dampens the movement of the fibrosa and the ventricularis with respect to one another during valve opening and closure. When proteoglycans are extracted, this damping effect is lost and "delamination" or separation of adjacent layers of cuspal connective tissue develops.[1,3,4] Another consequence of the extraction of proteoglycans is the formation of empty spaces that become filled with plasma proteins and formed elements of the blood, and eventually become sites of calcification.[3] Type IV cuspal perforations tend to develop in close association with calcific deposits.

Because collagen is the most important structural component of bioprosthetic heart valves, tissue failure in these devices must be regarded mainly as collagen failure. Tissue failure, that is, breakdown of collagen, can be mediated by different mechanisms (infection, poorly understood biochemical factors, purely mechanical factors) and can be localized in different areas of the cusps, thus resulting in the 4 types of tears and perforations observed in this study.

The contribution of bioprosthetic infection to cuspal perforations was evident in 4 of the bioprostheses, in which the resulting lesions had a characteristic morphology. It has been postulated that subclinical infection can contribute to bioprosthetic failure.[4] However, we have encountered only 1 example of this, and the infecting organisms were demonstrated in this bioprosthesis by transmission electron microscopy.[2]

The contribution of biochemical changes to the breakdown of collagen remains to be defined. It is known that treatment with aldehyde fixatives increases considerably the extent of collagen cross-linking and the resistance of collagen to attack by collagenases.[32,33] However, it is not known whether these modified properties are altered by severe degrees of mechanical disruption of the collagen fibrils. Furthermore, it is possible that the glutaraldehyde treatment increases the brittleness of collagen. As discussed in detail later, the morphologic patterns of localization of the cuspal lesions that we have observed can be interpreted in terms of the localization of mechanical forces of compressive flexure of collagen[34] during valve opening and closure.

Pathogenesis of Different Types of Tears and Perforations

Type I lesions. These lesions, defined as tears involving the free edge of the cusp, were the most common type of lesion in bioprostheses implanted in the mitral and in the aortic positions. They were more common in the right coronary cusp than in the other 2 cusps and were not related to bioprosthetic infection or calcification. Type I lesions are caused by breakage of collagen fibrils located along the free edge of the cusp. Such tears were found in each lateral third of the cusp in which the cuspal edge is thinner than in the central third (the latter is reinforced by the nodulus Arantii). The collagen along the free edge of the cusp is arranged parallel to this edge, extending from one commissure to the other. The mechanical forces of compressive flexure to which this collagen is subjected during valve opening and closure[34] are considered to be the main factors responsible for the development of type I tears. Such flexure-induced breakage of collagen would appear to be increased (over that in normal valves in situ) by 2 factors: treatment of the tissue with glutaraldehyde under pressure, and the mounting of the bioprosthesis on a stent. Fixation under presure decreased the collagen waviness or "crimping."[34] This collagen waviness serves the purpose of distributing the bending stresses more evenly than is the case with collagen that has been straightened out.[34]

The use of a flexible stent and the technique of placement of sutures anchoring the aortic wall to the Dacron covering of the stent have been considered to diminish the likelihood of cuspal tears.[4] These are thought to occur with greater frequency in bioprostheses with rigid stents than in those with flexible stents. Nevertheless, the contribution of the flexible stent in this regard has been questioned,[35] and we found type I tears to be the most common type of lesions in porcine aortic valve bioprostheses mounted in flexible stents. The nonexpanding nature of the bioprosthetic stent contrasts with the normal aortic valve ring, which undergoes expansion as the valve opens in vivo and in situ. The lack of expansion of the bioprosthetic stent increases the mechanical stresses borne by the cusps during opening and closure.[36–38]

The pattern of uneven opening of the cusps of porcine bioprostheses is also thought to contribute to the development of localized bending stresses. These cusps open unevenly, with the right coronary cusp tending to open less than the other 2 cusps (because of the cardiac muscle shelf that it contains). The degree to which the 3 cusps open is related to the characteristics of the flow through the valve.[39] Under conditions of low flow, the orifice created by the opening of these cusps tends to be triangular. Because of this, the free edges of the cusps undergo maximal bending not at the commissures but, instead, at points between the commissures and the junctions of the central and lateral thirds of the free edges (particularly in the right coronary cusp). Thus, the patterns of opening and closure of the cusps of porcine bioprostheses, together with the straightening of the waviness of the collagen fibrils, tend to result in bending stresses that become localized at certain points along the free edges. Therefore, tears that develop along the free edges of the cusps can be regarded as flexure lesions analogous to those that are related to "hinging" of the basal regions of the cusps.

Type II lesions. These lesions, defined as perforations parallel to the basal attachment of the cusp, were more uncommon than had been anticipated in light of the relatively minimal thicknesses of the basal regions of the cusps and the "hinging" motion reported to occur in these regions during cuspal opening and closure.[4] Separation of adjacent, parallel bundles of collagen plays an important role in the pathogenesis of type II lesions, as shown by scanning electron microscopic observations made on porcine bioprostheses failing in vitro during the course of extended durability testing. Such a separation of collagen bundles was not a feature of the other 3 types of lesions. The relatively high frequency of type II lesions in bioprostheses subjected to accelerated fatigue testing is probably related to the high speed of valve motion, which tends to maximize the "hinging" and to keep it more sharply localized to a given region. Our observations also suggest that formation of a fibrous sheath and covering of basal portions of bioprosthetic cusps by endothelial cells of host origin also protect against development of type II lesions.[40]

Type III lesions. These lesions, consisting of rounded or oval perforations involving central areas of the cusps, were more common in bioprostheses implanted in the aortic position than in those implanted in the mitral position. The loss of cuspal tissue in these lesions was associated either with infection or with severe degenerative changes.

Type IV lesions. These lesions develop as a consequence of bending stresses at the boundaries between highly rigid calcific deposits and adjacent areas of soft, degenerated collagen. Type IV lesions may progress to type III lesions, particularly in bioprostheses implanted in the aortic position. This possibility is suggested by the paucity of type IV lesions in aortic bioprostheses, a finding that could be interpreted as meaning that a small (type IV) perforation could expand and become a large (type III) perforation. Type IV lesions tended to be multiple and occurred more frequently in the noncoronary and left coronary cusps than in the right coronary cusp. The muscle shelf that extends into the proximal third of the right coronary cusp may have exerted a protective effect against the development of these lesions, possibly by providing additional structural support and by minimizing bending stresses in this cusp.

References

1. Ferrans VJ, Spray TL, Billingham ME, Roberts WC: Structural changes in glutaraldehyde-treated porcine heterografts used as substitute cardiac valves. Transmission and scanning electron microscopic observations in 12 patients. Am J Cardiol 41:1159, 1978.
2. Ferrans VJ, Boyce SW, Billingham ME, Spray TL, Roberts WC: Infection of glutaraldehyde-preserved porcine valve heterografts. Am J Cardiol 43:1123, 1979.
3. Ferrans VJ, Boyce SW, Billingham ME, Jones M, Ishihara T, Roberts WC: Calcific deposits in porcine bioprostheses: Structure and pathogenesis. Am J Cardiol 46:721, 1980.
4. Angell WW, Angell JD: Porcine valves. Prog Cardiovasc Dis 23:141, 1980.
5. Spray TL, Roberts WC: Structural changes in porcine xenografts used as substitute cardiac valves. Gross and histologic observations in 51 glutaraldehyde-preserved Hancock valves in 41 patients. Am J Cardiol 40:319, 1977.
6. Fishbein MC, Gissen SA, Collins JJ Jr, Barsamian EM, Cohn LH: Pathologic findings after cardiac valve replacement with glutaraldehyde-fixed porcine valves. Am J Cardiol 40:331, 1977.
7. Magilligan DJ Jr, Lewis JW Jr, Jara FM, Lee MW, Alam M, Riddle JM, Stein PD: Spontaneous degeneration of porcine bioprosthetic valves. Ann Thorac Surg 30:259, 1980.
8. Carpentier A, Deloche A, Relland J, Fabiani JN, Forman J, Camilleri JP, Soyer

R, Dubost C: Six-year follow-up of glutaraldehyde-preserved heterografts. With particular reference to the treatment of congenital valve malformation. J Thorac Cardiovasc Surg 68:771, 1974.
9. Gallucci V. Discussion to Carpentier et al.[8] J Thorac Cardiovasc Surg 68:782, 1974.
10. McIntosh CL, Michaelis LL, Morrow AG, Itscoitz SB, Redwood DR, Epstein SE: Atrioventricular valve replacement with the Hancock porcine xenograft: A five year clinical experience. Surgery 78:768, 1975.
11. Hannah H, Reis RL. Current status of porcine heterograft prostheses. A 5-year appraisal. Circulation 54 (Suppl III):27, 1976.
12. Cevèse PG, Gallucci V, Morea M, Volta SD, Fasoli G, Casarotto D: Heart valve replacement with the Hancock bioprosthesis. Analysis of long-term results. Circulation 56 (Suppl II):111, 1977.
13. Zuhdi N: The porcine aortic valve bioprosthesis: A significant alternative. Ann Thorac Surg 21:573, 1976.
14. Stinson EB, Griepp RB, Oyer PE, Shumway NE: Long-term experience with porcine aortic valve xenografts. J Thorac Cardiovasc Surg 73:54, 1977.
15. Housman LB, Pitt WA, Mazur JH, Litchford B, Gross SA: Mechanical failure (leaflet disruption) of a porcine aortic heterograft. Rare cause of acute aortic insufficiency. J Thorac Cardiovasc Surg 76:212, 1978.
16. Hetzer R, Hill JD, Kerth WJ, Wilson AJ, Adappa MG, Gerbode F: Thrombosis and degeneration of Hancock valves: Clinical and pathological findings. Ann Thorac Surg 26:317, 1978.
17. Brown JW, Dunn JM, Spooner E, Kirsh MM: Late spontaneous disruption of a porcine xenograft mitral valve. Clinical, hemodynamic, echocardiographic, and pathological findings. J Thorac Cardiovasc Surg 75:606, 1978.
18. Bloch WN Jr, Karcioglu Z, Felner JM, Miller JS, Symbas PN, Schlant RC: Idiopathic perforation of a porcine aortic bioprosthesis in the aortic position. Chest 74:579, 1978.
19. Oyer PE, Stinson EB, Reitz BA, Miller DC, Rossiter SJ, Shumway NE: Long-term evaluation of the porcine xenograft bioprosthesis. J Thorac Cardiovasc Surg 78:343, 1979.
20. Geha AS, Laks H, Stansel HC Jr, Cornhill JF, Kilman JW, Buckley MJ, Roberts WC: Late failure of porcine valve heterografts in children. J Thorac Cardiovasc Surg 78:351, 1979.
21. Magilligan DJ, Lewis JW, Jara FM, Lakier JB, Davila JC: Indications for reoperation after bioprosthetic valve implantation. Experience with the porcine xenograft valve. In: Bioprosthetic Cardiac Valves (F Sebening, WP Klövekorn, H Meisner, E Struck, Eds). Munich, Deutsches Herzzentrum, 1979, p 341.
22. Oyer PE, Stinson EB, Rossiter SJ, Miller DC, Reitz BA, Shumway NE: Extended experience with the Hancock xenograft bioprosthesis. In: Bioprosthetic Cardiac Valves (F Sebening, WP Klövekorn, H Meisner, E Struck, Eds). Munich, Deutsches Herzzentrum, 1979, p 47.
23. Bachet J, Bical O, Goudot B, Menu P, Richard T, Barbagelatta M, Guilmet D: Early structural failure of porcine xenografts in young patients. In: Bioprosthetic Cardiac Valves (F Sebening, WP Klövekorn, H Meisner, E Struck, Eds). Munich, Deutsches Herzzentrum, 1979, p 341.
24. Le Clerc JL, Deuvaert FE, Wellens F, Goffin Y, Primo G: A four year experience of bioprosthetic cardiac valve replacement. Early and late results. In: Bioprosthetic Cardiac Valves (F Sebening, WP Klövekorn, H Meisner, E Struck, Eds). Munich, Deutsches Herzzentrum, 1979, p 27.
25. Myerowitz PD, Lamberti JJ, Replogle RL, Schwarz D, Anagnostopoulos E:

Delayed complications following heterograft valve replacement. In: Bioprosthetic Cardiac Valves (F Sebening, WP Klövekorn, H Meisner, E Struck, Eds). Munich, Deutsches Herzzentrum, 1979, p 335.
26. Angell WW. A nine year experience with the Angell-Shiley xenograft and a comparative literature review of the porcine bioprosthesis versus the mechanical prosthesis. In: Bioprosthetic Cardiac Valves (F Sebening, WP Klövekorn, H Meisner, E Struck, Eds). Munich, Deutsches Herzzentrum, 1979, p 81.
27. Monties JR, Goudard A, Blin D, Mouly A, Henry JF, Deveze JL, Avierinos C, Mahieddine B, Medouakh M: 481 bioprosthetic valves. Early and middle term results. In: Bioprosthetic Cardiac Valves (F Sebening, WP Klövekorn, H Meisner, E Struck, Eds). Munich, Deutsches Herzzentrum, 1979, p 39.
28. Casarotto D, Bortolotti U, Thiene G, Gallucci V, Cevèse PG: Long-term results (from 5 to 7 years) with the Hancock S-G-P bioprosthesis. J Cardiovasc Surg 20:399, 1979.
29. Williams JB, Karp RB, Kriklin JW, Kouchoukos NT, Pacifico AD, Zorn GL Jr, Blackstone EH, Brown RN, Piantadosi S, Bradley EL: Considerations in selection and management of patients undergoing valve replacement with glutaraldehyde-fixed porcine bioprostheses. Ann Thorac Surg 30:247, 1980.
30. Sanders SP, Levy RJ, Freed MD, Norwood WI, Castaneda AR: Use of Hancock porcine xenografts in children and adolescents. Am J Cardiol 46:429, 1980.
31. Crupi G, Gibson D, Heard B, Lincoln C: Severe late failure of a porcine xenograft mitral valve: Clinical, echocardiographic, and pathological findings. Thorax 35:210, 1980.
32. Woodroof E: The chemistry and biology of aldehyde treated tissue heart valve xenografts. In: Tissue Heart Valves (MI Ionescu, Ed). London, Butterworths, 1979, p 347.
33. Harris ED Jr, Farrell ME: Resistance to collagenase: A characteristic of collagen fibrils cross-linked by formaldehyde. Biochim Biophys Acta 278:133, 1972.
34. Broom ND: Fatigue-induced damage in glutaraldehyde-preserved heart valve tissue. J Thorac Cardiovasc Surg 76:202, 1978.
35. Thomson FJ, Barratt-Boyes BG: The glutaraldehyde-treated heterograft valve. Some engineering observations. J Thorac Cardiovasc Surg 74:317, 1977.
36. Thubrikar M, Bosher LP, Nolan SP: The mechanism of opening of the aortic valve. J Thorac Cardiovasc Surg 77:863, 1979.
37. Thubrikar M, Nolan SP, Bosher LP, Deck JD: The cyclic changes and structure of the base of the aortic valve. Am Heart J 99:217, 1980.
38. Thubrikar M, Piepgrass WC, Deck JD, Nolan SP: Stresses of natural versus prosthetic aortic valve leaflets in vivo. Ann Thorac Surg 30:230, 1980.
39. Wright JTM: Hydrodynamic evaluation of tissue valves. In: Tissue Heart Valves (MI Ionescu, Ed). London, Butterworths, 1979, p 29.
40. Ishihara T, Ferrans VJ, Jones M, Boyce SW, Roberts WC: Occurrence and significance of endothelial cells in implanted porcine bioprosthetic valves. Am J Cardiol 48:443, 1981.

34

Pathologic Substrates of Porcine Valve Dysfunction

G. Thiene, E. Arbustini, U. Bortolotti, E. Talenti, A. Milano, M. Valente, G. Molin, V. Gallucci

In the early 1970s when we started using glutaraldehyde-preserved Hancock porcine bioprostheses for valve replacement,[1,2] we were aware that they would undergo structural changes. Thus, it appeared clear that a concomitant pathologic study of the explanted xenografts would be mandatory to assess the validity of these as bioprostheses as cardiac valve substitutes. Accordingly, a detailed morphologic study, including gross, x-ray, and histologic examinations, coupled more recently with electron microscopy, was carried out for each porcine valve explanted in our department or referred to us from other institutions, and it has been the subject of previous reports.[3–9] Pathologic data have been published by other centers, collecting initial experience, but little information is available on long-term modifications and ultimate fate of these bioprostheses.[10–19]

We herein analyze the substrates of early and late dysfunction of 129 glutaraldehyde-fixed porcine valves. This extensive experience allows a reliable appraisal of the various causes that adversely affect the performance and durability of porcine xenografts.

Materials and Methods

On hundred and twenty-nine glutaraldehyde-fixed porcine bioprostheses were available for pathologic examination. They were recovered from 114 patients, 57 females and 57 males, ranging in age at time of death or reoperation from 9–68 years (mean, 45.8).

From the Institutes of Pathological Anatomy, Cardiovascular Surgery, Radiology, and Mineralogy and Petrography, University of Padova, Padova, Italy.

This work has been supported in part by a grant of Consiglio Nazionale delle Ricerche, Italy.

The material has been divided into 2 groups according to the duration of function of the bioprostheses: less than 1 month (early explants, 51 BP), more than 1 month (from 2–138 months, mean, 55; late explants, 78 BP). All the explants have been submitted to gross anatomic examination and photographed on both aspects; the last 51 consecutive explants were also examined by x ray to disclose even minimal calcification. Multiple sections of each cusp were paraffin-embedded, sectioned at 7 μ in thickness and stained with hematoxylin-eosin, Weigert-van Gieson, alcian blue-periodic acid–Schiff and von Kossa. When necessary, histochemical reaction on frozen sections with Sudan III for lipid detection also was carried out.

In 19 explanted valves, small portions of the cusps were fixed with cold 2% glutaraldehyde in phosphate buffer (pH 7.2), postfixed in osmium tetroxide, dehydrated, and embedded in Epon. Ultrathin sections were cut and stained with uranyl acetate and lead citrate.

As a control group, 4 unimplanted and 2 unstented porcine valves were also submitted to ultrastructural examination. Finally, in order to identify the nature of the mineralization process, x-ray diffraction studies using the powder method were carried out on pulverized, dehydrated calcified leaflets. Other samples were embedded in epoxy resin, polished, coated with a 200 Å thick film of carbon, and submitted to electron microprobe analysis. Areas that were suspected of being calcified deposits were mapped for energy dispersive analysis.

Results

Early Explants

This group includes 51 bioprostheses from 43 patients, 18 males and 25 females, aged 9–68 years (mean, 50). All were necropsy observations of patients who died from 0–28 days after operation (mean, 6 days).

Thirty-five bioprostheses were implanted in the mitral position, 13 in the aortic position, and 3 in the tricuspid position. Complications were found in 25 valves (49%), 24 of which had been in the mitral position and only 1 in the aortic position ($p < 0.001$). Complications observed in the mitral position were single or multiple and consisted of left ventricular outflow tract obstruction in 13 cases (43.3%), thrombosis in 7 (23.3%), myocardial disruption in 6 (20%), cardiac rupture in 3 (10%), and paravalvular leak in 1 (3.3%) (Fig. 1).

Left ventricular outflow obstruction was caused by an incorrect insertion of the bioprosthesis in the mitral orifice, resulting in subaortic obstruction by a prosthetic strut. It was frequently worsened by a disproportion between the left ventricular cavity and the size of the prosthesis, and it was particularly observed in female patients with prevalent mitral stenosis (Fig.

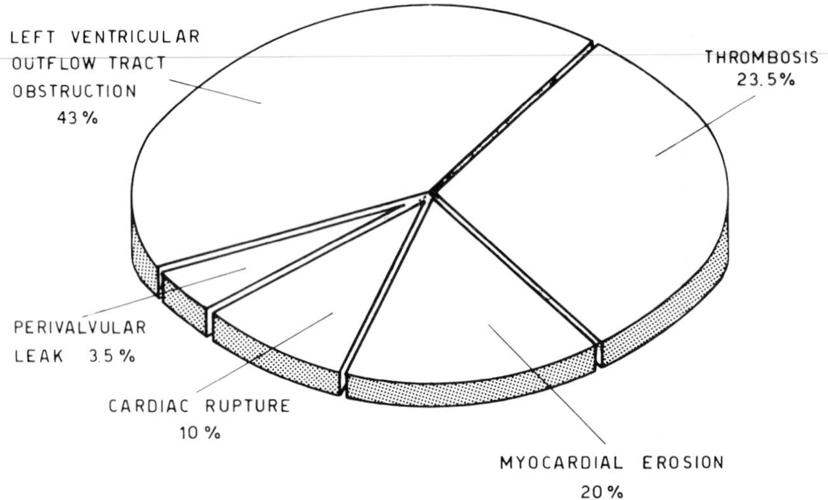

FIG. 1 Type and incidence of early complications observed after mitral valve replacement with porcine bioprostheses.

2). All these patients died of low cardiac output at a mean time of 2 days from operation, with signs of overt myocardial infarction in 2. This type of complication was also observed in 2 patients with a low profile bioprosthesis.

Myocardial disruption was present in 6 patients and was located at the posterolateral wall of the left ventricle. It consisted of an endomyocardial laceration that was located, in 4 cases, 2 cm below the mitral anulus, just opposite to the edge of one prosthetic strut, and, in 2, at the midventricular level, quite far from the device (Fig. 3).

Cardiac rupture occurred in 3 patients. In one it was a complication of a deep endomyocardial disruption and in the other 2 it was located at the left atrioventricular groove. Death, because of massive hemorrhage, occurred in all patients within 2 hours of implantation.

Early thrombus formation was noted in 7 cases. The thrombus lined the sewing ring in 5 (Fig. 4), was mural in 1, and filled the left auricle in 1. All patients were in chronic atrial fibrillation, had an enlarged left atrium, were not anticoagulated, and died at an average of 14 days from surgery with signs of low cardiac output. Three patients sustained a cerebral embolism postoperatively. No cusp-related thrombosis was noted in early explants.

The only complication observed in the aortic position consisted of obstruction of the right coronary artery ostium by 1 prosthetic strut, which caused a fatal myocardial infarction (Fig. 5).

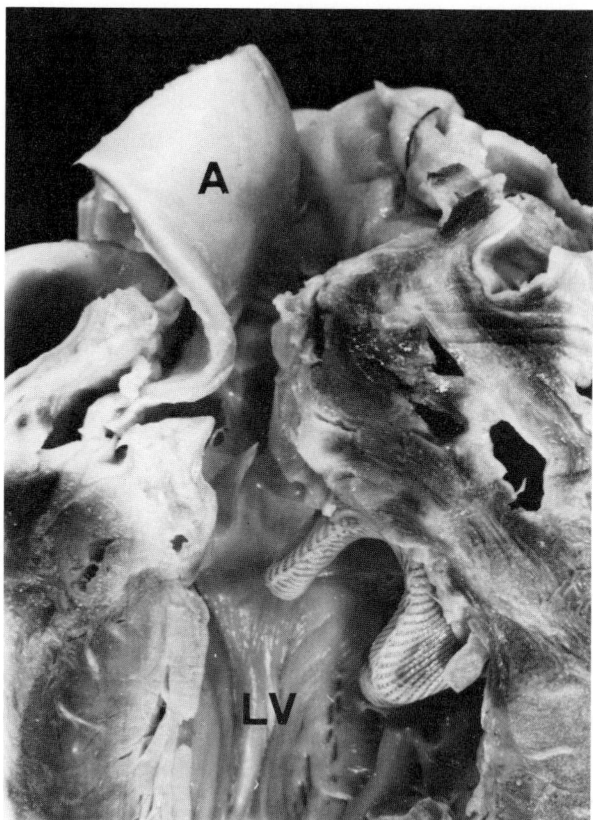

FIG. 2 Left ventricular outflow tract obstruction caused by porcine mitral valve in 58-year-old woman who died 24 h after operation for low cardiac output syndrome. Note 1 prosthetic strut just underneath aortic valve.

Late Explants

Included in this group are 78 bioprostheses removed from 71 patients, 39 males and 32 females. These bioprostheses had been in place from 2–138 months (mean, 55); 49 were mitral, 27 aortic, and 2 tricuspid. Twenty-seven heterografts were recovered at necropsy from 20 patients, with a mean time of function of 30 months; 51 were explanted at reoperation from 51 patients after an average interval of 67.5 months after implantation. Figure 6 shows the distribution of late explants according to the time of function.

Signs of dysfunction were found in 66 bioprostheses (85%): in 58 dysfunction was intrinsic to the tissue and in 8, extrinsic. The 12 heterografts that did not exhibit evidence of failure were removed from patients who died or were reoperated upon for causes unrelated to the bioprostheses.

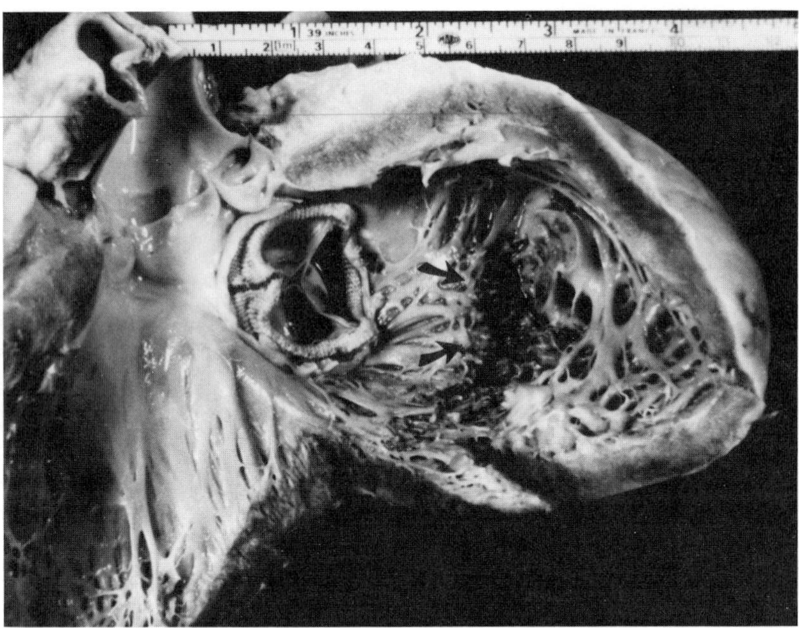

FIG. 3 Midventricular myocardial disruption (arrows) located far from prosthetic struts of low profile porcine mitral valve, implanted in 27-year-old woman who died 2 days following valve replacement with signs of low cardiac output.

Figure 7 summarizes the incidence of the various significant causes of prosthetic dysfunction: calcification accounted for 46% of cases, thrombosis for 16%, endocarditis for 12%, fibrous tissue overgrowth for 11%, paravalvular leak for 9%, and miscellaneous for 6%.

Endocarditis. Ten bioprostheses removed from 9 patients had evidence of infection. Seven had been in the mitral position and 3 in the aortic position, the time of function ranging from 2–86 months (mean, 37.5).

The microorganisms responsible for the infection were Gram negative in 3 patients (*Klebsiella pneumoniae, Enterobacter cloacae* and *Serratia marcescens*), Gram positive in 2 (*Staphylococcus aureus* and *Streptococcus viridans*), and fungi in 4 (*Candida* species in 3 and *Aspergillus fumigatus* in 1).

On gross inspection, the prostheses showed a polypoid, vegetative process involving the leaflets; in 1 patient with mitral endocarditis the infection extended to the anulus and created a paravalvular abscess and a periprosthetic leak.

Sepsis was the most frequent cause of death and was due to systemic dissemination of the friable vegetations. Prosthetic regurgitation occurred in 5 xenografts because of ulcerations and tears of the cusps; stenosis due to polypoid masses obstructing the prosthetic orifice was present in 2. Three

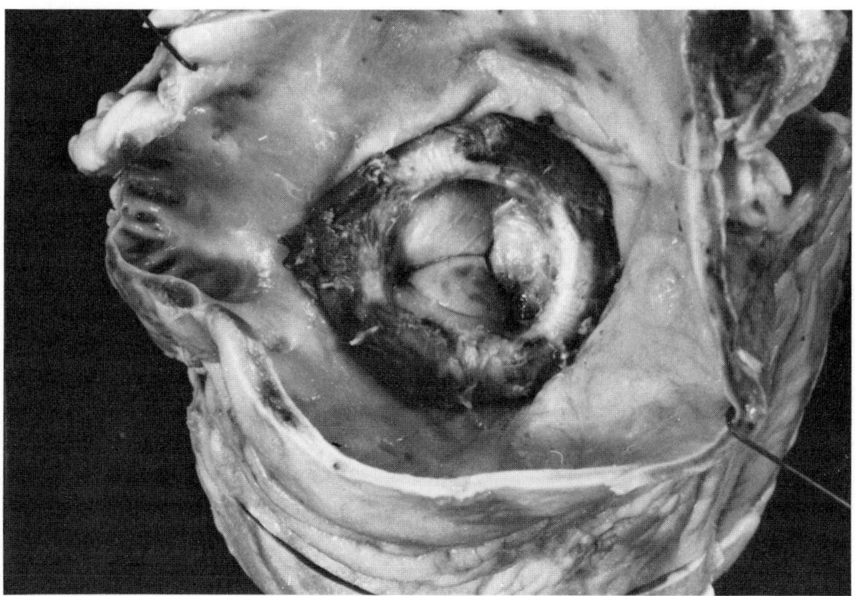

FIG. 4 Left atrial view of mitral bioprosthesis with anular thrombosis lining Dacron cloth of sewing ring. The patient, a 68-year-old woman, died 6 days after operation because of cerebral embolism.

infected valves had no evidence of dysfunction. Clusters of microorganisms and leukocytic infiltrates were observed deep in the cusp tissue in almost all cases; one bioprosthesis had the histologic features of a healed endocarditis.

Late thrombosis. Prosthetic-related thrombosis was found in 13 patients with 14 heterografts (12 mitral, 1 aortic, and 1 tricuspid), which had been in place from 26–138 months (average, 59.4). Thrombi filled one or more cusp sinuses in 6 BP (5 mitral and 1 aortic) (Fig. 8). Seven patients had evidence of left atrial mural thrombosis, caused by a calcified and stenotic prosthesis, and 1, with severe stenosis of a tricuspid xenograft, had a giant ball thrombus filling the right atrial cavity. Thrombosis was favored by atrial fibrillation (9 patients) and lack of anticoagulant treatment (8 patients). Systemic thromboembolic episodes occurred in 4 patients, being fatal in 1.

Histologically, thrombi filling the cusp sinuses usually appeared unorganized and the corresponding cusp did not exhibit significant changes (Fig. 8b), except in 1 case in which marked calcific degeneration was present.

Calcific degeneration. The main cause of late prosthetic failure was calcific degeneration, which, either isolated or in association with other factors, determined dysfunction in 35 patients with 37 bioprostheses (22 mitral, 14 aortic, and 1 tricuspid). The overall mean time of function was 68.5 ± 30 months. In only 13 patients were we able to find factors possibly predis-

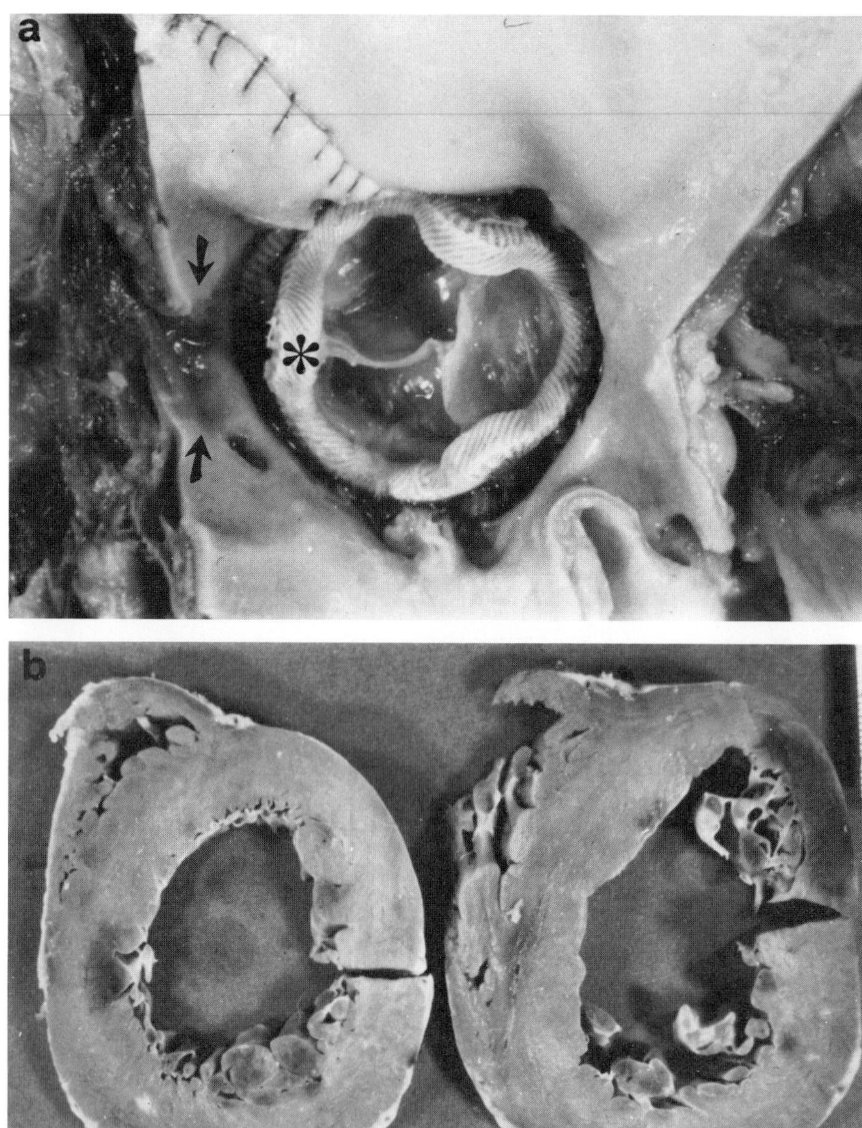

FIG. 5 A 58-year-old man died 3 days after aortic valve replacement with signs of myocardial infarction. At necropsy 1 prosthetic strut (asterisk) was noted to occlude the right coronary ostium (arrows), due to a malorientation of the heterograft (a). Cross-sections of the myocardium (b) show posterior myocardial infarction.

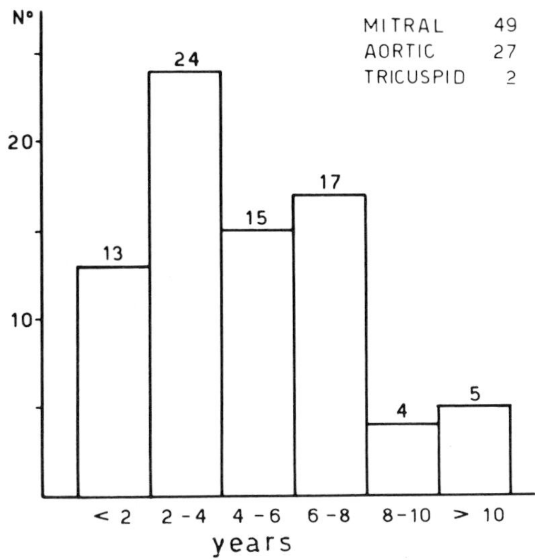

FIG. 6 Distribution of 78 late explants according to duration; 49 were mitral, 27 aortic and 2 tricuspid.

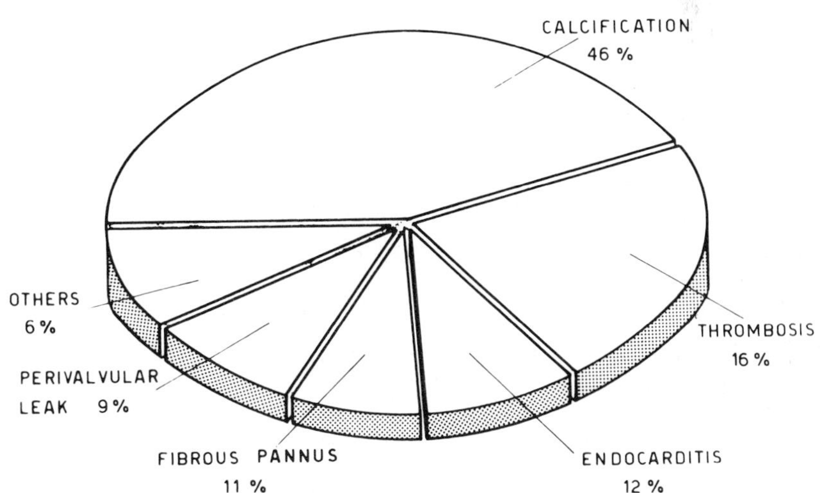

FIG. 7 Type and incidence of causes of late dysfunction observed in the 66 late malfunctioning bioprostheses.

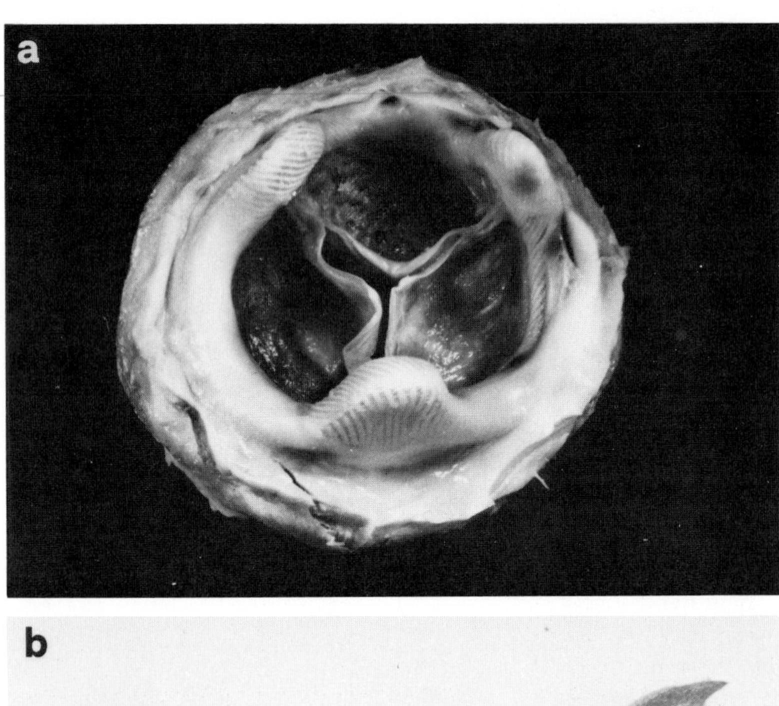

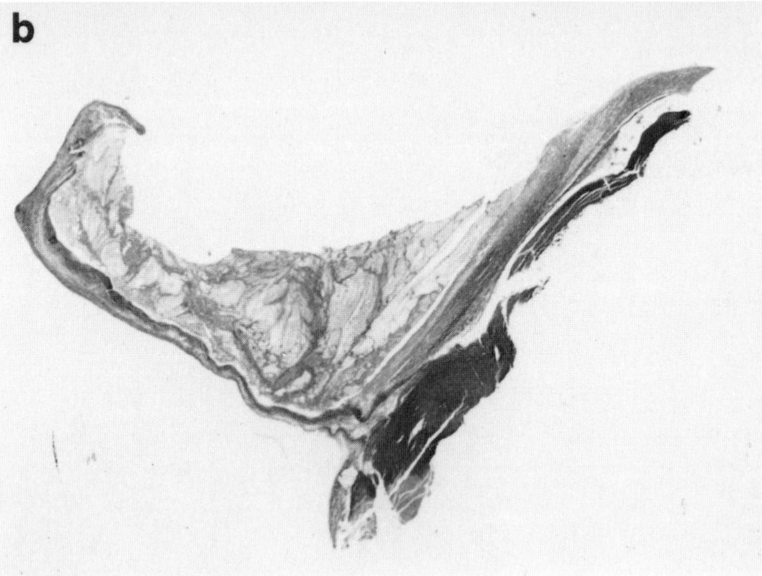

FIG. 8 A 57-year-old woman had fatal cerebral thromboembolism 40 months after mitral valve replacement. Postmortem examination revealed that 2 cusp sinuses were filled by thrombotic material (a). Histologic examination showed a nonorganized thrombus (b). Elastic-van Gieson stain, original magnification ×5.

TABLE I Calcific dysfunction

Age group	# explants	Duration (mo.)*
Young (<20 yrs.)	9	48 ± 20
Adult	28	75 ± 30

* $p < 0.001$.

posing to calcification: young age (<20 years at the time of valve replacement) in 8 patients, chronic renal failure in 2, pregnancy in 2, and healed endocarditis in 1. The 9 xenografts from the 8 young subjects failed as a consequence of calcification at an average of 48 ± 20 months, whereas 28 xenografts from adult patients (more than 20 years old at the time of valve replacement) failed at an average of 75 ± 27 months ($p < 0.001$) (Table I). In adult patients the mean time of function of aortic explants was 60 ± 20 months, compared to 85 ± 30 months for mitgral explants ($p < 0.05$) (Table II).

Study of the distribution of the bioprostheses into different time intervals following surgery disclosed an increasing incidence of calcification with time as the main cause of valve failure: 0% within the first 2 years, when endocarditis and paravalvular leak were prevalent; 43% between the second and the fourth year; 50% between the fourth and the sixth year; 64% between the sixth and the eighth year; and 75% longer than 8 years (Fig. 9).

Calcification resulted in bioprosthetic stenosis in 14 cases, in regurgitation in 16, and in both stenosis and regurgitation in 7. Malfunction due to calcification had a stenosis substrate when stiffness reduced leaflet pliability and regurgitation when disintegration of calcified cusps led to tears, fraying, and loss of substance. In flexible-stented bioprostheses, stenosis predominated in the mitral position and regurgitation in the aortic position. Interestingly, we observed that regurgitation of rigid-stented mitral valve was determined by isolated torn commissures due to selective calcium deposits. Impending detachement of pieces of calcific cusps was frequently observed,

TABLE II Calcific dysfunction in adults*

Type BP	# explants	Duration (mo.)†
Aortic	12	60 ± 20
Mitral	16	85 ± 30

* Older than 20 years at the time of implantation.
† $p < 0.05$.

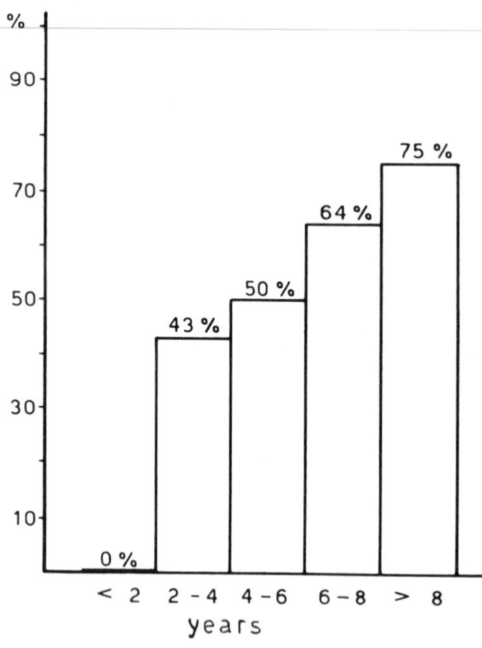

FIG. 9 Incidence of bioprosthetic dysfunction due to calcific degeneration increases with time.

mostly in aortic bioprotheses. "Wash out" of calcific fragments may be responsible for embolic events in the absence of prosthetic thrombosis (Fig. 10).

Fibrous tissue overgrowth. This complication caused severe reduction of the effective prosthetic orifice in 8 bioprostheses (6 mitral, 1 tricuspid, and 1 aortic) that had been in place from 37–129 months (mean, 83.1). It was isolated in 2 explants and was associated with cuspal calcific deposits in 6.

Pathologically, a fibrous sheath covered the atrial side of the leaflets in the atrioventricular position (Fig. 11) and the ventricular side in the aortic position.

Paravalvular leak. Seven bioprostheses were removed from 7 patients because of regurgitation due to a paravalvular leak: 5 were mitral and 2 aortic, and they were in place from 2–84 months (mean, 32.2). Only 1 case showed signs of intrinsic dysfunction because of cusp degeneration due to mild calcific deposits.

Miscellaneous changes. In 2 patients severe prosthetic regurgitation occurred 74 and 96 months after implantation; regurgitation due to a torn commissure was caused by massive lipid infiltration in the presence of only minimal calcific deposits detected by roentgenogram. One patient had evidence of mitral prosthetic regurgitation 53 months after surgery: bio-

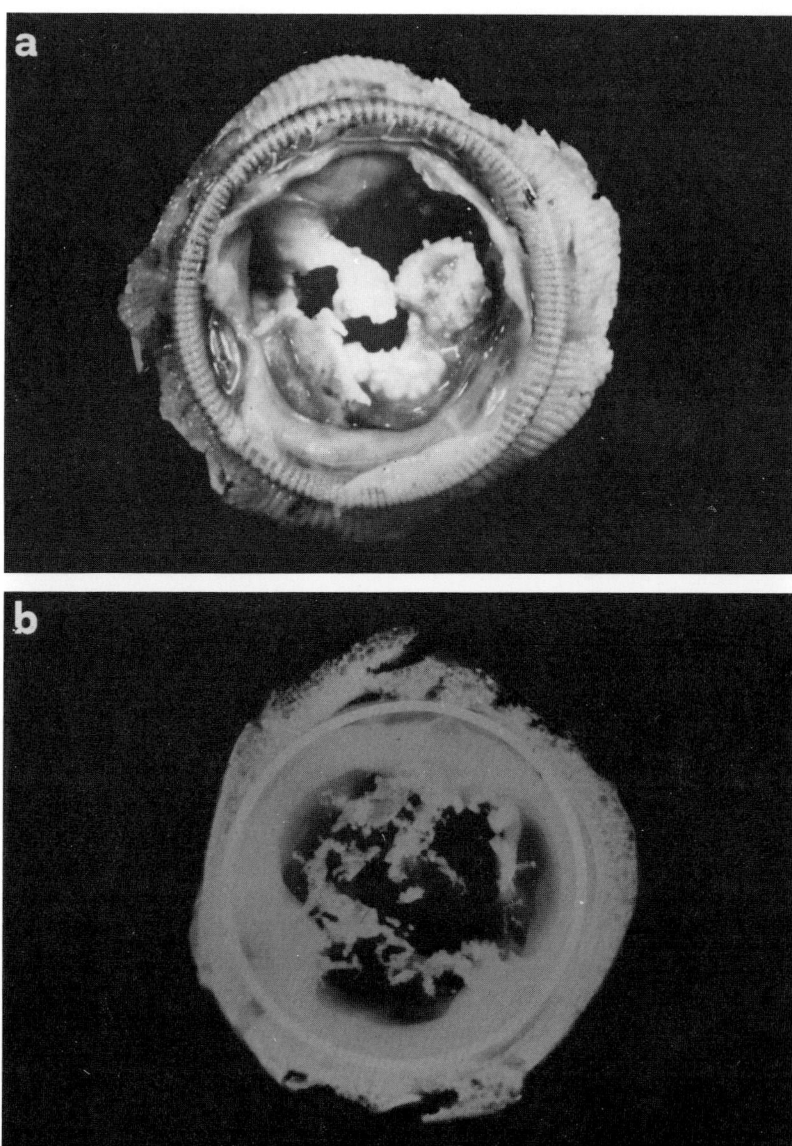

FIG. 10 A 51-year-old man was successfully reoperated upon for aortic bioprosthetic regurgitation 67 months after native valve replacement. (a) Gross view of the explanted xenograft shows fragmented cusps with loss of substance and impending detachment of pieces of leaflets. (b) X ray reveals marked calcific cusp degeneration.

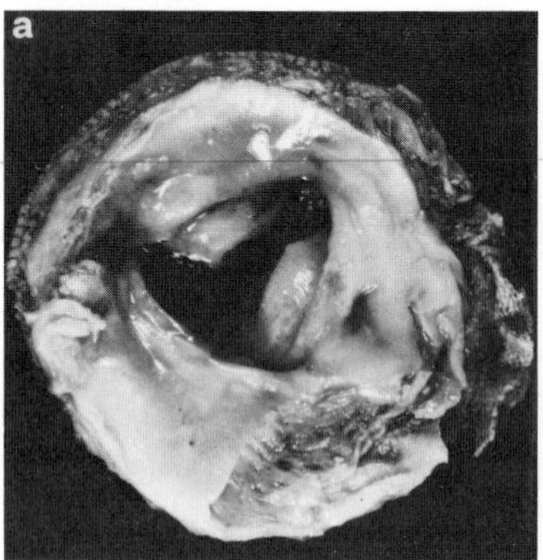
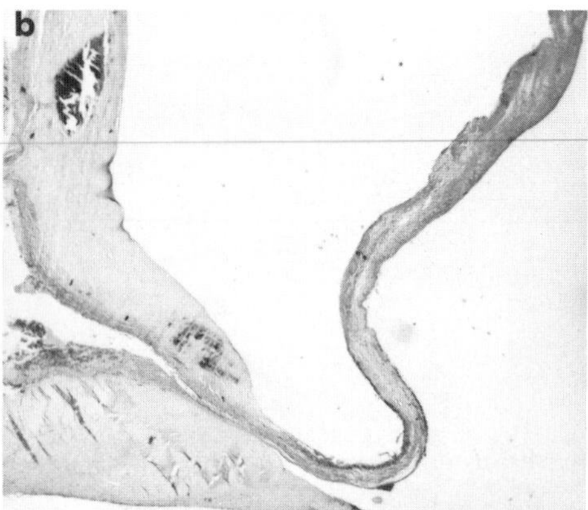

FIG. 11 A 47-year-old woman underwent excision of a mitral bioprosthesis 119 months after insertion. (a) Left atrial view of the explanted valve shows severe reduction of the effective mitral orifice due to fibrous pannus. (b) Histologic section of cusp shows a thick fibrous sheet partially covering atrial side of leaflet. Calcific deposition is present only at level of porcine aortic wall.

prosthetic dysfunction was caused by a large and isolated tear of the muscular ridge at the base of the right coronary cusp without calcium deposition. In another case, an aortic BP, which had been in place for 98 months, was replaced because of stenosis caused by a thick hematoma infiltrating the right coronary cusp. Finally, extrinsic dysfunction was found in 1 patient who died after reoperation for aortic bioprosthetic endocarditis. At necropsy, a deep, healed endocardial laceration was observed, corresponding to one of the struts of the noninfected mitral xenograft.

Histologic findings. Histologic examination of the cusp tissue only rarely added significant information to the gross examination. The endothelium appeared partially reconstructed by host cells. Fibrous pannus, when present, was constituted by an overgrowth of dense, partially vascularized fibrous tissue, 0.5–1.2 mm thick (Fig. 11b). Calcified deposits appeared intrinsic to the leaflet, usually involving the cusp layers in the form of the laminar or nodular infiltrates (Fig. 12a). Fibrin deposits occasionally lined both cuspal surfaces (Fig. 12b). Round cell inflammatory infiltrates were observed in some leaflets, but were limited to the outer layers in all but 2 cases (Fig. 12b). Lipid accumulation was marked in 3 cases and presented as clefts, like cholesterol needles, sometimes surrounded by foreign body inflammatory reaction (Fig. 12c). The muscle shelf of the right cusp appeared reduced in size and showed coagulated myofibers. Inflammatory infiltrates were frequent but usually limited to the base of the right cusp (Fig. 12d). Spots of hyaline material were an almost regular finding within the spongiosa. Intracuspal hemorrhage involved the valvular spongiosa in 4 cases,

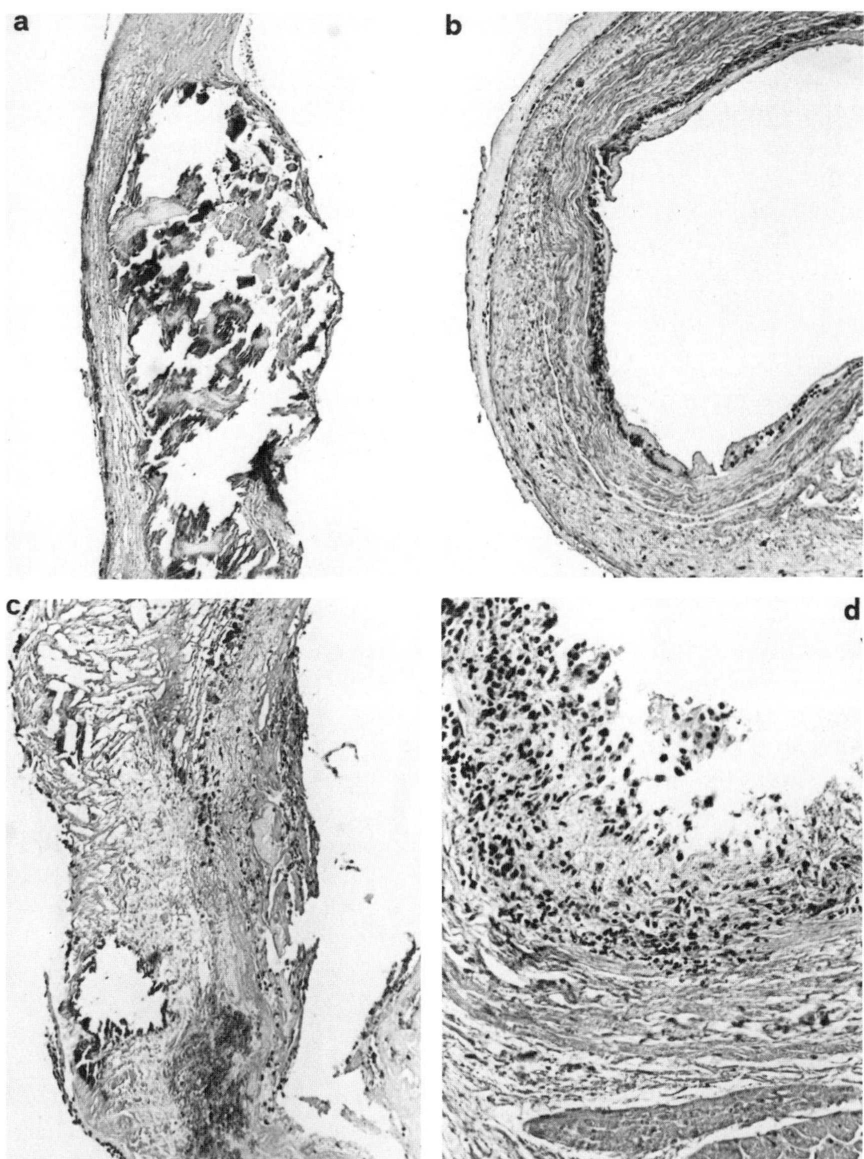

FIG. 12 Histologic aspects of late explants. (a) Intrinsic calcium deposits in cusp of mitral valve removed from a 39-year-old man, 125 months after implantation. ×48. (b) Fibrin films lining both surfaces of mitral xenograft that has been in place for 29 months in a 34-year-old woman. Left atrial thrombosis was detected at reoperation. Inflammatory infiltrates are confined in the surface of the fibrosa. ×75 (c) Calcification, hemorrhage and lipid accumulation, in the form of clefts, are present in 1 leaflet of a mitral heterograft in place for 114 months, removed from a 53-year-old woman. Note superficial fibrin deposition and inflammatory infiltrates. ×75. (d) Inflammatory infiltrates at base of right coronary cusp of mitral bioprosthesis removed from a 57-year-old woman, 64 months after implantation. H & E ×150.

and it was represented by accumulation of erythrocytes, macrophages, leukocytes, and fibrin strands.

Ultrastructural findings. In reporting the results of ultrastructural examination, we divided the material into 3 groups: unimplanted BP (control group), explants removed because of causes extrinsic or unrelated to the bioprosthesis (extrinsic valve dysfunction group), and valves explanted due to tissue failure (intrinsic valve dysfunction group).

Control group. This group encompasses 6 unimplanted bioprostheses (4 mounted and 2 unstented), each subjected to glutaraldehyde tanning. The endothelial layer appeared focally disrupted in the outflow surface and almost completely absent in the inflow surface. The fibroblasts and the residual endothelial cells showed various degrees of autolytic phenomena, consisting of loss of integrity of the cytoplasmic membranes and swelling of organelles, which were frequently extruded from the cells. The collagen fibrils were normal in structure and the matrix in the spongiosa was highly electron lucent. The muscle shelf of the right cusp also was examined and revealed severe autolytic changes with disruption of the structure of the sarcomeres.

Extrinsic valve dysfunction group. The 4 bioprostheses belonging to this group, all mitral, had been in place from 27–84 months (mean, 55) and were removed at reoperation for paravalvular leak[3] or at necropsy for valvular cardiomyopathy.[1] A superficial lining, including fibrin, platelets, and blood cell aggregates, was a regular finding. In the absence of endothelium, the fibrin strands appeared in direct contact with the subendothelial connective tissue. Most of the collagen fibrils showed a normal banding pattern (Fig. 13). Finely granular electron-dense material was present in all valvular layers and was thought to be insudated plasma proteins. Lipid droplets of variable size were interspersed among the collagen bundles in 3 cases. Porcine fibroblasts appeared generally well preserved, even in the latest explant. Microcalcification, not detected by x-ray examination, was observed either within the cytoplasm of fibroblasts or in the interstitial space.

Intrinsic valve dysfunction group. Fifteen valves (12 mitral and 3 aortic), in place from 26–137 months (mean, 80.5), were removed at surgery (12) or at necropsy (3) for severe dysfunction due to intrinsic tissue failure. Causes of failure were: massive calcification (12), endocarditis (1), isolated torn commissure (1), and large tear in the muscle shelf of the right cusp (1).

Both valvular surfaces were frequently bare of endothelium and were lined by fibrin and blood cells. The collagen fibrils had normal periodic banding in 11 BP and were focally disrupted in the others. The most prominent structural changes were observed in the porcine fibroblasts, which lost the integrity of cytoplasmic membranes and showed swollen or disrupted organelles. Cellular debris was a regular finding in the interstitium.

Lipid droplets were detected in 12 cases. In 8 they were rare and small; in 4, large in size and in number. In 2 cases the lipid infiltration had the features of cholesterol needles.

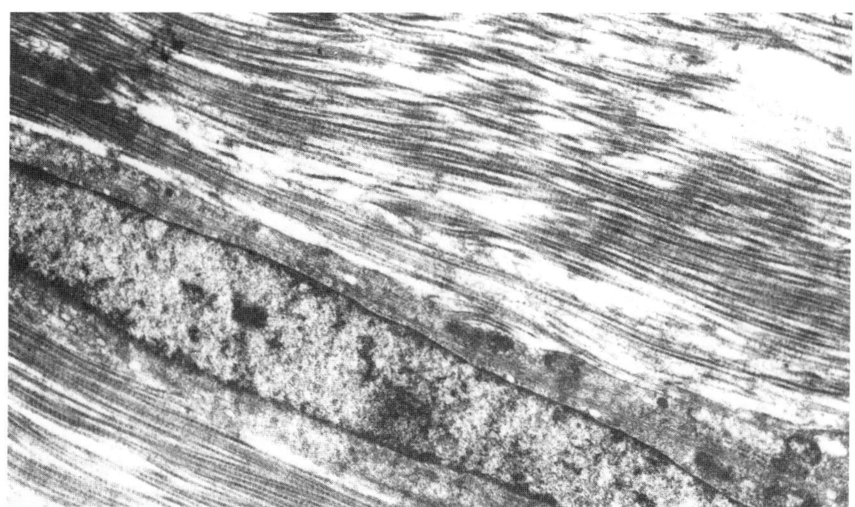

FIG. 13 Fairly well preserved collagen fibrils surrounding a native fibroblast from a mitral xenograft removed from a 53-year-old man, 27 months after implantation, because of paravalvular leak. Uranyl acetate and lead citrate, original magnification ×30,000.

In the 12 explants in which calcification was visible on gross examination, mineral deposition involved all the tissue components. When it was massive, no underlying tissue structures were recognizable. When it was minimal, calcium deposits were detected in the collagen fibrils as well as in the cytoplasm of fibroblasts and in the interstitial space. Collagen calcification appeared as a result of focal deposition of amorphous or needle-shaped electron-dense material along individual collagen fibrils. The collagen not involved in the mineralization process frequently preserved its periodicity, even in areas very close to calcific deposits. Cytoplasmic and interstitial calcifications consisted of bodies (calcospherules) variable in size and morphology. The smallest bodies were fully calcified spherules ranging in diameter from 0.2–0.5 μ. Larger calcospherules consisted of one or more targetlike dense layers constituted by radially arranged microneedle-shaped crystals; the core was both dense and electron lucent, containing, in this case, only sparse aggregates of microneedle crystals. Concentrically arranged plasma membranelike structures were observed around the calcific bodies. Aggregation of 2 or more calcospherules was also observed.

X-ray microanalysis revealed the presence of calcium and phosphorus with small amounts of chlorine and iron, suggesting that mineralization was mainly due to hydroxyapatite. X-ray diffraction showed the characteristic pattern of apatite crystals.

The case in which prosthetic dysfunction was caused by infective endocarditis showed severe collagen disruption and many granulocytes with pyknotic nuclei in valvular tissue. Finally, macrophages phagocytosing myofibrils were observed in the bioprosthesis with a tear at the muscle shelf of the right cusp; massive lipid accumulation accounted for the failure of the value with an isolated torn commissure.

Comment

Complications in the Early Postoperative Period

All the complications observed in the first 30 days following operation were extrinsic to the tissue valve, were most frequently observed in the mitral position, and were predominantly related to the high profile of the porcine bioprosthesis.

The obstruction of the left ventricular outflow tract, severe enough to cause low cardiac output and early fatal outcome, seems to depend upon the combination of different factors: 1) incorrect insertion of the device into the mitral orifice; 2) high profile of the porcine xenograft; and 3) disproportion between the size of the prosthesis and the left ventricular cavity, particularly evident in pure rheumatic mitral stenosis. A technical mistake, however, seems to be the major determinant of this complication, since it was observed even in patients receiving a low profile bioprosthesis.

A prosthesis and left ventricle disproportion appears to be the main cause of endomyocardial laceration when the tear corresponds to the edge of a prosthetic strut.[5] This complication may be extremely life-threatening, as witnessed by the case in which cardiac rupture occurred as a result of full-thickness erosion of the left ventricular wall. The pathogenesis of mid-ventricular disruption is still controversial, but most likely it is unrelated to the type of mitral bioprosthesis.[20–22]

Early thrombus formation is rare and always extrinsic to the cusp tissue. Left atrial or sewing ring thrombosis are the usual findings and are related to the presence of atrial fibrillation, dilation of left atrium and postoperative low output syndrome.[7,23–24] The lack of anticoagulant treatment in the early postoperative period also may contribute to the onset of thrombosis. Thrombogenicity of the Dacron cloth of the sewing ring, not yet lined by the host's neoendothelium, cannot be excluded as well. Early thrombi are not trivial, as documented by the occurrence of fatal cerebral thromboembolism in 3 of our patients.

Dysfunction of Late Explants

Prosthetic endocarditis is a rare condition that carries a high mortality.[25] From the pathologic viewpoint, endocarditis on porcine valves is usually an ulcerative and vegetative infection of the cusps, quite similar to that involving the natural aortic valves.[9] Clusters of microorganisms observed within the cusps are responsible for tissue necrosis with tears and perforations. As far as the type of microorganisms is concerned, it is remarkable that there was a high incidence, in our series, of fungal endocarditis and the occurrence of infection by *K. pneumoniae* and *S. marcescens,* which were absent in the recent review of the literature on porcine valve endocarditis made by Ferrans et al.[15] The severity of the disease is explained either by progressive disruption of the leaflets or by systemic embolization of the highly friable vegetations. Regurgitation may occur as the consequence of the tissue destruction and it has therefore a different substrate from regurgitation of mechanical prostheses, which is due to paravalvular leak caused by anular abscesses.[26] Stenosis is the consequence of orifice obstruction by septic polypoid masses.

Late thrombus formation also complicates valve replacement with porcine heterografts and occurs mainly in valves implanted in the mitral position. In contrast with early thrombosis, late thrombus formation is usually a cusp-related phenomenon, since it fills the cusp sinuses, with impairment of their motility.[7] Interestingly, late thrombi were not organized, most likely because the ventricular side of the mitral prosthesis is protected from host tissue ingrowth; therefore absence of organization may explain the friability of the thrombotic material, which may become a potential source of emboli. As far as the pathogenesis of late thrombosis, denuded surfaces described at scanning electron microscopy[17] might favor platelet aggregation and thrombus formation; thrombi also may be located in the atrial cavities, due to bioprosthetic stenosis with consequent blood stasis.[8]

Calcific degeneration of the cusp tissue represents the main cause of late bioprosthetic dysfunction. Calcific deposits wre initially noted at the commissures, where, despite a flexible stent, the hemodynamic stress seems to be still considerable. Isolated commissural calcification in rigid-stented mitral bioprostheses was responsible for torn commissures and valvular regurgitation without significant involvement of the remaining cusp tissue. In this regard, it should be remembered that the placement of a porcine "aortic" valve in the atrioventricular position is quite unnatural, with regard to the pressure load that these porcine cusps must face during ventricular systole.

Stenosis was the predominant feature in mitral prostheses, due to calcific stiffening of the cusp tissue; on the contrary, regurgitation due to tears and loss of substance of the cusps was prevalent in aortic prostheses and was most likely explained by progressive disintegration of the calcified tissue, with eggshell fragility. The "wash out" of calcific fragments might be responsible for embolic events in the absence of prosthetic thrombosis.

Our pathologic experience on explants from patients who were older than 20 years of age at the time of valve replacement indicates that calcific dysfunction occurs earlier in aortic than in mitral xenografts. This finding is in agreement with the clinical experience of Lakier et al,[27] who have observed a higher incidence of dysfunction in patients with aortic bioprostheses on follow-up from 60–89 months after operation. We were able to identify possible risk factors only in a few cases: young age is certainly a favoring factor, since calcification in this age group occurs significantly earlier than in older patients. Our data confirm the results recently reported on the early and severe calcific degeneration of porcine valves implanted in children.[6,28–33] Patients with chronic renal failure also have a high tendency to accelerated calcification of bioprostheses[28] and this was also confirmed in our series. Pregnancy is another factor that might favor mineralization of porcine valves, due to high calcium turnover in this condition. Our pathologic experience is limited to 2 women: 1 died 26 months after surgery, and 1 was successfully reoperated on after 82 months; in both patients the porcine valves exhibited stenotic dysfunction due to gross calcification. However, our clinical experience with patients who became pregnant after valve replacement with porcine valves suggests that the influence of pregnancy on bioprosthetic calcification remains unclear, at present, and needs further studies.[34]

In most of the patients of the present series, calcification was a primary phenomenon and accounted for nearly half of the causes of late bioprosthetic failure, increasing with the time intervals after operation, from 0% in the first 2 years, to 75% over 8 years. Thus, it is clear that calcific mineralization is a clue to the presence of a biodegradation process.

Sanders et al[31] detected high levels of γ-carboxyglutamic acid (GLA) in the cusps of calcified xenografts, but not in controls. According to these investigators, GLA-containing proteins, probably plasmatic in origin, might be the calcium-binding sites. Ferrans et al[16] showed that calcification also involves degenerated collagen fibrils. It is known that ϵ-amino groups of lysine and hydroxylysine of collagen fibrils may react with calcium phosphate groups, but they are usually blocked by proteoglycans and glycoproteins of the ground substance.[35–36] Ferrans et al[16] pointed out that the loss of ground substance during commercial processing may predispose to collagen calcification; although glutaraldehyde employed for preimplantation treatment reacts with the amino groups, the plasma proteins, insudated to replace proteoglycans, may reverse these linkages and, in addition, may provide new reactive residues.

Our electron microscopic observations suggest that calcification of the bioprosthesis is the result of calcium phosphate precipitation at nucleating sites, not only in collagen fibrils, but also in cellular debris and in so-called residual bodies. The calcific deposits involving cytoplasmic and interstitial noncollagen sites consisted of round or oval bodies with a light or electron-dense core surrounded by one or more electron-dense layers, formed by radially arranged microneedle-shaped crystals, and occasionally by a few concentric layers of cytoplasmic membranelike structures. These findings suggest that debris of cytoplasmic organelles, because of the affinity of the membrane phospholipids for calcium,[37] might be an additional early nucleating site of calcification, as seen in the calcific processes occurring in human aortic valves.[38] According to these observations, the autolytic phenomena observed in porcine connective cells, even in unimplanted valves should play a significant role in determining the morphogenesis of calcifications. The concentration of glutaraldehyde used in commercial treatment, while effective for collagen and cusp pliability preservation, might be too low to allow appropriate porcine cell fixation. The variability in the status of the native porcine valve possibly might be related to the nonstandardized time interval between the killing of the animals and the beginning of the preimplantation processes. The observation of well-preserved cellular components in some late, functioning bioprostheses gives further evidence of this variability.

The collagen had normal banding pattern in many calcific explants that had been in place for more than 10 years and periodicity was present also in fibrils close to the calcific deposits. We believe that primary calcification occurs independent of the degree of collagen degeneration and that the preimplantation status of the native porcine cells plays a determinant role in bioprosthetic durability.

Cusp lacerations and perforations were usually encountered at the sites of calcific deposits and were due to fragmentation of rigid leaflets. However, primary tears can occur, although rarely, in the absence of calcific deposition. In 1 of our cases, the substrate of cusp disruption was marked lipid accumulation due to insudation of plasma lipoproteins.[39] Another pathologic substrate, observed in 1 case, was a basal laceration of the right muscular leaflet in association with inflammatory infiltrates. Glutaraldehyde tanning, while effective in decreasing the antigenicity of the collagen, may leave free antigenic sites on the muscle cells.

Conclusions

The early complications observed after valve replacement with porcine valves were extrinsic to the valve tissue and mainly related to the implantation of the bioprothesis in the mitral position.

Calcification is the leading cause of long-term failure and it was accelerated in young patients and in valves implanted in the aortic position. Calcification accounted for cusp stiffness, causing stenosis, and for cusp tears, causing regurgitation.

It appears that the preimplantation status of native porcine valves may influence the morphogenesis of calcification and the long-term durability of bioprostheses. Further studies should be aimed at preventing calcification in order to enhance bioprosthetic performance.

References

1. Cévese PG, Gallucci V, Morea M, Dalla Volta S, Fasoli G, Casarotto D: Heart valve replacement with the Hancock bioprosthesis. Analysis of long-term results. Circulation 56 (Suppl. II):111, 1977.
2. Casarotto D, Bortolotti U, Thiene G, Gallucci V, Cévese PG: Long-term results (5 to 7 years) with the Hancock SGP bioprosthesis. J Cardiovasc Surg 20:399, 1979.
3. Bortolotti U, Gallucci V, Casarotto D, Thiene G: Fibrous tissue overgrowth on Hancock mitral xenografts. A cause of late prosthetic stenosis. Thorac Cardiovasc Surg 27:316, 1979.
4. Thiene G, Bortolotti U, Casarotto D, Valfré C, Gallucci V: Prosthesis-left ventricle disproportion in mitral valve replacement with the Hancock bioprosthesis: Pathologic observations. In: Bioprosthetic Cardiac Valves (F Sebening WP Klövekorn, H Meisner, E Struck, Eds). Munich, Deutsches Herzzentrum, 1979, p 357.
5. Bortolotti U, Thiene G, Casarotto D, Mazzucco A, Gallucci V: Left ventricular rupture following mitral valve replacement with a Hancock bioprosthesis. Chest 77:235, 1980.
6. Bortolotti U, Milano A, Mazzucco A, Gallucci V, Valente M, Del Maschio A, Valfré C, Thiene G: Alterazioni strutturali delle bioprotesi di Hancock applicate in età pediatrica. G Ital Cardiol 10:1520, 1980.
7. Thiene G, Bortolotti U, Panizzon G, Milano A, Gallucci V: Pathological substrates of thrombus formation after heart valve replacement with the Hancock bioprosthesis. J Thorac Cardiovasc Surg 80:414, 1980.
8. Bortolotti U, Thiene G: Calcification of porcine heterografts implanted in children. Chest 80:117, 1981.
9. Bortolotti U, Thiene G, Milano A, Panizzon G, Valente M, Gallucci V: Pathological study of infective endocarditis on Hancock porcine bioprostheses. J Thorac Cardiovasc Surg 81:934, 1981.
10. Carpentier A, Lemaigre G, Robert L, Carpentier S, Dubost C: Biological factors affecting long-term results of valvular bioprostheses. J Thorac Cardiovasc Surg 58:467, 1969.
11. Spray TL, Roberts WC: Structural changes in porcine xenografts used as substitute cardiac valves. Gross and histologic observations in 51 glutaraldehyde-preserved Hancock valves in 41 patients. Am J Cardiol 40:319, 1977.
12. Fishbein MC, Giessen SA, Collins JJ Jr, Barsamian EM, Cohn LH: Pathologic findings after cardiac valve replacement with glutaraldehyde-fixed porcine valves. Am J Cardiol 40:331, 1977.
13. Ferrans VJ, Spray TL, Billingham ME, Roberts WC: Structural changes in glutaraldehyde-treated porcine heterografts used as substitute cardiac valves. Transmission and scanning electron microscopic observations in 12 patients. Am J Cardiol 41:1161, 1978.
14. Ashraf M, Bloor CM: Structural alterations of the porcine heterograft after various durations of implantation. Am J Cardiol 41:1185, 1978.
15. Ferrans VJ, Boyce SW, Billingham ME, Spray TL, Roberts WC: Infection of glutaraldehyde-preserved porcine valve heterografts. Am J Cardiol 43:1123, 1979.
16. Ferrans VJ, Boyce SW, Billingham ME, Jones M, Ishihara T, Roberts WC: Calcific deposits in porcine bioprostheses: Structure and pathogenesis. Am J Cardiol 46:721, 1980.

17. Riddle JM, Magilligan DJ Jr, Stein PD: Surface morphology of degenerated porcine bioprosthetic valves four to seven years following implantation. J Thorac Cardiovas Surg 81:279, 1981.
18. Ishihara T, Ferrans VJ, Jones M, Boyce WS, Roberts WC: Occurrence and significance of endothelial cells in implanted porcine bioprosthetic valves. Am J Cardiol 48:443, 1981.
19. Ishihara T, Ferrans VJ, Boyce SW, Jones M, Roberts WC: Structure and classification of cuspal tears and perforations in porcine bioprosthetic cardiac valves implanted in patients. Am J Cardiol 48:665, 1981.
20. Miller DW Jr, Johnson DD, Ivey TD: Does preservation of the posterior chordae tendineae enhance survival during mitral valve replacement? Ann Thorac Surg 28:22, 1979.
21. Katske G, Golding LR, Tubbs RR, Loop FD: Posterior midventricular rupture after mitral valve replacement. Ann Thorac Surg 27;130, 1979.
22. Cobbs BW, Hatcher CR, Craver JM, Jones EL, Sewell CW: Transverse midventricular disruption after mitral valve replacement. Am Heart J 99:33, 1980.
23. Edmiston WA, Harrison EC, Duick GF, Parnassus W, Lau FYK: Thromboembolism in mitral porcine valve recipients. Am J Cardiol 41:508, 1978.
24. Hetzer R, Hill JD, Kerth WJ, Ansbro J, Adappa MG, Rodvien R, Kamm B, Gerbode F: Thromboembolic complications after mitral valve replacement with Hancock xenograf. J Thorac Cardiovasc Surg, 75:651, 1978.
25. Rossiter SJ, Stinson EB, Oyer PE, Miller DC, Schapira JN, Martin PR, Shumway NE: Prosthetic valve endocarditis. Comparison of heterograft tissue valves and mechanical valves. J Thorac Cardiovasc Surg 76:795, 1978.
26. Arnett EN, Roberts WC: Valve ring abscess in active infective endocarditis. Frequency, location and clues to clinical diagnosis from the study of 95 necropsy patients. Circulation 54:140, 1976.
27. Lakier JB, Khaja F, Magilligan DJ Jr, Goldstein S: Porcine xenograft valves. Long-term (60–89 month) follow-up. Circulation 62:313, 1980.
28. Kutsche LM, Oyer PE, Shumway NE, Baum D: An important complication of Hancock mitral valve replacement in children. Circulation 60 (Suppl I):98, 1979.
29. Silver MM, Pollock J, Silver MD, Williams WG, Trusler GA: Calcification in porcine xenograft valves in children. Am J Cardiol 45:685, 1980.
30. Thandroyen F, Whitton IN, Pirie D, Rogers MA, Mitha AS: Severe calcification of glutaraldehyde-preserved porcine xenografts in children. Am J Cardiol 45:690, 1980.
31. Sanders SP, Levy RJ, Freed MD, Norwood WI, Castaneda AR: Use of Hancock porcine xenografts in children and adolescents. Am J Cardiol 46:429, 1980.
32. Curcio CA, Commerford PJ, Rose AG, Stevens JE, Barnard MS: Calcification of glutaraldehyde-preserved porcine xenografts in young patients. J Thorac Cardiovas Surg 81:621, 1981.
33. Rocchini AP, Weesner KM, Heidelberger K, Keren D, Berhendt D, Rosenthal A: Porcine xenograft valve failure in children: An immunologic response. Circulation 64 (Suppl II):162, 1981.
34. Bortolotti U, Milano A, Mazzucco A, Valfré C, Russo R, Schivazappa L, Valente M, Thiene G, Gallucci V: Pregnancy in patients with a porcine bioprosthesis. Am J Cardiol 50:1051, 1982.
35. Glimcher MJ: Composition, structure and organization of bone and other mineralized tissues and the mechanism of calcification. In: Handbook of Physiology, Section 7, Endocrinology Vol. 7: Parathyroid Gland (RO Gleep, EB Astwood, GD Aurbach, SR Geiger, Eds). Washington, American Physiological Society, 1976, p 116.

36. Anderson JC: Glycoproteins of the connective tissue matrix. Int Rev Connect Tissue Res 7:251, 1976.
37. Wuthier RE: Lipids of matrix vesicles. Fed Proc 35:117, 1976.
38. Kim KM: Calcification of matrix vesicles in human aortic valve and aortic media. Fed Proc, 35:156, 1976.
39. Arbustini E, Bortolotti U, Valente M, Milano A, Gallucci V, Pennelli N, Thiene G: Cusp disruption by massive lipid infiltration. A rare cause of porcine valve dysfunction. J Thorac Cardiovasc Surg 84:(Nov), 1982.

35

Mode of Failure in 226 Explanted Biologic and Bioprosthetic Valves

A. Bodnar, D. N. Ross

Some recent publications reveal a growing concern about tissue failure, but most important of all, about early and late calcification in commercial porcine bioprosthetic valves.[1–3] Although follow-up studies on large clinical material show an acceptable performance of these valves for periods up to 5–7 years,[4,5] pathologic investigations describe several defective features of the porcine bioprosthesis, including collagen deterioration due to the manufacturing, surface lesions, as well as extracellular mineral depositions, leading to extrinsic or intrinsic calcification, respectively.[6,7] By definition, these pathologic studies do not report failure rate, only the mode of failure.

Similar criticism was directed at earlier generations of biologic valves, such as aortic homografts and fascia lata valves, when the medium-term clinical results and, especially, pathologic reports on failed valves became available. Although the ultimate failure of these valves caused only occasional fatal complications, the number of reoperations was substantial, and many surgeons abandoned using the early generations of biologic valves. However, at present the assessment of the long-term performances of these valves show an excellent patient survival over a 15-year-period in those patients whose original cardiac valve replacement was carried out using biologic valves, especially aortic homograft and pulmonary autograft valves.[8,9]

These is no comparably long follow-up information available on the current generation of bioprosthetic valves, making it very difficult to predict how the reported pathologic changes will affect the long-term survival of patients. The present study therefore focuses on biologic and bioprosthetic valves that failed. It compares the mode of failure in the early and in the current generation of valves, and it assesses 6 different types of biologic or bioprosthetic valves.

From the Department of Surgery, Cardiothoracic Institute, and the National Heart Hospital, London, England.

Materials and Methods

Two hundred and twenty-six biologic or bioprosthetic valves that were removed at reoperation or at autopsy at the National Heart Hospital, London, from 1963–1981 have been included in the study. The valves included aortic homograft, pulmonary autograft, autologous fascia lata, homologous dura mater, porcine aortic, and bovine pericardial valves (Table I).

Method of Preparation and Preservation of the Valves

Aortic homografts. The donor hearts were collected from mortuaries within 48 hours of death, and the dissected aortic valves were freeze-dried from 1963–1967, flash frozen in 1968–1969, both series being sterilized in ethylene oxide or by gamma irradiation. Since 1970 the homograft valves have been sterilized in antibiotic-antifungal mixtures and preserved in a nutrient medium for up to 8 weeks. All homografts involved in the present study were inserted into the aortic position as free, unsupported grafts. Details of preservation and surgical techniques have been published elsewhere.[10]

Pulmonary autografts. The patient's pulmonary valve was taken during cardiopulmonary bypass and inserted into the aortic position as a free, unsupported graft. The pulmonary valve and the main pulmonary artery was replaced using autologous fascia lata, or, more often, homograft aortic valves.[11]

Autologous fascia lata valves. A suitable strip of the patient's fascia lata was taken during cardiac surgery and it was mounted on the rigid metal Ionescu-Ross-Wooler stent.

The autologous material, pulmonary autograft or fascia lata, was never submitted to any chemical or antibiotic treatment.

Homologous dura mater valves. The human dura mater was collected as autopsy material, and the suitable parts of it were dissected and stored in

TABLE I Distribution of 226 explanted biologic or bioprosthetic valves

Type of valve	#	%	Period of insertion
Aortic hemografts	80	35	1963–
Pulmonary autografts	14	6	1966–
Fascia lata	58	26	1969–1971
Dura mater	33	15	1974–1977
Porcine aortic bioprostheses*	28	12	1975–
Bovine pericardial bioprostheses†	13	6	1978–
Total	226	100	

* Hancock standard valve and Carpentier-Edwards valve.
† Ross-Bentley bioprosthesis.

glycerol. The material was mounted on rigid metal stents identical to the ones used for fabricating the fascia lata valves. The mounted valves were sterilized in an antibiotic-antifungal mixture.[12]

Xenograft valves. The commerical valves (Hancock, Carpentier-Edwards, Ross-Bentley) have been processed and sterilized by the manufacturers, glutaraldehyde being the common primary fixative in all of them.

Classification of the Failure Mode

Valve failure was defined as a condition in which pathologic processes related to the valve required reoperation or caused the death of the patient. The pathologic changes were assessed as 1 or more of the following 6 conditions:

1. Surgical error and paravalvular leak. Some early failures in unsupported homograft and pulmonary autograft valves were apparently related to surgical technical error at insertion, and they were treated as paravalvular leaks that occurred with every type of stented valve.
2. Infection was defined as acute or subacute bacterial or fungal endocarditis on the inserted valve according to the NYHA definition.
3. Tissue fatigue involved attenuation, perforations, small tears, or gross ruptures on one or more of the cusps without clinical or pathologic evidence of infection.
4. Shrinkage was defined as shortening and/or thickening of one or more of the cusps.
5. Calcification was noted irrespective of whether it was extrinsic or intrinsic, macroscopically apparent, or detectable only by histology or in vitro x-ray examination.
6. Tissue growth onto the valve was observed only on porcine bioprostheses, and it consisted of a pannus formation that crept onto the biologic part of the valve and caused stenosis and/or incompetence.

Results

The overall results of the assessment are summarized in Table II.

The occurrence of the primary tissue failure was calculated as all failures less paravalvular leak/technical error and infection. The results are summarized in Table III.

Comment

The replacement cardiac valves currently in clinical use have several shortcomings. When the choice has to be made between mechanical and biologic or bioprosthetic valves, durability is considered to be the main

TABLE II Mode of failure in 226 explanted valves

Valve	Total explanted	Paravalvular leak & technical problems	Infection	Shrinkage	Tissue fatigue	Calcification	Tissue overgrowth
Homograft	80	22 (27.5%)	11 (13.7%)	8 (10%)	25 (31.2%)	14 (17.5%)	0
Pulmonary autograft	14	7 (50%)	2 (14.5%)	0	5 (35.7%)	0	0
Dura mater	33	8 (24.2%)	3 (9%)	0	21 (63.6%)	1 (3.03%)	0
Porcine bioprosthesis	28	9 (32.1%)	7 (25%)	0	5 (17.9%)	4 (14.3%)	6 (10.7%)
Bovine pericardial bioprosthesis	13	8 (61.5%)	4 (30.7%)	0	0	1 (7.6%)	0
Fascia lata	58	3 (5.1%)	7 (12.0%)	26 (44.83%)	17 (29.3%)	5 (8.6%)	0
Total	226						

TABLE III Primary tissue failure in 226 explanted valves

Valve	Total explanted	Primary tissue failure #	%	Period of insertion (yr)
Homograft	80	47	58.7	1–17
Pulmonary autograft	14	5	35.7	1–15
Fascia lata	58	48	82.7	1–12
Dura mater	33	22	66.6	1–7
Porcine aortic bioprosthesis*	28	9	32.1	1–7
Bovine pericardial bioprosthesis†	13	1	7.6	1–3

* Hancock standard and Carpentier-Edwards valves.
† Ross-Bentley valve.

advantage of the mechanical valves. Nevertheless, reoperation may become necessary because of the failure of mechanical prostheses, and the removal of the originally inserted prosthetic valve may have to be carried out for problems specifically related to mechanical prostheses, for example, gross thrombosis of the valve or hemolysis.[13] Such complications are practically unknown with biologic and bioprosthetic valves and have not been the cause of failure in any of the 226 valves assessed in the present study.

Paravalvular leaks and early or late infection are not unique to mechanical or biologic valves, and statistics on long-term follow-up studies have shown no difference in this respect between bioprosthetic and mechanical valves.[14,15] Ninety-one failures out of the 226 (40.3%) were due to paravalvular leak or bacterial or fungal endocarditis on the inserted valves, and the proportion of these complications was strikingly high in pulmonary autografts (64.5%), porcine bioprostheses (67.8%, including tissue overgrowth), and bovine pericardial bioprostheses (92.3%) involved in the present random study. Therefore it may be concluded that, at least with the present length of experience, about two thirds of the porcine bioprostheses had to be removed for reasons related not to the biologic part of the valve, but to problems generally encountered with replacement cardiac valves, and that tissue failure is only an occasional finding in bovine pericardial prostheses.

The 6 types of valves assessed by the study can be grouped as autologous (pulmonary autograft, fascia lata), homologous (aortic homograft, dura mater), and heterologous (porcine aortic and bovine pericardial valves) in origin. Since no specific pattern of failure is attributed to any of these 3 groups, it is suggested that immunologic reaction alone is not the most significant determinant of the fate of the biologic valves. A much higher proportion of primary tissue failure was observed in the autologous fascia lata than in the aortic homografts.

The definition "stented tissue valve" does not seem to describe a consistent group either. Three types of valve have been assessed from this group: stented fascia lata, dura mater, and bovine pericardial. Tear of one or more cusps was shown to be the major problem related to the stented dura mater valves, but shrinkage has never occurred, whereas shrinkage accounted for the failure of 44.8% of the fascia valves. Neither of these complications has been observed in stented bovine pericardial valves.

Calcification was not related specifically to the porcine aortic bioprosthesis and it was observed among all types of failed valves, the only exception being the pulmonary autografts. Pulmonary autografts have 5 important features that are partly or completely missing from the other 5 valves, as follows: 1) Autologous in origin; 2) there is no delay between harvesting and implantation; 3) there is no chemical treatment and/or storage involved; 4) there is no artificial part attached to the valve; and 5) since it is a semilunar valve, it is always inserted into the semilunar position.

The last 2 criteria are related to the flow characteristics and flow conditions of the valve, and they alone may determine calcification, as occurred in 8.62% of the stented fascia lata valves, which were autologous, inserted without delay, and given no chemical treatment. On the other hand, aortic homografts with ideal flow conditions equal to that of pulmonary autografts displayed calcification in 17.5% of the failed valves. These results support the theory that calcification in bioprosthetic valves can be caused by a variety of factors. They raise considerable doubts as well whether any chemical treatment, excellent though it may be, could eliminate calcification altogether. The difficulty of the problem is well illustrated by the surprisingly low incidence of calcification in the failed dura mater valves, although the material is not autologous, is not valvular in origin, is mounted on rigid stents, and is sterilized in antibiotics and stored in glycerol for weeks or months before clinical use.

In conclusion, it is suggested that in the majority of the bioprosthetic (porcine and bovine) valve failures reoperation had to be carried out because of paravalvular leak or infection, none of them characteristic of biologic or bioprosthetic valves. No specific pattern of failure was found in any one of the 6 types of valve assessed in the study. Calcification is not unique to porcine aortic bioprostheses, and its occurrence is negligible when compared to paravalvular leak and infection. The results also suggest that several different criteria will have to be fulfilled in the manufacture of the bioprosthetic valves if calcification is to be eliminated completely.

References

1. Sanders SP, Levy RJ, Freed MD, Norwood WI, Castaneda AR: Use of Hancock porcine xenografts in children and adolescents. Am J Cardiol 46:429, 1980.

2. Magilligan DJ, Lewis JW, Jara FM, Lee MW, Alam M, Riddle JM, Stein PD: Spontaneous degeneration of porcine bioprosthetic valves. Ann Thorac Surg 30:259, 1980.
3. Rose AG, Forman R, Bowens RM: Calcification of glutaraldehyde-fixed porcine xenograft. Thorax 33:111, 1978.
4. Oyer PE, Stinson EB, Reitz BA, Miller DC, Rossiter SJ, Shumway NE: Long-term evaluation of the porcine xenograft bioprosthesis. J Thorac Cardiovasc Surg 78:343, 1979.
5. Oyer PE, Miller DC, Stinson EB, Reitz BA, Moreno-Cabral RJ, Shumway NE: Clinical durability of the Hancock porcine bioprosthetic valve. J Thorac Cardiovasc Surg 80:824, 1980.
6. Spray TL, Roberts WC: Structural changes in porcine xenografts used as substitute cardiac valves. Am J Cardiol 40:319, 1977.
7. Ferrans VJ, Spray TL, Billingham ME, Roberts WC: Structural changes in glutaraldehyde-treated porcine xenografts used as substitute cardiac valves. Am J Cardiol 41:1159, 1978.
8. Wain WH, Greco R, Ignegeri A, Bodnar E, Ross DN: 15 years' experience with 615 homograft and autograft aortic valve replacements. Int J Artif Organs 3:169, 1980.
9. Bodnar E, Wain WH, Martelli V, Ross DN: Long-term performance of homograft and autograft valves. Artif Organs 4:20, 1980.
10. Ross DN, Martelli V, Wain WH: Allograft and autograft valves used for aortic valve replacement. In: Biological Tissue Valves, (MI Ionescu, Ed). London, Butterworth, 1979.
11. Ross DN: Replacement of aortic and mitral valve with a pulmonary autograft. Lancet 2:959, 1967.
12. Martelli V, Wain WH, Bodnar E, Ross DN: Mitral valve replacement with dura mater bioprosthesis. Artif Organs 4:163, 1980.
13. Hylen JC: Mechanical malfunction and thrombosis of prosthetic heart valves. Am J Cardiol 30:396, 1972.
14. Rossiter SJ, Stinson EB, Oyer PE, Miller DC, Schapira JN, Martin RP, Shumway NE: Prosthetic valve endocarditis. J Thorac Cardiovasc Surg 76:795, 1978.
15. Oyer PE, Stinson EB, Griepp RB, Shumway NE: Valve replacement with the Starr-Edwards and Hancock prostheses. Ann Surg 186:301, 1977.

SECTION VII

BIOPROSTHETIC BIOENGINEERING

36

The Unileaflet Heart Valve Bioprosthesis: New Concept

S. GABBAY, R. W. M. FRATER

A tanned xenograft pericardial unileaflet valve has been developed and tested in vitro in a pulse duplicator, in a fatigue tester, and in vivo in the mitral position in dogs. It combines the usual resistance to thromboembolism of bioprostheses with: 1) outstanding hemodynamic performance; 2) strut-free mounting system making for ease of use, and 3) an apparent resistance to calcification.

The benefits of a low incidence of thromboembolism without anticoagulants, good hemodynamics in the larger sizes, and reasonable durability have made bioprostheses the valve replacement of choice in many centers.[1–9] Active and successful efforts are being made to improve hemodynamics in the small sizes. Early calcification in children remains a serious problem[10–19] and has led many surgeons to give up the use of bioprostheses in the young. However, the alternative of using mechanical valves and permanent long-term anticoagulation in children, especially children in underdeveloped countries where chronic anticoagulation and long-term follow-up are extremely difficult, presents major drawbacks.

In our efforts to develop a valve that would be suitable for children as well as adults, we have attempted to improve the hemodynamic characteristics, especially for small-sized valves, and to understand the chemical and physical factors of the calcification process. The work has proceeded simultaneously along several paths. Tanned xenograft pericardium has been implanted in various canine cardiac locations. A unileaflet xenograft pericardial valve has been developed in which all movement resides in 1 leaflet. This design has been tested extensively in vitro and in vivo. Chemical treatments to prevent calcification are under trial.

From the Department of Cardiothoracic Surgery, The Albert Einstein College of Medicine and Montefiore Hospital and Medical Center, New York City, New York.

Materials and Methods

The valve, a single leaflet, made of calf pericardium, mounted on a flexible pericardium-covered stent, is shown in Fig. 1 (A, B, and C). The stent is made of Delrin with a wall thickness of 0.5–0.6 mm; it is highly flexible. The stent is entirely covered by tanned pericardium. At the base there is a Dacron sewing ring so designed that it holds the valve up into the atrium in the mitral position and at the ring level for the aortic position. After the bovine pericardium has been treated with glutaraldehyde, additional treatment is used to reduce the space between the collagen fibers in the hope of reducing calcification. The single cusp opens fully, giving a tubular passage for blood flow. Since the thickness of the covered stent is only 1 mm, the ratio between mounting and orifice size is extremely favorable.

Figure 2 illustrates the valve in the mitral position in a dog's heart shown from the inflow and outflow aspects. The absence of struts avoids the

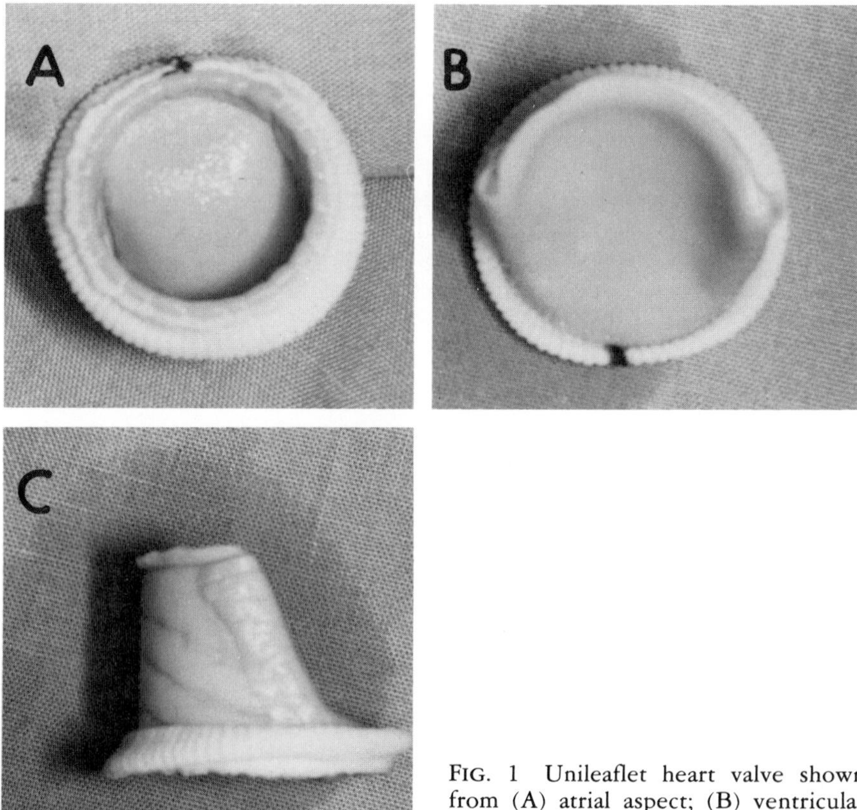

FIG. 1 Unileaflet heart valve shown from (A) atrial aspect; (B) ventricular aspect; (C) side.

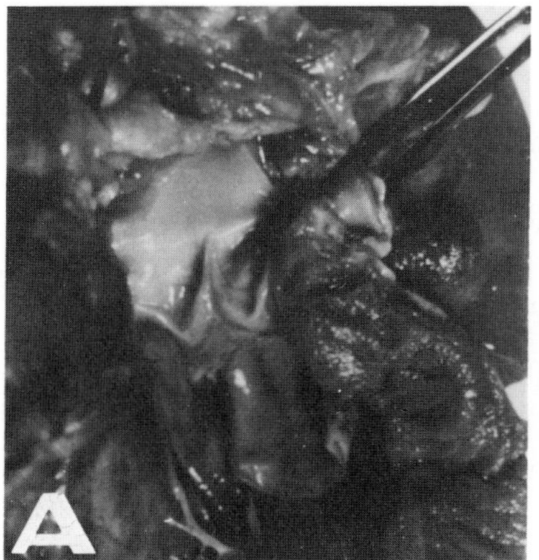

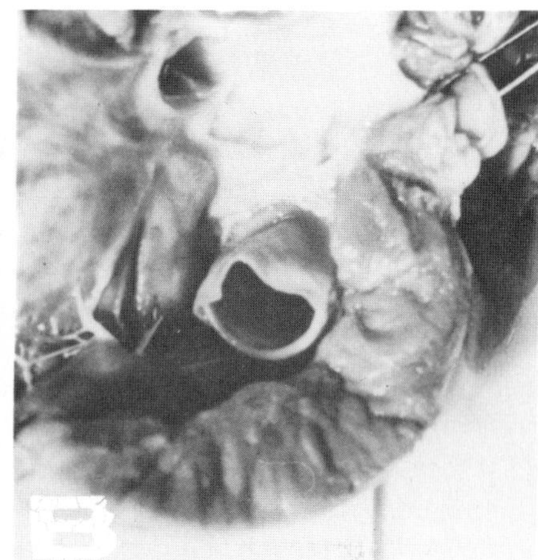

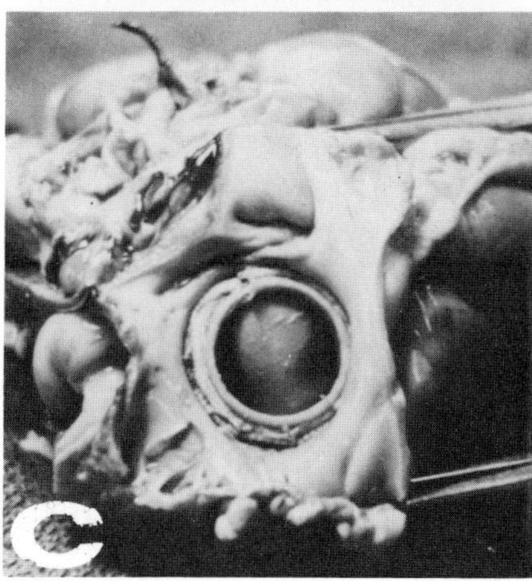

FIG. 2 Valve in mitral position of dog's heart. (A) Ventricular view of closed valve. Note that valve is away from aortic valve. (B) Ventricular view of opened valve. Wide opening of cusp can be appreciated. (C) Atrial view of closed valve.

danger of stent damage of the ventricular wall and leaves the ventricular outflow tract free of potential obstruction. Figure 3 shows the valve in the aortic position. The stent should face the noncoronary cusp to avoid ostial obstruction.

In Vitro Testing

Hemodynamic performance was tested in our pulse duplicator according to the methods we have previously described.[20,21] The valves were studied with pulsatile flow at different stroke volumes and heart rates in the aortic position and mitral position. Effective orifice areas, performance indices, and regurgitant fractions were calculated. Mean gradients were calculated at

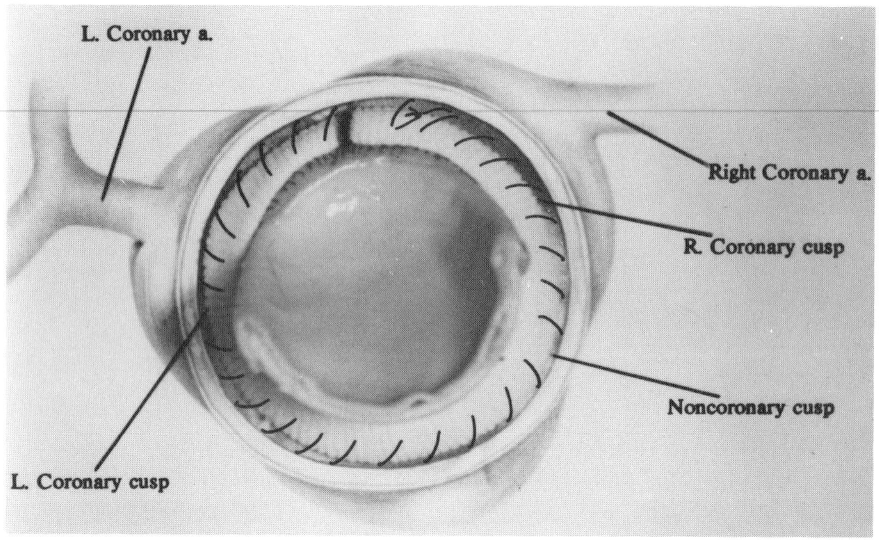

FIG. 3 Schematic view of unileaflet valve in aortic position. Note that stent should face noncoronary cusp.

flows equivalent to "cardiac outputs" of 5, 9, and 13 liters/min to imitate the clinical circumstances of rest and exercise conditions. Valves of mounting sizes 19 to 27 mm were tested at rest and exercise in the pulse duplicator.

Fatigue Testing

In vitro fatigue testing of bioprosthetic heart valves is not, at present, an absolute method to predict the time and mode of failure in vivo.[22,23] There is general agreement that accelerated testing of heart valves can screen defective designs in the development of a new valve. Comparative results can have significance if the different valves are tested in the same fatigue tester under the same conditions. We have developed a fatigue tester with the cooperation of Shelhigh (Hartsdale, NY). This fatigue tester works on the inertia principle, is mechanically very simple, and runs at speeds of 1,600 to 2,500 beats/min, with adjustable physiologic pressures (Fig. 4). It will be fully described elsewhere. Six valves were each tested at 1,800 beats/min in the fatigue tester.

In Vivo Study

The valves were placed in the mitral position in a series of dogs. Despite the tendency for infection, thrombosis, and bleeding in the early post-

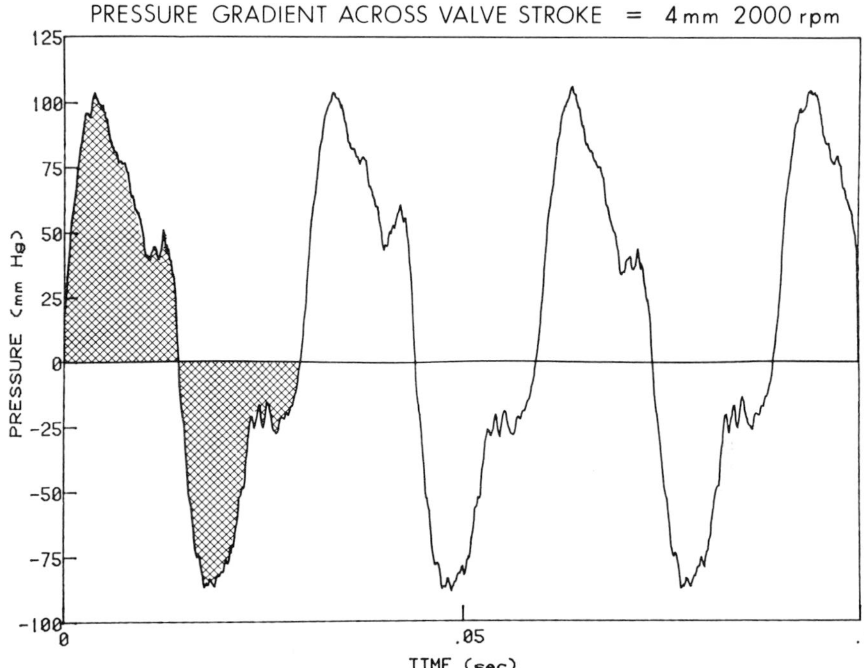

FIG. 4 Curves of pressure gradient across valve in fatigue tester at 2,000 beats/min. These curves show results of pressures measured from inflow and outflow of valve in chamber of fatigue tester.

operative period, described by others as drawbacks of the use of dogs for experimental cardiac surgery (24–28), we have developed routines that allow us to have satisfactory results (to be described elsewhere). In addition, from our experience of implanting xenograft pericardium in various parts of the canine heart and as a substitute for mitral chordae,[29,30] we have found that the rate of calcification in the mitral position is at least similar to, if not more rapid than, that occurring in children. In dogs, we have seen calcification in mitral chordae occurring in 4–12 months, whereas in children, tanned xenograft valves tend to calcify in 15–60 months.[10–11] If a valve does not calcify in the mitral position in dogs, it may well be suitable for children. The natural tachycardia and hypertension (by human standards) of the dog both subject the implanted valve to a severe test. Twenty-one animals underwent mitral valve replacement.

Echocardiography was done at 1 month, 5 months, and at the time of sacrifice to evaluate the excursion of the cusp.

For the in vitro studies, the valves used had mounting sizes 19, 21, 23, 25, and 27 mm. For in vivo implantation, the sizes used had 21 and 23 mm mounting diameters.

The thickness of fibrin deposits and the extent of collagen destruction were evaluated. The presence of infective endocarditis was also evaluated by histology and culture.[27]

Results

The pressure drop (ΔP) across each valve at the time of peak flow was plotted as a function of peak flow (Fig. 5a) for the aortic position and (Fig. 5b) for the mitral position. Table I summarizes the results. As can be seen for the mitral valves, even small valves (21 mm) had relatively little gradient at a "cardiac output" equivalent to 9 liters/min. Sizes 25 mm and larger present very low mean gradients at even higher outputs of 13 liters/min.

A common measure of the hydraulic merit of a valve is its effective orifice area (EOA). Table I shows the EOA based on the best fit through the data for the valve tested. Note the large EOA of the small valves: in our previous studies we found that the 25 mm size of the currently available valves had EOAs from 2.0–2.2 cm^2. Size 21 of the unileaflet has an EOA of approximately 1.90 in the mitral position and 2.13 in the aortic position. All the valves had a larger EOA in the aortic position than in the mitral position ($p < 0.01$).

Performance indices (PI) are shown in Table II. The PI reflects how well the external dimension of a valve is utilized in providing forward flow. The PIs were calculated from the EOA of the mitral and aortic positions. The PIs are from 0.50–0.61. For comparison, the PIs of porcine valves are 0.30 (Hancock) to 0.34 (Carpentier).[20,21]

Although excursion of the cusp is larger than usual, the regurgitant fraction (RF) is quite low, ranging from 0.63–5.8% in the aortic position and 2.5–9.8% in the mitral position (Table II). It is a closing volume and not a regurgitation. As can be seen in Table II, the smaller valves have more RF (closing volume). The difference between the aortic and mitral position can be explained by the closing pressure being higher in the mitral position and lower in the aortic position.

We have tested 6 valves (of the final design) in the accelerated tester for more than 200 million cycles each. There have been no signs of degeneration up to the moment. We are in the process of testing a larger number of valves and comparing them with other bioprostheses.

Animal Studies

Twenty-one dogs underwent mitral valve replacement. Ten deaths in less than 1 month were due to bleeding and infections, most occurring in the early phase of the study. Proper attention to certain procedures, to be described elsewhere, reduces the incidence of these complications. Of the

A

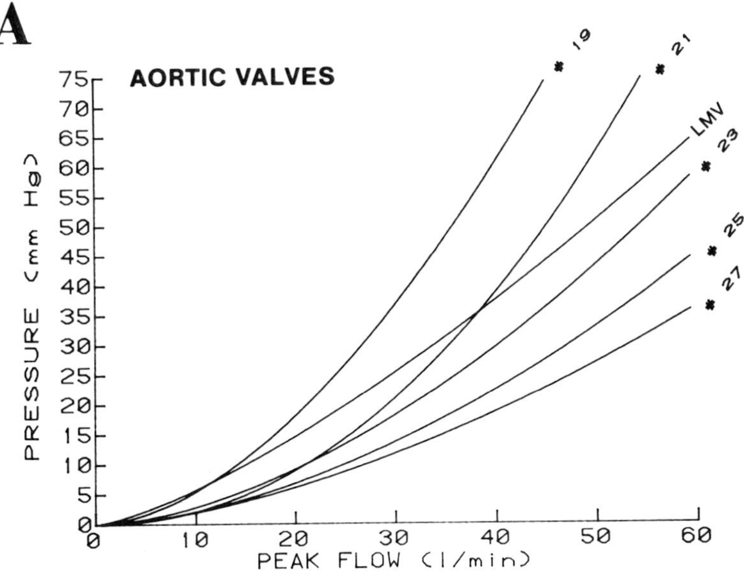

B

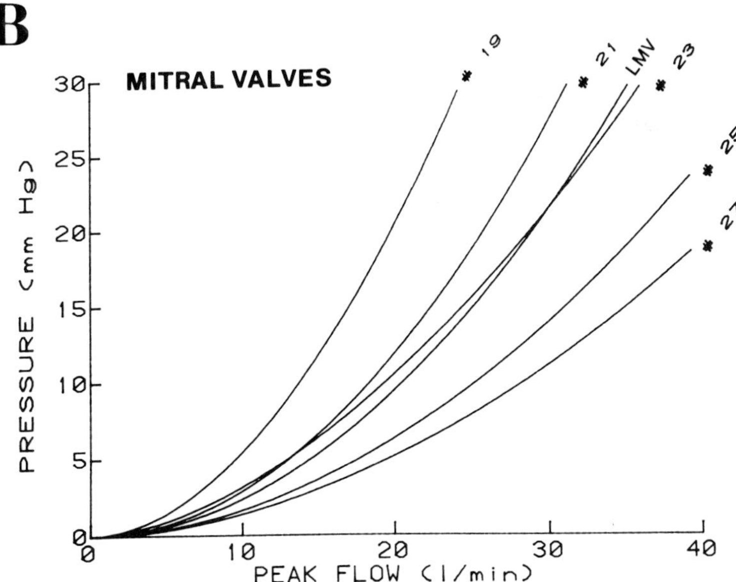

FIG. 5 (A) Peak pressure drops as function of peak flow of different sizes of valve in aortic position, compared with a leading mechanical valve (LMV) of 25 mm mounting diameter. (B) Peak pressure drop versus peak flow in mitral position compared with same mechanical valve (LMV).

TABLE I Effective orifice areas (EOAs) and mean gradients at "cardiac outputs" of 5, 9, and 13 liters/min

	Mitral				Aortic*
Size (mm)	EOAs (cm^2)	5 liters/min	9 liters/min	13 liters/min	EOAs (cm^2)
19	1.44 ± 0.03†	9.1	16.1	41.8	1.66 ± 0.11
21	1.90 ± 0.06	6.8	9.9	24.0	2.13 ± 0.03
23	2.11 ± 0.12	5.8	10.2	22.0	2.39 ± 0.14
25	2.62 ± 0.12	3.6	7.7	21.6	2.80 ± 0.18
27	2.88 ± 0.09	3.0	7.0	16.5	3.03 ± 0.23

* The mean gradient for the aortic position was not calculated.
† ± standard deviation.

11 long-term survivors, 5 remain alive, and 3 have been sacrificed at 6, 7, 13 months (1 after a thromboembolic episode). Two dogs died of endocarditis at 3½ and 2 months. One female dog accidentally became pregnant, and had no difficulty during the pregnancy. Nine months after valve insertion she delivered 13 healthy puppies, but unfortunately was found dead in the morning after delivery. Autopsy showed pulmonary edema and a chronic perivalvular dehiscence of at least 40% of the circumference of the anulus. Presumably with uterine contraction during the third stage of labor there was a sudden overwhelming increase in circulating blood volume (dog #4). This may have led to enlargement of the area of dehiscence. Another female dog (#21), to our surprise, was found to be pregnant 7 weeks after the valve replacement. This animal, which was pregnant at time of surgery, delivered 5 healthy puppies; at present mother and puppies are doing very well.

Six valves have been examined pathologically. In 5 there was no calcium on the moving cusp. In 1 dog dying of endocarditis the cusp showed some calcium on histologic examination. (It is known that biologic valves can

TABLE II Performance indices (PI) and regurgitation fraction (RF*)

	Mitral		Aortic	
Size	PI	RF (%)	PI	RF (%)
19	0.51	2.5	0.58	0.63
21	0.55	5.25	0.61	1.4
23	0.51	5.46	0.57	4.2
25	0.53	5.7	0.57	5.3
27	0.50	9.8	0.53	5.8

* Once the valve is closed the RF is practically nil and it is essentially a closing volume.

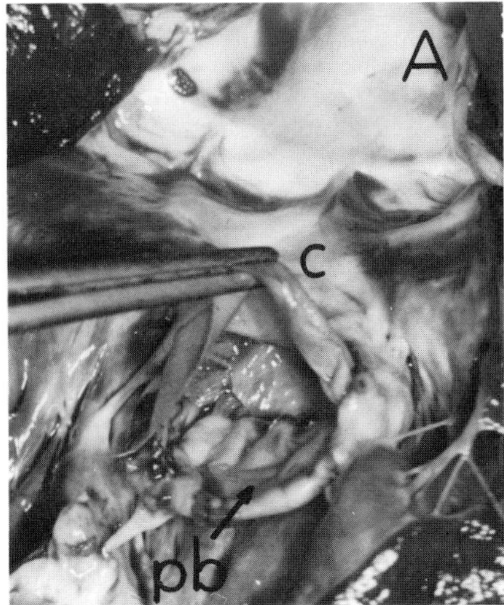

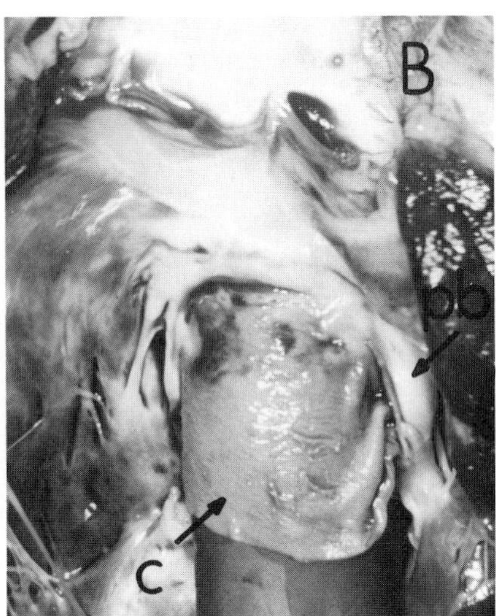

FIG. 6 Valve of dog #1, 13 months after implantation (earlier design). Note soft and clean cusp while nonmoving posterior baffle (PB) is heavily calcified without impairing valve function. (A) Cusp is elevated with forceps. Note that posterior baffle has hardened. (B) Side of PB is thickened. Note that opening of valve is still large.

calcify[31] early if infected). Calcification or chondroplastic metaplasia were found, however, in the nonmoving parts of the pericardium or in the posterior baffle of 3 valves. Figure 6 shows the valve of dog #1 (earlier design). Figure 7 shows the valve of dog #3 sacrificed after 7 months of implantation. The pregnant dog (#4) had calcium on the sewing ring of the valve and on the nonmoving parts of the pericardium. More extensive description of the pathologic and histologic results will be done in a separate publication. Echocardiograms have been done periodically on the long-term survivors and show complete excursion of the valve. Figure 8 shows echocardiograms at 1 month and at the time of sacrifice at 7 months after implantation (dog #3). There is full excursion of the cusp. Follow-up of this valve has been greatly facilitated by the ease of performing echocardiography. The single leaflet is easily recognized and since the opening of the valve is circular, the EOA can be readily measured.

Comment

The hemodynamic performance of bioprostheses is under constant improvement. The monoleaflet valve has excellent hemodynamic characteris-

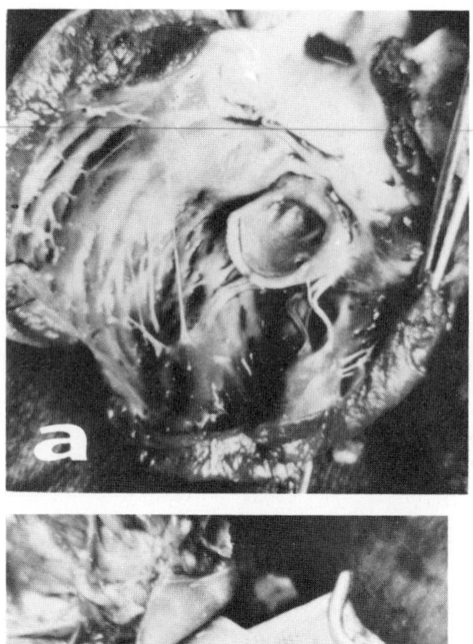

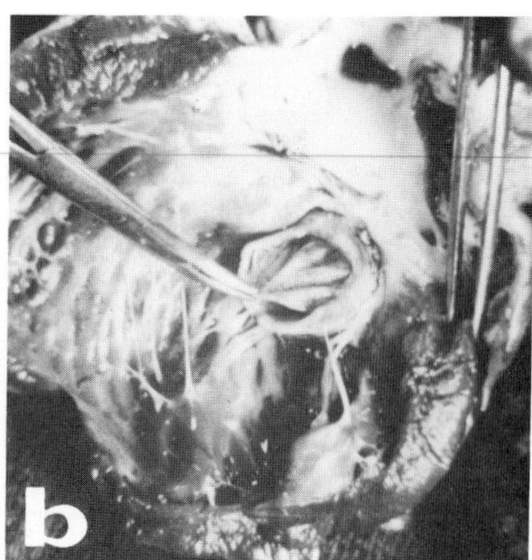

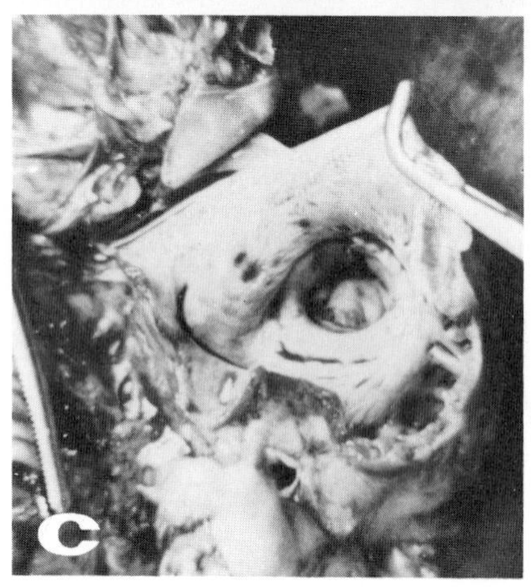

FIG. 7 Valve #3 sacrificed 7 months after implantation. (a) Valve from ventricular aspect. (b) Valve from ventricular aspect. Cusp is elevated with forceps. Note pliable cusp. (c) Valve from atrial aspect. Note perfect healing of anulus. No calcium was found on cusp.

tics; we feel that we are very close to the limit of what ratio can be obtained in terms of optimal internal/external diameter in a valve with a fixed ring. In an earlier experiment the unileaflet was used with a nonrigid prosthetic ring, but this resulted in stenosis because of severe contraction during healing. The diastolic expansion of the natural mitral ring can thus not be reproduced. Fortunately, an area 60% smaller than the maximal orifice area of the natural mitral valve can still allow high flow rates with modest gradients, especially with large valves. (The adult mitral anular area is 9–11 cm^2.[32,33] Indeed, patients with large bioprostheses in the mitral position have good tolerance to exercise.[1,3,5] The early degeneration of bioprostheses in children and young adults is a major concern in their use.[12,15,18,34] Most of the calcified valves have been in the mitral position,[10,11,14] with relatively few occurring in the aortic or tricuspid positions or in valved

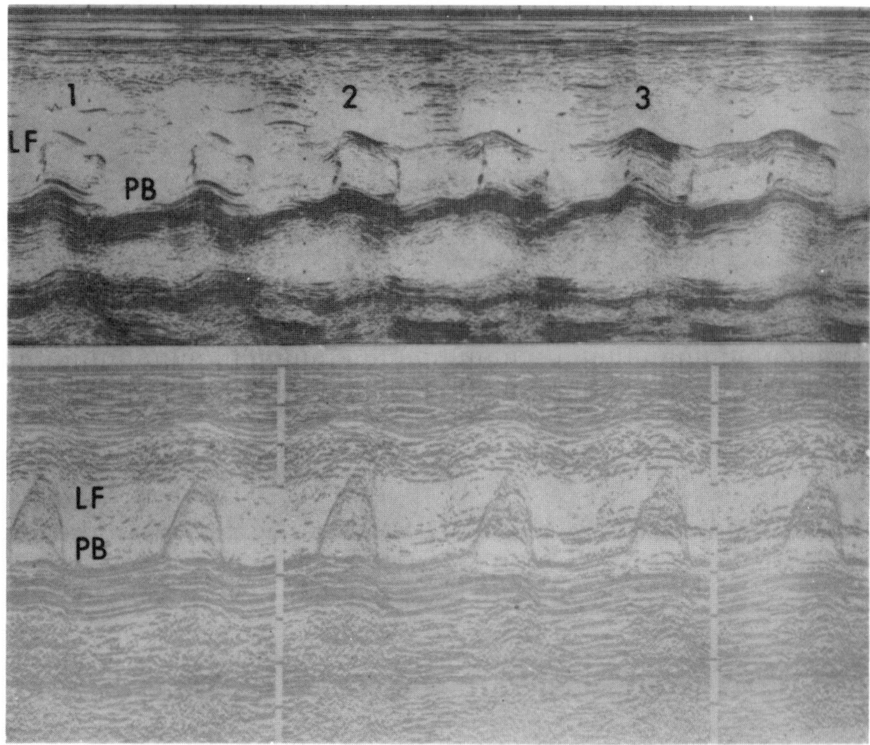

FIG. 8 (above) Echocardiogram of dog #3 taken with chest closed, 1 month after surgery (LF = leaflet, PB = posterior baffle). (below) Echocardiogram of same dog with open chest at time of sacrifice (7 months). Note complete excursion of cusp.

conduits. Of interest is the fact that some surgeons still find it appropriate to replace the calcified valve with another bioprosthesis.[4,16,18]

Mechanism of Calcification

There is no doubt that the high calcium turnover in children plays a critical role in early bioprosthetic calcification, but the mechanism is not clear. Several authors stress the fact that calcified bioprostheses contain large amounts of carboxyglutamic acid (GLA), a calcium-binding amino acid that is found also in calcified natural aortic valves.[10] The calcification is usually considered to be dystrophic, i.e., related to damage in the valve tissue. However, the calcification that is seen in children and that seen in patients on long-term hemodialysis for chronic renal failure have in common a high calcium turnover and may be considered to represent metastatic calcification.[35,36] In dialysis patients there is also calcification of soft tissues.[37] However, despite a classification as metastatic, the calcium in xenografts in such patients may be focally distributed. There clearly must be a host factor in xenograft calcification. Yet, many questions need answering. Why do valves in the mitral position calcify more than in the aortic position and much less commonly than in the tricuspid position or in conduits? The oxygen content of the blood might have some influence on this difference. Alternatively, the difference in pressure on the closed valve might be important: yet, bioprosthetic valvular calcification occurs more quickly and more often in children, who have lower diastolic pressures, than in adults, who have higher systolic pressures. From our experience with this unileaflet valve in dogs, we have concluded that, at least for this design, a large amount of motion in the xenograft tissue appears to protect against calcification, whereas immobility encourages it. We have observed this phenomenon in trileaflet xenograft valves in human beings in whom a cusp has, for one reason or another, been restricted in movement and has undergone calcification. This may be related to the vulnerability to platelet/fibrin deposition. Once the latter has occurred for whatever reason, including infection, then calcification is probably inevitable. There is no doubt about the relationship of infection in xenograft valves in patients and the tendency to calcification[31] and no doubt also that much of the platelet/fibrin thrombus formation seen in dogs is in reality the result of infection.[27] Failure of the unileaflet valve to calcify in the mitral position in the dog is encouraging. It may be that valves of this design have a low tendency to calcify in children. The high performance index also makes this valve a suitable device for children and for replacement of the aortic valve in patients with a small aortic root.

References

1. Lurie AJ, Bryant LE, Schechter FG: Hemodynamic assessment of the glutaraldehyde-preserved porcine heterograft in the aortic and mitral positions. Circulation 56:(Suppl 2):104, 1977.
2. Hetzer R, Hill JD, Kerth WJ, Ansbro J, Adappa MG, Rodvein R, Kamm B, Gerbody R: Thromboembolic complications after mitral valve replacement with Hancock xenograft. J Thorac Cardiovasc Surg 75:651–658, 1978.
3. Tandon AP, Smith DR, Ionescu MI: Hemodynamic evaluation of the Ionescu-Shiley pericardial xenograft in the mitral position. Am Heart J 95:595, 1978.
4. Wada J, Yokoyama M, Hashimoto A, Imai Y, Kitamura N, Takao A, Monna K: Long term follow-up of artificial valves in patients under 15 Years Old. Ann Thorac Surg 29:6, 1980.
5. McIntosh, CL, Michaelis LL, Morrow AG, Itscoitz SB, Redwood DR, Epstein SE: Atrioventricular valve replacement with the Hancock porcine xenograft: A five year clinicial experience. Surgery 78:768, 1975.
6. Ott DA, Coelho AT, Cooley DA, Reul GJ Jr: Ionescu-Shiley pericardial xenograft valve: Hemodynamic evaluation and early clinical follow-up of 326 patients. Cardiovas Dis 7:137, 1980.

7. Ionescu MI, Tandon AP, Mary DAS, Abid A: Heart valve replacement with the Ionescu-Shiley pericardial xenograft. J Thorac Cardiovasc Surg 73:31, 1977.
8. Pipkin RD, Buch WS, Fogarty TJ: Evaluation of aortic valve replacement with a porcine xenograft without long-term anticoagulation. J Thorac Cardiovasc Surg 71:179, 1976.
9. Stinson EB, Griepp RB, Shumway NE: Clinical experience with a porcine aortic valve xenograft for mitral valve replacement. Ann Thorac Surg 18:391, 1974.
10. Sanders SP, Levy RJ, Freed MD, Norwood WI, Castaneda AR: Use of Hancock porcine xenografts in children and adolescents. Am J Cardiol 46:429, 1980.
11. Thandroyen FR, Whitton IN, Duncan P, Rogers MA, Mitha AS: Severe calcification of glutaraldehyde-preserved porcine xenografts in children. Am J Cardiol 45:690, 1980.
12. Silver, MM, Pollock J, Silver MD, Williams WG, Trusler GA: Calcification of porcine xenografts in children. Am J Cardiol 45:685, 1980.
13. Geha AS, Laks H, Stansel HC, Cornhill JF, Kilman JW, Buckley MJ, Roberts WC: Late failure of porcine valve heterografts in children. J Thorac Cardiovasc Surg 78:351, 1979.
14. Ferrans VJ, Spray TL, Billingham ME, Roberts WC: Structural changes in glutaraldehyde-treated porcine heterografts used as substitute cardiac valves. Am J Cardiol 41:1159, 1978.
15. Ferrans VJ, Boyce SW, Billingham ME, Jones M, Ishihara T, Roberts WC: Calcific deposits in porcine bioprosthesis, structure and pathogenesis. Am J Cardiol 46:721, 1980.
16. Galloti FM Jr, Midgley FM, Shapiro SR, Perry LW, Ciaravella JM Jr, Scott LP: Mitral valve replacement in infants and children. Pediatrics 67:230, 1981.
17. Sade R, Ballenger JF, Hohn AR, Arrants JE, Riopel DA, Taylor AB: Cardiac valve replacement in children. Comparison of tissue with mechanical prostheses. J Thorac Cardiovasc Surg 78:123, 1979.
18. Hellberg K, Ruschewski W, de Vivie ER: Early stenosis and calcification of glutaraldehyde-preserved porcine xenografts in children. Thorac Cardiovasc Surg 29:369, 1981.
19. Williams JB, Karp RB, Kirklin JW, Kouchoukos NT, Pacifico AD, Zorn, GL Jr, Blackstone EH, Brown RN, Piantadosi S, Bradley EL: Considerations in selection and management of patients undergoing valve replacement with glutaraldehyde-fixed porcine bioprostheses. Ann Thorac Surg 30:247, 1980.
20. Gabbay S, McQueen DM, Yellin EL, Becker RM, Frater RWM: In vitro hydrodynamic comparison of the mitral valve prostheses at high flow rates. J Thorac Cardiovasc Surg, 76:771, 1978.
21. Gabbay S, McQueen DM, Yellin EL, Frater RWM: In vitro hydrodynamic comparison of mitral valve bioprostheses. Circulation 60 (Suppl 2):17, 1978.
22. Clark RE, Swanson WM, Kardos JL, Hagen RW, Beauchamp RA: Durability of prosthetic heart valves. Ann Thorac Surg 26:323, 1978.
23. Steinmetz GP Jr, May KJ Jr, Aueller V, Anderson HN, Merendino KA: An improved accelerated fatigue machine and pulse simulator for testing and developing prosthetic cardiac valves. J Thorac Cardiovasc Surg 47:186, 1964.
24. Williams WG, Kent G, Gunning AJ, Salt R, Spratt EH: Technique for cardiopulmonary bypass in the goat. Can. J. Surg. 19:254, 1976.
25. Baird RJ, Williams WG, Spratt EH, Cohoon WJ: Experimental homograft replacement of mitral valve. Can J Surg 12:144, 1969.
26. Fletcher WS, Rogers AL, Donaldson SS: Use of goat as experimental animal. Lab Anim Care 14:65, 1964.
27. Jones RD, Aksao M, Cross FS: Bacteremia and thrombus accumulation on prosthetic heart valves in the dog. J Surg Res 9:93, 1969.

28. Aasen AO, Resch F, Semb BJ, Dale J, Stadskleiv K, Lilleaasen P, Froysaker T: Development of a canine model for long-term studies after mitral valve replacement with the Hall-Kaster prosthesis. Eur Surg Res 12:199, 1980.
29. Shore D, Gabbay S, Yellin E, Frater RWM: Replacement of the anterior chordae of the mitral valve. Thorax 36:75, 1981.
30. Frater RWM, Gabbay S, Shore D, Strom J: Reproducible shortening and replacement of mitral valve chordae. Presented at the 19th Annual Meeting of the Society of Thoracic Surgeons, New Orleans, La., January 11–13, 1982.
31. Williams EH, Conti VR, Nishimura A, Stout LC, Ferrans V: Early calcific stenosis of aortic and mitral Ionescu-Shiley valves in a patient with bioprosthetic infection. J Thorac Cardiovasc Surg 82:391, 1981.
32. Rahlf G: Relative AV-insufficiency. Morphometric and morphologic investigation of the AV-valve apparatus. Thorac Cardiovasc Surg 29:338, 1981.
33. Ormiston JA, Shah PM, Tei C, Wong M: Size and motion of the mitral valve annulus in man. I. A two-dimensional echocardiographic method and findings in normal subjects. Circulation 64:113–120, 1981.
35. Lamberti JJ, Wainer BH, Fisher KA, Karunaraine HB, Al-Sadir J: Calcific stenosis of the porcine heterograft. Ann Thorac Surg 28:28, 1979.
36. Fishbein MC, Gissen SA, Collins JJ, Barsamian EM, Cohn LH: Pathologic findings after cardiac valve replacement with glutaraldehyde-fixed porcine valves. Am J Cardiol 40:331, 1977.
37. Kuzela DC, Huffer WE, Conger JD, Winter SD, Hammond WS: Soft tissue calcification in chronic dialysis patients. Am J Pathol 86:403, 1977.

37

Hancock II—An Improved Bioprosthesis

J. T. M. Wright, C. E. Eberhardt, M. L. Gibbs, T. Saul, C. B. Gilpin

Glutaraldehyde-fixed porcine bioprostheses first became commercially available in February 1970. Since that time, approximately 130,000 valves have been supplied to surgical centers in the United States, Europe, and other parts of the world. Initially the porcine tissue, fixed by the stabilized glutaraldehyde process, was mounted in rigid metal stents, but in 1971 a flexible polypropylene-stented valve was introduced.[1] The rationale for the flexible stent was to reduce the shock loading and hence stress level on the tissue during closure, and thus improve the longevity of the valve. As the surgical demand for the porcine valve grew, it became necessary to increase production rapidly. One method was to improve yield, and so the stent post profile was raised so that a slightly higher (but still small) percentage of valve tissue could be mounted in the stents.

Whereas the earlier formalin-fixed valves had been processed in a semirelaxed state by merely packing the cusps with rayon during fixation, the glutaraldehyde-processed valves were fixed at near physiologic pressures. This method produces well-formed valves with good coaptive properties, but requires highly skilled operators to produce cosmetically pleasing and functional bioprostheses, mainly because of the asymmetric shape of the valve tissue and the effects of the septal shelf associated with the right coronary cusp. This muscle bar (formed from the ventricular myocardium of the outflow tract) generally occupies a significant portion of the right coronary leaflet; it reduces the flow area of the valve and produces cosmetic disadvantages. However, testing has shown that valves produced by other laboratories, in which the cosmetic effects of the muscle bar have been minimized, possess no significant flow advantages.

During 1977 the modified orifice valve was introduced. In this valve the

From Hancock/Extracorporeal, Inc., Anaheim, California, and California State University, Long Beach, California.

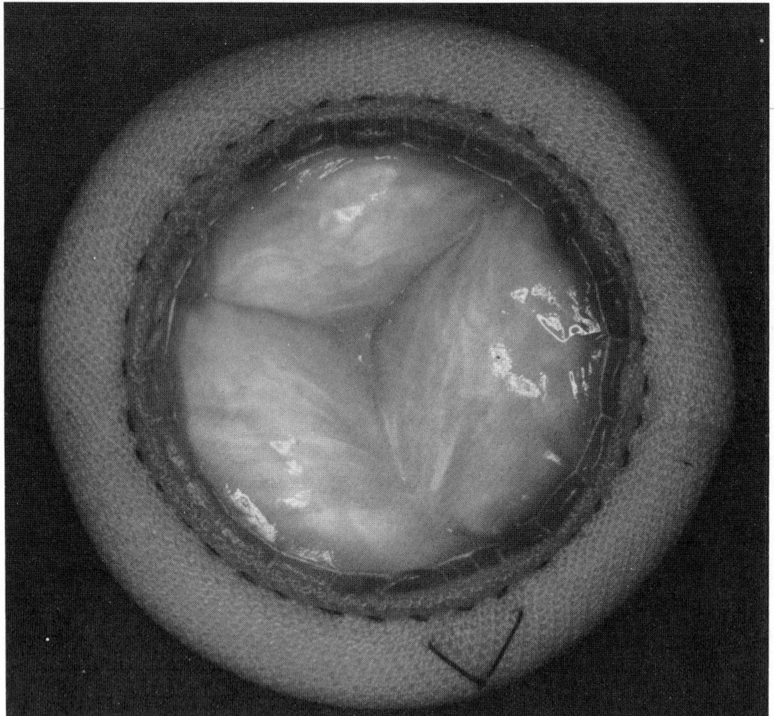

FIG. 1 Inflow aspect of a Hancock II mitral valve.

right coronary cusp was excised and replaced by the noncoronary cusp from a larger porcine valve. Extensive flow testing of the modified orifice valves demonstrated a 1 size advantage of flow area over that in conventional porcine valves. The modified orifice valve minimized one of the disadvantages of the standard porcine valve—adverse hydrodynamics in the small aortic root, but an increased stent post profile was necessary to accommodate the leaflet segment. However, a more serious drawback of tissue valves has generally emerged, in that durability is variable due to intrinsic calcification in certain patients, particularly children.[2]

To address these characteristics and to provide better surgical convenience features, an improved porcine bioprosthesis has been developed (Fig. 1). The integration of a newly developed fixation technique and a new stent form of different material results in a prosthesis with improved hydrodynamics and durability, a lower profile, and surgical advantages. These, combined with a calcification retardant[3] treatment, should result in a range of porcine bioprostheses with significant advantages to patients and surgeons alike.

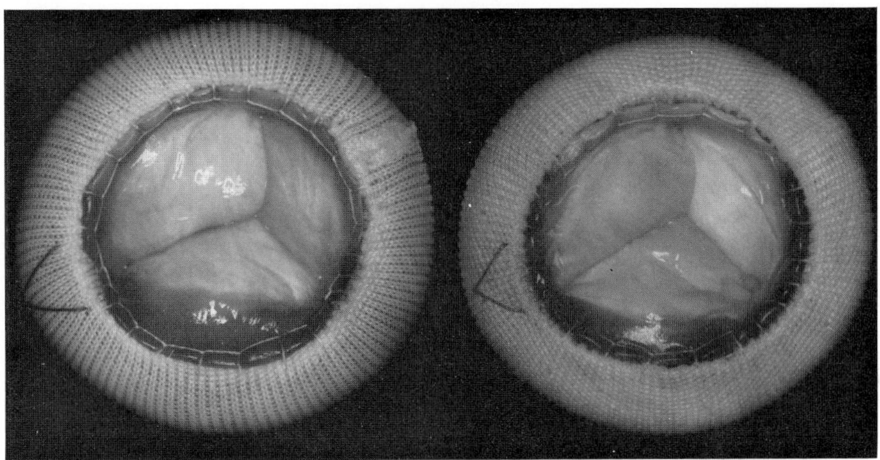

FIG. 2 Typical examples of (left) Hancock 342 mitral valve manufactured in 1978 and (right) similar valve manufactured in 1981. Note that the septal shelf has been reduced by improved tissue selection.

Fixation Technique

The appearance and effects of the septal shelf in the right coronary cusp of commercially produced porcine valves varies from valve to valve, depending upon the selection criteria and the shape of the stent. For example, Fig. 2 shows a typical Hancock 342 valve manufactured in 1978 with a moderately sized septal shelf. As quality assurance criteria developed, the acceptable size of the septal shelf was gradually reduced, as also shown in Fig. 2, which illustrates a typical Hancock 342 valve manufactured in 1981. Although the septal shelf had been reduced, it had not been eliminated. This raised the question, was the presence of the septal shelf in fixed valves due to the anatomy of the pig, or was it an artifact of the fixation method? A series of fixation experiments was undertaken and revealed that it was possible to fix valves without a septal shelf that extended into the valve orifice.

Meanwhile, the advantageous effects of fixing the valve leaflets at less than 2 mmHg had been demonstrated by Broom and Thomson.[4] These leaflets showed improved in vitro fatigue resistance.[5] Primary tissue failure due to tissue fatigue has seldom been reported with the Hancock valve. However, this may have been because durability is usually limited by intrinsic calcification. Thus, should an effective calcium retardant treatment be used, then the long-term fatigue resistance of the collagen would become an even more important factor in valve longevity.

Following the earlier experiments, a new fixation technique has been developed that results in the septal shelf being effectively eliminated from the valve orifice without resorting to a composite valve. In the new technique the leaflets are fixed at 1½ mmHg, thus ensuring retention of collagen crimp and providing improved valve geometry. Fig. 3 shows a typical example of a porcine valve fixed by the new method. Note that the orifice is circular in cross-section and the leaflets have good coaptation and appearance. This technique ensures that the architectural capabilities of the porcine valve are fully exploited with regard to fatigue resistance and hydrodynamic performance.

Stent

The polypropylene stent has proved to be acceptable over a 10 year period as a clinically effective support mechanism for the Hancock valve. The inflow aspects of the stents were made rigid by the incorporation of a metallic radiographic marker ring, and aortic and mitral valves were differ-

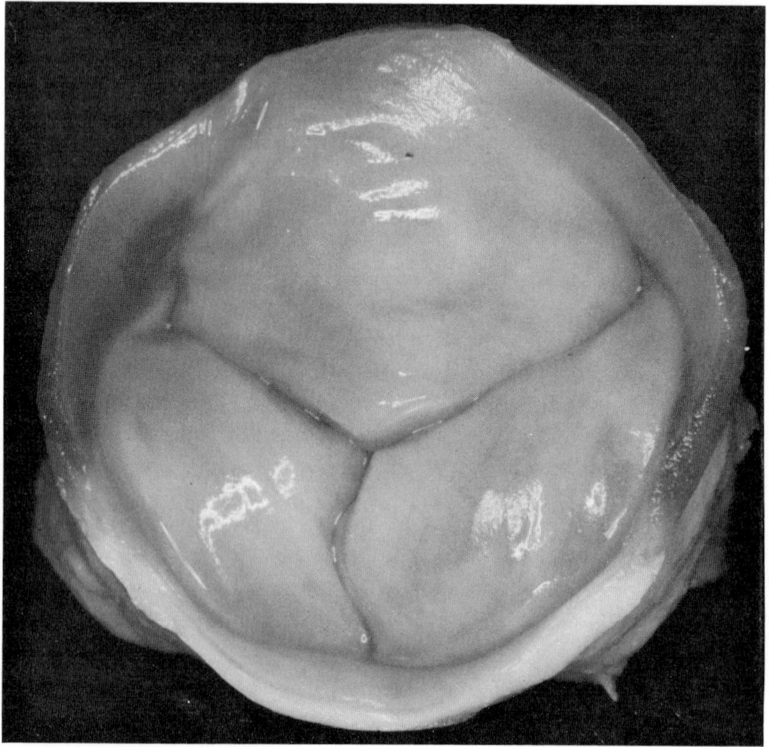

FIG. 3 Porcine valve fixed by the new fixation method.

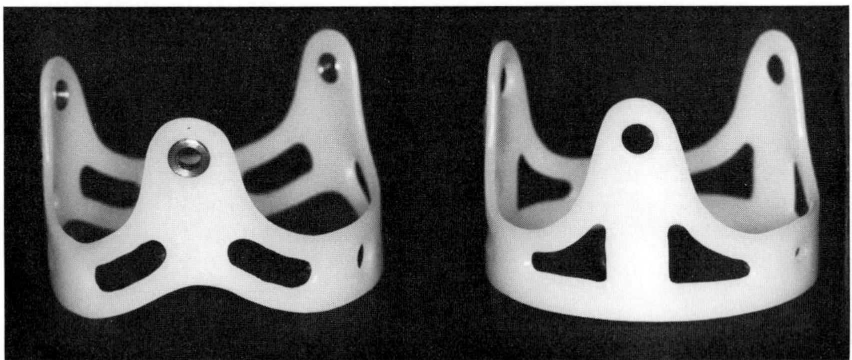

FIG. 4 Stents of the Hancock II. (Left) Aortic stent, (Right) mitral stent. Radiographic markers are not shown on mitral stent.

entiated mainly by the sewing ring configuration. The design was such that the stressed members of the stent were relatively small in width and thick in cross-section. This, coupled with the noncircular form of the coronary outflow rails and the mechanical properties of polypropylene, led to a stent with a less than ideal ratio of inside to outside diameter. Additionally, inward migration of the polypropylene stent posts has occasionally been observed.[6–8] This may be caused by the use of an oversized valve in a patient, the effects of tissue ingrowth in the stent cloth, or to creep of the polypropylene stent.

In designing the stent of the Hancock II valve, the advantageous features of the clinically proved polypropylene stent and covering techniques, combined with those of the low pressure-fixed tissue, and other valve experiences were incorporated with several novel features.

The new stents of the aortic and mitral valves (Fig. 4) are constructed from acetal resin (Delrin), a material with excellent fatigue, tensile, and creep properties. Delrin was successfully used for the occluder disc of the early series of Björk-Shiley mechanical heart valves[9] and the stent for the Angell-Shiley porcine bioprosthesis.[10] The higher stiffness modulus, and the tensile, fatigue, and creep characteristics of Delrin relative to polypropylene made it possible to reduce significantly the wall thickness of the new stents compared to those in Hancock models 242, 250, and 342 made from polypropylene. However, the flexibility of the stent posts was not significantly changed, since it proved to be clinically successful. The reduced wall thickness of the Hancock II stent allows the fitting of a larger porcine valve with a consequential increase in effective orifice area. The profile of the Hancock II stent is 2 mm lower than that of the polypropylene stent.

In the aortic valve configuration, the inflow aspect of the stent is profiled to conform closely to the natural anulus, whereas in the mitral valve the inflow aspect is flat for the same reason. Titanium radiopaque markers are placed close to the apex of the stent posts to allow radiographic visualization of the relationship of the stent posts both to one another and to the aortic or ventricular wall where this should be in question. The asymmetrical configuration of the commissure posts corresponds to the normal anatomy of the valve leaflets. The stents are covered with a Dacron knitted polyester fabric, and the suture ring of the mitral valves contains polyester felt, which provides a resilient cushion with low needle penetration and suture drag forces. The aortic valves are fitted with scalloped sewing rings, which enable the valves to be mounted within the anulus or in the supra-anular position. Thus, in some circumstances larger aortic valves may be used, and they may be especially beneficial in the case of patients with an abnormally small aortic root.

Stiffness of Stent

One important criterion in designing the Hancock II stent was to match closely the force/deflection characteristics of the stent posts with those of the Hancock 250 modified orifice valve and the 242/342 standard valve stents. This was done because these characteristics had proved to give good clinical results, with a low incidence of primary tissue failure.[11]

The test method to evaluate the stiffness characteristics used a 3 lever system that simultaneously applied a force normal to each of the 3 stent posts. The Instron testing machine measured the mean force/displacement characteristics of the stent. The results are shown in Fig. 5.

Statistically each of the sizes of Hancock II stent has force/displacement characteristics within 12.5% of those of Hancock 250, 242/342 stents of the same size at a confidence level of 99%. Therefore the tissue loading characteristics of the new porcine valve are substantially equivalent to those of the Hancock 250 and 242/342 valves.

Finite Stress Analysis

A comprehensive finite stress analysis of the mitral and aortic stents was carried out using MCAUTO model generation package Fastdraw 3, and ANSYS (Swanson Analysis Systems Inc.) finite element analysis package.

The computer model was used to determine stent post stiffness, the stress contours, and the maximum stress levels. Mitral stents 27 and 33 mm and aortic stent 27 mm mounting diameter were modeled.

The procedure was done in 3 steps. Step 1 consisted of laying out the boundaries as a flat pattern in 2 dimensions. Next the mesh was added.

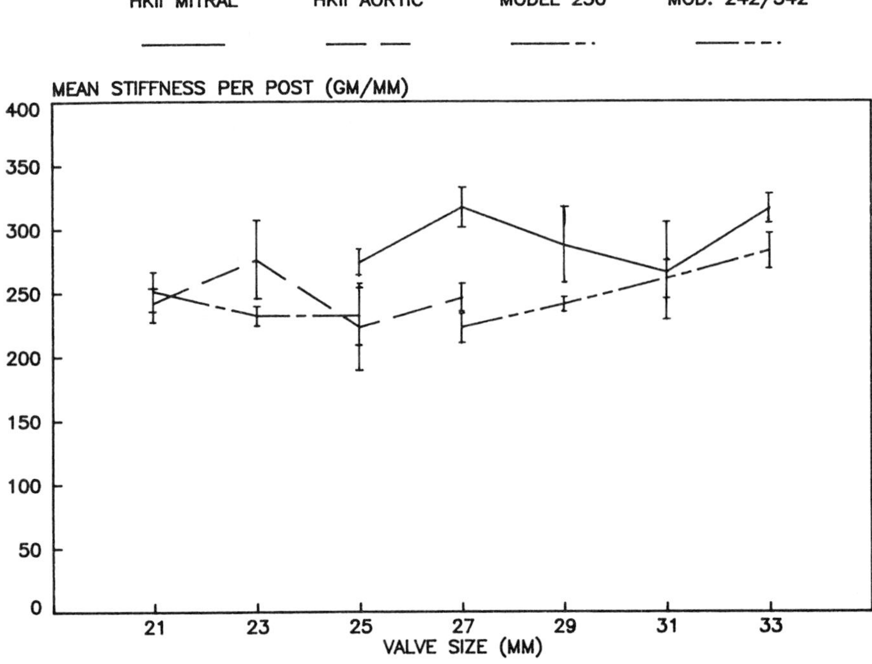

FIG. 5 Stent post force/displacement characteristics of Hancock 250 and 242/342 and Hancock II mitral and aortic valves.

When meshing the 3-dimensional (3-D) stent as a flat pattern, it was necessary to insure that the mesh was generated in such a way that all elements had at least 1 side that was parallel to the Z axis in the 3-D model and that a row of elements aligned in the Z direction had the same width. The flat pattern was then transposed into cylindrical coordinates so that the Z direction remained the same and the X direction, parallel to the base, was transposed into r, θ (Fig. 6). This ensured that no warping occurred in the model as a result of transposition.

The analysis system chosen for this model was ANSYS. "STIF 63" was used to model the Delrin stent, a quadrilateral shell element consisting of 4 nodes, each with 6 degrees of freedom. The element was used with both the extra displacement shapes and Zienkiewicz in-plant rotation options, active.

The mitral models consisted of 1085 nodes, 961 "STIF 63" elements, and 24 "STIF 4" elements. The aortic modeling procedure was similar to that used on the mitral model but elements were refined in the higher stress areas. The final model consisted of 896 nodes and 778 elements.

The forces exerted by the valve tissue on the stent are complex. Therefore it was necessary to lump the action of the tissue into a set of boundary

AORTIC MODEL

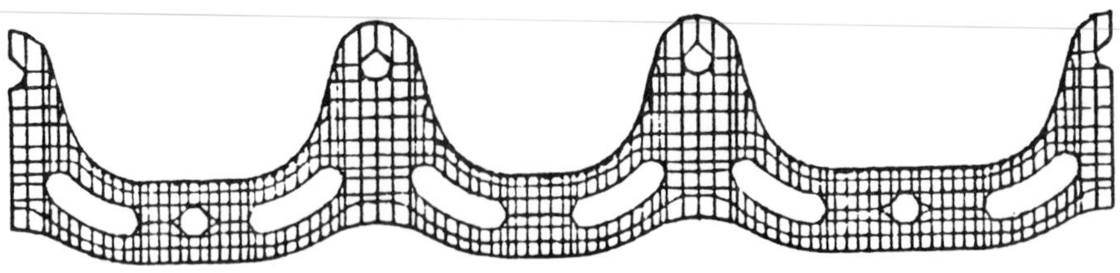

FLAT PATTERN

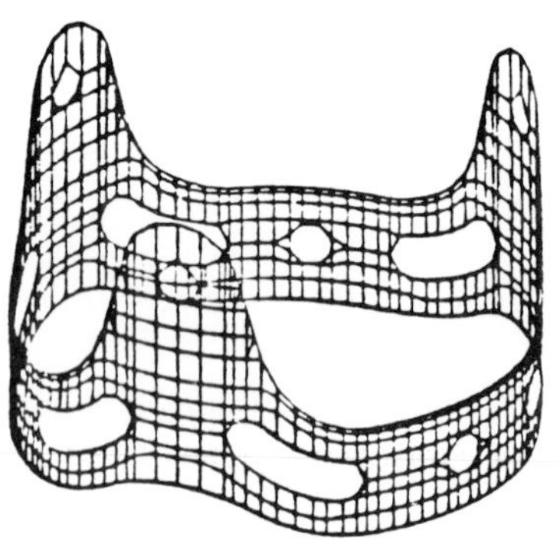

FINAL MODEL

FIG. 6 Flat pattern and final model used for finite element stress analysis of aortic stent.

conditions that would give a simplified but conservative approximation of the tissue forces on the stent. The following assumptions were used:

1. The peak load seen by the stent arises from the back pressure across the valve while it is closed.
2. The load is not distributed around the perimeter of the cusp, but acts as a point load whose action is along the coaptive ridge and is distributed among the 3 posts.
3. The load is transferred to each post in proportion to the area of cusps it supports and the center of coaption is concentric within the stent.

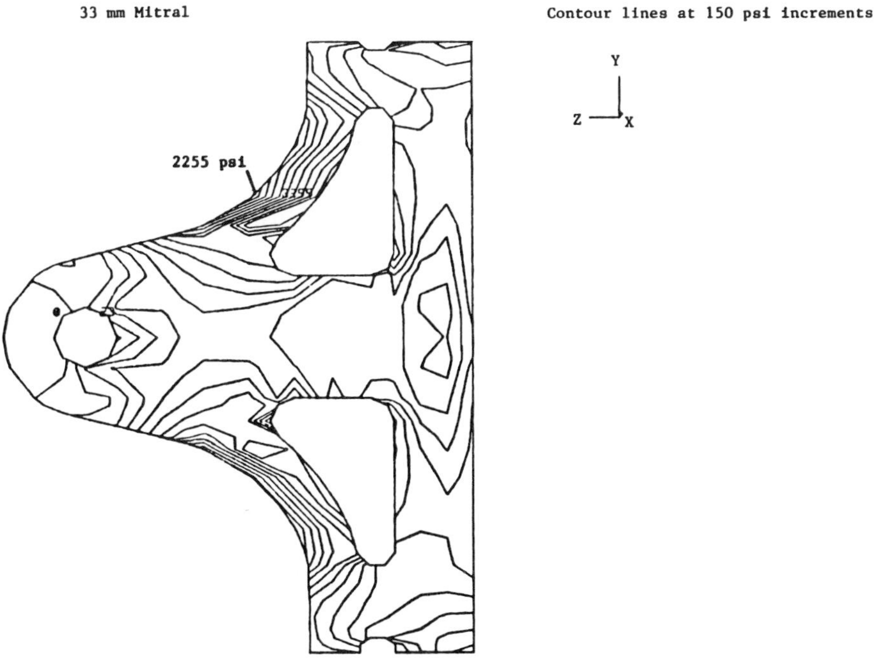

33 mm Mitral

Contour lines at 150 psi increments

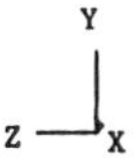

2255 psi

FIG. 7 Stress contours for LR posts of 33 mm mitral stents.

4. The commissures have angular orientations of 135° (right), 120° (left), 105° (noncoronary), which corresponds to the stent posts.
5. The valve will be mounted so that the point of attachment of the coaptive ridge will be centered in the radiopaque eyelet; the force at the commissure was applied at a vertical angle of 60° which corresponds to the angle of the main fiber reinforcement of the porcine leaflet.

The stent force/displacement predictions of the computer model agreed closely with those measurements made on actual stents (within 12%). This finding enhanced our confidence in the model and subsequent results.

The maximum local stress levels found were 2,069 psi for the 27 mm mitral and 2,255 psi for the 33 mm mitral (Fig. 7), both with a back pressure of 120 mmHg. Under a back pressure of 100 mmHg, the 27 mm aortic valve had a maximum stress of 2,021 psi (Fig. 8). These figures all represent worst case equivalent nodal stresses, since the more distributed loading characteristics found in actual valves should produce lower stresses. This notwithstanding, the stress levels predicted by the computer model were well within the mechanical properties of Delrin 500 with regard to fatigue limit, strain, tensile strength, and creep characteristics.

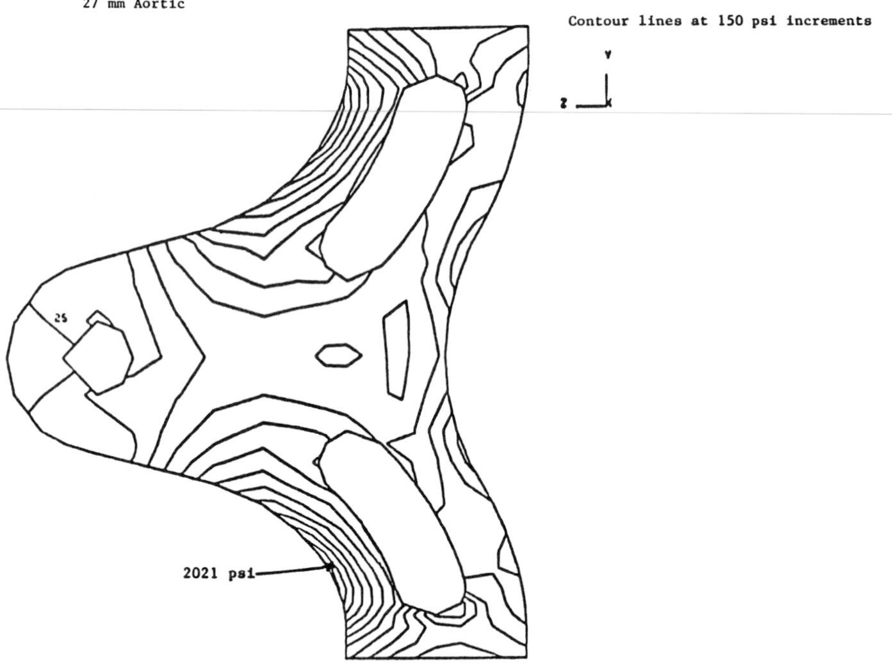

FIG. 8 Stress contours for LR post of 27 mm aortic stent.

Static Creep of Cloth-Covered Stents

Creep tests were performed on 27 mm cloth-covered 342R stents (made of polypropylene) and Hancock II stents (made of Delrin). The stents were pushed into a snug fit cylindrical fixture that prevented any circular deformation as the stent post was loaded. Only the LR post was loaded. For the 342R stent, load was applied by looping a stiff wire around the end of the post through the cloth. For the Hancock II stent, the wire was pushed through the cloth and the titanium radiographic marker. Loads of 20, 40, and 80 g were applied to the free end of the wire. These loads were chosen to bracket the expected deflection due to service load.

The test fixtures were loaded into ATS creep frames and the temperature maintained at 37 ± 0.5°C. Measurements of deflection with time were recorded, using a measuring cathetometer accurate to ±0.01 mm. The total deflection of the stents with time is shown in Figs. 9 and 10. Figure 11 gives the creep deflection data. Creep deflection was determined by subtracting initial deflection from total deflection. It can be seen that the Delrin stents had enhanced creep resistance.

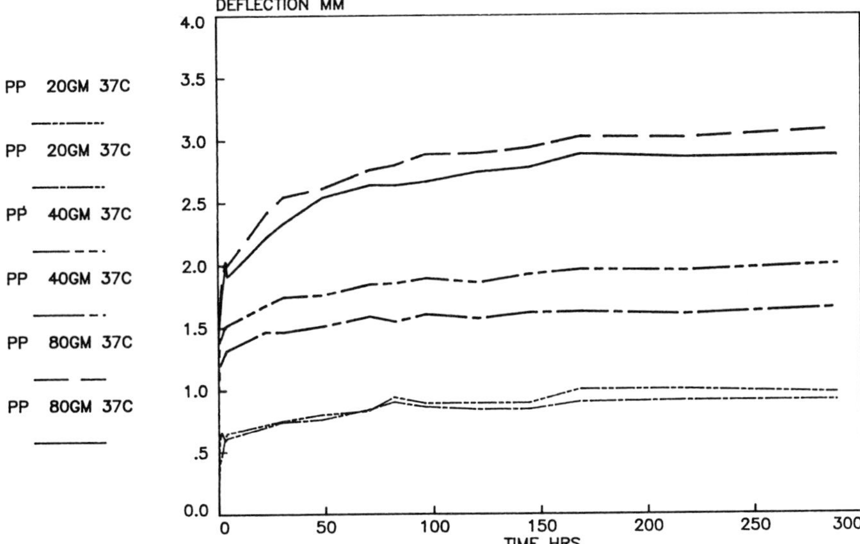

FIG. 9 Deflection under static load for 27 mm polypropylene covered stent.

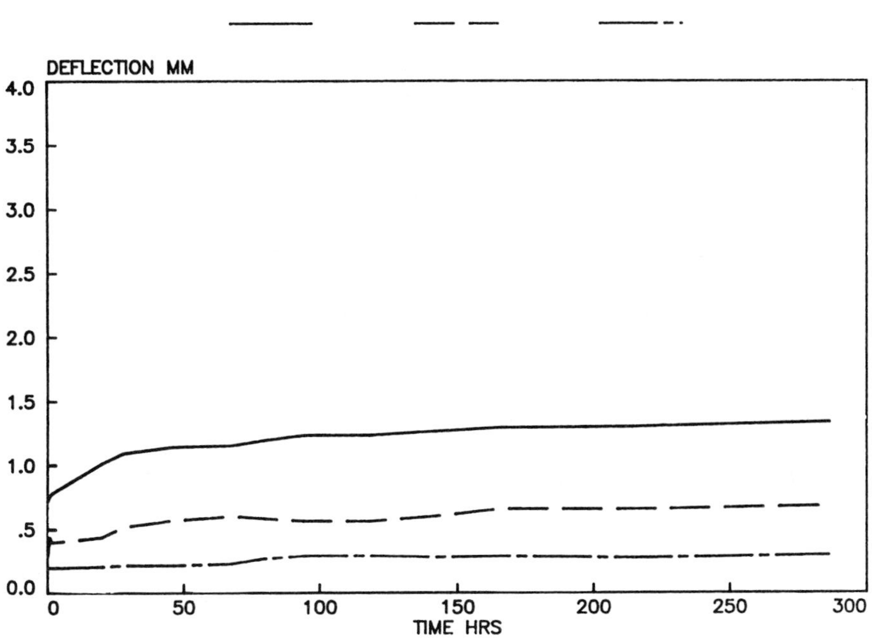

FIG. 10 Deflection under static load for 27 mm Delrin Hancock II covered stent.

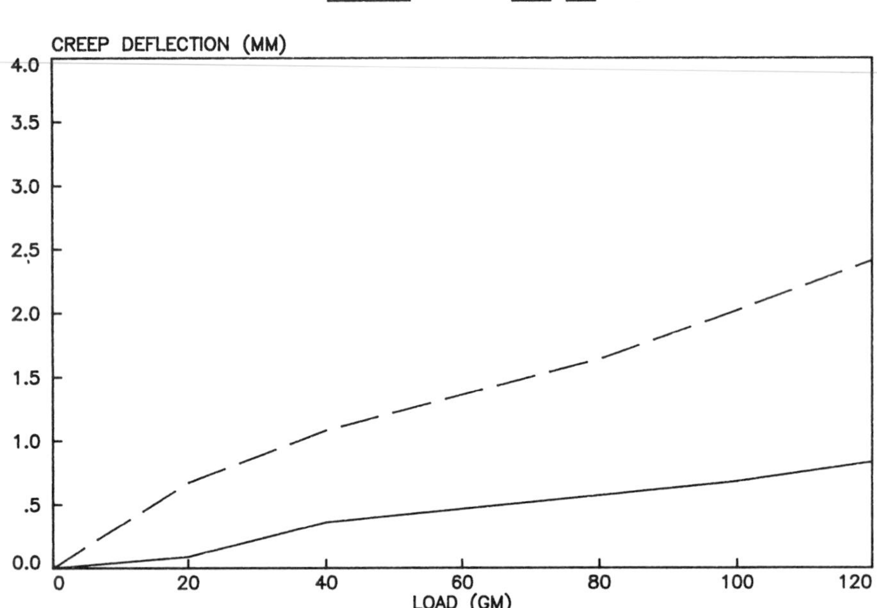

FIG. 11 Creep deflection of cloth-covered 27 mm Delrin and polypropylene stents at 137 hours and 37°C.

Static Creep of Polypropylene and Delrin

Creep tests were performed on American Society for Testing Materials (ASTM) standard flat dog bone specimens. The specimen was a 2 inch gauge length with a nominal cross-section of 0.122 × 0.513 inches. Tests were performed on ATS creep machines with ATS transducer extensometers. The extensometers provided continuous data that are plotted on strip chart Perkin-Elmer recorders. Temperature was controlled at 37 ± 0.5°C, 45 ± 0.5°C, and 55 ± 0.5°C. Specimens were run at 3 temperatures in order to determine the temperature shift factor for 10 year creep prediction. Specimens were tested with induced tensile stresses of 2,000, 1,000, and 500 psi. Most data were terminated at 300 hours but samples at 37°C and 1,000 psi were run in excess of 1,000 hours.

A typical result is shown in Fig. 12, in which strain is plotted against time at stress levels of 500, 1,000, and 2,000 psi at 37°C for Delrin and polypropylene. It may be seen that Delrin at 2,000 psi behaves similarly to polypropylene at 500 psi. This finding was repeated at 45 and 55°C.

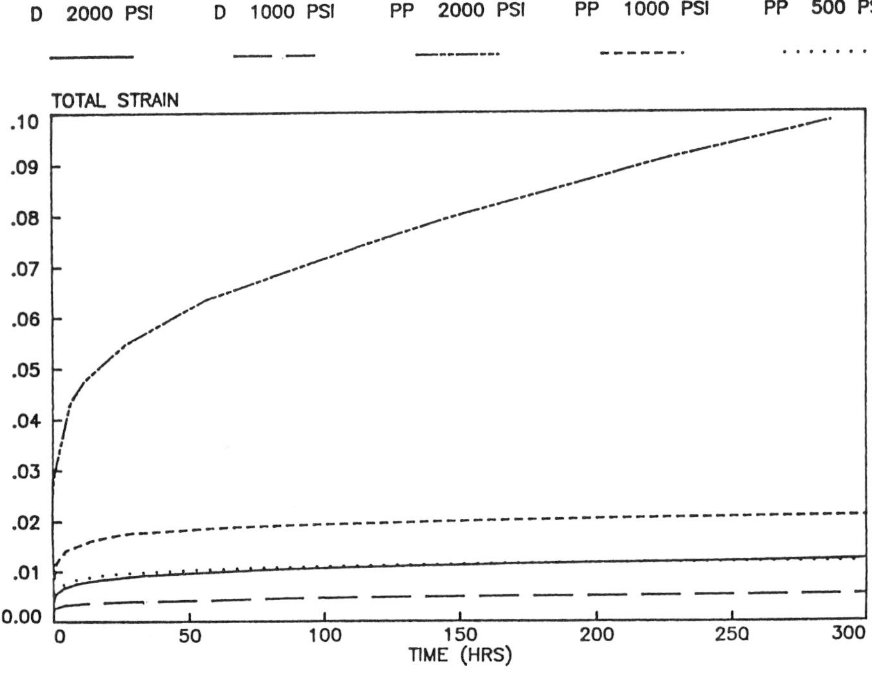

FIG. 12 Total strain of ASTM dog bone Delrin and polypropylene specimens under static loading.

Dynamic Creep of Polypropylene and Delrin

Dynamic creep (fatigue) tests were performed on the same type samples as used for static creep. All testing to date was done at 37°C at 1 Hz with R = 0.1 and R = 0.01. R is the ratio of minimum to maximum applied stress. For R = −1, samples were machined from bars with 0.5 inch gauge length and 0.5 inch diameter. Testing was performed in a model 810 MTS closed loop hydraulic test machine. All testing was under load control using sinusoidal loading. Data were taken by a digital data acquisition system. The data accumulated were of several types. One was to determine the maximum and minimum strains for each fatigue cycle and to relate this to time (similar in form to static creep but determined under dynamic conditions). The second was to determine creep compliance in the first second (i.e., from 1 Hz) as it was affected by the number of fatigue cycles. These data were collected at the end of 1, 10, 100, 1,000, and higher cycles. The third was to determine the effect of temperature in order to determine a temperature shift factor for dynamic creep.

One of the main purposes of this study was to predict long-term (10 year) dynamic creep characteristics of stents. This can be done in the following sequence:

1. Determine static creep data for materials used in the stents. With at least 2 independent methods, calculate the 10-year creep strain. If these 2 methods give consistent creep strains, go to the next step.
2. Determine enough dynamic creep data to verify 2 independent methods of calculating long-term dynamic creep from static creep. If this is successful, use the calculated 10 year dynamic creep values and go to the next step. If not, use static creep results in the next step.
3. Determine an equivalent stress behavior of stents when loaded to deflections observed in service. Maximum stress would be used as a very conservative worst case.
4. Use the results of 1 and/or 2 at the equivalent stress in 3 to calculate 10 year dynamic creep of stents.

Once the material characteristics in 1 and 2 are determined, any new stent designs can be evaluated either by experimentally determining an equivalent stress or by calculating it if the finite element models are available. The following will discuss each of these 4 steps.

Static Creep Strain of Polypropylene and Delrin

Two methods have been chosen to calculate long-term creep behavior. They are a logarithmic regression and the WFL temperature shift factor.

Regression. For polymers, logarithmic regression is of the form E = Eo + AtB, where Eo, A, and B are determined constants and t is time. For these regression formulas to work, it is necessary for the mechanism of creep not to change with time. This is usually true after some initial time; thus, it is a good idea to try several initial times and check the consistency. The results are summarized in Table I.

WFL Temperature Shift Factor. This method of long-term prediction presumes that the mechanism of creep is the same at the temperatures considered. If this is true, then a temperature shift factor can be determined and long-term creep calculated at low temperture from short-term creep at high temperatures. In this method the modulus, E, is determined at various times from $E = \sigma/\epsilon$ where σ is stress, and ϵ is strain.

Log E -vs- log t is then plotted. The curves are then shifted in time, and if the two curves are reasonably superimposed a shift factor can be calculated. For both polypropylene and Delrin, the curves do superimpose and shift factors were calculated. Results are given in Table I.

Note there is good agreement between the WFL temperature shift factor and regression methods. Thus step (4) is satisfied.

TABLE I Ten year post creep predictions on size 27 mm cloth-covered stents

Stent	Predicted stent post creep (mm)	
	By regression analysis method	By WFL temperature shift method
Model 342 polypropylene	0.8–1.0	1.0 at a stress of 1,000 psi (7 year prediction)
Hancock II Delrin	0.3	0.2 at 1,000 psi

Dynamic Creep Strain of Polypropylene and Delrin

Two methods have been chosen to calculate long-term dynamic creep data. The first is the Boltzmann superposition principle. The second is to perform a cycle by cycle calculation of strain, taking into account the change in creep compliance with fatigue.

Boltzmann method. The Boltzmann superimposition method assumes that the creep strains of 2 or more stresses are the sum of strains that result from each of these stresses acting independently (but is risky to apply without other support for absolute dynamic creep strain calculations). It was assumed that polypropylene could be modeled by the extended Voight-Kelvin model. The collected static creep data were fitted by computer to this model to determine a family of relaxation times for the polymers. These were then used to calculate the expected creep curve. It appears that the Boltzmann method overestimates the amount of creep actually observed for up to 100,000 cycles at 1 Hz and 37°C. The dynamic creep strain at a given stress appears to be somewhat less than 75% of the static creep strain at the same stress. The Boltzmann method calculates the dynamic strain to be about 75% of the static creep strain.

Creep Compliance Method. This method uses experimentally determined creep compliance to calculate, by numerical computer integration over all cycles, the total strain. For materials that exhibit fatigue softening, such as polypropylene and possibly Delrin, the relaxation time decreases. Therefore in the part of the cycle with low stress there is a greater recovery than predicted by Boltzmann. Thus, the dynamic creep strain is less. For materials that exhibit fatigue hardening, there is greater dynamic creep strain than predicted by Boltzmann. For tests on polypropylene and Delrin at cycles up to 100,000, this method agreed with experimental data very well.

These results give the clear indication that static creep overestimates dynamic creep, that the Boltzmann method slightly overestimates dynamic creep and that the creep compliance method gives fairly close results. At this time, it appears that a dynamic creep of 75% of static creep could be used to estimate long-term behavior. The actual values will probably be considerably less. Dynamic creep of polypropylene at 10 years appears to be between 47% and 56% of static creep.

Equivalent Stress of Stents

Finite element stress analysis indicates the Hancock II maximum local stresses to be just over 2,000 psi. Because the stent has a complex loading, an attempt was made to correlate the observed creep deflection data of the stents with the creep strain data of the material tests. If an equivalent load concept can be developed, then it will be possible to predict the long-term dynamic creep characteristics of the stents. Compare the data in Figs. 8 and 11. Visual observation suggests that the 342R stent made of polypropylene loaded to produce 1 mm of deflection would act as an equivalent mean stress of about 1,200 psi. This also looks like an equivalent mean stress for the Delrin stents.

Manufacturing Techniques used for Hancock II

Stents are machined from implantable grade Delrin 500 and subjected to normal quality assurance acceptance criteria. Radiographic eyelets are attached and the cloth covering applied, using the same material and techniques as the standard Hancock valve. However, the mitral sewing cushions contain Dacron felt rather than a silicone rubber, and the scalloped aortic sewing cushion is composed solely of cloth layers. Fixed valves are mounted in the stent using the same method as in the Hancock 242/342 valves. Immediately before valve holders are applied, the valves are flow tested. Valves are also chemically treated in the T6 calcification retardant solution, after which they are sterilized and packed.

Accelerated Fatigue Studies

A group of 10 Hancock II valves were durability tested in the Hancock accelerated fatigue testers. The rigs were run at approximately 1,200 cycles/min, and the test liquid was buffered electrolyte at 37°C. Near physiologic back pressures (80–120 mmHg) were applied to the valve during the closed portion of the simulated cardiac cycle. Pressures were adjusted and recorded on a weekly basis. Each valve was examined visually and macroscopically at the initiation of the tests, and every 25 million cycles until the termination of testing at 100 million cycles. In addition, an additional 6 low pressure valves, mounted in polypropylene stents, were also tested, as were a group of standard Hancock valves of the same size range. The latter were used as control valves in this study.

The results showed that individually and as a group the low pressure-fixed valves showed less fatigue damage at the completion of the studies than did the standard valves. Those low pressure valves mounted in Delrin stents showed even less damage to the leaflets than did those valves mounted in polypropylene stents. In the Hancock II the stent form is such that leaflet contact between the leaflet and the stent rail is minimal. However, leaflet abrasion from the stent rail is one well-documented artifact of the accelerated fatigue tester used by us. A thin coating of silicone rubber is routinely applied to the stent rail bias strip to minimize this damage. However, even this coating does not entirely eliminate this trauma, which is virtually never seen in explanted clinical prostheses.

Flow Characteristics

The pulsatile flow characteristics of the range of Hancock II valves (multiple samples for each size) were measured using a pulse duplicator.[12] Valves

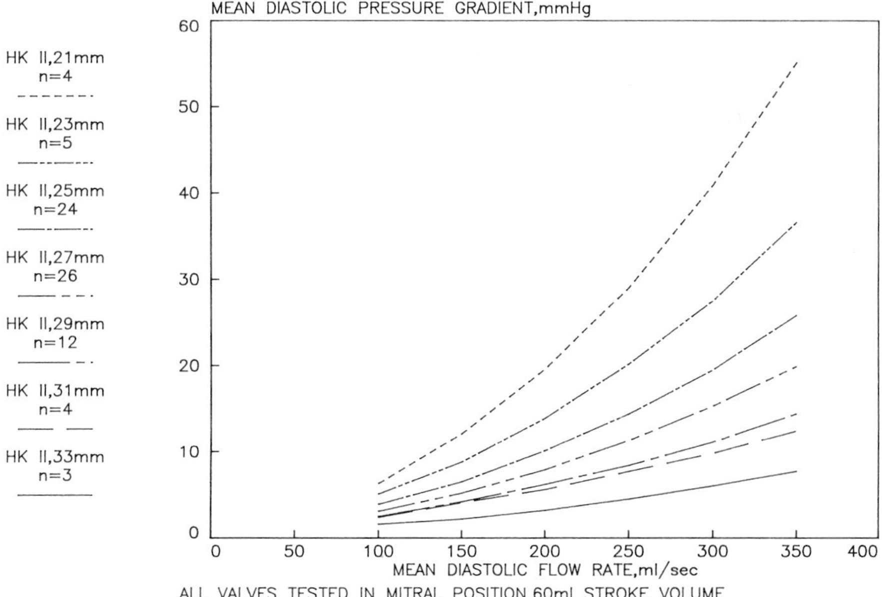

FIG. 13 Variation of mean pressure gradient with mean pulsatile flow rate for typical Hancock II valves. All valves tested in the mitral position, 60 ml stroke volume.

TABLE II Hancock II valve—hydrodynamic data

Hancock II size style, (#)	Effective orifice area, cm^2, at 300 ml/sec (37.9)	% regurgitation at 100 beats/min 60 ml stroke (#)	Minimum peak pulsatile flow to open last cusp, ml/sec (#)
21 mm aortic (7)	1.25 ± 0.10	≤calibration (0.1) (6)	42 ± 17 (6)
23 mm aortic (8)	1.53 ± 0.11	0.7 ± 0.6 (8)	88 ± 34 (8)
25 mm aortic & mitral (26)	1.77 ± 0.15	1.15 ± 0.9 (23)	93 ± 28 (23)
27 mm aortic & mitral (28)	2.02 ± 0.30	1.3 ± 1.2 (24)	106 ± 36 (26)
29 mm mitral (13)	2.38 ± 0.10	1.9 ± 1.2 (10)	128 ± 39 (10)
31 mm mitral (7)	2.58 ± 0.12	3.2 ± 1.6 (7)	173 ± 43 (7)
33 mm mitral (7)	3.00 ± 0.24	2.3 ± 1.2 (6)	160 ± 51 (6)

were tested only in the mitral position, although slightly lower gradients are recorded in the aortic position of the pulse duplicator due to pressure recovery effects. Measurements were made of mean pulsatile pressure gradients at various mean pulsatile flow rates over the range 100–350 ml/sec. The regurgitation and leaflet function were also measured using the same test rig, which had a stroke volume of 60 ml. The test liquid was buffered electrolyte at room temperature. Previous experience has shown that the viscosity of the test liquid has an almost negligible effect on the pulsatile pressure gradients of tissue heart valves.[13]

The results of the pressure gradient studies are shown in Fig. 13. The effective orifice areas of the Hancock II, calculated from Gorlin and Gorlin[14] are listed in Table II. Regurgitation levels, expressed as a percentage of regurgitation of the 60 ml stroke volume and minimum peak pulsatile flow to open the stiffest leaflets, are also listed in Table II.

Several hundred consecutive production valves have been tested on the Hancock single pass flow tester.[15] This device measures the effective orifice area of the valve at a pressure gradient of 20 mmHg. The results are listed in Table III.

Conclusions

Hancock II is the result of an extensive development program involving new fixation techniques, material research, and the incorporation of specific surgical requirements. The new tissue fixation method results in a valve virtually without a septal shelf, and yet with good geometry and collagen crimp retention. This should provide clinical advantages of enhanced durability and improved hemodynamic characteristics.

The stent design results from an extensive material and finite element stress analysis and has a lower profile, a flexible anulus, and a nominal improvement in creep resistance. Long-term (10 year) predictions for inward post migration are approximately 1/3 mm, which would have a negligible effect on valve performance.

TABLE III Single pass flow test results on consecutive production Hancock II valves

Size	Effective orifice area,* cm^2	Sample size
21	1.36 ± 0.13	21
23	1.74 ± 0.11	31
25	2.04 ± 0.17	109
27	2.38 ± 0.14	103
29	2.82 ± 0.20	87
31	3.12 ± 0.27	53
33	3.58 ± 0.15	14

* Calculated from Gorlin and Gorlin at a Δp of 20 mmHg.

In vitro accelerated fatigue data demonstrated little or no damage at 100 million cycles under arduous test conditions. This result compares favorably with similar studies of high pressure-fixed valves, especially in the septal shelf area.

Pulsatile flow studies show that the Hancock II valves have increased effective orifice areas, which are approximately equal to 1 size gain. However, because the aortic valves may be mounted in the supraanular position more readily than previous porcine valves, larger valves may be utilized in some patients.

References

1. Reis RL, Hancock WD, Yarbrough JW, Glancy DL, Morrow AG: The flexible stent. J Thorac Cardiovasc Surg 62:683, 1971.
2. Kutsche LM, Oyer PE, Shumway NE, Baum D: An important complication of Hancock mitral valve replacement in children. Circulation 60:98, 1979.
3. Lentz DJ, Pollock EM, Olsen DB, Andrews EJ: Inhibition of mineralization of glutaraldehyde-fixed Hancock xenograft tissue. In: Proceedings of the International Symposium on Cardiac Bioprostheses, Rome, 1982, Yorke Medical Books, New York, 1982, p 306.
4. Broom ND, Thomson FJ: Influence of fixation conditions on the performance of glutaraldehyde-treated porcine aortic valves: Towards a more scientific basis. Thorax 34:166, 1979.
5. Broom ND: An 'in vitro' study of mechanical fatigue in glutaraldehyde-treated porcine aortic tissue. Biomaterials 1:3, 1980.
6. Salomon NW, Copeland JG, Goldman S, Larson DF: Unusual complication of the Hancock porcine heterograft. Strut compression in the aortic root. J Thorac Cardiovasc Surg 77:294, 1979.
7. Magilligan DJ, Fisher E, Alam M: Hemolytic anemia with porcine xenograft aortic and mitral valves. J Thorac Cardiovasc Surg 79:628, 1980.
8. Borkon AM, McIntosh CL, Jones M, Roberts WC, Morrow AG: Inward stent-post bending of a porcine bioprostheses in the mitral position. J Thorac Cardiovasc Surg 83:105, 1982.
9. Björk VO: A new central-flow tilting disc valve: J Thorac Cardiovasc Surg 60:355, 1970.
10. Angell WW, Angell JD, Sywak A, Kosek JC: The tissue valve as a superior cardiac valve replacement. Surgery 82:875, 1977.
11. Oyer PE, Miller DC, Stinson EB, Reitz BA, Moreno-Cabral RJ, Shumway NE: Clinical durability of the Hancock porcine bioprosthetic valve. J Thorac Cardiovasc Surg 80:824, 1980.
12. Wright JTM, Brown MC: A method for measuring the mean pressure gradient across prosthetic heart valves under in vitro pulsatile flow conditions. Med Instrum 11:110, 1977.
13. Wright JT: Hydrodynamic evaluation of tissue heart valves. In: Tissue Heart Valves (MI Ionescu, Ed). London; Butterworths, 1979, p 31.
14. Cohen MV, Gorlin R: Modified orifice equation for the calculation of mitral valve area. Am Heart J 84:839, 1972.
15. Wright JTM, Derby CF, Hammond P, Myers DJ, Snyder S: A new method for measuring the flow characteristics of porcine xenograft heart valves under production conditions. Proceedings of the Association for the Advancement of Medical Instrumentation, 15th Annual Meeting, 1980, p 240.

38

Design and Stress Analysis of Bioprosthetic Valves in Vivo

M. J. THUBRIKAR, J. R. SKINNER, S. P. NOLAN

We investigated the design, dynamics, and stresses of bioprosthetic valves in the aortic position in calves. Heart valve bioprostheses have been in clinical use for several years, and the development of new bioprostheses as well as the improvement of existing ones still continues. Most bioprostheses currently in use in human beings produce a small (clinically acceptable) pressure drop; there is no significant danger of catastrophic failure of bioprosthetic valves, which are not antigenically rejected. The problem with bioprosthetic valves is the calcification and subsequent immobilization of the leaflets during their clinical life. At the present time, there is a need for a new generation of valves that will not calcify and that will be as efficient and durable as the natural heart valve. To this end, it is necessary to have knowledge of fundamental properties, such as design, behavior, and stresses in vivo and to understand how these properties influence the efficiency and durability of bioprosthetic valves.

Materials and Methods

Geometric design and dynamic behavior were investigated for 3 Carpentier-Edwards porcine valves (CE), 4 Hancock porcine valves (H), and 4 Ionescu-Shiley pericardial valves (IS), and the stresses were investigated for 2 CE valves. To determine the geometry, 3 radiopaque markers (1.5 mm × 1.5 mm, 14 mg weight) were placed on 1 leaflet in the circumferential direction, 3 markers were placed on another leaflet in the radial

---

From the Department of Surgery, University of Virginia Medical Center, Charlottesville, Virginia.

This work was supported by NIH Grant HL-17969.

direction, and 3 markers were placed on 3 stent posts at the level of the leaflet free edge. These valves, each of 23 mm mounting diameter, were implanted in the aortic position in calves during cardiopulmonary bypass. The calves were allowed to recover and were studied 8–15 days postoperatively. During the study, the calves were anesthetized and positioned under the x-ray tube. The movement of the markers during fluoroscopy was recorded on videotape at 60 fields per second. The recording was done in 2 projections. In the first projection, a perfect side view of the leaflet was obtained by keeping the x-ray tube perpendicular to the axis of the aorta and by adjusting the position of the calf so that the 2 markers on the stent posts were superimposed on each other. This projection was used for measuring design parameters directly. In CE valves, this projection was used also to determine the angle of rotation of the leaflet and the length of the zone of flexion. These measurements are required for calculation of the stresses in CE valves. In the second projection, a top view of the BPV was obtained by keeping the x-ray beam parallel to the aortic axis. This projection was used for determining the movement and configuration of the leaflets and the movement of the stent posts. In CE valves this projection was used also to determine the angle of rotation in the circumferential direction of the leaflet and to determine leaflet curvature. These parameters were required for calculating the stresses in these valves. To eliminate any error that might occur from the movement of the BPV toward or away from the x-ray source during each cardiac cycle, these 2 projections were recorded again after turning the calf 180° on its spinal axis. Electrocardiographic and systemic pressure were recorded during the fluoroscopy. For CE valves the pressure gradient across the leaflets was recorded during diastole and during systole. The videotape was displayed on a television screen in a stop-motion mode, and the marker positions were copied on transparent acetate paper. The marker positions were noted field by field for 3 consecutive cardiac cycles in each projection.

The design of BPV was determined as 1) the bottom surface angle α, 2) the free edge angle ϕ, 3) the radius of the commissures Rc, 4) the radius of the bases Rb, and 5) the valve height H. The details of the marker placement and of the design parameters have been reported by us elsewhere.[1,2] The dynamics of the leaflet were studied in terms of the distance between the markers at the center of the free edge of the 2 leaflets. The flexibility of the stent post was measured in terms of change in the distance between the markers on the stent posts.

For CE valves, additional data required for computation of stresses were obtained as follows. The calves were sacrificed after the study and the valves were removed. The geometry of the valves in diastole was determined from the silicone mold of the closed valve, prepared at diastolic pressure. In systole, the geometry was determined from the in vivo marker-fluoroscopic studies, as described earlier. The stress-strain properties of the leaflets were determined using an Instron tensile-testing machine. These properties were determined in the circumferential or radial direction of the leaflet, depending upon whether the leaflet had markers in the circumferential or the radial direction. The stress-strain curves were used to determine the stresses in the leaflets.

Results

Dynamics of the Leaflets and Stent Posts

For each of the CE, H, and IS valves, the typical behavior of the leaflet and of the stent posts is shown in Fig. 1. During the opening and closing of each of the valves, leaflet displacement occurred rapidly, indicating that opening to a full orifice and complete closure of the valve were achieved in less than 33 msec. For all of the valves, there was no significant motion of the leaflets during systole, indicating that there was no change in the size of the orifice during systole. This observation is different from that of the natural aortic vavle, in which the size of the orifice decreases slowly during systole.[3,4] Flexibility of the stent posts was determined from the change in the perimeter of a triangle formed by the markers on the posts in the commissural region. There was no significant change in the commissure perimeter during a cardiac cycle, indicating that none of the stent posts of any of the valves were flexible. Although it is not possible, with the present technique, to detect high frequency vibrations of the stent posts, using the same technique we have demonstrated that the commissure perimeter of the natural aortic valve decreases from systole to diastole.[3,4] These observations were the same for the 18, 24, and 24 cardiac cycles analyzed for CE, H, and IS valves, respectively. During these studies the aortic blood pressure ranged from 135/105–85/65 mmHg, the heart rate from 110–140 beats/min and the systolic pressure gradient across the valve ranged from 5–10 mmHg.

Design of the Bioprostheses

For all of the valves, the design parameters were measured in mid-diastole and were compared with those of the natural aortic valve. The design parameters α, ϕ, Rb/Rc, and H/Rc were, respectively, 8°, 44°, 1.1, and 1.55 for the CE valve; 1°, 56°, 1.43, and 2.0 for the H valve; α undetermined, 16°, 0.95, and 1.2 for the IS valve; and 20°, 32°, 1.2, and 1.4 for the natural aortic valve.[1,2] Thus, in their designs, CE, H, and IS valves were different from each other and also from the natural valve. The differences in their design are diagrammatically illustrated in Fig. 2. In all of the bioprostheses, there were no significant changes in the design parameters during

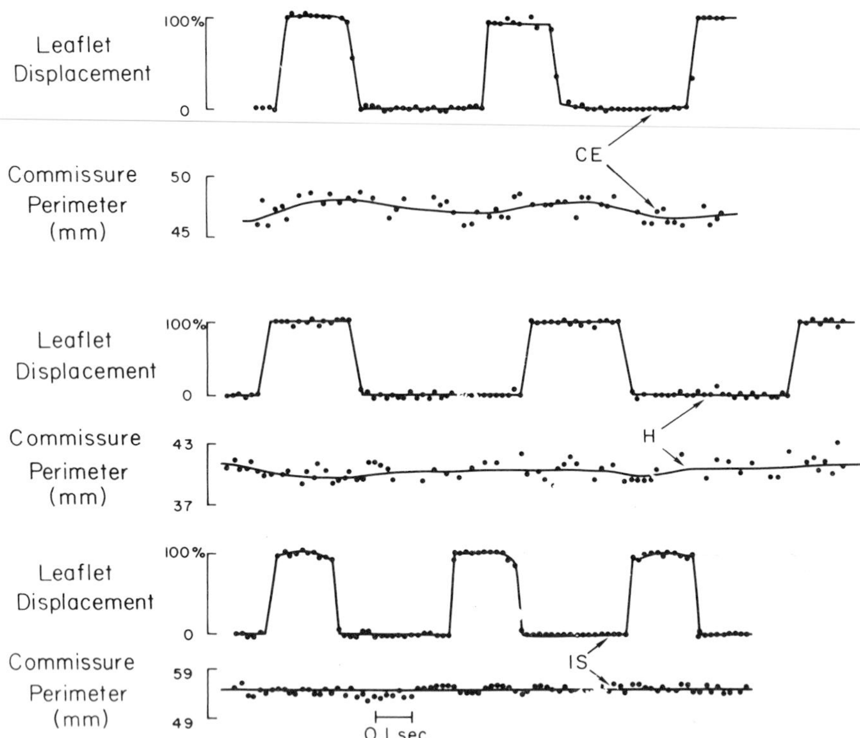

FIG. 1 Leaflet displacement and commissure perimeter plotted against time for 3 continuous cardiac cycles for CE, H, and IS valves. Leaflet displacement is measured as distance between the 2 leaflets, where maximum distance represents 100% displacement, and minimum distance represents 0% displacement. Commissure perimeter is plotted as perimeter of triangle formed by 3 markers on stent posts. Each data point is obtained from single videofield. All valves opened and closed in less than 33 ms; stent posts of all the valves showed no significant flexibility during cardiac cycle.

a cardiac cycle. Each value of the design parameter was obtained from 12−18 videofields taken from a total of 3 cardiac cycles. The leaflets of the CE and H valves were cylindrical, but those of the IS valves were spherical.

In all of the valves maximum flexion occurred along the leaflet attachment as the leaflets moved from the diastolic to the systolic position and back.

Stress in the Bioprosthesis

Although stress was analyzed for 2 CE valves only, the methodology used and the conclusions drawn apply qualitatively to all 3 types of bioprostheses.

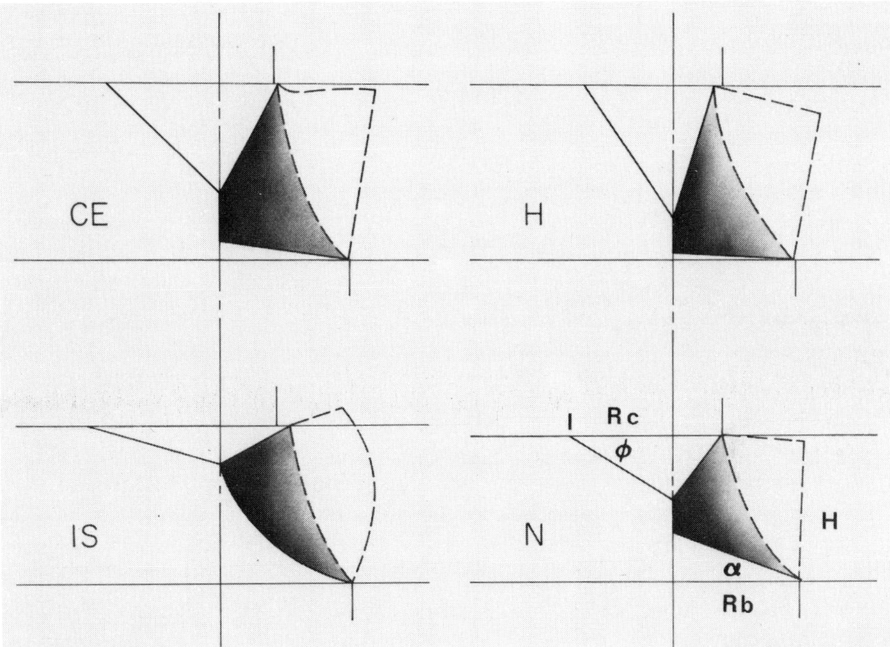

FIG. 2 Diagrammatic presentation of leaflets' side view of CE, H, IS, and N (natural aortic) valves, indicating differences in their design parameters α, ϕ, Rc, Rb, and H.

In diastole. The leaflet is treated as a cylindrical shell across which the pressure gradient is present from the inside of the cylinder to the outside. Membrane stress in the circumferential direction of the leaflet is given by

$$\frac{(P_a - P_v)R_d}{T}$$

and in the radial direction by

$$\frac{(P_a - P_v)R_d}{2T}$$

where P_a, P_v, R_d, and T represent pressure in the aorta, pressure in the ventricle, radius of the leaflet, and thickness of the leaflet, respectively.

P_a and P_v were measured in vivo, and R_d and T were measured in vitro. The membrane stress was 33 and 28 (10^5 dynes/cm^2) circumferentially and 17 and 14 (10^5 dynes/cm^2) radially for these 2 valves. This is the only stress present in diastole and therefore it represents the total stress in the leaflet.[5]

In systole. There is a small pressure gradient across the leaflet in systole which induces small membrane stress. However, the configuration of the leaflet changes from diastole to systole, and this change induces large bending stress in the leaflet. The total stress is obtained by vectorial summation of the membrane stress and the bending stress. At the center of the leaflet, the membrane stress in the circumferential direction was 2 and 1.6 (10^5 dynes/cm^2) for the 2 valves. Bending strain is given by

$$\frac{T}{2R_m} + \frac{T}{2R_d}$$

where R_m is the radius of the leaflet in this region.

To obtain the total stress, membrane stress (σ_m) was plotted on the stress-strain curve (Fig. 3), and bending strain (ϵ_m) was plotted on both sides of the membrane stress, since the bending strain is compressive in half the thickness of the leaflet and tensile in the other half. The total stress was +38 (10^5 dynes/cm^2) on the aortic surface and −7.3 (10^5 dynes/cm^2) on the ventricular surface for one valve and +26 and −3.7 (10^5 dynes/cm^2) for the other. Hence, small compressive stress, indicated by the negative sign, occurs on the ventricular side of the leaflet. The details of the stress analysis are reported elsewhere.[5] There is no bending, and therefore no bending stress, in the radial direction. Membrane stress in the radial direction was 1 and 0.8 (10^5 dynes/cm^2) for the 2 valves.

Using a similar procedure, stress was calculated in a region 3−4 mm from the leaflet attachment. In this region, the total stress in the radial direction was −1 and −0.7 (10^5 dynes/cm^2) for the 2 valves. In the circumferential direction, the total stress was −5.9 (10^5 dynes/cm^2) on the aortic surface and −0.3 (10^5 dynes/cm^2) on the ventricular surface for one valve and −3.7 and +0.7 (10^5 dynes/cm^2) for the other.

At the attachment. The stresses at the attachment of the leaflet were most important, since maximum flexion in systole occurred in this region. Bending strain was determined from the model of deformation illustrated in Fig. 4. From the angle of rotation θ and the length of the zone of flexion Y, the radius R of the bend was determined and the bending strain was computed as T/2R. The strain was plotted on both sides of the origin on the stress-strain curve, and the stress was determined. At the commissures, the stress was −131 (10^5 dynes/cm^2) on the aortic side and +131 (10^5 dynes/cm^2) on the ventricular side in one valve and −109 and +109 (10^5 dynes/cm^2) in the other. At the base, the stress was −5.2 (10^5 dynes/cm^2) on the aortic side and +5.2 (10^5 dynes/cm^2) on the ventricular side in one valve and −5.6 and +5.6 (10^5 dynes/cm^2) in the other.

Figure 5 shows the summary of total stress in the entire leaflet of 1 valve.

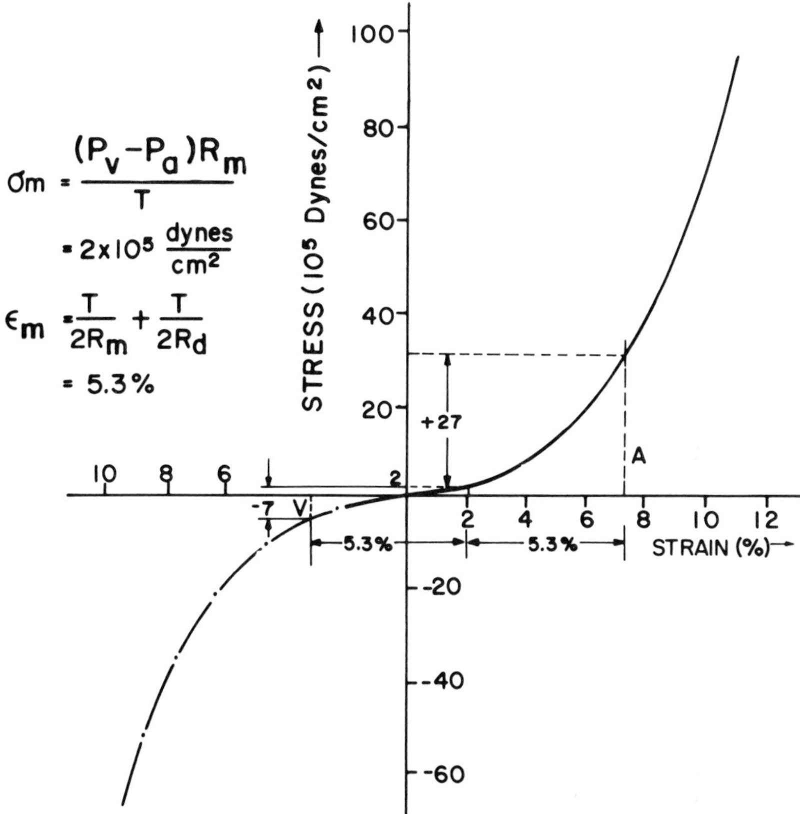

FIG. 3 Illustration of superimposition principle used to obtain total stress. Typical stress-strain curve in circumferential direction of CE valve leaflet is shown. Curve in compressive stress region was not (it cannot be) determined experimentally, but was taken as mirror image of curve in tensile stress region. Membrane stress (σ_m) was plotted on curve, and bending strain (ϵ_m) was superimposed on both sides of σ_m to obtain total stress. Bending stress +27 and −7 (10^5 dynes/cm^2) was corrected for Poisson's effect before adding to σ_m to obtain total stress. Bending strain is superimposed on both sides of membrane stress because strain is compressive for half the leaflet thickness and tensile for other half. Superimposition gives distribution of total stress through thickness of leaflet. See Thubrikar et al[5] for more details.

The highest compressive stress occurred in systole along the leaflet attachment on the aortic side of the leaflet, and the stress was maximum at the upper point of leaflet attachment, decreasing toward the base. Since this stress is directly related to the degree of flexion and to the properties of the leaflet, the stress is likely to be the same in all bioprostheses that have similar flexion behavior and leaflet properties.

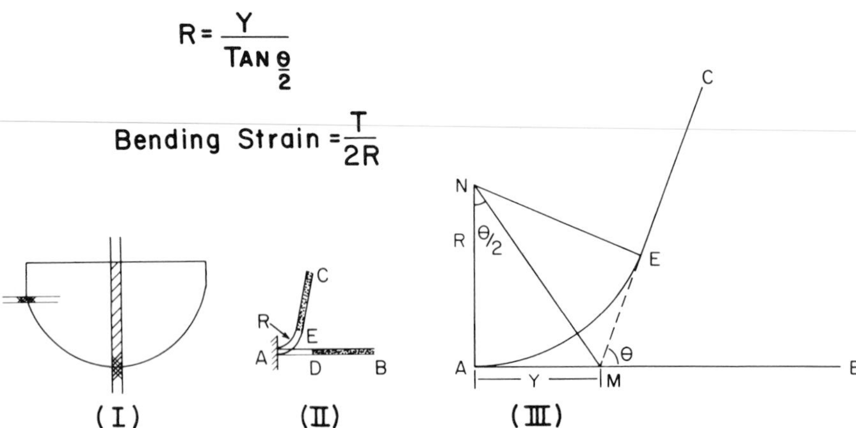

FIG. 4 A model of bending deformation to calculate bending strain at leaflet attachment. (I) Leaflet showing the 2 typical areas of attachment. (II) Leaflet strip corresponding to area of attachment shown in I. Leaflet ADB in diastole moves to position AEC in systole, so that region AD is bent to AE. (III) Radius R of the bend is given by $Y/\tan(\theta/2)$. Angle of rotation θ and zone of flexion Y were measured in vivo.

Comment

All 3 types of valves (CE, H, and IS) opened and closed rapidly in the aortic position in calves (Fig. 1). This is an interesting observation, particularly since the leaflets of the porcine valves (CE and H) have a different thickness than those of the pericardial valve (IS), and the 3 types of valves also have different designs. In patients, porcine valves were observed to show rapid opening and closing behavior in the aortic position,[6] as well as in the mitral position.[7] However, movement of only 1 or 2 cusps in the tricuspid position in dogs[8] and sequential opening of the cusps in in vitro flow chambers have also been observed.[9,10] Hence, the opening and closing of the valve depends upon the flow conditions. Stent posts of all of the valves were found to be inflexible (Fig. 1). IS valves were known to have inflexible stent posts, but the stent posts of H valves were thought to be flexible.[11,12] Thomson and Barratt-Boyes[13] however, have reported that in vitro stent posts of H valves showed very little movement (0.2 mm for 33 size valve) at physiologic pressure. Such small movements and high frequency vibrations of the posts will not be detected by the technique employed in the present study.

The design of all 3 types of bioprosthetic valves were different from each other and from the natural aortic valve (Fig. 2), despite the fact that all of the bioprostheses were expected to perform the same function. It was

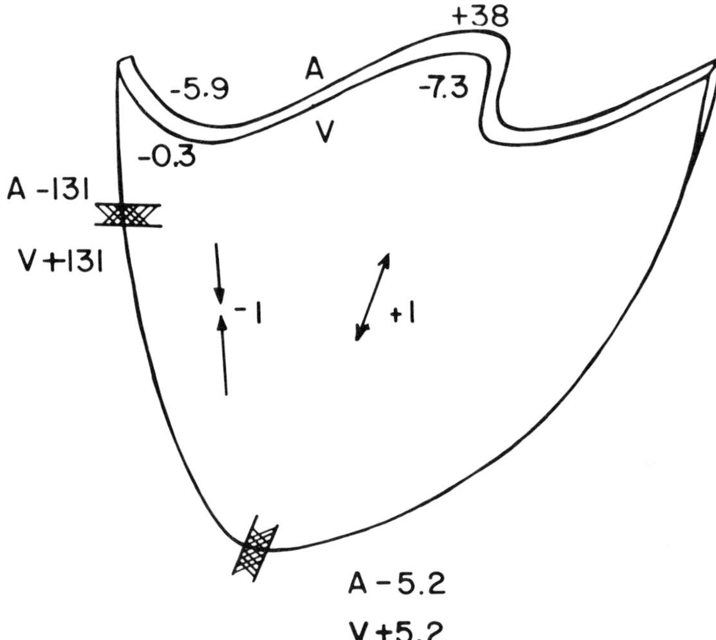

FIG. 5 Summary of total stress in entire leaflet of bioprosthetic valve in systole. (A) aortic surface; (V) ventricular surface. Negative sign indicates compressive stress. Positive sign indicates tensile stress. Large compressive stresses occur along leaflet attachment on aortic surface.

inevitable, though, that such varied designs were developed, since the design of the natural aortic valve was not known until recently.[1]

There are no published reports of stress analysis of bioprosthetic valves that correspond to their behavior in vivo. Stress analysis of a trileaflet valve made of Avcothane polymer has been performed from a design point of view, which does not necessarily apply to the functioning valve in vivo.[14] There are reports on stress analysis in vitro of the human aortic valve[15] and of the natural porcine aortic valve,[16] but these analyses apply to stress only in diastole and do not take into account the configurational changes that occur in vivo. The present study elucidates a simplified method of stress analysis which corresponds to the actual behavior of the valve in vivo. The method employed is similar to that used previously to analyze the in vivo stress in natural aortic valve.[17]

For computing the stress in diastole, we have used standard equations of equilibrium for cylindrical geometry. The leaflets of the porcine bioprosthesis are cylindrical in their load-bearing portion, as demonstrated by the shape of silicone molds made from these valves. The stress values presented for bioprosthetic valves are in close agreement with those of Robel[18] and Gould et al[15] for human valves in diastole. For computing the stress in systole, it was proposed that small membrane stress occurs due to a small pressure gradient across the leaflet, that large bending stress occurs due to changes in the configuration of the leaflet from diastole to systole, and that the total stress is a summation of the 2. This procedure ignores any influence of membrane and bending stress on each other. Consideration of such an influence complicates the analysis greatly and therefore may not be justified, unless it can also account for the inhomogeneity of the leaflet. Thus, the method presented here is adequate for an estimate of the stress values. At the attachment, membrane stress was considered negligible, and bending stress equalled total stress. This is justified on the basis that in systole the leaflet geometry at the attachment is quite complex, and the small radius of bend and small gradient across the leaflet make the membrane stress negligible, at the same time that bending stress is intensified. It should be emphasized that the stress in systole is computed from the geometry of the leaflet, which is determined from the markers. The markers do not represent a continuous geometry. Rather, a smoothed geometry, corresponding to the least stressful conditions, is obtained through the multiple markers. If there are any kinks in the leaflet, the stress would be even greater than those reported.

The present study has demonstrated that bioprosthetic valves have designs and dynamics that differ from those of the natural valve. Consequently, bioprosthetic valves have greater stresses than do natural valves. The stresses are greatest where the greatest flexion occurs, namely, along the leaflet attachment, and they are compressive on the aortic surface. Broom[19] demonstrated that, in vitro, the leaflets are unable to sustain compressive stresses. We[17] demonstrated that the natural valve minimizes compressive stress by virtue of its design and properties. Therefore in bioprosthetic valves the stress failure of leaflets should be expected to occur along the attachment. In another study,[20] we have observed that in bioprosthetic valves the leaflets show calcification that begins in the area of attachment, suggesting that stress plays an important role in initiating calcification. Hence, the longevity of BPV is compromised by increased stress, which occurs by virtue of design, dynamics, and properties that are different from those of the natural valve. In conclusion, in order to increase the durability of BPV, their design and properties should be changed to match those of the natural valve.

References

1. Thubrikar M, Piepgrass WC, Shaner TW, Nolan SP: The design of the normal aortic valve. Am J Physiol 241:H795, 1981.

2. Thubrikar M, Skinner JR, Aouad J, Finkelmeier BA, Nolan SP: Analysis of the design and dynamics of aortic bioprostheses *in vivo.* J Thorac Cardiovasc Surg 84:282, 1982.
3. Thubrikar M, Harry R, Nolan SP: Normal aortic valve function in dogs. Am J Cardiol 40:563, 1977.
4. Thubrikar M, Bosher LP, Nolan SP: The mechanism of opening of the aortic valve. J Thorac Cardiovasc Surg 77:863, 1979.
5. Thubrikar M, Skinner JR, Eppink RT, Nolan SP: Stress analysis of porcine bioprosthetic heart valves *in vivo.* J Biomed Mater Res 16:(Nov), 1982.
6. Bloch WN Jr, Felner JM, Schlant RC, Symbas PN, Jones EL: The echocardiogram of the porcine aortic bioprostheses in the aortic position. Chest 72:640, 1977.
7. Harston WE Jr, Robertson RM, Friesinger GC: Echocardiographic evaluation of porcine heterograft valves in the mitral and aortic positions. Am Heart J 96:448, 1978.
8. Imamura E, Kaye MP, Davis GD: Radiographic assessment of leaflet motion of Gore-Tex laminate trileaflet valves and Hancock xenograft in tricuspid position of dogs. Circulation 56:1053, 1977.
9. Walker DK, Scotten LN, Modi VJ, Brownlee RT: *In vitro* assessment of mitral valve prostheses. J Thorac Cardiovasc Surg 79:680, 1980.
10. Rainer WG, Christopher RA, Sadler TR Jr, Hilgenberg AD: Dynamic behavior of prosthetic aortic tissue valves as viewed by high-speed cinematography. Ann Thorac Surg 28:274, 1979.
11. Reis RL, Hancock WD, Yarbrough JW, Glancy DL, Morrow AG: The flexible stent: A new concept in the fabrication of tissue heart valve prostheses. J Thorac Cardiovasc Surg 62:683, 1971.
12. Zuhdi N, Hawley W, Voehl V, Hancock W, Carey J, Greer A: Porcine aortic valves as replacements for human heart valves. Ann Thorac Surg 17:479, 1974.
13. Thomson FJ, Barratt-Boyes BG: The glutaraldehyde-treated heterograft valve: Some engineering observations. J Thorac Cardiovasc Surg 74:317, 1977.
14. Ghista DN, Reul H: Optimal prosthetic aortic leaflet valve: Design parameters and longevity analysis: Development of the Avcothane-51 leaflet valve based on the optimum design analysis. J Biomech 10:313, 1977.
15. Gould PL, Cataloglu A, Dhatt G, Chattopadhyay A, Clark RE: Stress analysis of the human aortic valve. Comput Struct 3:377, 1973.
16. Chong M, Missirlis YF: Aortic valve mechanics—Part II: A stress analysis of the porcine aortic valve leaflets in diastole. Biomater Med Devices Artif Organs 6:225, 1978.
17. Thubrikar M, Peipgrass WC, Deck JD, Nolan SP: Stresses of natural vs. prosthetic aortic valve leaflets *in vivo.* Ann Thorac Surg 30:230, 1980.
18. Robel SB: Structural mechanics of the aortic valve, In: Prosthetic Replacement of the Aortic Valve (LR Sauvage, RF Viggers, K Berger, SB Robel, PN Sawyer, SJ Wood, Eds). Springfield, Ill., Charles C Thomas, 1972.
19. Broom ND: An *in vitro* study of mechanical fatigue in glutaraldehyde-treated porcine aortic valve tissue. Biomaterials 1:3, 1980.
20. Deck JD, Thubrikar MJ, Nolan SP, Aouad J: Role of mechanical stress in calcification of bioprostheses. In: International Symposium on Cardiac Bioprostheses, Rome, 1982, Yorke Medical Books, New York, 1982, p 293.

39

In Vitro Comparison of the Newer Heart Valve Bioprostheses in the Mitral and Aortic Positions

S. Gabbay, R. W. M. Frater

Bioprostheses are the valve replacements of choice in many centers, surgeons being satisfied with the low incidence of thromboembolism, the ability to avoid anticoagulants, and the finding that the hemodynamics and durability are acceptable both per se and when compared with the performance of the mechanical alternatives.[1-5] Imperfect hemodynamics are an acknowledged problem of bioprostheses. With both mechanical and bioprosthetic heart valves, exercise tolerance has been shown to be inadequate, even though resting hemodynamics are adequate.[6-10] In vitro studies have clearly shown the stenotic behavior of prosthetic valves at high flow rates.[11,12]

Porcine valves have been improved hemodynamically, but the need to support the natural porcine aortic valve from inside a stent imposes finite limits on the possible improvements. The Ionescu-Shiley pericardial xenograft valve has proved to have better hemodynamics.[11-13] The ability to manufacture a valve using xenograft tissue, as opposed to mounting a harvested natural valve, is the key to this improvement.

There is a strong drive on the part of the manufacturers to improve the hemodynamic performance of bioprostheses to fit the need for a valve good for the small aortic root and for a valve that can tolerate the high flow rates of exercise. Most of the in vitro comparative studies of heart valve prostheses in pulse duplicators have been done in the aortic position[14,15] or in the mitral position separately.[16,17] All our published studies were done in the mitral position,[11,12] which we found very convenient in our pulse duplicator. Lately, we have made some changes in the aortic impedance system of our tester to make both mitral and aortic studies more convenient.

From the Albert Einstein College of Medicine and Montefiore Hospital and Medical Center, New York City, New York.

In this study we have compared 3 new pericardial xenograft bioprostheses with the old Ionescu-Shiley pericardial xenograft valve and with the Carpentier-Edwards porcine aortic xenograft valve. We have attempted to determine: 1) how much hemodynamic improvement is provided by the new designs; 2) how do these valves compare with each other; and 3) whether or not there is a difference between the performances of the same valves in the mitral and in the aortic positions.

Materials and Methods

Figure 1 shows the modifications made in our pulse duplicator. The changes essentially relate to the aortic chamber and include: 1) a characteristic linear resistance (Rc); 2) an aortic compliance (C), and 3) variable linear peripheral resistance (Rp). The compliance and resistance were calculated to duplicate the natural human aortic impedance.[18]

Figure 2 shows the curves of mitral and aortic flows as well as the pressure curves. Note the resemblance of the curves to the natural human physiologic pressures: the pressure responses of this aortic system are similar to those seen in nature, especially while simulating exercise. The mean aortic pressure is 70–90 mmHg at flows simulating a "cardiac output" of 5 liters/min; this pressure rises to, but does not exceed, 180 mmHg at flows simulating 15 liters/min "cardiac output", which is very similar to the normal human response to exercise.

The valves were tested in the mitral and aortic positions at different stroke volumes and heart rates. The hydrodynamic characteristics of each valve were analyzed using the pressure drop at the time of peak flow as a function of peak pulsatile flow. The rationale for this approach was discussed previously.[11,12] We have found that using the peak to peak flow method is equivalent to using mean pressure drop as a function of the square root of the mean flow squared during pulsatile flow, as well as using pressure drop as a function of flow during steady flow.

Mean pressure drop was measured at flows simulating "cardiac outputs" of 5, 9, and 12.5 liters/min, to evaluate the tolerance of the valves to flows simulating exercise.

An effective orifice area (EOA) is calculated using the hydraulic formula, with a discharge coefficient of 1.[11,12] The ratio of flow (ml/s) and pressure drop (mmHg) used to compute the EOA is based on the best fit through the data.

The performance index (PI) is the ratio of EOA over the measured mounting area. Since the EOA of bioprostheses increases with flow,[12] we have calculated the EOA based on each set of data (Q, AP) and plotted it as a function of flow.

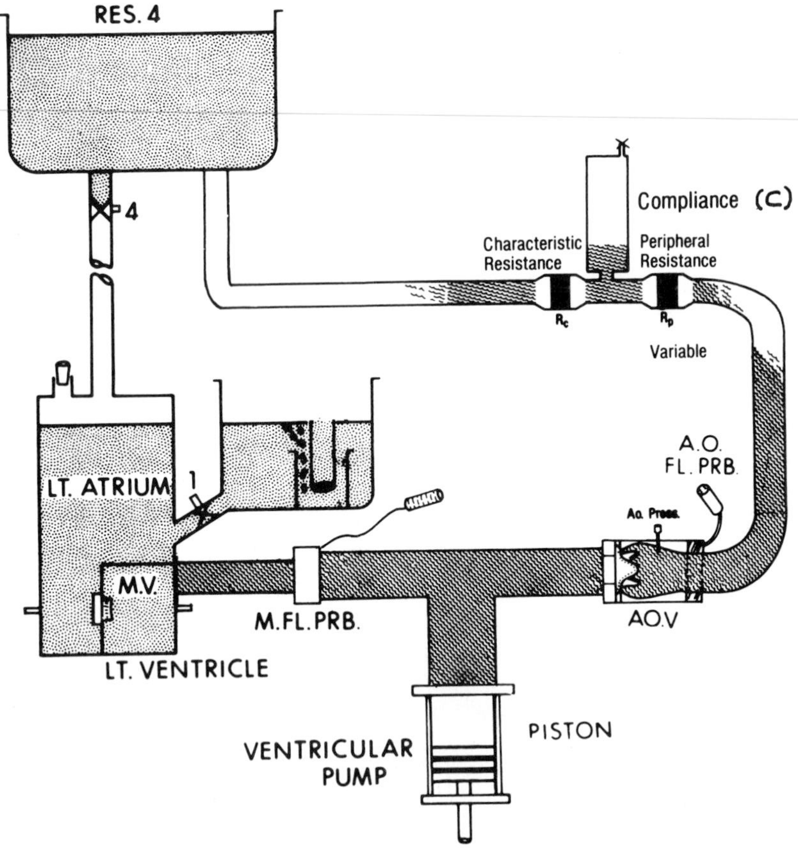

FIG. 1 Pulse duplicator. Changes relate to aortic system, which has impedance similar to that of human aorta. Note characteristic linear resistance (RC); aortic compliance (C); variable linear peripheral resistance (RP); mitral flow probe (M.Fl.Prb); mitral valve (MV); aortic valve (Ao.V.); aortic flow probe (Ao.Fl.Prb).

The statistical significance of differences in pressure drops and EOA were determined by Student's *t* test.

The valves were divided into 3 groups with 21 mm (small), 25–26 mm (medium), and 29–31 mm (large) mounting diameters. The group of large valves was not tested in the aortic position for obvious reasons. The valves were supplied by the manufacturers (Carpentier-Edwards porcine valves and Edwards pericardial valves by American-Edwards, Santa Ana, CA; Ionescu-Shiley valves, the current and the new, by Shiley Laboratories, Irvine, CA; Hancock pericardial valve by Hancock Laboratories, Anaheim, CA). These valves are shown in Fig. 3 and described in Table I.

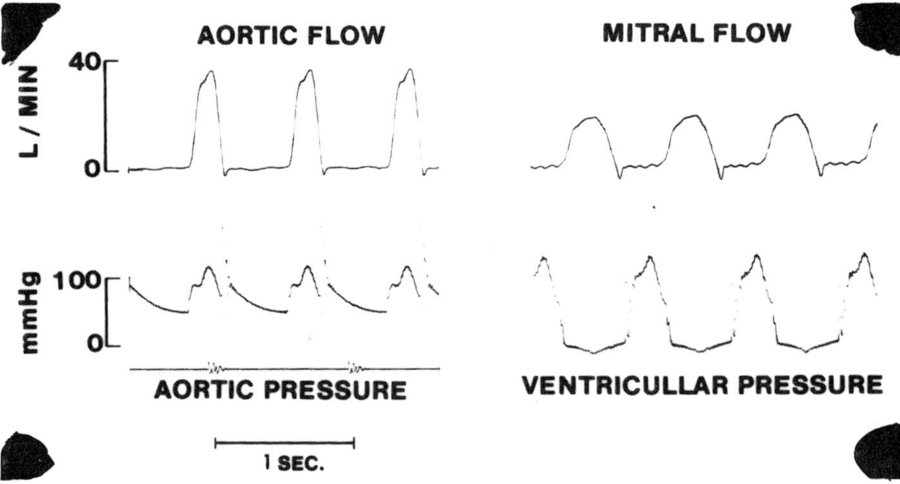

FIG. 2 Typical curves of aortic and ventricular pressures, and mitral and aortic flows. Note that aortic pressure curves are very similar to physiologic human pressure curves.

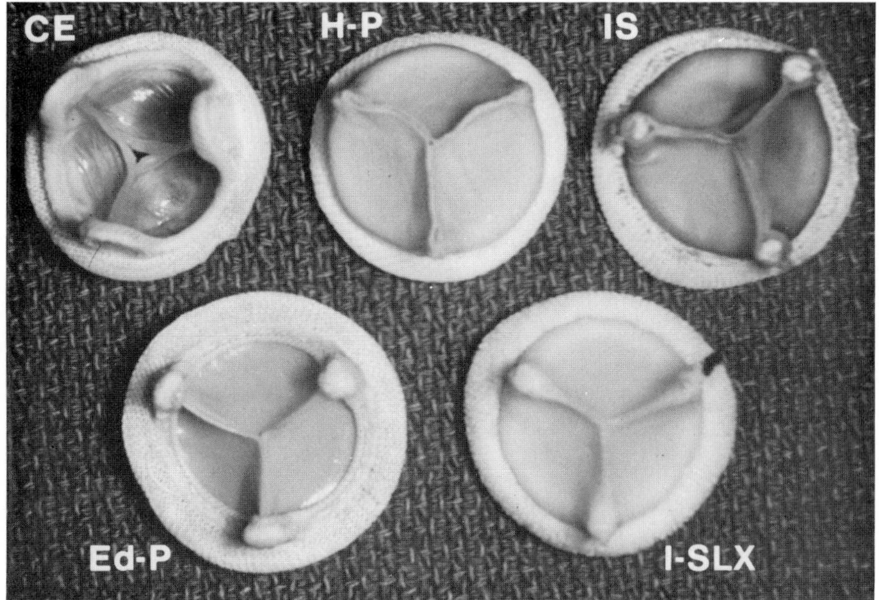

FIG. 3 Valve tested. Medium size group. C-E = Carpentier-Edwards; I-S = Ionescu-Shiley (current); I-SLX = Ionescu-Shiley (new); Ed-P = Edwards pericardial; H-P = Hancock pericardial.

TABLE I Description of valves tested

Valve	Size mounting	Orifice: Diameter* (mm)	Orifice: Area* (cm^2)	Mounting area (cm^2)	Ratio of orifice to mounting area
Small					
Carpentier-Edwards	21	18	2.54	3.46	0.73
Ionescu-Shiley	21	17.4	2.37	3.46	0.68
Ionescu-Shiley (new)	21	17	2.37	3.46	0.68
Edwards pericardial	21	20	3.14	3.46	0.90
Hancock pericardial	21	18	2.54	3.46	0.73
Medium					
Carpentier-Edwards	25	21	3.46	4.90	0.70
Ionescu-Shiley	25	21.4	3.60	4.90	0.73
Ionescu-Shiley (new)	25	21	3.46	4.90	0.70
Edwards pericardial	25	24.5	4.71	4.90	0.96
Hancock pericardial	26	2.14	3.63	5.30	0.68
Large					
Carpentier-Edwards	29	24.5	4.71	6.60	0.71
Ionescu-Shiley	29	25.4	5.05	6.60	0.76
Ionescu-Shiley (new)	31	27	5.72	7.54	0.75
Edwards pericardial	29	28	6.15	6.60	0.93
Hancock pericardial	29	24	4.52	6.60	0.68
Hancock pericardial	31	28.5	6.37	7.54	0.84

* Internal diameter at the base of the valve.

Results

Mitral Position

Figure 4 and Table II summarize the results for the pressure drops for the valves tested in the mitral position. For the small and medium sizes, the Hancock pericardial valve was significantly ($p < 0.001$) less stenotic than the other valves, with the Edwards pericardial valve ranking second. The small new Ionescu-Shiley pericardial valve showed no significant* improvement over the current model but the medium and large sizes showed significant improvement ($p < 0.001$). In the group of large valves, the Edwards pericardial valve performed the best, followed in order by the new Ionescu-Shiley, the Hancock (there being no statistical difference between the latter 2), and the old Ionescu-Shiley. The porcine Carpentier-Edwards was the most stenotic valve in all the groups: in fact the large porcine valve is more stenotic than some of the new medium-sized valves, and the medium-sized porcine behaves like a small size of the new valves.

The mean pressure drops were measured at "cardiac outputs" equivalent to 5, 9, and 12.5 liters/min to evaluate the behavior of the different valves at resting flow rates and flows simulating exercise. For the most stenotic of the medium-sized valves, Carpentier-Edwards porcine, the mean pressure drop was 12 mmHg at "cardiac output" of 5 liters/min, 17.5 mmHg at 9 liters/min, and 30 mmHg at 12.5 liters/min. Significant exercise would not be possible with this valve. For the least stenotic valve, Hancock pericardial, the mean pressure drop was 4.9 mmHg at 5 liters/min, 9.2 mmHg at 9 liters/min, and 15 mmHg at 12.5 liters/min. Modest exercise would be possible with this valve. For the group of large valves, the Carpentier-Edwards porcine valve continues to show critical pressure drops but the new valves have modest pressure drops that would permit some exercise.

It is important to mention that most patients who come to surgery for mitral stenosis have mean gradients between 10–18 mmHg at resting cardiac outputs. A mean gradient of 30 mmHg across the mitral valve would be incompatible with life.

Aortic Position

In the aortic position, the ranking stays the same but the differences become less significant: in both small- and medium-sized groups, the Edwards pericardial valve and the new Ionescu-Shiley valve behave more sim-

* We were advised by the manufacturer that the size 21 (new) tested was an imperfect design. Another valve was supplied and tested. Indeed, the latter showed a 15% increase in the EOA over the current Ionescu-Shiley 21 valve.

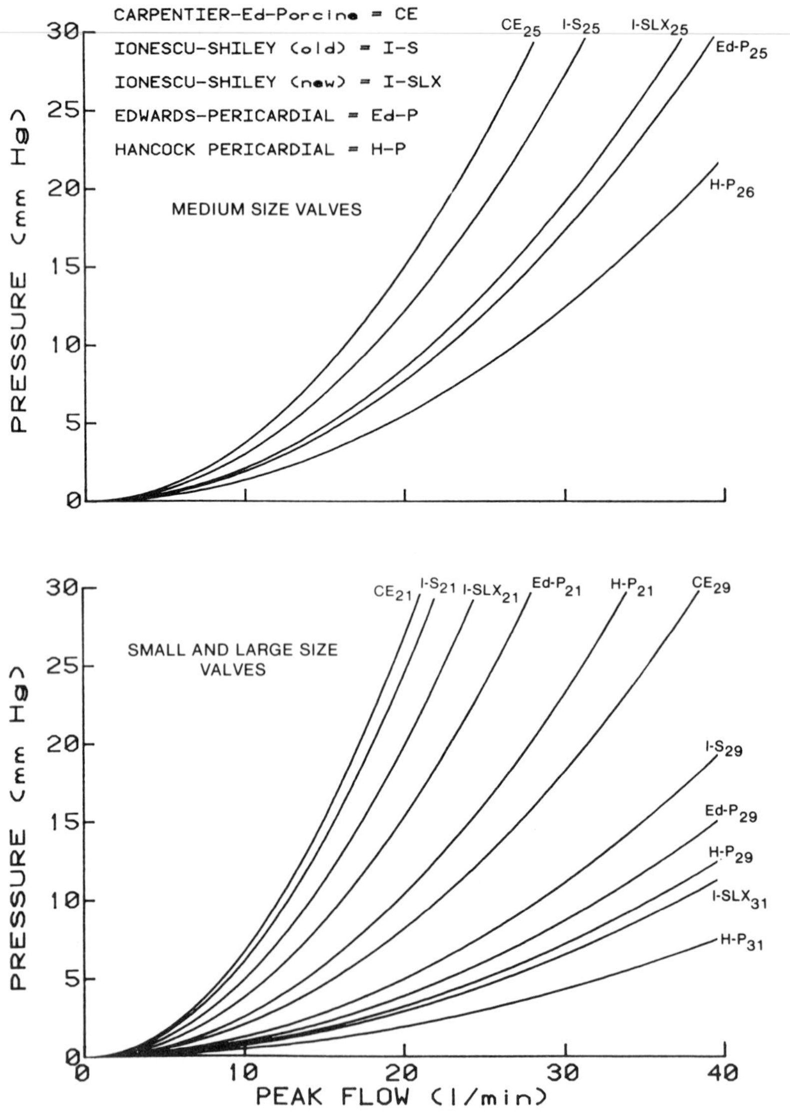

FIG. 4 Mitral position: Pressure drop versus peak flow. Note that performance of current medium size valves is similar to that of new small valves, and that C-E-29 has performance equivalent to that of new medium size valves.

TABLE II Comparison of parameters of the mitral valves

Valve	Range of EOA* (cm^2)	Mean EOA (cm^2)	PI	Mean gradient at "cardiac output" equivalent to 5 liters/min.	9 liters/min.	12.5 liters/min.
Small						
Carpentier-Edwards	1.06–1.25	1.16	0.33	24.6 mmHg	36.3 mmHg	—
Ionescu-Shiley	1.09–1.30	1.20	0.34	23.5	31.4	—
Ionescu-Shiley (new)	1.22–1.39	1.30	0.37	16.5	22.5	—
Edwards pericardial	1.36–1.62	1.50	0.43	15.0	19.7	—
Hancock pericardial	1.59–2.01	1.84	0.53	9.1	15.	—
Medium						
Carpentier-Edwards	1.42–1.71	1.59	0.32	12.0	17.5	30.
Ionescu-Shiley	1.27–1.78	1.60	0.32	11.0	22.1	29.8
Ionescu-Shiley (new)	1.81–2.19	2.02	0.41	9.3	14.5	23.8
Edwards pericardial	2.17–2.39	2.30	0.46	7.8	13.4	16.7
Hancock pericardial	2.07–2.74	2.51	0.47	4.9	9.2	15.
Large						
Carpentier-Edwards	1.56–2.31	2.13	0.32	6.17	12.4	20.8
Ionescu-Shiley	2.22–3.02	2.7	0.40	4.9	9.4	11.4
Ionescu-Shiley (new 31)	2.38–3.67	3.36	0.44	4.0	5.9	7.5
Edwards pericardial	2.83–3.21	3.08	0.46	2.8	7.1	10.
Hancock pericardial	1.81–3.36	2.84	0.43	4.4	7.1	10.
Hancock pericardial (31)	2.43–4.08	3.30	0.43	4.0	5.1	7.0

* As observed in previous studies and in this one, the EOA of the bioprosthesis increases with increased flow.
† All 29 mm unless otherwise mentioned.

ilarly. Obviously, the maximum peak gradient is much higher for all valves because of the higher peak flows (Fig. 5). Table III shows the mean gradients achieved at 5, 9, and 12.5 liters/min "cardiac output."

Effective Orifice Area

Mitral position. Table II compares the EOA based on the best fit through the data for the mitral group; since within certain limits the EOA is variable with the flow, a range of EOA is given for each valve. The EOA of the different groups were significantly different. In the small and medium sizes, the EOA of the Hancock is significantly better than that of the others ($p < 0.001$) and 50% greater than that of the old Ionescu-Shiley valve. The new Ionescu-Shiley valve shows a significant 30% improvement over the old one in the larger sizes but not in the 21 mm size.

Aortic position. For the aortic position, again the ranking is the same but the differences between the Edwards pericardial valve and the Ionescu-Shiley valve become insignificant. All valves have an EOA 5−15% greater in the aortic position than in the mitral position.

Performance Index

Mitral position. The performance index (PI) reflects how well the external dimension of a valve is utilized in providing forward flow. The Carpentier-Edwards porcine valve has the lowest PI (0.32) of all the sizes and the best PI was that of the Hancock 21 valve (0.53). In our previous studies[11,12], no biologic valve was found to have a PI more than 0.41.

Aortic position. In the aortic position the valves performed slightly better. For example, the PI of the Hancock 21 valve increased to 0.57.

Comment

This study shows that the biologic valves still have room for hemodynamic improvement. The new Ionescu-Shiley valve is an improvement over the previous design in larger sizes but not, unfortunately, in the small sizes. The Hancock pericardial valve has the largest opening in the small sizes. The pressure drops achieved by most of the small- and medium-sized valves in mitral and aortic positions are indicative of stenosis, but for the new devices these pressure drops are not critical for resting cardiac outputs. For even modest exercise, however, all remain excessively obstructive. The small Carpentier-Edwards porcine valve in the aortic position has a mean gradient of 29.5 mmHg at 5 liters/min (cardiac output), and of 51 mmHg at cardiac output of 9 liters/min. At higher flows of 12.5 liters/min, the mean gradient goes to 76 mmHg. The Ionescu-Shiley 21 (current)

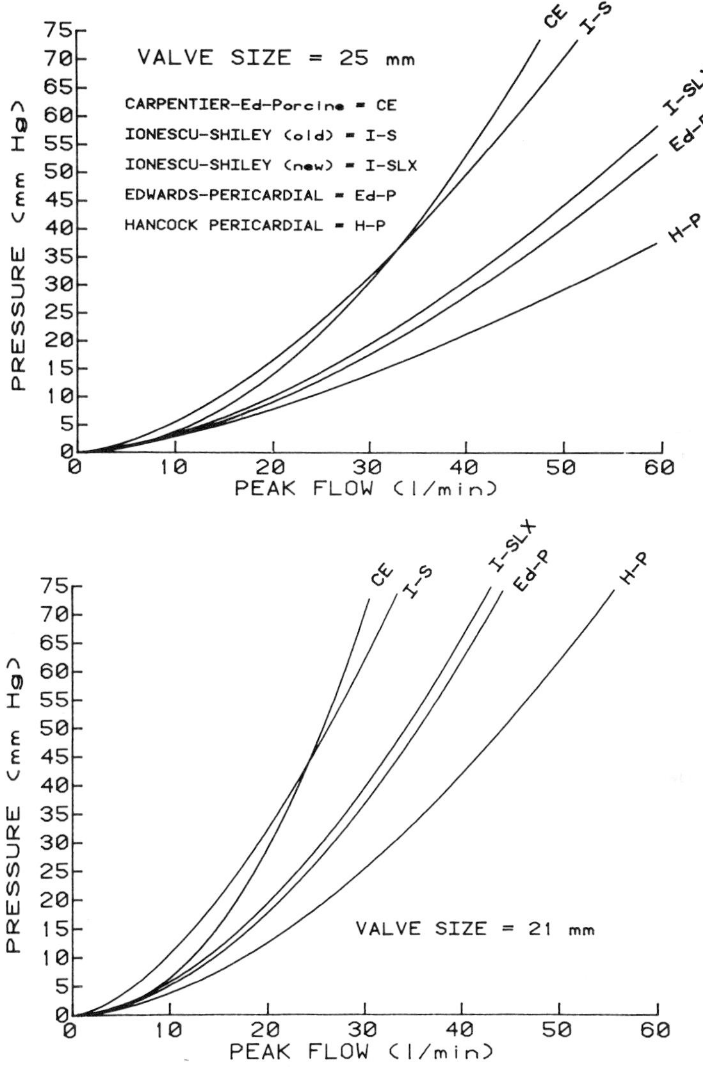

FIG. 5 Aortic position: Pressure drop as a function of peak flow. Same pattern is observed.

is not significantly better. The small Hancock pericardial valve in the aortic position has very acceptable gradients of 10, 21.4, and 31 mmHg, even at high flow rates.

The left ventricle can handle quite high pressure drops and it is difficult to define an acceptable gradient for an aortic valve. Mean gradients of 10 or 20 mmHg across aortic valves are acceptable, especially at higher flow rates.

TABLE III Comparison results in the aortic position

Valve	Range of EOA (cm^2)	Mean EOA (cm^2)	PI	Mean gradient* at "cardiac output" equivalent to		
				5 liters/min	9 liters/min	12.5 liters/min
Small						
Carpentier-Edwards	1.13–1.25	1.20	0.34	29.5 mmHg	51 mmHg	76 mmHg
Ionescu-Shiley	1.16–1.41	1.25	0.36	29	50	75
Ionescu-Shiley (new)	1.49–1.70	1.59	0.45	22.2	39.2	53
Edwards pericardial	1.55–1.76	1.64	0.47	22.8	41.3	73
Hancock pericardial	1.85–2.15	1.99	0.57	10	21.4	31
Medium						
Carpentier-Edwards	1.67–1.91	1.76	0.35	16.7	32	54
Ionescu-Shiley	1.61–2.02	1.84	0.37	19	32	48
Ionescu-Shiley (new)	1.91–2.44	2.30	0.46	11.3	22	33
Edwards pericardial	2.08–2.63	2.34	0.47	5.4	18.3	25
Hancock pericardial	2.31–3.08	2.80	0.52	8.3	16.8	23.8

* These gradients are probably higher than they would be in a patient at an equivalent cardiac output, because the ratio of systole to diastole in the duplicator is set at 3:6 at all flow and pulse rates, whereas in nature it would be closer to 1:1 at high rates.

Gradients that reach 20 mmHg in the mitral position are clearly not tolerable.

The question of the comparative performance of the same valve in the aortic and mitral positions is an interesting one. The peak flow and the peak gradient achieved in the aortic position, with the same setting of stroke volume and rate (Fig. 2), are inevitably higher than those in the mitral position. We have previously commented on the rise in EOA seen when transvalvular flows are increased.[12] Thus, it is not surprising that the EOA are larger in the aortic position. The systolic-diastolic ratio in our studies was maintained at a 30–60% ratio even at higher rates. This is not strictly comparable with what happens in nature and further studies are under way to define these questions more precisely.

The PI of these new valves has clearly improved. What PI should the "ideal" valve have? The healthy mitral valve has a potential diastolic area of 9–11 cm^2.[19] As a result, low gradients are recorded even in exercise. It is, in fact, probable that less than the whole mitral orifice is used.

Echocardiographically, the normal valve has a diastolic area of 4–6 cm^2.[20] Assuming that an ideal valve for the mitral position should have a mean gradient of less than 10 mmHg at high flow rates (12–15 liters/min), and that size 25 is the smallest reasonable size for adults in the mitral position, then the PI for the "ideal" valve should be 0.61, giving an area of 3.0 cm^2. This level is reached or closely approached in the larger sizes of all but the Carpentier-Edwards porcine bioprostheses. It has not been achieved in the smaller sizes. Of course, the use of these devices cannot be considered apart from durability, tendency to calcification, thromboembolism, and ease of use. With regard to the last factor, the Edwards pericardial xenograft has significantly shorter struts, making it attractive to the surgeon.

Conclusions

The porcine valvular bioprosthesis was significantly stenotic in all sizes. All the new pericardial valvular bioprostheses showed improvement over the current bioprosthetic designs. At high flow rates in the small and medium sizes, most of the biologic valves are still stenotic. If the pericardial valves will prove to have satisfactory durability, they will replace the porcine xenograft valves.

References

1. McIntosh CL, Michaelis LL, Morrow AG, Itscoitz SB, Redwood DR, Epstein SE: Atrioventricular valve replacement with the Hancock porcine xenograft: A five year clinical experience. Surgery 78:768, 1975.
2. Pipkin RD, Buch WS, Fogarty TJ: Evaluation of aortic valve replacement with a

porcine xenograft without long term anticoagulation. J Thorac Cardiovasc Surg 71:179, 1976.

3. Stinson EB, Griepp RB, Shumway NE: Clinical experience with a porcine aortic valve xenograft for mitral valve replacement. Ann Thorac Surg 18:391, 1974.
4. Galioto FM Jr., Midgley FM, Shapiro SR, Perry LW, Ciaravella JM Jr., Scott LP III: Mitral valve replacement in infants and children. Pediatrics 67:230, 1981.
5. Hetzer R, Hill JD, Kerth WJ, Ansboro J, Adappa MG, Rodvein R, Kamm B, Gerbode R: Thromboembolic complications after mitral valve replacement with Hancock xenograft. J Thorac Cardiovasc Surg 75:651, 1978.
6. Hellberg K, Ruschewski W, de Vivie ER: Early stenosis and calcification of glutaraldehyde-preserved porcine xenografts in children. Thorac Cardiovasc Surg 29:369, 1981.
7. Wada J, Yokoyama M, Hashimoto A, Imai Y, Kitamura N, Takao A, Monna K: Long-term follow-up of artificial valves in patients under 15 years old. Ann Thorac Surg 29:6, 1980.
8. Magilligan DJ Jr, Lewis JW Jr, Jara FM, Lee MW, Alam M, Riddle JM, Stein PD: Spontaneous degeneration of porcine bioprosthetic valves. Ann Thorac Surg 30:259, 1980.
9. Chaitman BR, Bonan R, Lepage G, Tubau JF, David PR, Dyrda I, Grondon CM: Hemodynamic evaluation of the Carpentier-Edwards porcine xenograft. Circulation 60:1170, 1979.
10. Wiltrakis MG, Rahimtoola SH, Harlan BJ, De Mots H: Diastolic rumbles with porcine heterograft prosthesis in the atrioventricular position. Normal or abnormal prosthesis? Chest 74:411, 1978.
11. Gabbay S, McQueen DM, Yellin EL, Becker RM, Frater RWM: In vitro hydrodynamic comparison of mitral valve prostheses at high flow rates. J Thorac Cardiovasc Surg 76:771, 1978.
12. Gabbay S, McQueen DM, Yellin EL, Frater RWM: In vitro hydrodynamic comparison of mitral valve bioprostheses. Circulation 60,(Suppl 2):17, 1978.
13. Becker RM, Strom J, Frishman W, Oka Y, Lin YT, Yellin EL, Frater RWM: Hemodynamic performance of the Ionescu-Shiley valve prosthesis. J Thorac Cardiovasc Surg 80:613, 1980.
14. Hauf E, Chalant C, Hahn C, Cosyns J, Pouleur H, Pollet J, Lefevre J, Charlier A: Comparative study of in vitro hydrodynamic behavior between three differently designed fascia lata valves and the Starr-Edwards prosthesis in aortic position. Eur Surg Res 5:37, 1973.
15. Björk VO, Olin C: A hydrodynamic comparison between the new tilting disc aortic valve prosthesis (Björk-Shiley) and the corresponding prostheses of Starr-Edwards, Kay-Shiley, Smeloff-Cutter and Wada-Cutter in the pulse duplicator. Scand J Thorac Cardiovasc Surg 4:31, 1970.
16. Scotten LN, Racca RG, Nugent AH, Walker DK, Brownlee RT: New tilting disc cardiac valve prostheses in vitro comparison of their hydrodynamic performance in the mitral position. J Thorac Cardiovasc Surg 82:136, 1981.
17. Wright JTM, Temple LJ: An improved method for determining the flow characteristics of prosthetic mitral heart valves. Thorax 26:81, 1971.
18. Gabbay S, Strom J, Frater RWM: Comparison of rigid and flexible pulse duplicator chambers for testing heart valves. Proceedings of the Association for Advancement of Medical Instrumentation, 16th Annual Meeting, 1981, p 45.
19. Rahlf G: Relative AV-insufficiency-morphometric and morphologic investigation of the AV-valve apparatus. Thorac Cardiovasc Surg 29:388, 1981.
20. Ormiston JA, Shah PM, Tei C, Wong M: Size and motion of the mitral valve annulus in man. I. A two-dimensional echocardiographic method and findings in normal subjects. Circulation 64:713, 1981.

40

In Vitro and In Vivo Assessment of the Flow Characteristics of the Xenomedica Porcine Xenograft

F. F. A. HENDRIKS, M. TURINA, H. A. HUYSMANS

Glutaraldehyde-preserved porcine bioprostheses are used for the replacement of human heart valves with increasing frequency. The lower risk of thromboembolism, even with possible avoidance of anticoagulation therapy, the theoretical merit of central orifice flow, and the acceptable hydrodynamic performance make it the prosthesis of choice in many cases. There is continuing research and redesigning of the valves, aimed at increasing their durability, avoiding early (stress- or other factor-induced) calcification and reducing the considerable transvalvular pressure gradients, especially for the small aortic models. Only recently Xenomedica AG in Switzerland introduced a new type of low pressure glutaraldehyde-preserved low profile porcine bioprosthesis. We have subjected this valve to a series of in vivo and in vitro tests. Applying pulsatile perfusion flow in an in vitro test setup (flow 0−13 liters/min using either saline or blood [30% Ht] as a perfusate), the hydrodynamic performance of aortic prostheses (20, 22, and 26 mm diameter supra-anular and 24 and 26 mm with conventional sewing rings) and mitral prostheses (25, 27, and 29 mm diameter) was assessed. In the supra-anular model the base of the sewing ring is placed at the level of the inflow orifice. In the flow tester the valves were mounted in a leak-tight housing specially constructed for all different valve sizes. Transvalvular pressure gradients at different flows, were measured using high fidelity pressure tip transducers directly proximal and distal to the valves. Flow through the valves was governed by a roller pump with a pulse duplicator and measured with an electromagnetic flow probe placed 2 cm above the valves. Regurgitating flow was read from the flow tracing.

From the Department of Thoracic Surgery, Leiden University Medical Center, Leiden, The Netherlands, and the Department of Cardiovascular Surgery, University Hospital, Zurich, Switzerland.

In 2 dogs and 2 pigs (± 40 kg weight) 25 mm diameter mitral valves were implanted. The pig experiments were unsuccessful, because the relatively large-sized valve, although low in profile (11 mm stent height), almost completely obstructed the outflow tract of the small ventricle. A smaller sized mitral model was not available at that time. In the dog experiments postoperative data could be obtained. Transvalvular pressure gradients were measured at different cardiac outputs.

Materials and Methods

A schematic drawing of the flow testing apparatus is given in Fig. 1. The temperature of the recirculating perfusate was kept at 37°C by means of a heat exchanger in the perfusate reservoir. Mitral valves were perfused with either saline or blood. In our hands no major difference was found in transvalvular gradients of the valves tested using either of the 2 perfusates. Therefore aortic prostheses were tested using only saline as a perfusate. In addition, the colorless perfusate allowed imaging of the valve behavior through a laparoscope positioned just above the valve. Transvalvular gradients (ΔP) were read at peak flow, and effective orifice areas were calculated according to the Gorlin formula[1] adapted for valvular prostheses by Gabbay et al.[2]

Results

Figure 2 shows an original recording of the in vitro measurement of the transvalvular gradient of a 20 mm aortic bioprosthesis. In Figs. 3 and 4, ΔP values for all mitral and aortic valves tested are plotted over the perfusion flow range. In Table I the gradients measured at 13 liters/min flow are given together with the calculated effective orifice areas. The maximum opening area of some of the valves was estimated by planimetry of segments of a film that was recorded while the valve was perfused (10 liters/min, saline perfusion). This calculated opening area (COA) is added to the data in Table I.

The amount of regurgitation was negligible for all valves (<2% of forward flow at a pressure difference of >80 mmHg). The results of an experiment with 1 dog are given in Table II.

Comment

The recently introduced Xenomedica porcine valvular bioprosthesis presents modifications over other porcine valves in the use for the past 10

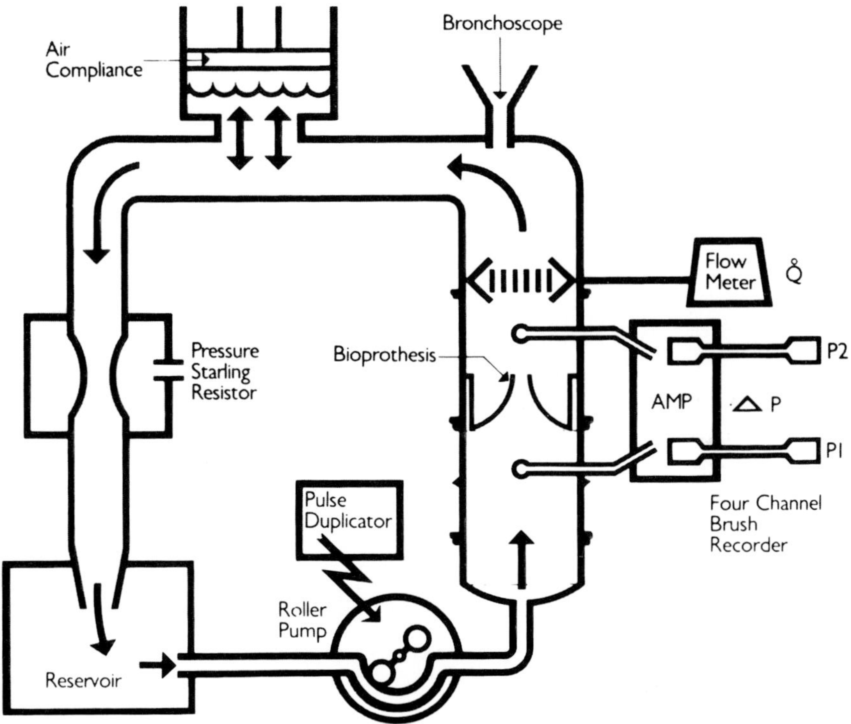

FIG. 1 Flow testing apparatus for in vitro assessment of hydrodynamic performance of valvular prostheses.

years. It has a low profile to decrease left ventricular protrusion markedly. Although low in profile, it induces no strain in the original porcine valve. Low pressure glutaraldehyde fixation (<10 cm water) preserves natural collagen structure and tissue elasticity[3] and possibly increases durability and decreases stress-mediated calcification. A limited pressure during fixation, however, is needed to assure coaptation of the valve leaflets. Stress at commissural junctions and sinuses is minimized in this valve prosthesis by the use of a creepless semirigid acetal copolymer stent. Carpentier et al[4] have only recently described the new techniques used to improve the design of the Carpentier-Edwards valvular bioprosthesis. The techniques of preservation and mounting of their valves are in many ways comparable to the procedures used by Xenomedica. The transvalvular gradients for the Xenomedica valves, measured in this study, compare well with those described for the improved Carpentier-Edwards valves. At a steady flow of 15 liters/min a transvalvular pressure gradient of, for example, 11.7 mmHg was found for the 21 mm diameter aortic valve.[4] Because in our setup 13

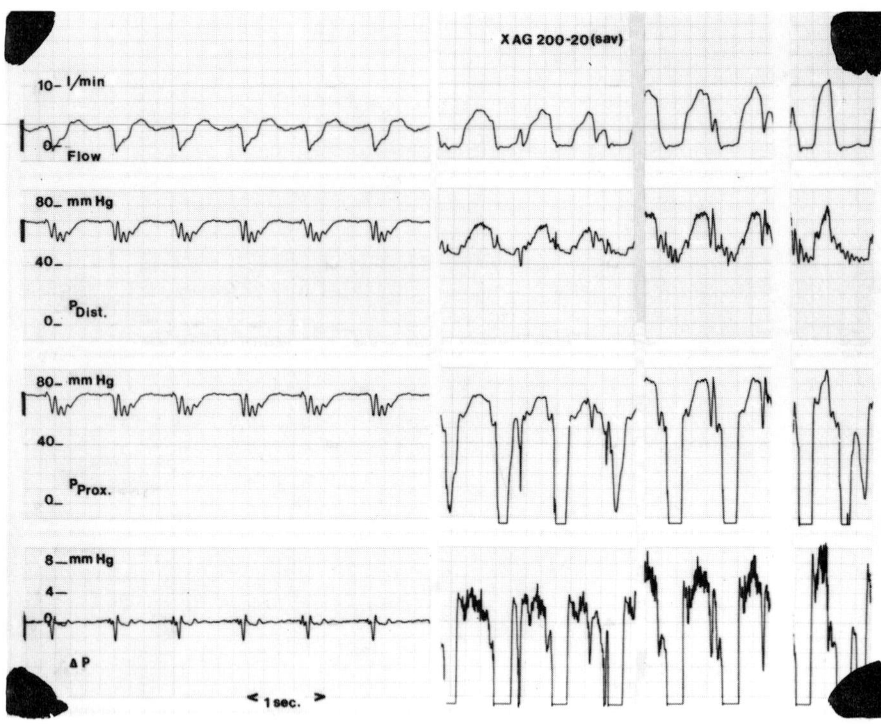

FIG. 2 Original recording of flow (upper tracing), distal pressure (second tracing), proximal pressure (third tracing,) and pressure difference (lower tracing) for a 20 mm diameter Xenomedica aortic bioprosthesis. Left part of recording shows that no pressure gradient was found perfusing the housing without a bioprosthesis.

liters/min is the maximum flow that can be achieved, comparison of gradients to flow beyond 13 liters/min cannot be given.

It was to be expected that in our setup no difference was found between "supra-anular" valves and valves with conventional sewing rings; the housing for the valves was constructed in such a way that only the stent and the valve were in the perfusion stream. In clinical implants the advantage consists of the option to replace the aortic valve with a larger-sized bioprosthesis (if supra-anular), since the prosthesis is fixed through the sewing ring above the original aortic anulus rather than inside it.

The calculated effective orifice areas for the mitral valves tested in this study are in the same range as the data presented by Gabbay et al[2] for the Hancock modified orifice prosthesis. It was a striking finding that an increased valvular diameter did not lead to markedly decreased gradients to flow for the mitral valves tested in this study. Although the differences were

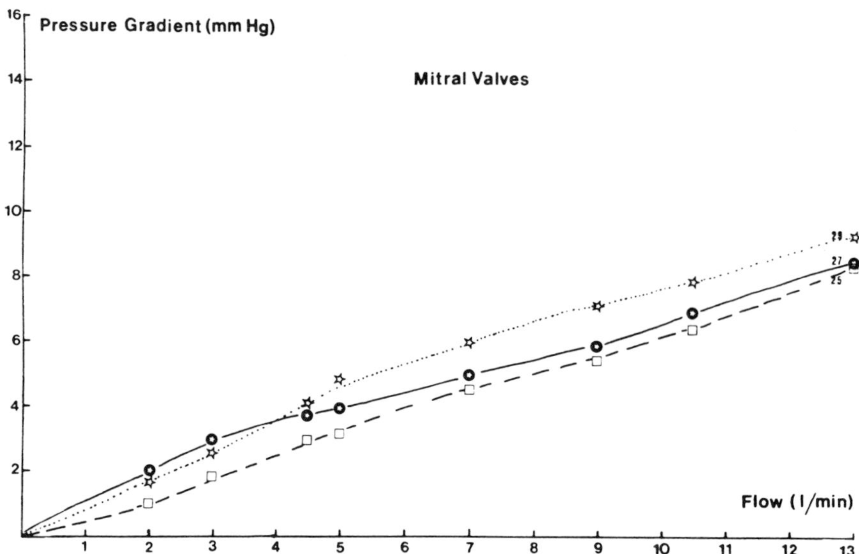

FIG. 3 Pressure gradients at different flows for 25 mm (---), 27 mm (——), and 29 mm (...) diameter Xenomedica mitral valve prosthesis.

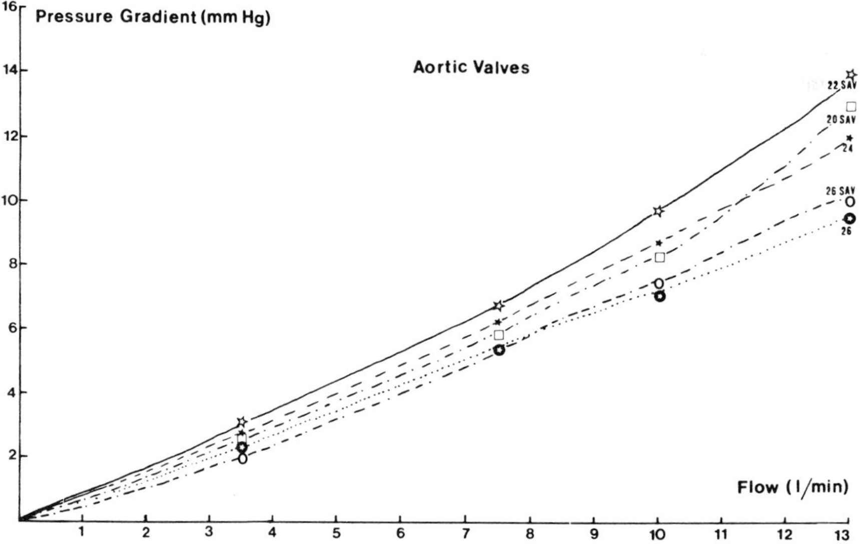

FIG. 4 Pressure gradients at different flows for 20 mm supra-anular (SAV) (-·-·), 22 mm SAV (——), 24 mm (---), 26 mm SAV (--·---·), and 26 mm conventional (· · ·) Xenomedica aortic valve bioprosthesis.

TABLE I Transvalvular pressure gradients (ΔP) at 13 liters/min perfusion flow*

Valve	Size (mm)	ΔP (mmHg)	EOA (cm^2)	COA (cm^2)
Aortic	20 SAV†	12.7	1.18	0.81
	22 SAV	13.7	1.13	0.94
	24	11.7	1.23	1.20
	26 SAV	9.8	1.34	1.35
	26	9.2	1.38	—
Mitral	25	8	1.48	1.32
	27	8	1.48	—
	29	9	1.40	—

* Effective orifice area was calculated from EOA = Q(ml/sec) $51.6\sqrt{\Delta P}$, and orifice area was obtained from planimetry at maximum opening (10 liters/min flow) (COA).
† SAV: supra-anular valve.

small (~1 mmHg for a flow of 13 liters/min) it seems obvious that increasing the valve diameter does not guarantee a decreased resistance to flow. Slight differences in the original valve construction, in the fixation procedure and in the mounting of the valve might influence the hydrodynamic behavior of the valve.

In the dog experiments we found pressure gradients in the range expected from the in vitro data, although the calculated effective orifice area for this 25 mm mitral valve prosthesis was somewhat larger than that for the 25 mm diameter tested in vitro.

Meanwhile, more than 30 clinical implants with the Xenomedica mitral and aortic porcine bioprosthesis have been performed in our institution. Several hundreds of these valves have been implanted clinically in several centers in Europe in the last 6 months. So far no complications have been reported.

TABLE II Transvalvular gradients (ΔP) and effective orifice area (Gorlin) for a 25 mm diameter mitral valve prosthesis in a 43 kg dog

	Heart rate (min^{-1})	Cardiac output (liters/min)	P (mmHg)	EOA (cm^2)
Preoperative	170	3.96	—	—
Directly	160	4.43	5.0	2.0
1 day postoperative	160	5.48	7.0	2.1
2 days postoperative	167	5.43	7.0	1.8

References

1. Gorlin R, Gorlin SG: Hydraulic formula for calculation of the area of the stenotic mitral valve, other cardiac valves, and central circulatory shunts. Am Heart J 41:1, 1951.
2. Gabbay S, McQueen DM, Yellin EL, Becker RM, Frater RWM: In vitro hydrodynamic comparison of mitral valve prostheses at high flow rates. J Thorac Cardiovasc Surg 76:771, 1978.
3. Broom ND, Thomson FJ: Influence of fixation conditions on the performance of glutaraldehyde-treated porcine aortic valves: Towards a more scientific basis. Thorax 34:166, 1979.
4. Carpentier A, Dubost C, Lane E, Nashef A, Carpentier S, Relland J, Deloche A, Fabiani JN, Chauvaud S, Perier P, Maxwell S: Continuing improvements in valvular bioprostheses. J Thorac Cardiovasc Surg 83:27, 1982.

41

The Structure/Function Relationship of Fresh and Glutaraldehyde-Fixed Aortic Valve Leaflets

N. Broom, G. W. Christie

The leaflets of natural aortic valves are highly differentiated connective tissue structures made up of the basic constituents—collagen, elastin, and glycosaminoglycans. As with all connective tissues, the specialization for a particular function is achieved by variations both in the relative amounts of each basic constituent and by variations in the morphologic arrangement.

Two factors can be identified as being central to the functional efficiency of aortic valve leaflets. Firstly, they must be capable of closing under minimal reverse pressure to ensure that the closed valve is fully competent. Secondly, the pressure difference across the closed valve gives rise to large stresses in the leaflets and, thus, the fibrous arrangement within the leaflets must be capable of distributing this load to the sinus boundary.

The functional requirements of the aortic valve are reflected in the morphology of the leaflet tissue. Although there have been many earlier studies of leaflet morphology, the relationship of the morphology to valve function is not yet fully understood.

It may be reasonably assumed that the aortic valve is optimally adapted to perform its purpose. However, when the aortic valve is fixed in glutaraldehyde, mounted on a frame, and implanted at some other site in the heart, such optimality will almost certainly be lost. It is hoped that by obtaining a more precise description of the morphology of aortic heart valves and, in particular, by relating that morphology to aortic valve function, a clearer picture will emerge of how fixation with glutaraldehyde and stent mounting alters the functional efficiency of the original structure.

This paper reviews what is currently known about leaflet morphology,

---

From the School of Engineering, University of Auckland, Auckland, New Zealand.

and then a computer model is utilized for clarifying the functional requirements of leaflets and determining how the physical properties of the tissue influence the valve function. Experiments are reported that show how the various structural elements of the leaflet contribute to its function. From this composite viewpoint, a picture is produced of the structure/function relationship for natural aortic valves. How the fixation with glutaraldehyde modifies the leaflet function is also investigated experimentally. High speed cine photography is employed to compare the in vitro function of high and low pressure-fixed porcine xenografts.

Previous Studies of Aortic Valve Leaflet Morphology

In the most recently reported studies of aortic valve morphology[1–3] 3 major structural layers have been identified. On the ventricular side, there is a layer of elastin fibers, on the aortic side, a layer of collagen fibers, and between these there is a loose connective tissue with a high content of glycosaminoglycans. The 2 outer layers are in each case covered with a thin layer of endothelial cells that are presumed to perform no mechanical function. The 2 fibrous layers, the elastin layer being termed the *ventricularis* and the collagen layer the *fibrosa,* can be readily identified by staining.[4]

This view of the structure is relatively simple. As noted by both Clark and Finke[3] and Sauren et al,[1] the ventricularis, although predominantly elastin, does appear to contain small quantities of collagen; Sauren et al[1] also identify a thin elastin layer lying above the fibrosa on the aortic side of the leaflet. Nevertheless, although the fine details of the structure of these 3 fundamental layers have not yet been determined, there is broad concurrence on their basic composition.

Of considerable importance is the fibrous arrangement within each of these layers. In the ventricularis, Sauren et al[1] found the elastin to be arbitrarily oriented in porcine aortic valves. However, Mohri et al[4] found the elastin layer in human valves to be arranged predominantly perpendicular to the free margin; Mohri et al's observations were in accord with those of Clark and Finke.[3]

There is more general agreement that the predominant alignment of collagen in the fibrosa is parallel with the free margin, although Sauren et al[1] apparently found collagen arranged perpendicular to the free margin. Clark and Finke[3] found a gradation of the collagen fiber diameters: the coarsest fibers lay near the aortic side and the finest on the interior side of the fibrosa. In addition, larger reinforcing bundles of collagen have been noted by various workers.[1,3,5] These bundles appear to radiate from the commissural area as a clearly discernible array and coalesce near the leaflet belly region, with similar large bundles radiating from points near the sinus boundary.

The central layer of loose connective tissue with a high content of mucopolysaccharide does not appear to have any clearly discernible structure and as yet its function remains uncertain. Mohri et al[4] have postulated that it may lubricate the relative movement of the fibrosa and ventricularis.

The coaptational part of the leaflet appears to have a fibrous arrangement that differs from that of the noncoaptational part. Although most authors have found this zone to be noticeably thinner than the rest of the leaflet, measurements made by Clark and Finke[3] of human aortic leaflets in the stressed state indicated that the coaptational part of the leaflet was substantially thicker than the remainder.

Within the fibrosa, the collagen is found to be arranged in planar arrays of crimped fibers.[5] Broom[5] has demonstrated that the characteristic stress-strain curve of microtensile samples taken parallel with the collagen fiber direction correlates closely with changes in the crimped waveform of the collagen layers on the application of a uniaxial stress. It is well known that collagen fibers have only a small intrinsic extensibility compared to elastin; hence, the circumferential compliance of the leaflet tissue would have to be primarily accounted for by the geometrical changes in the crimp arrangement rather than by significant stretching of the collagen fibers themselves. This is illustrated in Fig. 1. The approximately sinusoidal crimp can be characterized by the ratio of the amplitude, a, to the periodicity, P. The strain obtained as a function of the crimp parameter, a/P, is shown together with the measured values of a/P from Normaski interference micrographs. It is apparent that the straightening of the crimp alone accounts for the majority of the circumferential compliance. The remainder (approximately 3%) may be due to the intrinsic compliance of collagen fibers.

A further significant and consistently observable feature of the morphology of the fibrosa is its "corrugated" arrangement. These corrugations, which were first noted by Mohri et al,[4] produce a visible "rippling" of the aortic aspect of the leaflet. They are best seen on thin cross-sections stained to differentiate collagen and elastin. In stained sections, such as those studied by Mohri et al,[4] it is apparent that the fibrosa is corrugated and the ventricularis is not. The ridges of the corrugations are approximately parallel with the collagen fiber bundles in the fibrosa.

Clark and Finke[3] suggest that the corrugations on the aortic surface are due to large collagen bundles lying immediately below the endothelial layers on the aortic aspect. Sauren et al[1] theorize that the corrugations (variously referred to as invaginations, striations, and ripples) might act as hinges with the purpose of reducing bending stress during leaflet motions.

The tissue compliance in the radial direction (perpendicular to the free margin) is very much greater than that in the circumferential direction.[6–8] This means that the aortic leaflet tissue exhibits a very pronounced degree of elastic anisotropy. The strains possible in the radial direction are con-

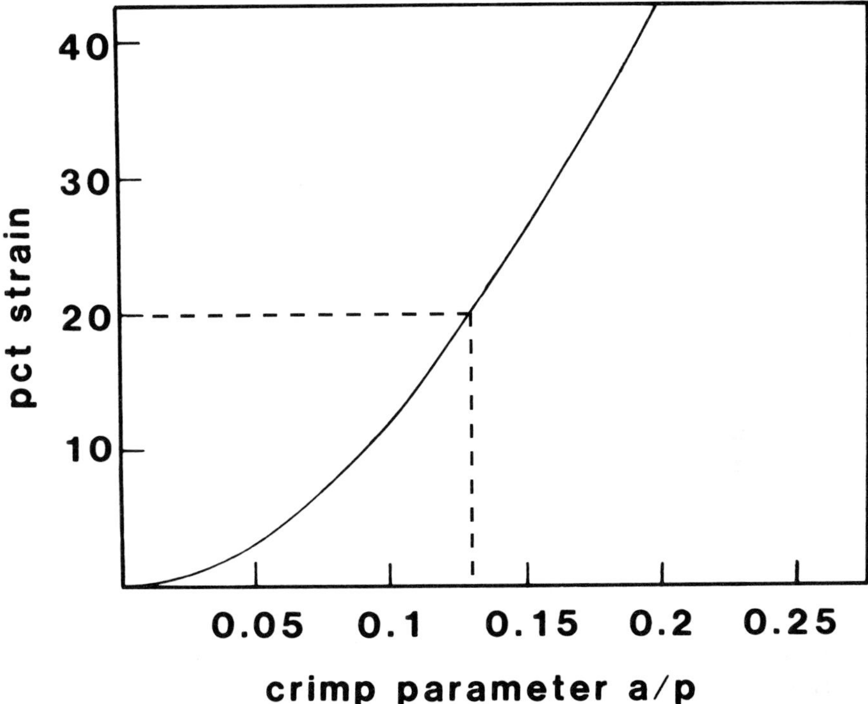

FIG. 1 Computed strain as function of crimp parameter a/P assuming geometry of sine wave.

siderably in excess of those that could be accounted for by any geometrical rearrangement of collagen crimp; therefore an alternative explanation must be sought. Sauren et al[1] postulate that the large radial compliance is due to the high intrinsic extensibility of the elastin-rich ventricularis.

There appears to be therefore a general acceptance of the concept that the aortic valve leaflet is composed of 3 reasonably distinct structural layers, the subdivision being based on the relative abundance of the fibrous proteins and glycosaminoglycans. Within each layer there may be further substructure, although there is no general concurrence on this point at the present time. There appears to be a conflict of opinion on the fibrous directionality in the ventricularis; it is described as arbitrarily arranged by Sauren et al[1] and as radially arranged by Mohri et al[4] and Clark and Finke.[3] In the fibrosa Sauren et al[1] report finding radially aligned collagen, whereas no other studies have commented on this feature. All studies have noted the corrugations of the fibrosa, although there is no uniformly consistent description of this feature.

Mechanical Requirements of an Aortic Valve Leaflet

The theoretic basis of this computer-based analysis has been discussed in detail by Christie[9] and Christie and Medland.[10] The leaflet deformation and the stress within the tissue can be calculated directly with greater reliability and generality than it can be measured using currently available experimental techniques. Within the computer-based method, no theoretic limitations are placed on the magnitude of the deformations that the leaflets may undergo or on the types of materials that can be considered.

The collagen fibers are aligned in an approximately circumferential direction within the leaflet. This gives the natural leaflets a very considerable degree of elastic anisotropy. The question is: in what way is such an arrangement of fibrous tissue beneficial to heart valve functions? To study this question in more detail, a series of aortic valve models were calculated, each being identical in terms of pressure loading and valvular geometry.

The first model used tissue with isotropic elastic properties. That is, the material compliance had no directional properties. When a back pressure is exerted on a valve with isotropic leaflets, the leaflets show virtually no tendency to move radially inward and form a coaptive seal. This is illustrated in Fig. 2(a), where a single leaflet is shown from the side along a line through the commissures. The configuration shown using the broken lines is the undistorted position of the leaflet, whereas the solid lines show the deformed position of the leaflet under a pressure of 16 kilopascal (kPa). The cross-hatched area is the coaptation area; the stresses are indicated by lines, the length of which gives the stress magnitude.

If, however, the material compliance in the circumferential direction is progressively reduced with all other model parameters held constant, the results given in Fig. 2(b)–(d) are obtained. With the progressive reduction in circumferential compliance, there is a concomitant increase in the coaptation area and a decrease in the stress magnitudes near the commissures.

Previous theoretic analyses[10] have shown that any isotropic leaflet with aortic valve geometry, irrespective of its material compliance, exhibits the same behavior displayed by the model in Fig. 2a. Effective valve closure has been achieved only when the circumferential compliance is substantially less than the radial compliance. The relatively inextensible collagen fibers substantially restrict the natural tendency of the leaflets to respond to a pressure applied to the aortic aspect of the valve by bulging down into the ventricle. Furthermore, in addition to bulging toward the ventricle when under pressure, isotropic leaflets show a tendency to move radially outward. This motion is precisely the opposite of that required to effect a completely competent valve closure.

By reducing the circumferential compliance with fibers of low extensibility, the downward bulging of the leaflet is greatly restricted and a considerable inward radial motion results. The net effect is a large increase in the

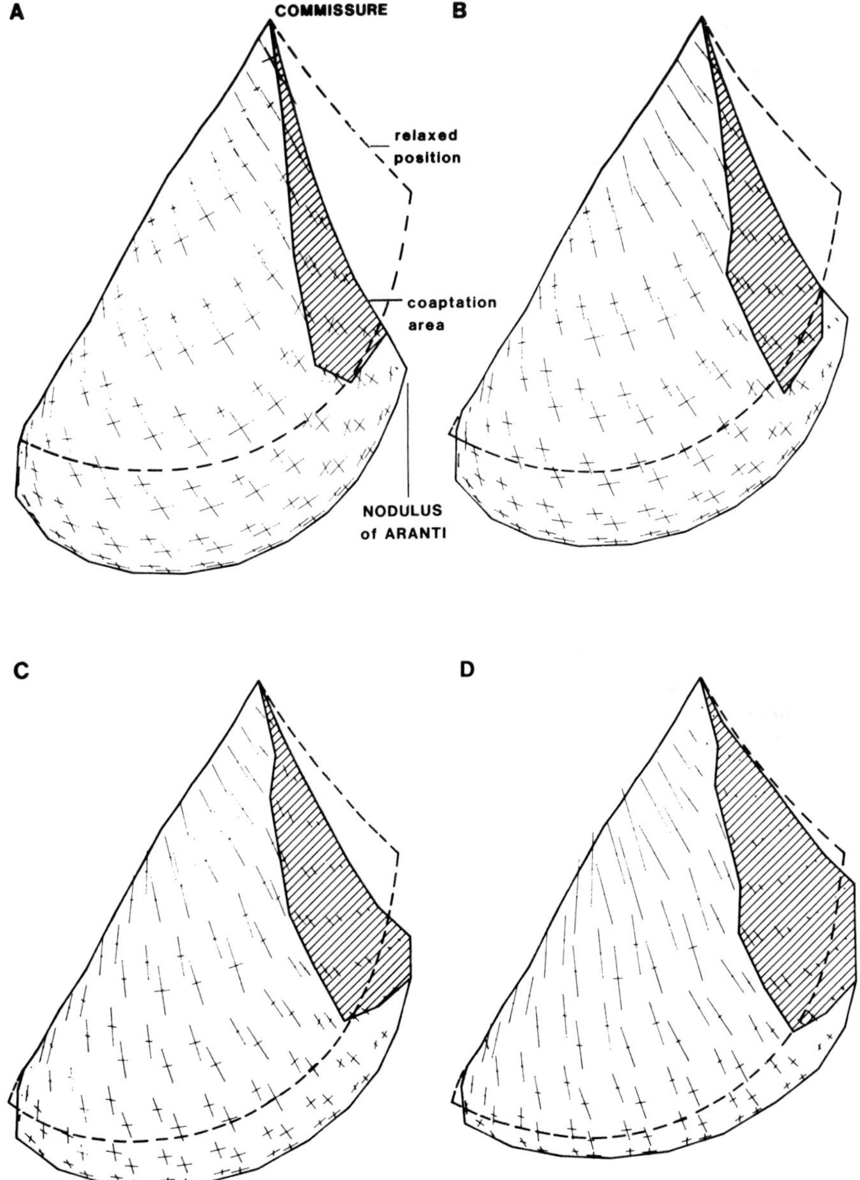

FIG. 2 Computed side views of modeled aortic heart valve leaflet: (A) elastically isotropic tissue; (B)–(D) illustrate effect of increasing the ratio of the radial to circumferential compliance.

coaptational area with a high degree of area redundancy, this being essential if the risk of regurgitation is to be minimized.

We may conclude that low circumferential compliance and large radial compliance are essential features of aortic leaflet tissue. The greater the relative difference between their compliances, the greater the advantage accrued by the valve in terms of functional efficiency and margin of safety. By inference, any restriction on the radial compliance, such as that that may result from the presence of radially aligned collagen fibers, could be expected to be disadvantageous to the functional performance of the valve and, hence, unlikely to be found.

The model studies are also significant in that they provide interesting insight into the orientation of the stress in aortic valve leaflets. It is generally supposed that connective tissues respond to stress by reinforcing themselves in the direction of stress and reabsorbing material aligned where little stress is present. Such behavior has been well demonstrated in the growth of bone under stress. Thus, the leaflets of aortic valves, which are repeatedly subjected to considerable stress during diastole, should exhibit a fiber arrangement that optimizes the transmission of load to supporting structures at the leaflet periphery.

The stresses in the isotropic leaflet show a marked alignment in the circumferential direction; the greatest stresses are near the commissures. As the circumferential compliance is reduced, there is an increase in the circumferential stress and a reduction in the radial stress component. It may be further observed that, as the coaptational area increases, the leaflet-free margin receives greater support; this is reflected by a significant drop in stress in the coaptive margin. This analysis therefore predicts that the tissue need not be as thick in the coaptational part of the leaflet as in the noncoaptational, an observation in harmony with the observation of Sauren et al[1] but contrary to the results of Clark and Finke.[3]

We note in passing that if the leaflet does adapt its load-bearing capacity to the stress and if the stress is low on the coaptational part of the leaflet, any fabrication error that brings part of the coaptational region into the noncoaptational part will expose to very high stresses tissue that has adapted its structure to carry only low stresses.

Experimental Study of Load-Bearing Elements in Aortic Leaflets

In order to elucidate the function roles of the different layers comprising the leaflet cross-section, we conducted a variety of tensile loading experiments on radial and circumferential samples of tissue removed from fresh porcine aortic leaflets. Load/strain curves were obtained from these samples both before and following severing of the fibrosa or ventricularis with a sharp blade. With the procedure, it was possible to differentiate between the load carried by either layer and then relate the functional role of each layer to its own particular configuration of fibers.

Circumferential Compliance and Its Structural Origin

Typical load/strain curves for intact circumferential samples are shown in Fig. 3(a) and (b). The initial, highly compliant region of the curve up to about 20% strain is followed rapidly by strain-locking, i.e., a sharp rise in load with increased strain. The reload curve following severing of the fibrosa or the ventricularis (Fig. 3) was similar in form to that obtained from the intact tissue and displaced only a small fraction along the strain axis. This suggested that both the fibrosa and the ventricularis were participating in

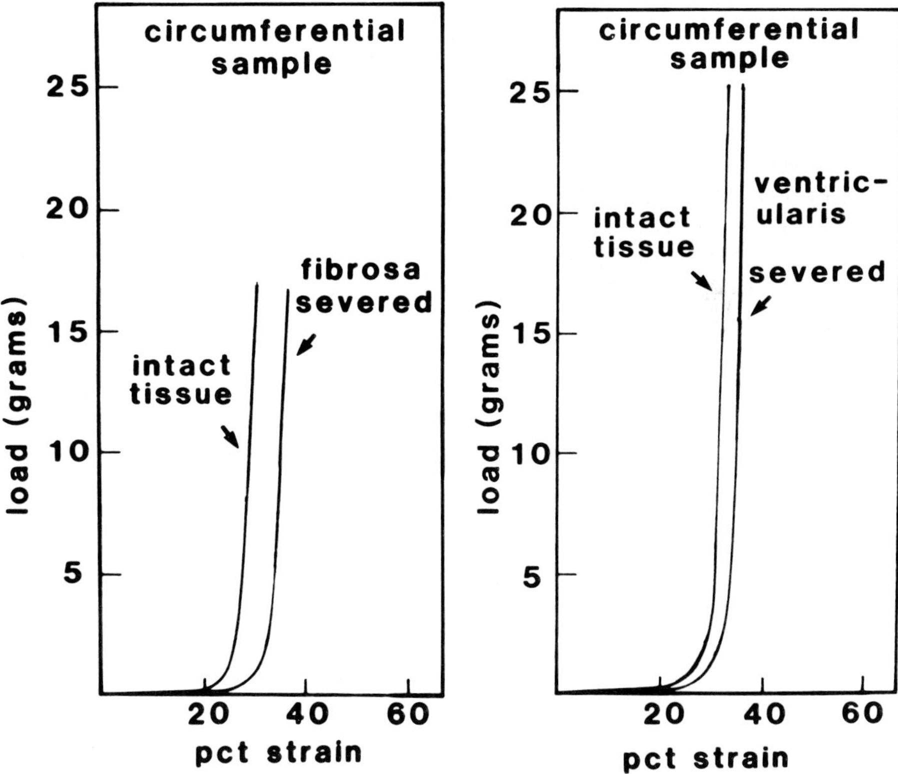

FIG. 3 (left) Load/strain response from fresh circumferential strip of porcine aortic leaflet before and following severing of fibrosa; (right) load/strain response from fresh circumferential strip of porcine aortic leaflet before and following severing of ventricularis.

circumferential loadbearing in the leaflet. A severing of either layer results in an immediate transference of load to the other with little increase in tissue compliance. The rapid decrease in compliance beyond about 20% strain arises from the presence of crimped collagen fibers aligned nearly circumferentially in both the fibrosa and ventricularis. Extension of these fibers beyond the region at which this crimp is largely straightened accounts for the observed rapid loss of compliance.[5] Hence, we conclude that the circumferential compliance in the leaflet is governed primarily by the presence of circumferential collagen. Because a greater proportion of collagen is present in the fibrosa, the bulk of the circumferential loading in the leaflet will be carried by this layer.

Radial Compliance and its Structural Origin

The fully relaxed radial sections of fresh tissue exhibited the familiar deep corrugations in the fibrosa (Fig. 4, top). Following loading in tension, these corrugations were considerably reduced in amplitude and the ventricularis, already smooth, simply extended (Fig. 4, bottom). Load/strain curves for intact radial sections are given in Fig. 5. Strains well in excess of 70% were observed in these radial sections. The reload curves obtained following severing of the fibrosa were almost identical to those from the intact tissue, whereas severing of the ventricularis resulted in a dramatic increase in compliance at extensions well beyond those at which strain locking was observed in the intact tissue (Fig. 5). Thus we can conclude that it is the ventricularis and not the fibrosa that constitutes the primary load-bearing layer in the radial direction of the leaflet.

Structurally, the elastin in the ventricularis provides this radial compliance. Here the elastin fibers, at least in the central belly of the fully relaxed fresh leaflet, are arranged as a diffuse multilayered meshwork but with a predominant radial alignment. In response to tensile loading in the radial direction this meshwork becomes increasingly realigned radially. The initial high compliance reflects an increasing straightening of the irregular elastin meshwork and the increased stiffness with increasing deformation arising from the axial loading of the realigned fibers.

We found no evidence of any radially orientated collagen in the ventricularis: all collagen observed in this layer was approximately circumferential. This ventricularis collagen tended also to occur as discrete aggregates compared to the more continuous sheetlike arrays in the fibrosa.

Glutaraldehyde Fixation Studies

In considering the general concept of glutaraldehyde fixation of tissue valves, we believe that as a working principle it is essential to retain as far as

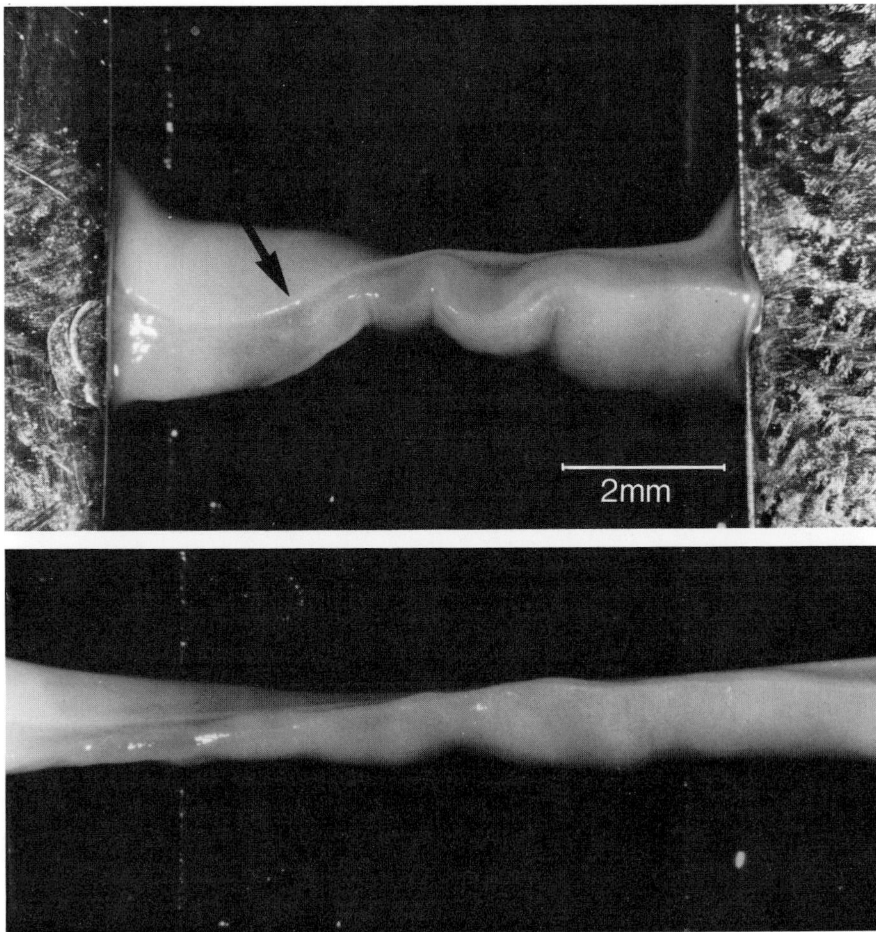

FIG. 4 (top) Radial strip from fresh porcine aortic leaflet. Note corrugations in fibrosa in contrast to the smooth ventricularis (arrow); (bottom) Radial strip as in above deformed in tissue to greater than 70% strain.

possible in the fixed tissue those structural characteristics exhibited by the fresh tissue.

Quite apart from such variables as glutaraldehyde concentration, temperature of fixation, pH, and chemical modifications of the basic fixative formula, the pressure to which the whole valve is subjected during fixation is now known to influence dramatically the mechanical properties of the leaflet tissue. Although much less is known about the ability of glutaraldehyde to permanently cross-link elastin structures,[11] it has been shown that this

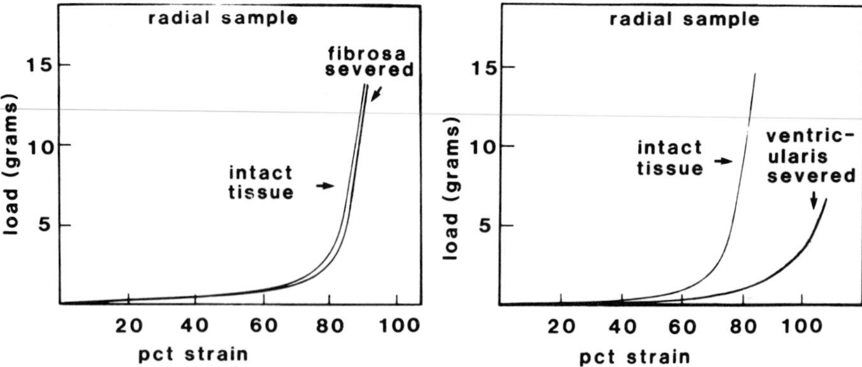

FIG. 5 (left) Load/strain response from fresh radial strip of porcine aortic leaflet before and following severing of fibrosa; (right) load/strain response from fresh radial strip of porcine aortic leaflet before and following severing of ventricularis.

fixative captures permanently the geometry of the leaflet collagen, as determined by the pressure loading on the valve, and that this in turn determines very largely the circumferential compliance of the fixed leaflets,[12,13]

The initial high compliance characteristic of the stress/strain curve, being related directly to large changes in the collagen crimp geometry, means that quite small pressures applied to the whole valve during fixation will significantly affect the circumferential compliance of the fixed leaflets. Thus, in order to retain as much as possible the full crimp geometry present in the fresh tisssue, fixation must be carried out with the valve at nearly 0 pressure.

Most recently, we have investigated the effect of glutaraldehyde fixation on the radial compliance. Tissue fixed in its relaxed condition demonstrates a definite loss of compliance (Fig. 6, left). For example, comparing strains at the rather arbitrary load of 50 g, there is a decrease in compliance of about 23% in the fixed tissue. Fixation of tissue loaded into the strain-locked region results in a greatly reduced radial compliance on reloading compared to the tissue fixed at 0 load (Fig. 6, right).

Severing of the fibrosa of radial sections obtained from leaflets fixed in their relaxed state had only a minor influence on the load/strain response (Fig. 7). Thus, it is the cross-linking of components in the ventricularis rather than those in the fibrosa that determines the radial compliance of the fixed leaflet.

These studies therefore demonstrate the important role of fixation pressure in determining both the circumferential and radial mechanical properties of the leaflets. These in turn have a direct influence on whole valve function and this will be discussed next.

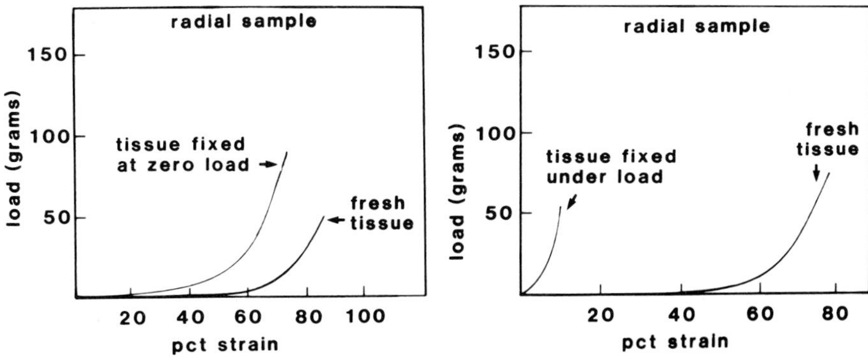

FIG. 6 (left) Load/strain response from a radial strip of porcine aortic leaflet before and following fixation in its fully relaxed state; (right) load/strain response from radial strip of porcine aortic leaflet before and following fixation in loaded state.

High Speed Cine Studies of Glutaraldehyde-Fixed Whole Valves In Vitro

A pulse duplicator that realistically represented the pulsatile flow conditions at the aortic position was used to compare the leaflet motion of the high and low pressure-fixed valves. The valves used were 27 mm (nominal diameter) Carpentier-Edwards porcine bioprostheses and were of clinical quality.

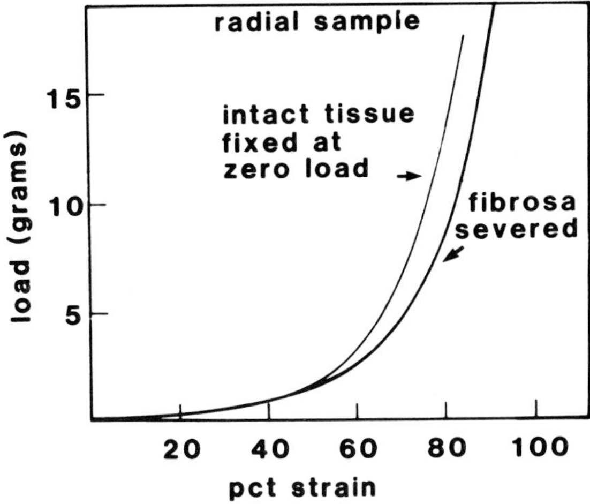

FIG. 7 Load/strain response from radial strip of porcine aortic leaflet fixed in its fully relaxed state but before and following severing of fibrosa.

The pulse rate was 72 beats/min and the flow rate was 5.5 liters/min. The fluid medium used was Ringer's solution at room temperature. Moderate film speeds of 300 frames/sec were found to be adequate for the purposes of illustrating the differences in leaflet motion between the high and low pressure-fixed valves. The results, showing only the closure phase, are given in Fig. 8 for the high pressure and low pressure valves, respectively.

In the high pressure-fixed valve the leaflets respond to the changing flow conditions via a series of localized points of high surface curvature separating regions of only minimal flexure. This behavior is particularly prominent at the leaflet-free margins closer to the commissures. No such sites can be identified in the leaflets of the low pressure-fixed valve. Instead, movement occurs via a sequence of gentle curvature changes spreading progressively across the whole leaflet. No one region of the leaflet appeared to be subjected to any localized concentration of strain.

Earlier studies[5,12] demonstrated that these sites of high curvature or "kinks" are a consequence of the crimp in the collagen being eliminated through high pressure fixation. Furthermore, accelerated fatigue studies conducted on both glutaraldehyde-fixed porcine mitral leaflet tissue[13] and high and low pressure-fixed porcine aortic leaflet tissue[5] have demonstrated a greatly increased susceptibility to fatigue disruption of the collagen in regions where there is a concentration of compressive stress: namely, those kink sites in the high pressure-fixed valves.

Similar high speed cine studies of stent-mounted aortic valve allografts have failed to show any evidence of any localized areas of high curvature; it may be inferred that the presence of "kinks" is a characteristic of the high pressure valve but not of glutaraldehyde-fixed valves generally. On the basis of available evidence, it may be concluded that low pressure-fixed valves should show an increase in longevity in vivo. In particular there should be a significant reduction in tissue disruption near the commissures where the "kinks" in the high pressure valve are most commonly found.

Relationship of Aortic Valve Leaflet Morphology to Function

It is now possible to combine the complementary theoretic and experimental studies to produce what appears to be a consistent structure/function relationship for aortic heart valve leaflets. We believe that, although the picture is not yet complete, it does offer a clarification of our current understanding of why aortic leaflets have their particular form and why that form is advantageous to whole valves.

Such a viewpoint is useful for other reasons. Firstly, it provides us with a basis for deciding whether a given feature of leaflet morphology is a general feature of all valves or whether it is better attributed to the small anatomic variations that occur within any biologic population. The second advantage to be gained from developing a model for leaflet structure is the

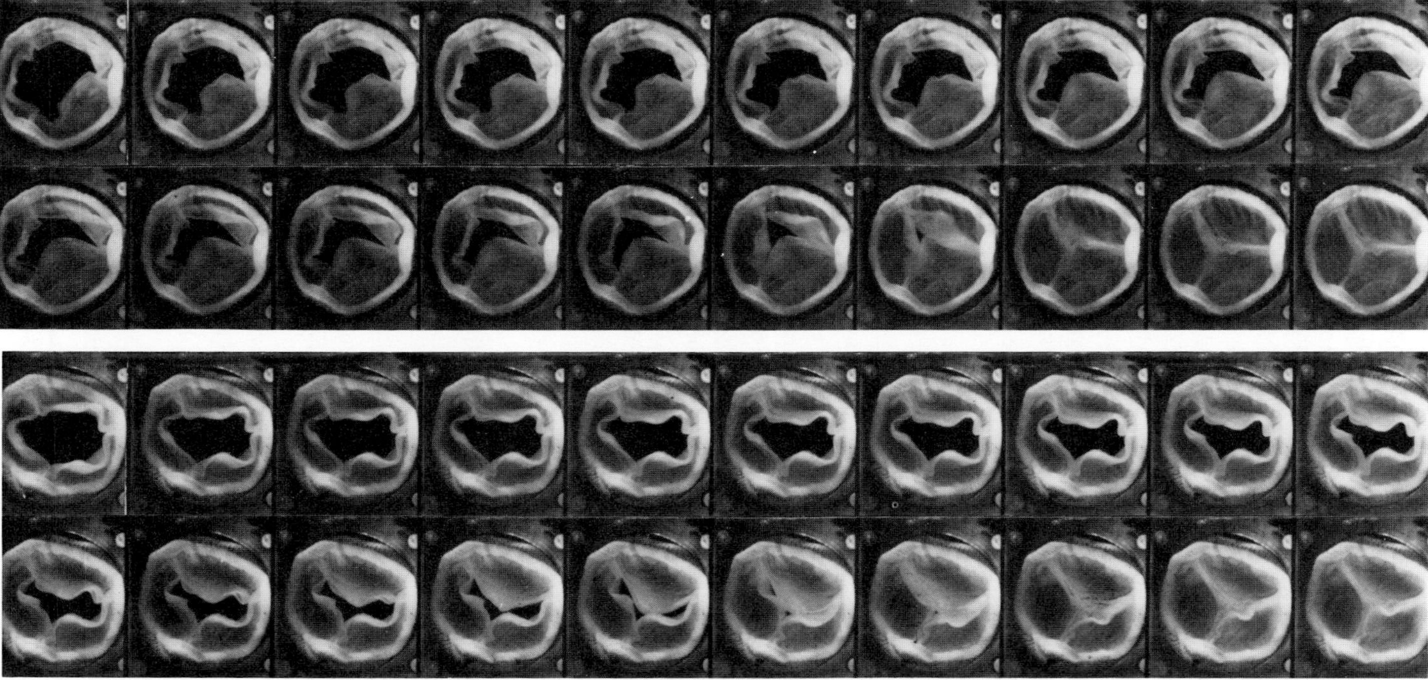

FIG. 8 Cine film sequence showing closure phase of 2 Carpentier-Edwards porcine bioprostheses: (top) high pressure-fixed valve; (bottom) low pressure-fixed valve.

instructive insight it offers when interpreting how any geometric or biochemical manipulation is likely to affect the whole valve function.

We may summarize the leaflet morphology by a simple model. There are 3 major layers, which are differentiated primarily by their material composition, fibrous arrangement, and mechanical function.

The principal load-bearing layer is the fibrosa, which is composed almost entirely of circumferentially aligned planar sheets of collagen. We theorize that these planar sheets of crimped collagen are responsible for transmitting stress from the noncoaptional part of the leaflet to different parts of the aortic wall. The fibrosa has corrugation crests aligned circumferentially to prevent the destruction of its structural integrity when undergoing very large radial strains.

The ventricularis is predominantly composed of elastin with small isolated bundles of collagen interspersed within it. The collagen is arranged approximately circumferentially while the elastin shows a slight predominance of radial alignment in the relaxed state and a marked rearrangement toward radial alignment as the radial strain is increased. This dependence of elastin arrangement on strain may explain some of the divergence of opinion on elastin alignment evident in the earlier studies.

How the fibrosa and ventricularis are attached to each other is not clear, although an attachment is easily demonstrated experimentally. The attachment is by no means as strong as bonding *within* the 2 main fibrous layers; it is relatively easy mechanically to delaminate the fibrosa from the ventricularis. This question is of importance when considering the long-term effects of glutaraldehyde fixation on valvular longevity.

The voids between the corrugated fibrosa and the relatively flat ventricularis are filled by loose connective tissue, as may be readily seen in radial cross-sections. At the present time, the mechanical function of this intermediate layer (termed the spongiosa) is not clear. At least 4 possible functions have been ascribed to it, being: 1) void filling; 2) fibrosa/ventricularis bonding; 3) interlayer lubrication; and 4) viscous damper for energy dissipation. All 4 seem plausible possibilities, especially as the mechanical properties of the spongiosa are probably nearer to those of a viscous fluid than a fibrous solid and, further, there must be a significant rearrangement of the spongiosa as the fibrosa corrugations are repeatedly flattened and retracted.

The overall leaflet thickness reduction of 50% in going from the relaxed to the stressed state in human aortic valve leaflet, as reported by Clark and Finke,[3] would appear to be accounted for by the reduction in amplitude of the corrugations as the leaflet is stretched radially. Therefore the thickness change is partially made up from the reduction that always accompanies in-plane stretching of any material and partially from geometric rearrangements within the leaflet.

The experiments on radially aligned microtensile samples fixed in a relaxed state with glutaraldehyde indicate that the fractional loss of radial compliance compare to that of fresh tissue is substantially larger than that found for similar circumferentially aligned samples. It should be emphasized, however, that current "reduced" pressure-fixed porcine bioprostheses have been fixed while the valve is closed. This means the radial strains are close to the maximum they will obtain when fixation takes place and hence the compliance loss should not adversely affect valvular competence. We also note in passing that fixation of elastin is not yet well understood: Fung[11] has shown that pure samples of elastin do not appear to be completely fixed by glutaraldehyde and that some elastin contraction occurs after fixation when fixation has been carried out in a stressed state.

The differences between the thickness and possibly also the fibrous arrangement of the tissue in the low stress coaptional and the high stress noncoaptional parts of the leaflet are significant. It is therefore essential that the natural boundaries of these 2 apparently different tissue structures be carefully preserved during fabrication of stent-mounted aortic valves.

References

1. Sauren AAHJ, Kuijpers W, VanStreenhoven AA, Veldpaus FE: Aortic valve histology and its relation to mechanics—preliminary report. J Biomech 13:97, 1980.
2. Ferrans VJ, Spray TL, Billingham ME, Roberts WC: Structural changes in porcine xenografts used as substitute cardiac valves. Am J Cardiol 41:1159, 1978.
3. Clark RE, Finke EH: Scanning electron microscopy of human aortic leaflets in stressed and relaxed states. J Thorac Cardiovasc Surg 67:792, 1974.
4. Mohri H, Reichenback DD, Merendino KA: Biology of homologous and heterologous aortic valves. In: Biological Tissue in Heart Valve Replacement (MI Ionescu, DN Ross, GH Wooler, Eds). London, Butterworths, 1972, p 137.
5. Broom ND: An "in vitro" study of mechanical fatigue in glutaraldehyde-treated porcine aortic valve tissue. Biomaterials 1:3, 1980.
6. Tan AJK: Tensile behaviour of aortic heart-valve leaflets and sterilization effects. Masters Dissertation, University of Auckland, New Zealand, 1974.
7. Clark RE: Stress-strain characteristics of fresh and frozen human aortic and mitral leaflets and chordae tendineae. J Thorac Cardiovasc Surg 66:202, 1973.
8. Missirlis YE, Chong M: Aortic valve mechanics—Part I: Material properties of natural porcine aortic valves. J Bioeng 2:287, 1978.
9. Christie GW: Analysis of the mechanics of bioprosthetic heart valves. Doctoral Dissertation, University of Auckland, New Zealand, 1982.
10. Christie GW, Medland IC: A non-linear finite element stress analysis of bioprosthetic heart valves. In: Finite Elements in Biomechanics (RH Gallagher, BR Simon, PC Johnson, JF Gross, Eds). New York, John Wiley, 1982.
11. Fung YC: Biomechanics—Mechanical Properties of Living Tissue. New York, Springer-Verlag, 1981, Chapter 7.
12. Broom ND, Thomson FJ: Influence of fixation conditions on the performance of glutaraldehyde-treated porcine aortic valves: Towards a more scientific basis. Thorax 34:166, 1979.
13. Broom ND: Simultaneous morphological and stress/strain studies on the fibrous components in wet heart valve leaflet tissue. Connect Tissue Res 6:37, 1978.

SECTION VIII

LONG-TERM FOLLOW-UP

42

Bioprostheses in the Tricuspid Position Versus Valvuloplasty and Mechanical Valves

D. Blin, M. Mostefa, J. E. Kara, J. E. Touze, A. Mouly, F. Langlet, A. Goudard, J. R. Monties

Between September 1972 and February 1982, we operated upon 302 patients for tricuspid valve disease; there were 186 females and 116 males, the average age was 41 years (range, 5–70 years).

Of the 302 operations, 200 involved the tricuspid and mitral valves (TM) and 89 involved the tricuspid, mitral, and aortic valves (TMA). Only 12 operations were performed on the tricuspid valve alone (T) and 1 on tricuspid and aortic valves.

Operative therapy of the tricuspid valve consisted of 169 bioprosthesis replacements, 111 anuloplasties, and 22 mechanical valve implantations. The different types of prostheses and anuloplasties are listed in Table I. Follow-up and analysis of results were performed automatically by means of an original Progiciel (SESAME), which we composed on an IBM computer (4342 model 2).

Myocardial protection was achieved by the following techniques: moderate hypothermic coronary perfusion (1972–1976); general hypothermia, with aortic cross clamping and local hypothermia (1977–1978), and associated with cardioplegia (1979–1982).

Postoperatively, patients received heparin intravenously through an electric syringe. After the initial 48 hours, heparin was replaced by Calciparin for 45 days. If at the end of that time the patient displayed sinus rhythm and had not received a mechanical valve, anticoagulants were used for 3 months or until the patient was put on antiaggregates. If not, the patients were put on anticoagulants for life.

From the Hôpital Salvator, Marseille, France.

TABLE I Type of tricuspid valve repair

Valve	#
Anuloplasty	
De Vega	72
Kay	5
Carpentier	34
Total	111
Bioprosthesis	
Carpentier	89
Hancock	58
Angell	22
Total	169
Mechanical	
Beall	12
Björk	9
Braunwald	1
Total	22

Results

Operative Mortality

The overall mortality rate was 10.9% (Table II). This rate varied according to the following factors: 1. The associated valvulopathies were TM: 7.5% (15/200): TMA: 17.9% (16/89): T: 16.7% (2/12). 2. The circumstances of the operation included planned first operation: 9% (20/225); semiemergency: 14.2% (1/7); emergency: 47% (8/17); first reoperation: 5.7% (2/35); second reoperation: 25% (2/8); third reoperation: 50% (1/2). (Semiemergency means that the patient could not wait 1 week and emergency, that he could not wait 1 day). 3. The date of operation (and therefore the type of myocardial protection (Fig. 1): 1972–1976: 16.9% (11/65); 1977–1978: 11.8% (9/76); 1979–1982: 8.9% (14/157). 4. The right ven-

TABLE II Operative mortality

Valves repaired	# operations	Deaths	%
Tricuspid and mitral	200	15	7.5
Tricuspid, mitral, aortic	89	16	17.9
Tricuspid	12	2	16.7
Tricuspid and aortic	1	0	0
Total	302	33	10.9

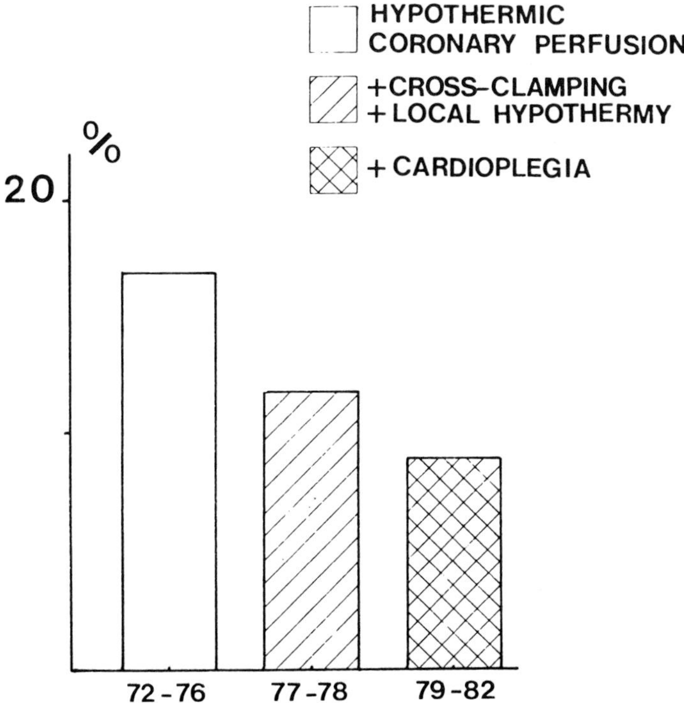

FIG. 1 Operative mortality (%) for tricuspid valve replacement for each time period based on different forms of myocardial protection.

tricular peak systolic pressure (RVSP) was less than 60 mmHg in 2.8% and more than 60 mmHg in 18%.

Operative mortality was not influenced by age or tricuspid bioprosthetic valve replacement (10%) or anuloplasty (9.9%). Cases involving mechanical valve implantation were higher (22.7%) but were operated upon early in the series.

Long-term Survival

Overall survival up to 9 years was projected to be 47.7%. It was noted that survival depended on several factors:

1. The type of the tricuspid repair: up to 7 years, survival was 63.6% for anuloplasties as opposed to 48% for bioprosthesic implantations and 39.7% for mechanical valves.
2. The valvulopathy corrected along with tricuspid repair: although operative mortality was higher for triple valve operations, survival

appeared to be the same regardless of whether the operation was TM or TMA (up to 7 years, TM, 49.7%; TMA, 44.5%).

3. The age at time of operation: survival rate was much lower for patients younger than age 19 years (25%) than for adults (50%) or patients older than 60 years.
4. The age and the type of tricuspid repair: survival rate up to 5 years is the same for young patients implanted with tricuspid bioprosthesis (54.6%) as for those undergoing anuloplasty (49%). On the other hand, survival rate is higher for adult and elderly patients undergoing anuloplasty (67.3%) than for those implanted with bioprostheses (55.2%).
5. The preoperative RVSP (Fig. 2): survival rate was much lower for patients displaying severe (RVSP > 60 mmHg) pulmonary hypertension (22.6%) than for those with moderate hypertension (RVSP < 60 mmHg; 64.2% up to 8 years).
6. The circumstances of the tricuspid repair: survival rate for patients undergoing a planned first intervention was 49% up to 7 years as opposed to 40% for patients undergoing tricuspid repair during a reoperation on an emergency basis.
7. The postoperative electrocardiograph rhythm: survival up to 8 years

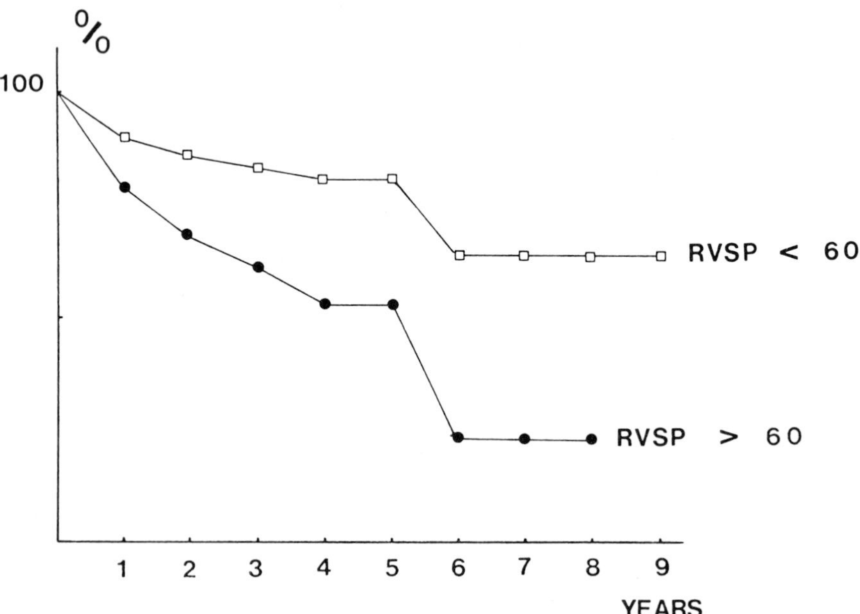

FIG. 2 Actuarial calculation of long-term survival after tricuspid valve replacement divided according to preoperative right ventricular peak systolic pressure (<60 or >60 mmHg).

was exactly the same regardless of rhythm, or 54.8% for atrial fibrillation and 54.2% for sinus rhythm.

There were a total of 53 late deaths: 13 from unknown causes, 9 noncardiac, 16 related to the valvular prosthesis (28%), and 15 caused by myocardial failure (27%).

Reoperations

The causes of bioprosthetic tricuspid reoperation (10/169) were because the valve was too small, because of calcification of the valve, and because of calcification or degeneration of the tricuspid and mitral bioprostheses. Six reoperations were performed on young patients (age <19) and 4 patients were reoperated on for a recurrent valvulopathy (1), endocarditis (1), or dysfunction of another prosthesis (2).

Of 22 patients with a mechanical tricuspid valve, 5 were reoperated on for thrombosis (4 Björk and 1 Beall), 2 for dysfunction (Beall). Of the 111 patients who underwent anuloplasties, 3 had to be reoperated on, because of failure of the anuloplasty alone (1) or associated with dysfunction of another prosthesis (2).

The rate of reoperation on the tricuspid depended on the type of tricuspid repair: mechanical valve, 7.9% per patient year; bioprostheses in young patients, 7.8% per patient year and none in adults; anuloplasties 0.6% per patient year.

Postoperative Rhythm

Correction of valvulopathies resulted in an improvement of heart rhythm but there was a difference according to the type of tricuspid repair (Fig. 3). The number of patients with chronic atrial fibrillation decreased significantly ($p < 0.01$) from 75% preoperatively to 55% postoperatively with no significant difference between the kind of operation. Likewise, the rate of sinus rhythm increased from 23.7% preoperatively to 35.6%, but there was a significant difference ($p < 0.001$) in the rate of postoperative atrioventricular block (AVB) according to the type of tricuspid repair.

The AVB rate was 12.7% in tricuspid replacement (bioprosthetic or mechanical) as opposed to 1.6% in cases of anuloplasty. However, we did decrease the incidence of postoperative AVB by modifying the tricuspid resection technique. Complete resection of the 3 leaflets of the tricuspid resulted in 14.8% of postoperative AVB, whereas keeping the septal leaflet and attaching the prosthesis to it, reduced the rate of AVB to 6.7%.

Finally, in order to compare the results of the bioprosthetic group and the anuloplasty group, we attempted to determine if the 2 groups were identical in regard to risk factors. The only significant difference found was the

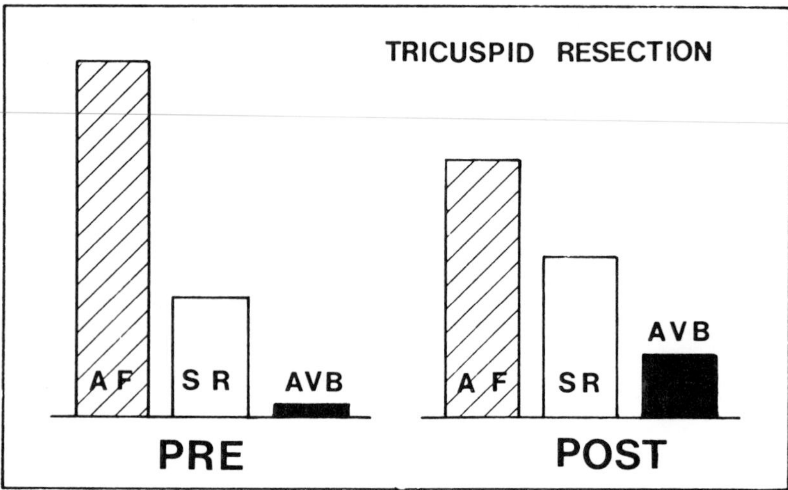

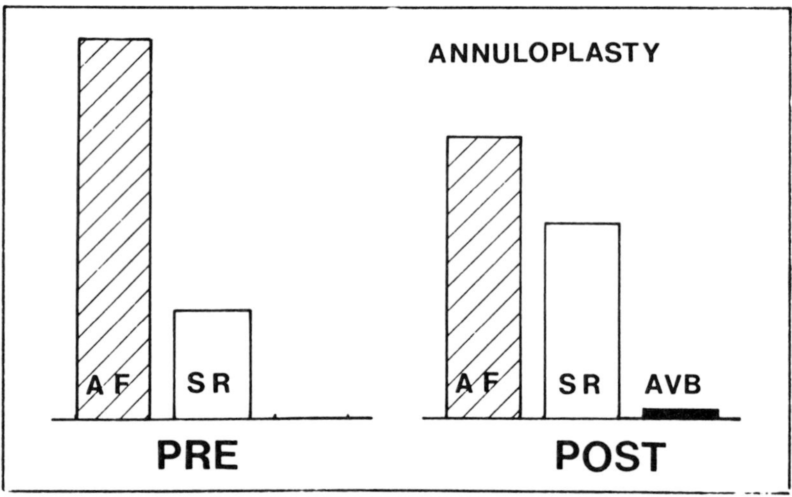

FIG. 3 Comparison of pre- and postoperative cardiac rhythms divided according to valve resection or repair. AF: atrial fibrillation; SR: sinus rhythm; AVB: atrioventricular block. Scale is 0 to 100%.

higher rate of reoperations and emergencies in the bioprosthetic group ($p < 0.02$).

Comment

Tricuspid replacement by mechanical valve appears to be the least effective alternative, although the high number of Beall valves used accounted for most of the bad results. Indeed operative mortality, late mortality, and rate of AVB and of reoperation are higher than for both the bioprosthetic and anuloplasty groups.

Tricuspid replacement by bioprosthesis, although subsequent operative mortality and survival is the same as for anuloplasty, results in a much higher rate of postoperative AVB and a high rate of reoperations in young patients.

Anuloplasty would therefore seem to be the most acceptable technique in view of both survival and AVB rate.

We have not yet been able to determine if there is any difference between bioprostheses and anuloplasties as far as long-term clinical results are concerned (rather than survival rate).

In this study it was not possible to attribute the degree of responsibility to each factor in the final results, as for example the responsibility of age or the associated valvulopathies.

Conclusion

For several years our policy has been to try whenever possible to conserve the tricuspid valve, and, in the rare case in which that is impossible, to replace the tricuspid valve by a bioprosthesis, keeping the septal leaflet intact to prevent postoperative AVB.

43

The Role of Porcine Heterografts in a 14-Year Experience with Tricuspid Valve Replacement

F. Wellens, P. Van Dale, F. E. Deuvaert, J. L. Leclerc, G. Primo

Tricuspid valve surgery remains one of the challenging problems in the treatment of the patient with valvular heart disease. Diagnosis, indications, and surgical technical methods to be used in cases of tricuspid valve dysfunction are still controversial.[1–4] When a tricuspid valve lesion has to be treated, a conservative repair is always preferable.[1,5–7] Nevertheless, tricuspid valve replacement (TVR) is a necessity in some cases.

The high rate of prosthetic complications in the tricuspid position makes the choice of the type of prosthesis another critical problem. Particularly high incidences of thrombotic occlusions with tilting disc[8–15] and ball valves[2,16–18] have been reported.

A rather limited number of reports of tricuspid bioprosthetic replacements have been published. However, these valves may undergo progressive degeneration[19–22] and eventual reoperation carries a high risk in this patient group.

This study was undertaken to compare the results of mechanical versus porcine bioprosthetic TVR.

Patients and Methods

Between January 1967 and June 1981, 139 patients underwent TVR and 93, a tricuspid anuloplasty in the Department of Cardiac Surgery of the University of Brussels. During the same period, 1,346 patients had single or combined mitral valve replacement (MVR) and 286 had a mitral commis-

---

From the Division of Cardiac Surgery, Hopital Universitaire Brugmann, Brussels, Belgium.

surotomy (MC). Five patients had TVR for congenital lesions, 2 for endocarditis, and 132 patients presented with postrheumatic (organic or functional) lesions. Patient data related to the type of prothesis implanted are summarized in Table I.

All operations were performed via median sternotomy and with a standard cardiopulmonary bypass technique with hemodilution and several types of bubble oxygenators. Until 1974, normothermia was used together with intermittent aortic cross clamping or direct coronary perfusion. From 1975, systemic hypothermia (25–30°C) has been introduced together with selective deep myocardial hypothermia[23] and later (1977) cold cardioplegia (30 mEq K^+/liter). All the procedures were then performed during a single cross-clamp period.

From 1967 until 1975, Kay-Shiley (KS), Björk-Shiley (BS), and Smeloff-Cutter (SC) prostheses were implanted. Hancock (H) and Carpentier-Edwards (CE) porcine heterografts (mean size 33 mm) were used from 1975 until 1980, and St. Jude Medical (SJM) prosthesis from January 1979 until June 1981 (Table II).

Tricuspid valve replacement was routinely performed in every instance of tricuspid valve surgery up until 1975 but from 1972 on, pre-bypass digital assessment of the tricuspid valve and external constriction of the tricuspid anulus with our previously described method[6] were used to guide the choice between TVR and constrictive anuloplasty with a bicuspidalization technique.

All the resected valves were available for pathology. Clinical examination at regular intervals in the outpatient clinic or by the referring cardiologist or by the family physician provided the follow-up data. No patient was lost to follow-up.

Anticoagulation

Anticoagulation with warfarin was initiated 48–72 hours postoperatively in every patient. All the patients with left- or right-sided mechanical valves were indefinitely maintained under this regimen. In the patients with bioprostheses who were in sinus rhythm anticoagulation was as a rule discontinued after 3 months.

Four prognostic factors and their eventual influence on early and late death were examined: previous valve surgery, type of lesion, number of valves replaced, and functional class.

Results

Patient populations were very similar in the mechanical (group I) and bioprosthesis groups (group II) as listed in Fig. 1. Ninety-seven percent of

TABLE I Data on patients with tricuspid valve replacement related to the type of prosthesis implanted

Type of prosthesis	# Pts	Early death	Late death	Survivors	Patient follow-up (mo)	Mean follow-up	Number of prosthesis implanted	Valve follow-up (mo)	Mean follow-up
Group I									
Kay-Shiley	15	2	11	2	992	70	15	838	60
Björk-Shiley	23	4	7	12	1558	82	23	1390	73
Saint Jude Medical	11	2	2	7	108	12	13	144	13
Smeloff-Cutter	27	7	10	10	1233	62	31	1450	63
Group II									
Hancock	29	6	4	19	1152	50	29	1152	50
Carpentier-Edwards	34	3	4	27	972	36	35	972	36

TABLE II Tricuspid valve replacement: causes of late death

Cause	Group I (61 survivors)					Group II (54 survivors)		
	KS	BS	SJM	SC	Total	H	CE	Total
Myocardial failure	4	1		3	8	2	2	4
Arrhythmia	1			3	4			
Cerebral embolism		1		1	2	2		2
Tricuspid valve thrombosis	3	3	1	3	10			
Hemorrhage (anticoagulants)		1			1		1	1
Prosthetic endocarditis	1				1			
Noncardiac			1		1		1	1
Not documented	2	1			3			
Total	11	7	2	10	30	4	4	8
% per patient year follow-up					9			4.5

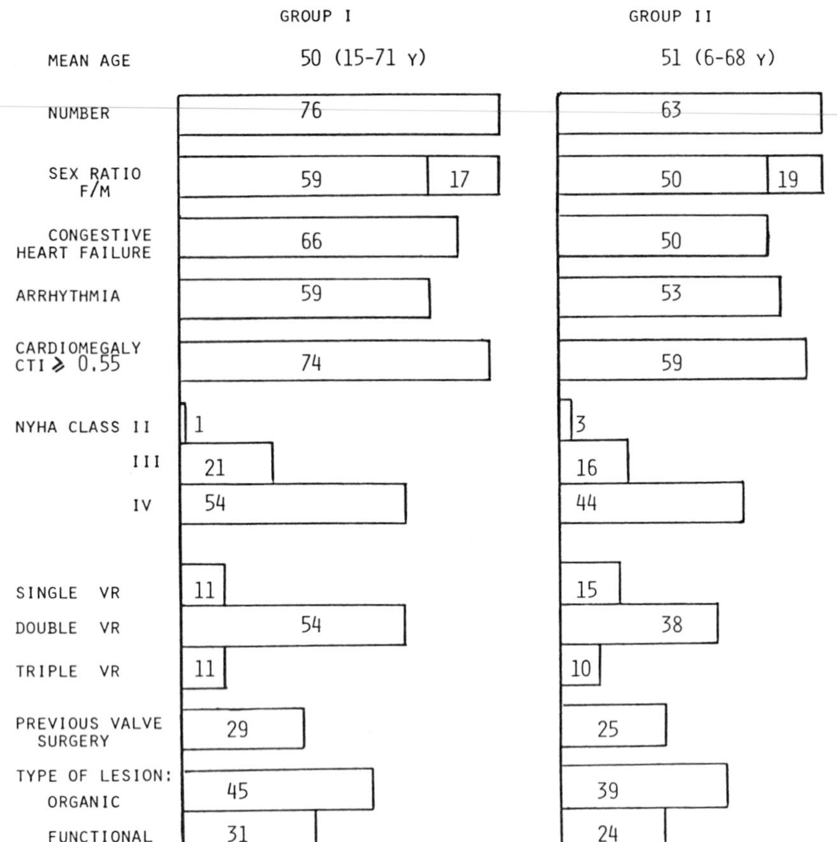

FIG. 1 Tricuspid valve replacement. Clinical data comparing group I (mechanical prostheses) and group II (bioprostheses).

the patients admitted for TVR were NYHA class III (38/139) or class IV (97/139). Previous valve surgery had been done in 39% of the patients (54/139). The tricuspid lesion was organic in 61% and functional in 39%, the congenital lesions being considered as organic. Early mortality for single TVR was 15%, for double valve replacement (VR), 20%, and for triple VR, 14%. In the valves classified as functional, pathology showed in all cases signs of secondary mucoid degeneration. These valves were clearly distinct from valves presenting histologic lesions of rheumatic disease.

Group I consisted of 76 patients receiving 82 mechanical prostheses (SJM, 13; BS, 23; KS, 15, SC, 31) and 1 CE bioprosthesis in the tricuspid position. Organic lesions were present in 45 and functional lesions, in 31 patients. Twenty-one patients were class III and 54 were class IV. Previous valve surgery was done in 29 patients.

Eleven patients underwent single TVR, which in 1 case was associated with an open mitral commissurotomy (OMC). All the others had previous left-sided valve surgery, and MVR in 6, aortic valve replacement (AVR) MVR in 4. In 54 patients a double VR was performed (MVR-TVR, 53, AVR-TVR, 1). In this subgroup 16 patients had 1 or repeated previous MC, associated in 3 with a tricuspid anuloplasty (TA). One had a previous AVR. Eleven patients had a triple VR and only 1 had a previous OMC.

Early mortality in group I was 20% (15/76). Two patients were class III and 13 were class IV. Previous valve surgery, functional tricuspid lesion, and functional class IV all influenced early mortality ($p < 0.01$). Low cardiac output and respiratory failure were the main causes of operative death. There was 1 valve-related death in this group after emergency reoperation for an acute thrombosis of a BS tricuspid valve prosthesis.

Four patients needed reoperation for bleeding. Nine patients needed temporary pacemaker support and 1 required a definitive pacemaker for complete postoperative atrioventricular (AV) block. Two nonfatal embolic accidents occurred with permanent neurologic disorders.

Complete follow-up was 3,822 patients months (average, 63 months) and ranged between 6 months and 14 years. The late mortality rate based on the original number of operated patients was 39% (30/76), representing an incidence of 9.4% per patient year follow-up. Actuarial survival at 5 years is 53% and at 10 years, 42% (Fig. 2).

The causes of late death and their relationship to the type of valve prosthesis implanted are summarized in Table II. Late tricuspid valve throm-

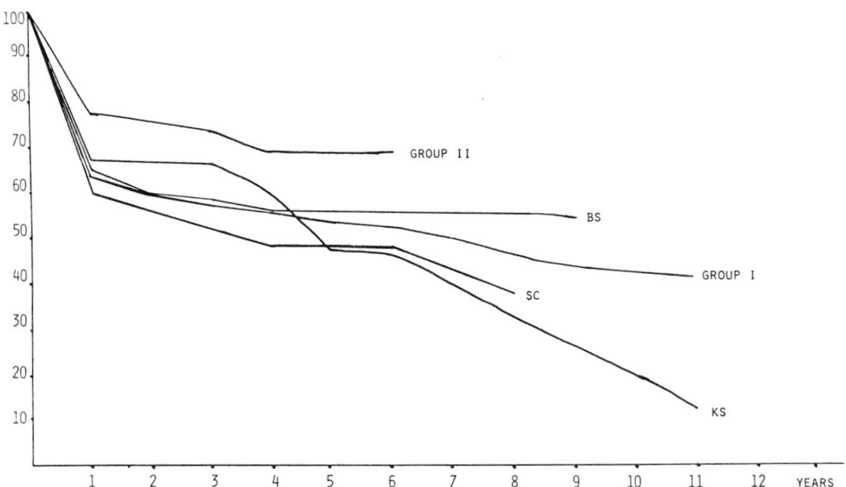

FIG. 2 Comparison of actuarial survival. Mechanical (group I) and bioprostheses (group II) valves: Björk-Shiley (BS) Smeloff-Cutter (SC), and Kay-Shiley (KS).

bosis related to the type of prosthesis. Seventeen events occurred in 14 patients; all but 1 had adequate anticoagulation. These events were confirmed at reoperation and autopsy and by angiography in 1 patient. It was the main cause of death in 8 patients. Six patients could be reoperated upon with 2 early postoperative deaths. In 1 of these patients a CE bioprosthesis was implanted.

Thrombosis occurred between 4 months and 10 years postimplantation. Gross examination showed acute thrombotic occlusion in 4 BS, 1 SJM, 1 KS, and 1 SC valve prosthesis, and occurred a mean of 18 months postimplantation (Fig. 3). In 8 SC and 2 KS prostheses an obstructing organized pannus formation was found, a mean of 90 months postimplantation. This complication was responsible for 33% of the late deaths in group I, with an incidence of thrombosis of 5.3% per patient year follow-up.

Group II contained 63 patients, with 29 H and 34 CE prostheses implanted. Organic lesions were present in 39 patients and functional lesions in 24. Previous valve surgery was performed in 25 patients (40%).

Fifteen patients underwent single TVR. Ten patients had undergone previous valve surgery (MVR, 6; MVR-TA, 1; OMC, 1; AVR-MVR-TA, 1; AVR-MVR, 1). Three other patients presented with Ebstein's anomaly and 2 with tricuspid endocarditis. Double VR was performed in 38 patients (MVR-TVR, 36; AVR-TVR, 2) with bioprosthetic implantation in the aortic and mitral positions in 90%. Fifteen patients had previous valve surgery (MVR, 1; MVR-TA, 1; AVR, 1; AVR-MVR, 1; MC, 10; OMC-TA, 1).

In 10 patients a triple VR was performed with 75% bioprosthetic im-

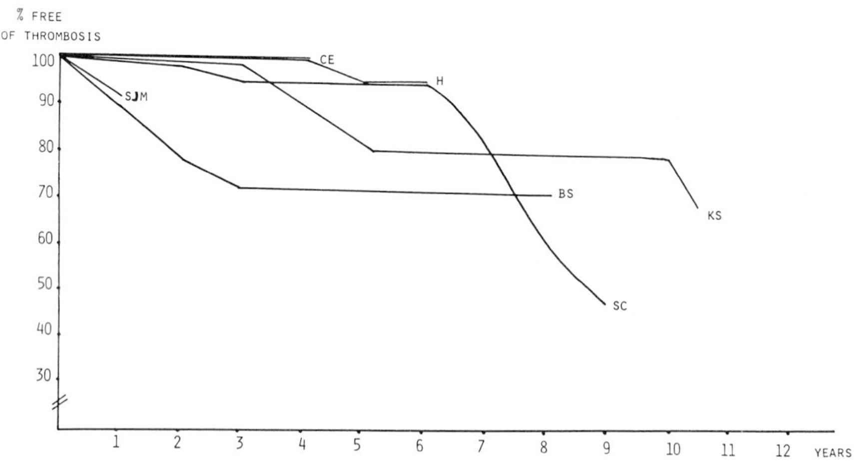

FIG. 3 Actuarial comparison of probability of freedom from thrombosis in patients with Carpentier-Edwards (CE), Hancock (H), St. Jude Medical (SJM), Kay-Shiley (KS), Björk-Shiley (BS), and Smeloff-Cutter (SC) valves.

plantation in the left-sided positions (Table II). Only 1 patient had a previously closed MC.

Early mortality rate was 14% (9/63), all class IV patients (9/44). Of the prognostic factors reviewed, only functional class IV approached significance ($p < 0.07$). Myocardial failure, arrhythmias, and respiratory failure accounted for 8 of 9 early deaths. One patient died of diffuse uncontrollable bleeding and 4 others had reoperation for bleeding. Twelve patients needed temporary pacemaker support and 1 had a permanent pacemaker implanted at operation. One patient suffered from a nonfatal cerebral event leaving permanent neurologic disorders. Complete follow-up was 2,124 patient months, with a mean duration of 40 months per patient and ranged from 12 to 80 months. The late mortality rate based on the total number of operated patients was 13% (8/63), representing a late mortality annual rate of 4.5% per patient year follow-up, which is statistically significant compared to group I ($p < 0.005$). The causes of late death are summarized in Table II.

The 5-year actuarial survival of the operated group is 73%, (Fig. 2), most patients improving by 1 or 2 functional classes (Fig. 4). Eleven of the 46 current survivors do not have any anticoagulant treatment; 8 are in sinus rhythm, 2 in atrial fibrillation, and 1 is on a pacemaker.

Major late complications are summarized in Table III. Two of the 3 patients with systemic emboli had a mechanical valve implanted previously (1 Starr-Edwards and 1 SC mitral prosthesis) and were on full anticoagulation treatment. Definitive pacemaker implantation was performed in 5

	GROUP I (N=31)		GROUP II (N=46)	
	PRE	POST	PRE	POST
I	0	2	0	18
II	1	23	3	21
III	12	4	16	6
IV	18	2	27	1

FIG. 4 Pre- and postoperative NYHA functional classification of survivors after mechanical (group I) and bioprosthetic (group II) TVR.

TABLE III Tricuspid valve replacement: late complications

Complications	Group I (n = 61)	% PPYFU*	Group II (n = 54)	% PPYFU*
Embolic event	5	1.6	3	1.65
Lethal	2	0.62	1	0.55
Prosthetic endocarditis	3	0.94		
Lethal	1	0.31		
Hemorrhagic complications (anticoagulant treatment)	17	5.3	4	2.2
Lethal	1	0.3	1	0.55
Pacemaker implantation	1	0.3	5	2.8
Left-sided valve dysfunction	4	1.25	1	0.55
Lethal	2	0.62		

* PPFYU: % per patient year follow-up.

patients, in 2 for complete postoperative AV block and in 3 for sick sinus syndrome.

Late tricuspid valve thrombosis occurred only once. This patient underwent an emergency reoperation for primary tissue failure of a bioprosthetic mitral prosthesis at 48 months, which was replaced by a SJM prosthesis. The right atrium was found to be filled with a fresh thrombus covering a completely normally functioning bioprosthesis. Right atrial thrombectomy was performed and the bioprosthesis was left in place. Two years postoperatively, this patient has no evidence of tricuspid valve dysfunction.

Comment

In the past years marked improvement in the results of valve surgery has been attributed to improved perioperative management and to the introduction of myocardial protection techniques; with early mortality rate in the range of 3% for AVR, 5% for MVR, and 9% for nontricuspid multiple VR. Nevertheless, overall early mortality for isolated and for combined TVR does not follow this general trend. Indeed, early mortality in group I was 20% and it was 14% in group II. Group II presented a cohort of more recently operated patients and included also 5 patients with nonrheumatic lesions, 3 in class II. Even in the recently operated subgroup of the SJM valve patients, early mortality remained relatively high (2/11).

Two factors influencing early mortality were the preoperative functional class (22 of the 24 early deaths were class IV patients) and TVR for functional tricuspid insufficiency. These 2 factors are causally related and other authors have found identical results.[14,24,25]

This high mortality rate for TVR in rheumatic patients can be attributed to long-standing and severe myocardial dysfunction. It results in terminal congestive heart failure, cardiomegaly, atrial fibrillation, pulmonary hypertension, and preoperative multiple organ failure of cardiac origin. These overall results attest the need for earlier valvular correction[2,6,16,23,26] before irreversible myocardial damage occurs. Even patients surviving the operation will have a poor prognosis, with persisting high morbidity and mortality of myocardial origin. Because of the rather disappointing results with TVR using mechanical valves, a certain reluctance to treat these lesions has grown with time, which has probably resulted in a less than optimal approach to the patient with a tricuspid valve condition.

Our experience with the mechanical valve group demonstrates the unfavorable long-term results, with a survival rate of 53% at 5 years. Stephenson et al,[25] MacManus et al,[2] Rhodes et al,[26] Peterffy et al,[27] Jugdutt et al,[16] and Schoevaerdts et al[14] report similar results in their respective patient populations. The suboptimal performance of several mechanical prostheses in tricuspid position was clearly demonstrated in these series. Only Stephenson et al[25] did not encounter any tricuspid valve-related complication in their 8 year follow-up (mean 44 months).

In our series the annual late mortality rate of 9.4% per patient year in group I contrasts sharply with the 4.5% per patient year rate in group II ($p < 0.005$). This striking difference can be attributed to 2 factors. In group I late tricuspid valve thrombosis accounted for an annual mortality rate of 3% per patient year against a 0 late mortality rate in group II. Better diagnosis and earlier treatment of concomitant arrhythmias in patients with valve lesions and chronic myocardial dysfunction seems to be the other favorable factor. The higher incidence of pacemaker implantation in group II (Table III) is probably related to a more aggressive approach of arrhythmias and conduction disturbances.

In the analysis of the performance of the mechanical valves in tricuspid position, the striking complication is the high incidence of thrombotic valve obstruction, even with a correct anticoagulation regimen.

The BS tilting disc prosthesis was implanted in 23 patients and presented a very high early thrombosis rate (Fig. 2). Five patients presented a thrombotic obstruction in the first 24 months postimplantation, in 3 with concomitant mitral BS thrombosis. Afterward, the probability for valve thrombosis remained at the 2 year level. The 8 year survival rate is better than in the KS and SC subgroup.

The annual thrombosis incidence of 4.3% per patient year in a mean follow-up of 6 years is slightly higher than the 3.2% rate (mean follow-up 4.9 years) quoted by Petterffy et al[27] in their 51 survivors. We disagree with these authors, who have described this complication as "relatively benign."

In our series there were 3 thrombosis-related sudden deaths, and 2 other patients survived reoperation. Both survivors had late pannus formation on their tricuspid SC prosthesis, with another late death. Several other authors report on thrombosis of the BS prosthesis in the tricuspid position[8,28,29,11,12,14] occurring often more insidiously than the well recognized acute thrombosis of this prosthesis in the left-sided positions. In our opinion, our results and those from the literature suggest that the BS tilting disc prosthesis is not an ideal valve substitute in the tricuspid position.

Follow-up with the bileaflet SJM prosthesis is too short for definitive conclusions. Nevertheless, in a series of 11 surviving patients, 1 tricuspid valve thrombosis occurred 12 months postoperatively when anticoagulant treatment was discontinued for 48 hours for elective gastrointestinal surgery. The patient died suddenly on the 4th postoperative day, while on intravenous heparin therapy. Autopsy confirmed complete thrombosis blocking the 2 leaflets of the prosthesis. Bowen et al[10] reported also another case of SJM valve thrombosis in a young patient who survived reoperation with implantation of a CE prosthesis.

Caged ball prostheses also do not represent a satisfactory alternative for TVR. The frequently used SE prosthesis has been reported to have poor early and late survival rates when implanted in the tricuspid position.[2,5,15,16,18,24] Again, late thrombotic obstruction has been relatively frequently reported. Mechanisms of obstruction of ball valve prosthesis have been suggested by Sanfelippo et al[24] and Vander Veer et al.[18]

In our center the SC ball valve prosthesis was the prosthesis most frequently implanted in the AV position from 1970 until 1975. Thirty-one SC prostheses were implanted in the tricuspid position in that period. The 5 year survival rate did not differ much from the other mechanical valves used (Fig. 1) but the prosthesis remained relatively free from thrombotic complications up to 7 years postoperatively. From that time on, a high incidence of thrombotic pannus formation occurred, with an associated high morbidity and mortality resulting in a low 9 year survival rate of 35%. Pannus formation was found nearly exclusively on the ventricular side of the prosthesis, interfering with the normal motion of the poppet.

The high early and late mortality rate together with the high annual probability of thrombosis (7.4% per patient year) makes the SC valve an unsuitable device for TVR. Our experience reinforces the suggestions of the Mayo Clinic group,[24] after their extensive experience with the SE valve, that the ball valve prosthesis, more than other mechanical valve types, offers a valuable alternative in cases of TVR.

TVR with bioprosthesis has been performed for more than 10 years. Most authors used the commercially available H and CE porcine bioprostheses; others used fresh aortic allografts[30] or porcine heterografts prepared in their laboratories before commercialization.[31,32] Our experience starts in 1975, with the implantation of porcine heterografts in all positions.

The overall results, with a cumulative survival of 181 valve years (mean, 40 months) are much better in comparison with the results of the mechanical valve group. There was no significant difference between the results of the H and the more recently used CE prosthesis. As already mentioned, early mortality in this more recently operated group remained relatively high (14%) but is not prosthesis related.

A more extensive use of temporary pacemaker support was necessary in the postoperative period. Rhodes et al[26] reported a similar experience. The use of deep selective myocardial cooling and later on cardioplegia could be the causative factor for the temporary conduction and rhythm disturbances.

The 5 year actuarial survival (early mortality included) was significantly better in group II, with 73% compared to 53% in group I (Fig. 1), and is clearly valve related due to absence of fatal valve thrombosis in group II (Fig. 2). Our results correlate very well with those of Rhodes et al,[26] who also compared mechanical versus porcine heterograft TVR in triple VR. Most of the group II survivors enjoy a relatively uncomplicated life, most of them being class I or II (Fig. 3).

Hemodynamic performance of the porcine bioprostheses in tricuspid position is very acceptable as proved by postoperative catheterization studies of Carpentier et al,[31] Mikaeloff et al,[32] and Rhodes et al.[26]

With 80% bioprosthetic VR in the left-sided positions in group II, overall late valve-related complications were lower in this group (Table III). Eleven of the 46 survivors (24%) are at the present time without any anticoagulant treatment. This decreases considerably the nonfatal hemorrhagic complications, without an increase in thromboembolic incidence.

Only 1 tricuspid thrombotic obstruction occurred, probably secondary to a low cardiac output state in the patient with a degenerated mitral bioprosthesis. After right atrial thrombectomy, the tricuspid bioprosthesis appeared to be completely normal and was left in place.

The most serious concern when selecting a bioprosthesis for implantation is its durability. Rapid calcification and degeneration in the tricuspid position was recently described in young animal models.[28] Large series of TVR with bioprosthesis have not been published but all authors report a lesser degree of valve degeneration in the right-sided position than in mitral and aortic positions.[4,16,19,20,21,29,31] Our personal experience with a total of 1,000 porcine heterografts implanted during that period and a 7 year follow-up accounts for a primary valve failure rate of 0.65% per patient year follow-up, whereas we did not encounter any clinical evidence of primary valve failure in the tricuspid position, including 5 patients younger than 18 years of age. Indeed, very favorable results up to 9 years with bioprosthetic TVR in children were recently reported,[21] contrasting with the early valve degeneration and calcification in the left-sided position in this young age group.

Beside the low incidence of valve degeneration in the tricuspid position, bioprostheses seem to be less prone to valve thrombosis even without anticoagulants, as shown by our experience and others. Nevertheless, Carpentier et al[31] reported another case of nonfatal thrombosis and Zudhi[33] reported on 2 tricuspid valve thromboses in his review of 20,000 implanted H prostheses without mentioning the total number of TVR in this series.

The advantages of porcine bioprostheses, i.e., decreased risk of thromboembolism, the lesser need for anticoagulants, the efficient hemodynamic performance, and the excellent durability in the tricuspid position makes this type of prosthesis the most suitable in all cases of TVR, children included. In spite of the possibility of late valve degeneration, we now implant porcine bioprostheses in all instances of TVR, speculating that bioprosthetic valve degeneration is slow and correctable on an elective basis and with a lower mortality than acute or subacute mechanical valve thrombosis.

References

1. Grondin P, Meere C, Limet R, Lopez-Bescos L, Delcan JL, Rivera R: Carpentier's annulus and De Vega's annuloplasty. The end of the tricuspid challenge. J Thorac Cardiovasc Surg 70:852, 1975.
2. MacManus Q, Grunkemeier G, Starr A: Late results of triple valve replacement: A 14-year review. Ann Thorac Surg 25:402, 1978.
3. Magilligan DJ, Lewis JW Jr, Jara FM, Lee MW, Alam M, Riddle JM, Stein PD: Spontaneous degeneration of porcine bioprosthetic valves. Ann Thorac Surg 30:259, 1980.
4. McIntosh CL, Michaelis LL, Morrow AG, Itscoitz SB, Redwood DR, Epstein SE: Atrio-ventricular valve replacement with the Hancock porcine xenograft: A five-year clinical experience. Surgery 78:768, 1975.
5. Baxter RH, Bain WH, Rankin RJ, Turner MA, Escarous AE, Thomson RM, Lorimer AR, Lawrie TD: Tricuspid valve replacement. A five-year appraisal. Thorax 30:158, 1975.
6. Cham B, Le Clerc JL, Primo G: Resultats immediats et a long terme de la chirurgie de la valve tricuspide. A propos de 62 cas operes. Acta Cardiol 31:277, 1976.
7. Duran CMG, Pomar JL, Colman T, Figueroa A, Revuelta JM, Ubago JL: Is tricuspid valve repair necessary? J Thorac Cardiovasc Surg 80:849, 1980.
8. Azpitarte J, de Vega NG, Santalla A, Rabago P, Rabago G: Thrombotic obstruction of Björk-Shiley tricuspid valve prosthesis. Acta Cardiol 30:419, 1975.
9. Bourdillon PDV, Sharratt GP: Malfunction of Björk-Shiley valve prosthesis in tricuspid position. Br Heart J 38:1149, 1976.
10. Bowen TE, Tri TB, Wortham DC: Thrombosis of a St. Jude Medical tricuspid prosthesis. Case report. J Thorac Cardiovasc Surg 82:257, 1981.
11. Cokkinos DV, Voridis E, Bakoulas G, Theodossiou A, Skalkeas GD: Thrombosis of two high-flow prosthetic valves. J Thorac Cardiovasc Surg 62:947, 1971.
12. Messmer BJ, Okies EJ, Hallman G, Cooley DA: Mitral valve replacement with the Björk-Shiley tilting disc prosthesis. J Thorac Cardiovasc Surg 62:938, 1971.
13. Peterffy A, Henze A, Savidge GF, Landou C, Björk VO: Late thrombotic malfunction of the Björk-Shiley tilting disc valve in the tricuspid position. Principles for recognition and management. Scand J Thorac Cardiovasc Surg 14:33, 1980.
14. Schoevaerdts JC, Jaumin P, Piret L, Kremer R, Ponlot R, Chalant CH: Tricuspid valve surgery. J Cardiovasc Surg 18:397, 1977.

15. Ben-Ismail M, Abid F, Sirinelle A, Curran Y: Thromboses tardives sur protheses tricuspidiennes. A propos de 6 cases. Arch Mal Coeur 74:289, 1981.
16. Jugdutt BI, Fraser RS, Lee SJK, Rossall RE, Callaghan JC: Long-term survival after tricuspid valve replacement. Results with seven different prostheses. J Thorac Cardiovasc Surg 74:20, 1977.
17. Samaan HA, Murali R: Acute tricuspid valve obstruction following the use of ball valve prosthesis. Thorax 25:334, 1970.
18. Vander Veer JB Jr, Rhyneer GS, Hodam RP: Obstruction of tricuspid ball valve prosthesis. Circulation 43(Suppl I):62, 1971.
19. Davila JC, Magilligan DJ Jr, Lewis JW Jr: Is the Hancock porcine valve the best cardiac valve substitute today. Ann Thorac Surg 26:303, 1978.
20. Dunn JM: Porcine valve durability in children. Ann Thorac Surg 32:357, 1981.
21. Hetzer RJ, Hill JD, Kerth WJ, Wilson AJ, Adappa MG, Gerbode G: Thrombosis and degeneration of Hancock valves. Clinical and pathological findings. Ann Thorac Surg 26:317, 1978.
22. Oyer PE, Miller DC, Stinson EB, Shumway N: Clinical durability of the Hancock porcine bioprosthetic valve. J Thorac Cardiovasc Surg 80:824, 1980.
23. Primo G, Cham B, LeClerc JL: Hypothermie selective profonde pour la protection peroperatoire du myocarde ischemique. Bull Acad Med Belg 131:265, 1976.
24. Sanfelippo PM, Giulani ER, Danielson GR, Wallace RB, Pluth JR, McGoon DC: Tricuspid valve prosthetic replacement. Early and late results with the Starr-Edwards prosthesis. J Thorac Cardiovasc Surg 71:441, 1976.
25. Stephenson LW, Kouchoukos NT, Kirklin JW: Triple valve replacement: An analysis of eight years experience. Ann Thorac Surg 23:327, 1977.
26. Rhodes GR, McIntosh CL, Redwood DR, Itscoitz SB, Epstein S: Clinical and hemodynamic results following triple valve replacement: Mechanical vs porcine xenograft prostheses. Circulation 56(Suppl II):122, 1977.
27. Petterffy A, Henze A, Jonasson R, Björk VO: Clinical evaluation of the Björk-Shiley tilting disc valve in the tricuspid position. Early and late results in 10 isolated and 51 combined cases. Scand J Thorac Cardiovasc Surg 12:179, 1978.
28. Barnhart GR, Hones M, Ishihara T, Rose DM, Chavez AM, Ferrans V: Degeneration and calcification of bioprosthetic cardiac valves. Am J Pathol 106:136, 1982.
29. Moreno-Cabral RJ, McNamara JJ, Mammiya RT, Brainard SC, Chung GK: Acute thrombotic obstruction with Björk-Shiley valves. J Thorac Cardiovasc Surg 75:321, 1978.
30. Mikaeloff Ph, Convert G, Fleurette J, Silie M, Didier-Laurent JF, Van Haecke P: Remplacement de la valve tricuspide par homogreffe valvulaire aortique. Resultats cliniques et hemodynamiques a plus de 5 ans. Nouv Presse Med 10:1131, 1981.
31. Carpentier A, Deloche A, Relland J, Fabiani JN, Forman J, Camilleri JP, Soyer R, Dubost C: Six-year followup of glutaraldehyde preserved heterografts. J Thorac Cardiovasc Surg 68:771, 1974.
32. Mikaeloff Ph, Delahaye JP, Convert G, Van Haecke P, Amouroux C, Boivin J: Resultats precoces et tardifs des triples remplacements valvulaires. Utilisation d'une bioprothese en position tricuspidienne. Arch Mal Coeur 74:719, 1981.
33. Zudhi N: The porcine aortic valve prosthesis. Ann Thorac Surg 21:573, 1976.

44

Patient Prosthesis Mismatch in the Tricuspid Position: The Rationale for an Oval Pericardial Tricuspid Valve

S. WESTABY, R. KARP

To date, no valve prosthesis has proved to be entirely satisfactory in the tricuspid position. Mechanical prostheses are subject to sudden thrombosis or late tissue encapsulation, often with fatal consequences, and early calcification causing degeneration of porcine heterografts has prevented their widespread acceptance as a suitable alternative. In addition to these well known complications of tricuspid valve replacement, a recent study by the authors and colleagues at the University of Alabama revealed 2 important factors that contribute to the dismal long-term outlook for these patients but which are not specifically related to the type of prosthesis inserted (Table I). One hundred and six patients had a total of 109 tricuspid prostheses, usually as part of double or triple valve replacement. There were 76 mechanical valves and 33 porcine heterografts with 9 valve failures in all, 7 from thrombosis or obstruction of a mechanical prosthesis and 2 from degeneration of a heterograft. Notably, however, 41% of patients, although improved in functional status, suffered continuing or worsened right heart failure with clinically evident venous hypertension requiring diuretic therapy. This finding is compatible with the experimental studies of McIntosh et al[1] whose patients with porcine heterografts in the tricuspid position showed a greater transvalvular gradient after valve replacement than before. Rahimtoolah[2] has brought attention to patient-prosthesis mismatch on the left side of the heart and our evidence suggests that restrictive valve prostheses are an even greater problem on the right.

Next, we found that, actuarially, late heart block requiring pacemaker

From the Department of Thoracic Surgery, Harefield Hospital, Harefield, England, and The Department of Cardiothoracic Surgery, University of Alabama, Birmingham, Alabama.

TABLE I Late complications of tricuspid valve replacement

	# prostheses	Complications #	Complications %
Related to type of prosthesis			
Mechanical valve thrombosis or pannus obstruction	76	7	9
Porcine heterograft degeneration	33	2	6
Unrelated to type of prosthesis			
Late heart block after mitral and tricuspid valve replacement			20*
Chronic right heart failure			41

* Actuarial percentage in 10 years.

insertion occurs in about 20% of patients with both mitral and tricuspid prostheses after 10 years. In adults often the largest available prosthesis is inserted into the naturally elliptic anulus, causing distortion of the right ventricular inlet and inlet septum. Pressure of adjacent rigid valve stents then causes fibrosis in the region of the His bundle. Paradoxically therefore many patients require a larger, less restrictive prosthesis yet larger valves appear to predispose to equally serious late sequelae.

We consider that the effective orifice areas of even the largest size of current valve prosthesis are inadequate for tricuspid valve replacement in many adults and that this may contribute to the observed late complications of chronic right heart failure and thrombotic occlusion. We therefore investigated this hypothesis and, considering the normal tricuspid valve morphology, designed a purpose-built ideal tricuspid prosthesis.

Materials and Methods

Tricuspid and mitral valve dimensions were measured in 160 postmortem hearts from adults both with and without congestive heart failure. Valve circumference was measured by opening and lying the valve ring flat, thereby minimizing the effect of systolic contracture after death. Circularized orifice area was derived from this valve and although the tricuspid orifice is elliptic in shape, circularized dimensions were appropriate for comparison with circular valve prostheses. Multivariate analysis was then used to relate tricuspid valve orifice area to age, sex, race, height, weight, body surface area, the presence of congestive cardiac failure, and mitral valve orifice area.

We then obtained the manufacturers' stated orifice area for their largest valve prostheses (not the in vivo calculated area).

We studied the morphology of the normal tricuspid valve and reviewed the late results and complications of tricuspid valve replacement at the

University of Alabama (to be published elsewhere) in order to determine those valve-related problems that limit a satisfactory long-term outcome. We then designed an "ideal" tricuspid prosthesis and obtained preliminary in vitro tests on a prototype valve.

Results

Mean circularized tricuspid and mitral valve orifice areas for adult males and females with and without congestive cardiac failure are shown in Table II. Multivariate analysis showed only sex and congestive cardiac failure to have important relationships to tricuspid valve size. Correlation coefficients showed other variables, including body surface area, height, and weight, to be poorly related. This therefore allows us to state a mean figure for adult tricuspid valve orifice area for males and females with and without congestive cardiac failure and use them as a guide for valve replacement as repair. Additionally the relationship between mitral and tricuspid orifice areas was noted, the tricuspid exceeding the mitral by about a third in normal persons and even more in patients with congestive cardiac failure.

Table III shows the orifice areas of the largest available prostheses. Comparison with our valves for adult tricuspid orifice area shows that most are restrictive even at rest, a finding that might be expected from our clinical findings. Further reduction of the orifice by tissue ingrowth serves to increase the tendency for obstruction or thrombosis.

As stated, the late results of tricuspid replacement were notable for mechanical valve dysfunction and persistence or sometimes worsening of right heart failure. Porcine heterografts seem less prone to the first but not to the second problem and it is likely that both were the result of a limiting prosthetic orifice area. The native tricuspid valve is elliptic, and certainly not round. Since the size of a prosthesis inserted into any anulus is in part determined by the smallest diameter of the anulus, it is feasible that an oval prosthesis could give a greater effective orifice area without the potential

TABLE II Calculated mean mitral and tricuspid valve orifice areas* in adult human hearts with and without congestive cardiac failure

Valve	Sex	Normal (cm^2)	Congestive cardiac failure (cm^2)
Mitral	Male	8.33 (1.98)†	9.21 (2.13)
	Female	6.66 (1.26)	7.58 (1.55)
Tricuspid	Male	11.50 (2.72)	12.56 (2.94)
	Female	8.75 (1.74)	10.54 (2.07)

* Circularized for comparison with circular prostheses.
† Standard deviation.

TABLE III Manufacturers stated orifice area for largest valve prostheses

Valve	Size	Orifice area (cm^2)
Carpentier-Edwards	35	7.34
Ionescu-Shiley	33	6.79
Hancock	33	5.50
St. Jude	31	5.15
Björk-Shiley	35	4.60
Lillehei-Kastor	31	4.58
Starr-Edwards mitral	34	3.66

problems of inserting larger round prostheses, namely, distortion of the right ventricular inlet and septum and pressure as an adjacent prosthetic mitral ring if present. We therefore designed an oval tricuspid prosthesis with the following features (Fig. 1):

1. A flexible plastic oval stent, the shape of which is similar to the Carpentier ring. This shape should fit the native anulus without distortion and both its configuration and flexibility should reduce the tendency to fixation and pressure on the crux of the heart. A degree of flexibility also improves the cusp-loading characteristics.
2. A trileaflet valve with porcine pericardial leaflets. These have good opening characteristics, are fully competent within the degree of stent flexibility, and offer little resistance to flow when tested on the pulse duplicator. Pericardium is used to construct the leaflets, since of necessity they are of different shape, to fit the oval orifice. As with other tissue valves, there is less likelihood of thrombosis or embolism and long-term anticoagulants can be avoided. Also, there is some

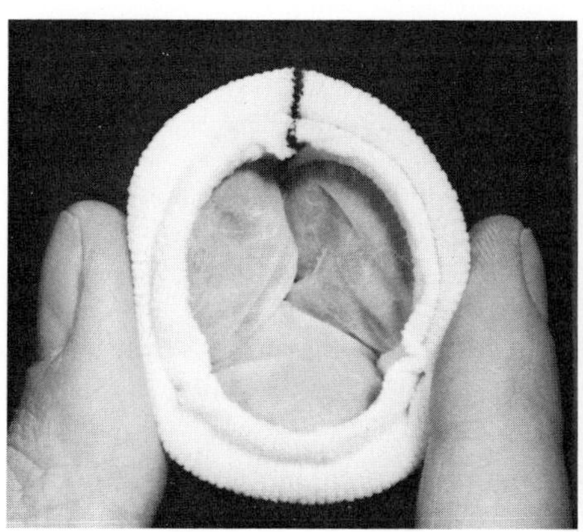
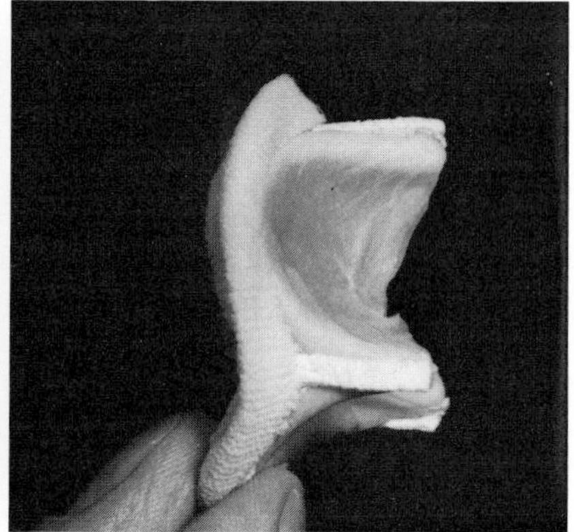

FIG 1. Oval tricuspid valve with flexible stent.

evidence that the tendency to calcification and degeneration are less on the right side, although durability is of less importance than the risk of sudden death.[3]

Comment

There can be no doubt that tricuspid valve repair, where appropriate, is the better alternative to valve replacement. Indeed many surgeons avoid tricuspid replacement altogether because of the well-known valve-related complications. However, valve repair cannot substitute for replacement in certain congenital anomalies, such as Ebstein's malformation, and acquired disorders, including endocarditis, traumatic disruption, and severe organic rheumatic valve disease. Of the currently available prostheses porcine heterografts give the best overall results and if one believes that the poor results of valve replacement are in part due to a restrictive prosthetic orifice area this is not surprising, since their orifice area is better than most mechanical valves. Nevertheless, it is desirable to maximize the orifice area and this can be achieved for the tricuspid position by a change in valve shape from circular to oval. The native anulus is elliptic and increasingly so during systole when the maximum force is placed on the tissue sewing ring junction as the anulus attempts to become elliptic and is resisted by a circular prosthesis. Lemole et al[4] first described the hemodynamic advantages of an oval prosthesis in the mitral position. Considering the anatomic factors determining the size of an atrioventricular prosthetic valve as 1) the smallest diameter of the native anulus, 2) ventricular volume, and 3) encroachment of the struts or cage on the outflow tract, an oval valve can provide an orifice area up to 30% greater than a round prosthesis according to the following formulas:

$$A = \pi r^2 \text{ for a circle}$$
$$A_a = \pi ab \text{ for an ellipse}$$

where $a = r$ and $b = r_L$.
thus:

$$\frac{A}{A_L} = \frac{\pi r^2}{\pi r \cdot r_L} = \frac{\text{short axis}}{\text{long axis}} \text{ or } \frac{1}{1.3}$$

Our design is based on theoretic considerations following an attempt to determine the reasons for valve failure in this position. We have shown that by comparison with normal tricuspid valves and more especially those from patients with congestive cardiac failure, existing prostheses must be restrictive at best. These conclusions are supported by the clinical findings of ourselves and others. Whether or not an oval pericardial prosthesis will improve the results of tricuspid valve replacement remains to be seen.

References

1. McIntosh CL, Michaelis LI, Morrow AG, Itscoitz SB, Redwood DR, Epstein SE: Atrioventricular valve replacement with the Hancock porcine xenograft: A five-year clinical experience. Surgery 78:768–775, 1975.
2. Rahimtoola SH: The problem of valve prosthesis-patient mismatch. Circulation 58:20–24, 1978.
3. Dunn JM: Porcine valve durability in children. Ann Thorac Surg 32:357–368, 1981.
4. Lemole AM, Weiting DW, Cooley DA: In vitro and in vivo flow patterns of mitral valve prostheses: Development of an elliptical valve. Trans Am Soc Artif Intern Organs 15:200–205, 1969.

The Porcine Bioprosthesis: Failure Rates in the Elderly

D. F. Pupello, L. N. Bessone, R. H. Blank, E. Lopez-Cuenca, S. P. Hiro, G. Ebra

Long-term durability of the porcine bioprosthesis has yet to be clearly defined, even though excellent results have been obtained for up to 7 years postimplantation.[1] Although there is ample documentation of accelerated failure rates in the very young,[2-4] age-related failure rates of bioprostheses in the elderly has not previously been addressed. Improving results and refinements in prosthetic devices have led to a more aggressive surgical approach in the older age group.[5] With this in mind, we have elected to examine our experience using porcine bioprostheses in patients older than 70 years of age.

Patients and Methods

From September 1974 to December 1981, 252 valves were implanted in 235 patients 70 years of age and older. There were 124 men and 111 women. Ages ranged from 70–88 years with a mean of 73.9 years. Preoperatively, 110 patients were NYHA class III (46.8%) and 125 were class IV (53.2%). Fifteen patients had emergency operative procedures (6.4%) and 6 patients had had previous implantation of a prosthesis. Patients were categorized according to the type of procedure performed, i.e., group I: isolated aortic valve replacement, 80 patients, (34%); group II, mitral valve replacement, 47 patients, (20%); group III: combined procedures (double valve, revascularization, or aneurysmectomy), 108 patients, (46%). All patients in the early portion of this series received Hancock bioprostheses. Since May 1978, there has been an equal distribution of

From the Tampa General Hospital, Tampa, Florida.

Hancock and Carpentier-Edwards prostheses. The distribution of patients by age at the time of surgery is given in Fig. 1.

All patients receive warfarin for 6 weeks postoperatively. Selected patients were then given medication indefinitely, i.e., patients with a left atrial thrombus at the time of surgery, patients who sustain a postoperative arterial embolus, and patients with anatomic changes that would predispose to clot formation.

Operative Technique and Follow-up Data

Our operative technique has been described previously.[6] It consists of a midsternal approach, routine caval and aortic cannulation with moderate systemic hypothermia (26–28°C). Relatively low flow rates are employed, (35–55 ml/kg/min). Myocardial preservation was achieved in the early portion of the series with local deep hypothermia. Since 1978, cold hyperkalemic cardioplegia (2–4°C) has been employed.

Follow-up data were obtained by contacting each patient or their primary

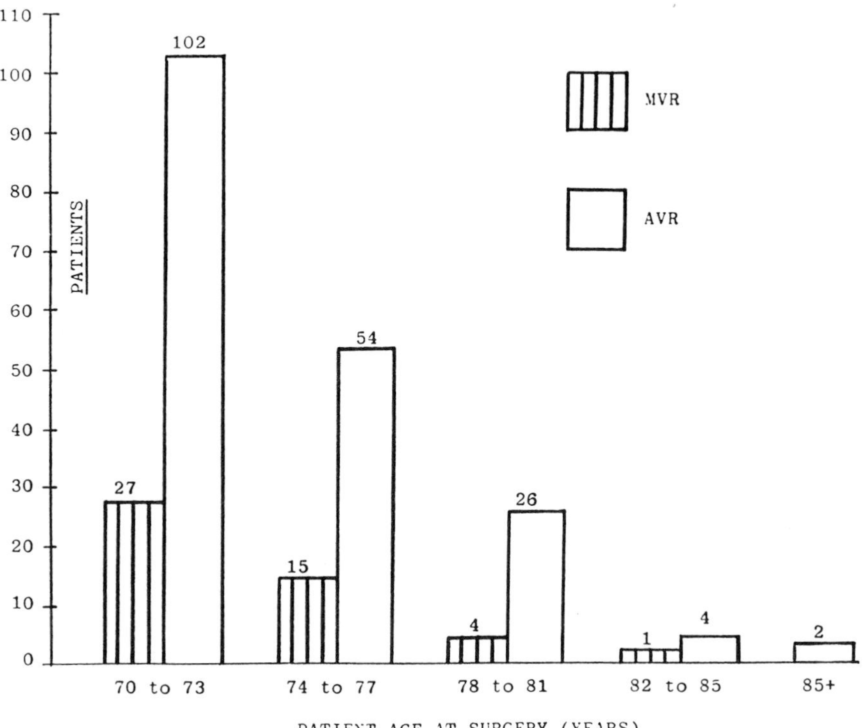

FIG. 1 Distribution of 235 patients by age group at time of surgery.

physician during the last 60 days of the study. A comprehensive questionnaire was completed assessing the clinical status and these data were subjected to computer-assisted analysis. The distribution of the 201 hospital survivors by postoperative years of follow-up is shown in Fig. 2. Follow-up data extend from 1−87 months with 6,517 months (543 patient years) of cumulative follow-up. Mean follow-up was 27.7 months.

Definition of Valve Failure

Criteria for valve failure was similar to that previously reported by Oyer et al[7] and is described as follows:

1. Valvular thrombosis resulting in reoperation or death
2. Development of a new regurgitant murmur
3. Infective endocarditis resulting in reoperation or death
4. Valvular dysfunction (confirmed) resulting in reoperation or death. Two types have been described:
   a. Spontaneous sterile degeneration[8] or "primary tissue failure" was defined as valve failure secondary to fibrosis, calcification with or without leaflet disruption, in the absence of any clinical, microscopic, or bacteriologic evidence of endocarditis
   b. Intrinsic stenosis denotes valve failure secondary to an unacceptable resting gradient even though gross and microscopic findings were normal.

Analysis of Data

Actuarial survival curves for patients were constructed for group I (aortic valve replacement), group II (mitral valve replacement), and group III

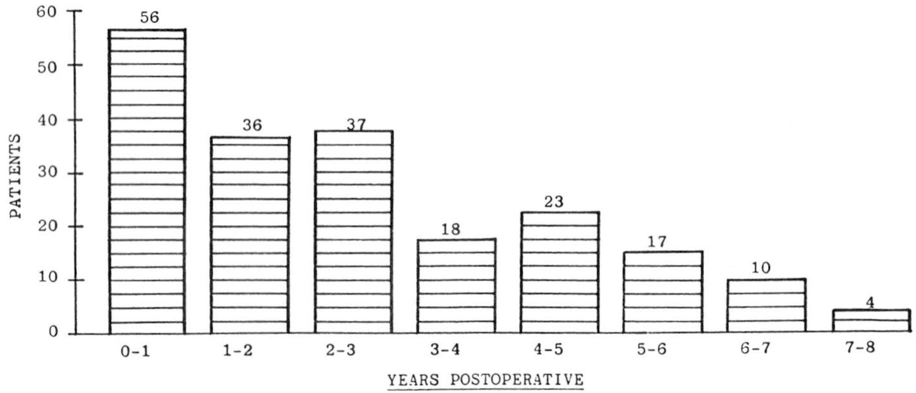

FIG. 2 Distribution of 201 hospital survivors by postoperative years of follow-up.

(combined procedures), using the method of Grunkemeyer and Starr.[9] Actuarial analysis for each patient group was plotted for 5 years postoperatively. Data points were applied only if associated with standard errors of the mean <5%.

Results

Patient Survival

Thirty-four patients died within 30 days of surgery (14.5% 30 day mortality). Two hundred and one patients (211 bioprostheses) were subjected to detailed follow-up and analysis. There have been 36 late deaths (17.9%) and 165 patients were alive at the completion of the study period. Seven patients (3.5%) were lost to follow-up, 12 patients (6%) had cardiac-related deaths, 5 patients had noncardiac-related deaths, and 12 patients died of unknown causes, all of whom are included in the actuarial curves. The 5 year survival for the isolated aortic group was 66.8%, for the mitral group, 51.8%, and for the combined group, 62.1%. Overall patient survival at 5 years for all groups was 61.6% (Fig. 3). Functional improvement post-

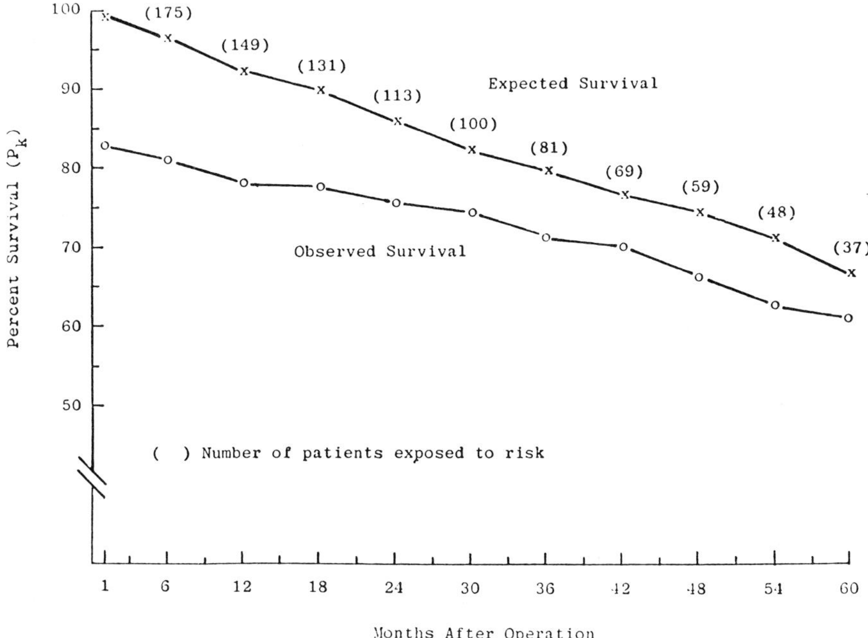

FIG. 3 Observed survival curve for all patients in the study. Compared to "Commissioners Standard Ordinary Mortality Table" matched for sex and age.

operatively has been impressive with 124 patients in class I (64.2%), ͻ8 patients in class II (30.1%), and 11 patients in class III (5.7%) (Fig. 4).

Bioprosthesis Failure

Four of the 211 valves at risk failed (1.9%). The percent of valves free of failure was plotted actuarially in Fig. 5. The linearized rate of overall bioprosthesis failure is 0.7% per patient year (543 patients years). Only 1 valve fulfilled the criteria for primary tissue failure (76 months), resulting in a linearized incidence of primary tissue failure of 0.18% per patient-year. The 2 remaining valve failures had active endocarditis confirmed at reoperation. The probability of freedom from valve failure from all causes determined by the actuarial method is 98.8% ± 2% at 5 years postoperatively. At 66 months, 96% of valves are free of failure.

Comment

The feasibility of operating upon an elderly patient population with an acceptable operative risk has been previously documented.[5] The 30 day mortality of 14.5% is approximately triple that of our previous report and probably reflects a larger number of combined operative procedures, surgi-

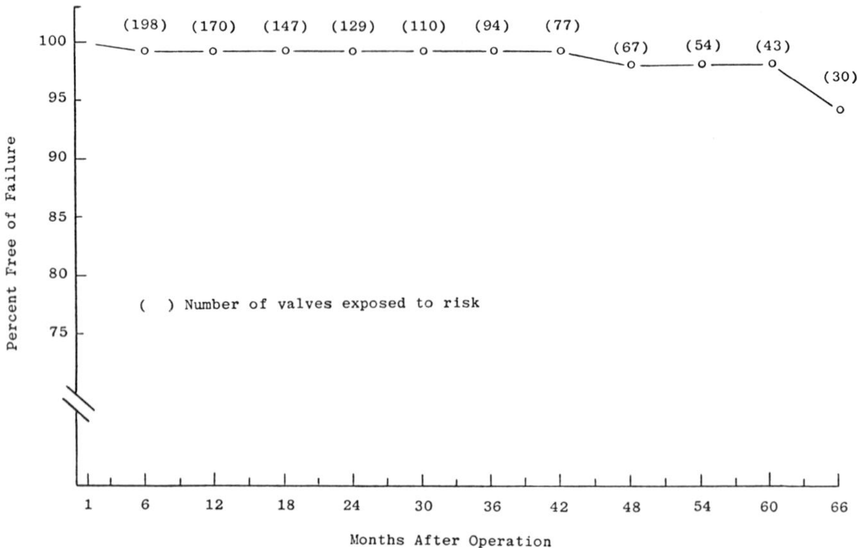

FIG. 4 Survival curve plotted actuarially for bioprostheses "at risk" to 66 months postoperatively.

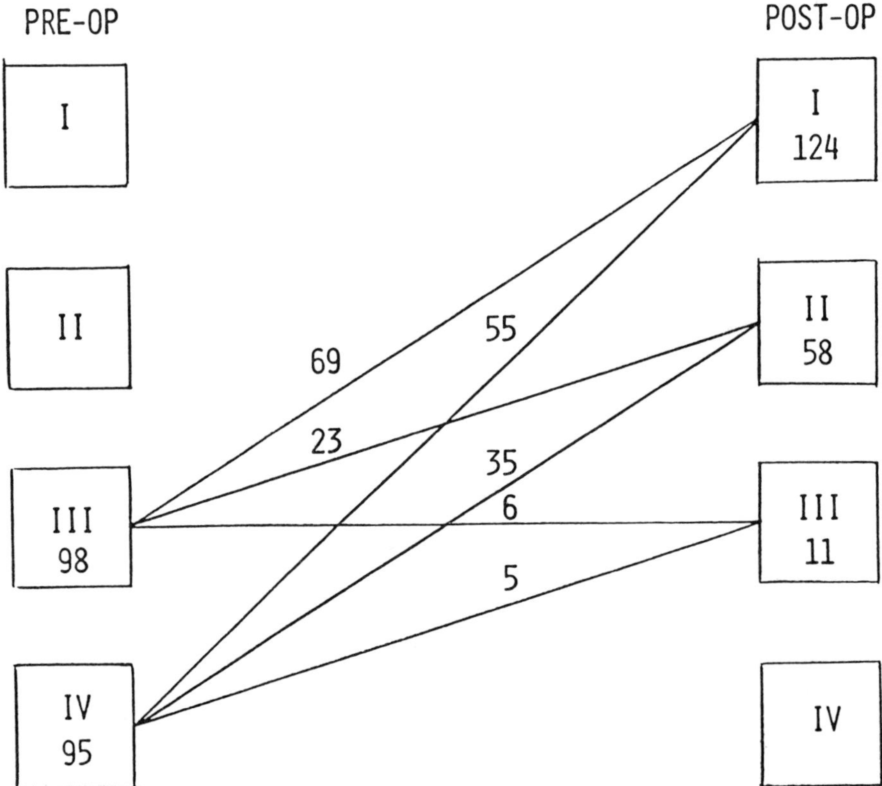

FIG. 5 Pre- and postoperative NYHA functional classification.

cal emergencies,[15] and reoperations. In addition, the majority of mitral valve patients had regurgitant lesions on the basis of coronary artery disease, a combination that carries a rather poor prognosis.[10]

The topic of age-related durability of the porcine bioprosthesis is an important issue. Relatively high rates of primary tissue failure in children have influenced several authors, prematurely and perhaps inappropriately, to refrain from using the porcine bioprosthesis in other age groups. Although the numbers are still limited, the linearized valve failure rate from all causes in this study (0.7% per patient year) is significantly lower than failure rates for patients less than 35 years of age as reported by Magilligan.[4] Similar findings have been reported by Oyer et al[7] for patients less than 15 years of age (9.8% per patient year) and more recently by Geha et al[11] in patients younger than 20 years of age. The only case of primary tissue failure in this cohort of patients occurred at 76 months, resulting in a linearized incidence of primary tissue failure of 0.18% per patient year. This valve demonstrated gross calcification and leaflet destruction. Microscopic examination showed loss of endothelium, disruption of collagen bundles, and punctate calcification. Only 2 of the 211 patients "at risk" developed endocarditis, confirmed at reoperation. This failure rate is comparable to that reported for patients who develop endocarditis with mechanical prostheses. One valve was removed at 6 months for unacceptable resting gradient even though anatomically and microscopically it was normal. This specimen was included among valve failures and for the sake of uniformity it is termed "intrinsic stenosis."[7]

The probability of freedom from valve failure from all causes determined by the actuarial method is 98.8% ± 2% at 5 years postoperatively and 96% at 5.5 years. These data therefore suggest a relatively low failure rate for the porcine bioprosthesis from all causes in elderly patients. Primary tissue failure is a rare event and appears related to calcification of the valve tissue either as a primary or secondary event.

Hydraulic function, except for extremely small devices, has been acceptable; most patients do not require anticoagulants (71.9% in this study) and thromboembolism is relatively low, even in the absence of long-term oral anticoagulation. The incidence of endocarditis has not been higher than reported in similar studies of patients with mechanical prostheses and failure of the porcine bioprosthesis, when it occurs, is usually gradual and not catastrophic. The data suggest that failure rates of the porcine bioprosthesis in older patients are significantly lower than in the younger patient population and warrants continued use of the porcine bioprosthesis in older patients.

Conclusions

The failure rate of the porcine bioprosthesis from all causes is low in elderly patients and significantly less than in younger patient populations. Valve replacement can be accomplished in elderly patients with acceptable morbidity and mortality. The porcine bioprosthesis remains the valve of choice in older patients.

References

1. Cohn LH, Mudge GH, Pratter F, Collins JJ: Five to eight year follow-up of patients undergoing porcine heart valve replacement. N Engl J Med 304:258, 1981.
2. Geha AS, Laks H, Stangel HC, Cornhill JF Kelman JW, Buckley MJ, Roberts WC: Late failure of porcine heterografts in children. J Thorac Cardiovasc Surg 78:351, 1979.
3. Silver MM, Pollock J, Silver MD, William WG, Trusler GA: Calcification in porcine xenograft valves in children. Am J Cardiol 45:685, 1980.

4. Magilligan DJ, Lewis JW, Jara FM, Lee MW, Alam M, Riddle JM, Stein PD: Spontaneous degeneration of porcine bioprosthetic valves. Ann Thorac Surg 30:259, 1980.
5. Bessone LN, Pupello DF, Blank RH, Harrison EE, Sbar S: Valve replacement in patients over 70 years. Ann Thorac Surg 24:417, 1977.
6. Pupello DF, Blank RH, Bessone LN, et al: Local deep hypothermia for combined valvular and coronary heart disease. Ann Thorac Surg 21:508, 1976.
7. Oyer PE, Miller DC, Stinson EB, Reitz BA, Moreno-Cabral RJ, Shumway NE: Clinical durability of the Hancock porcine-bioprosthetic valve. J Thorac Cardiovasc Surg 80:824, 1980.
8. Angell WW, Angell JD, Kosek JC: Twelve year experience with glutaraldehyde-preserved porcine xenografts. J Thorac Cardiovasc Surg 83:493, 1982.
9. Grunkemeier GL, Starr A: Actuarial analysis of surgical results. Rationale and method. Ann Thorac Surg 24:404, 1977.
10. Hildner FJ, Javier RP, Cohen LS: Myocardial dysfunction associated with valvular heart disease. N Engl J Med 288:194, 1973.
11. Geha AS, Hammond GL, Laks H, Stansel HC, Glenn WW: Factors affecting performance and thromboembolism after porcine xenograft cardiac valve replacement. J Thorac Cardiovasc Surg 83:337, 1982.

46

Causes of Valve Failure and Indications for Reoperation After Bioprosthetic Cardiac Valve Replacement

W. P. KLÖVEKORN, E. STRUCK, K. HOLPER, H. MEISNER, F. SEBENING

Since 1974, glutaraldehyde-preserved porcine bioprosthetic valves have been used in increasing numbers for cardiac valve substitutes at the German Heart Center in Munich. The following study is a review of our experience concerning causes of valve failure and indications for reoperation after bioprosthetic cardiac valve replacement.

Patients and Methods

Between April 1974 and February 1982, a total of 1,915 heart valve substitutes were implanted in 1,602 patients. Of these, 874 were mechanical valves (Björk-Shiley) and 1,041 porcine bioprostheses (Hancock and Carpentier-Edwards). From June 1976 to February 1982, a total of 27 patients required reoperation because of 31 bioprosthetic valve failures.

Our use of bioprostheses was originally limited to patients in whom anticoagulation was contraindicated, mainly children and patients from countries where reliable anticoagulation appeared to be impossible. As can be seen in Fig. 1, from 1976 on, bioprostheses were used more frequently and in 1979 more than 90% of all valves implanted were bioprostheses. Mechanical valves were only used in some special cases. In the last 2 years, we have reached relatively well balanced relationship between mechanical and bioprosthetic valve implants.

From the Department of Cardiovascular Surgery, German Heart Center, Munich, West Germany.

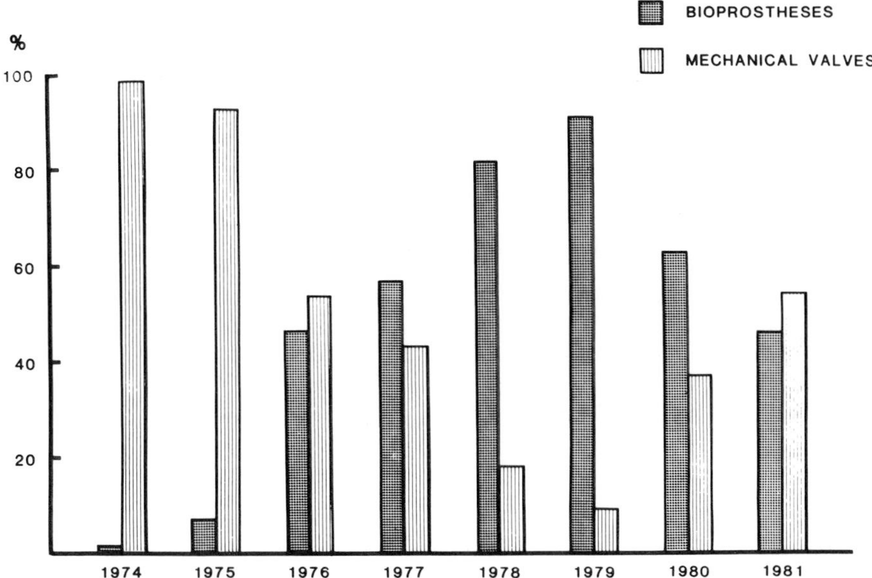

FIG. 1 Comparative use of bioprostheses and mechanical valves from 1974–1981.

Results

Our mean observation time after bioprosthetic valve replacement is 3.6 years, for a total of 2,943 patient years. Until March 1982, 185 bioprostheses were implanted for more than 60 months.

Causes of reoperation after bioprosthetic valve replacement in 27 patients (31 valves) are summarized in Table I.

Bioprosthetic valve *bacterial endocarditis* was the most frequent cause of valve failure (14 patients, 17 valves). There were 10 males and 4 females in whom 7 aortic, 9 mitral, and 1 tricuspid valves were affected. The mean age of this patient group was 47.4 ± 8.8 years. Reoperation was done 26.4 ± 21.2 months after first implantation.

Bioprosthetic valve *degeneration* necessitating reoperation was seen in 9 valves, 8 patients (6 males and 2 females). Six aortic and 3 mitral valves were affected. The mean age of this patient group was 32.3 ± 13.7 years, significantly ($p < 0.005$) lower than in patients with endocarditis. The interval between first implantation and reoperation was 50.6 ± 16.0 months, which is nearly twice as long as in the endocarditis group ($p < 0.01$).

In 5 patients (2 males, 3 females) with 2 aortic and 3 mitral valves a reoperation became necessary after 9.2 ± 8.3 months because of severe hemodynamic impairment due to a *paravalvular leak.* In all of these patients there was no evidence of bacterial endocarditis or degeneration and the bioprosthesis appeared normal at reoperation.

TABLE I Causes of reoperation in 27 patients (31 valves) after bioprosthetic valve replacement

Cause of reoperation	# pts (M/F)	Age (yr)	Time (mo)	Valves	Valve position		
					Aortic	Mitral	Tricuspid
Endocarditis	14 10/4	47.4 ± 8.8	26.4 ± 21.2	17	7	9	1
Degeneration	8 6/2	32.3* ± 13.7	50.6† ± 16.0	9	6	3	0
Paravalvular leak	5 2/3	41.4 ± 17.3	9.2‡ ± 8.3	5	2	3	0

* $p < 0.005$.
† $p < 0.01$.
‡ $p < 0.001$.

Of the 31 bioprostheses that required reoperation, there were 21 Hancock and 10 Carpentier-Edwards valves. Since in the total patient group with bioprostheses Hancock and Carpentier-Edwards valves were used in nearly 2:1 relationship, the failure rate equals closely the frequency of implantation of the 2 valve types. At reoperation, 17 bioprostheses were exchanged for Björk-Shiley valves. In 1 case a St. Jude valve was used and in 13 a new bioprosthesis was implanted or the old one refixated.

Twenty-five out of 27 patients survived the reoperation. In the 2 patients who died, an acute bacterial endocarditis necessitated reoperation on an emergency basis and death was caused by sepsis.

Comment

Excellent early results, a low rate of thromboembolism, and good hemodynamic performance, as well as favorable reports by others, stimulated our enthusiasm for the use of porcine bioprostheses. Since there are increasing recent reports about late bioprosthetic valve malfunction due to tissue degeneration or bacterial endocarditis, we have evaluated our results with more than 1,000 bioprostheses implanted during the last 7 years.

When we look at the causes of reoperation after bioprosthetic valve replacement (Fig. 2), we can see that bacterial endocarditis is a permanent threat for the patient. In our series, endocarditis and paravalvular leaks were the only causes for reoperation until 1979. The incidence was 1–4 cases per

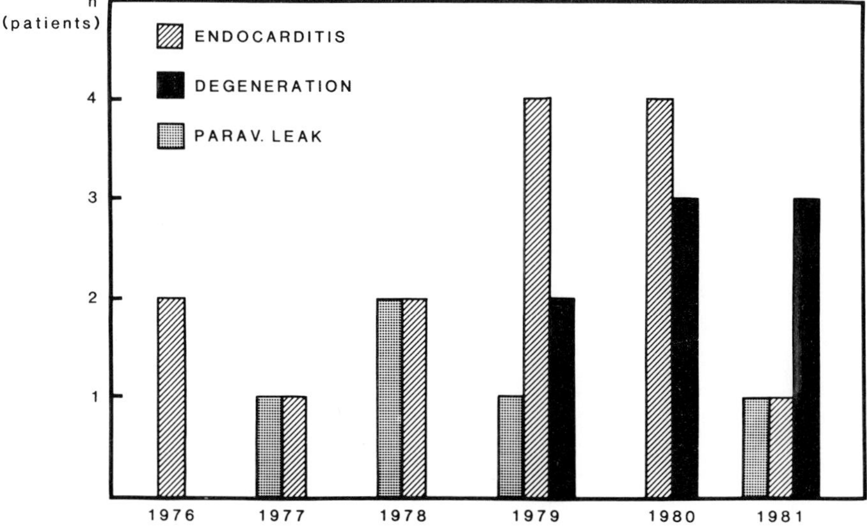

FIG. 2 Causes of reoperation after bioprosthetic valve replacement.

year and no increase could be found with increasing numbers of patients. As could be expected from reports by others, we also had to reoperate upon patients with bioprosthetic valve malfunction due to tisssue degeneration and calcification of the leaflets. We first saw those patients in 1979, nearly 5 years after we had started to use bioprostheses. The incidence in the last 3 years was 2–3 patients per year but only 185 valves have an observable time of more than 60 months.

When we look at the relationship of complications to patient age (Fig. 3), we can see that the incidence of tissue degeneration is more frequent in younger patients. Bacterial endocarditis, however, shows only a clear correlation with the numerical distribution of bioprostheses in relation to patient age. Since the highest number of valves was implanted in patients between 40 and 50 years of age, the incidence of bacterial endocarditis is also the highest in this age group. There is no correlation between patient age and the incidence of paravalvular leaks that were not caused by endocarditis.

When we look at the relationship of complications to the period of time the bioprosthesis had been implanted (Fig. 4), it becomes evident that the incidence of bacterial endocarditis is higher in the first 2 years following

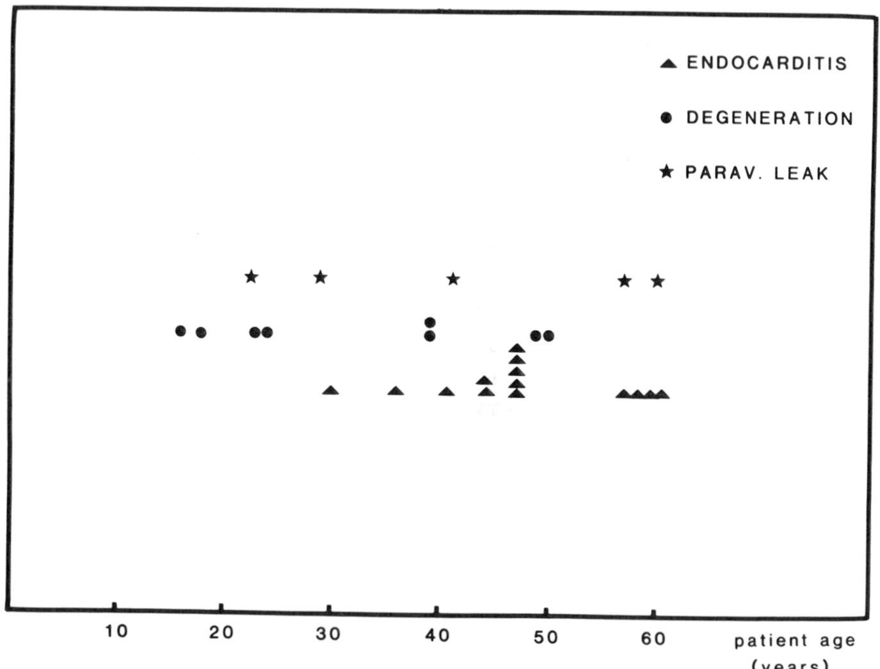

FIG. 3 Relationship of complications to patient age.

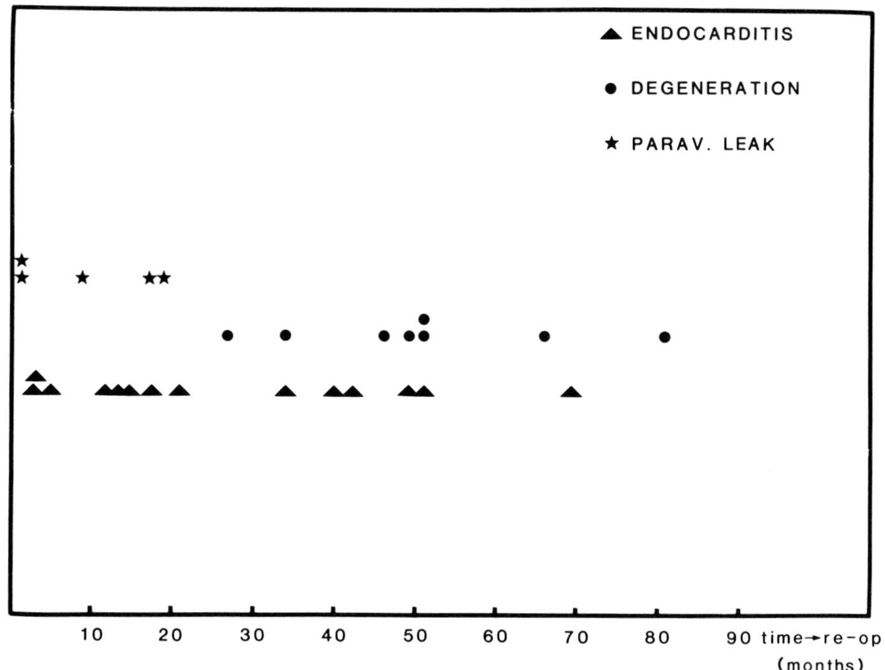

FIG. 4 Relationship of complications to time after implantation of bioprosthesis.

implantation, whereas tissue degeneration is a typical late complication. All paravalvular leaks without signs of endocarditis appeared rather early.

In 11 out of 14 patients reoperated upon because of bacterial endocarditis, the infecting organism could be identified (Table II). Except for 2 patients who died from sepsis, all other patients survived without recurrence of endocarditis regardless of whether a mechanical or bioprosthetic valve was used at reoperation. Whereas patients with valve degeneration show clinical signs of valvular stenosis, patients with bacterial endocarditis develop symptoms of valvular insufficiency which are reflected in the pathologic findings at reoperation. In almost all cases leaflet destruction and/or paravalvular leak are present.

Conclusions

From our experience, we have drawn the following conclusions for the use of bioprosthetic and mechanical valves:

1. Bioprostheses should be used in older patients (>50 years) with sinus rhythm.

TABLE II Summary of data from 14 patients reoperated on after bioprosthetic valve replacement because of bacterial endocarditis

Patient	Sex	Age (yrs)	Type of valve + position	Type of valve used at reoperation*	Pathologic findings	Infecting organism	Result
1	F	30	CE 29 Mitral	BS 31	Paravalvular leak leaflet destruction*	?	Survived
2	M	47	CE 27 Aortic	BS 27	Paravalvular leak vegetations	Staphylococcus epidermidis	Survived
3	M	47	HC 29 Aortic	BS 27	Paravalvular leak vegetations	?	Survived
4	M	57	CE 29 Aortic CE 31 Mitral	CE 29 Aortic HC 29	No pathologic changes! Mitral valve vegetations	Staphylococcus epidermidis	Survived
5	F	47	HC 31 Mitral	HC 31	Leaflet destruction vegetations	Klebsiella pneumoniae	Survived
6	F	59	HC 25 Aortic	HC 25 (same valve!)	Anular abscess	Streptococcus faecalis	Survived
7	M	44	CE 29 Aortic CE 31 Mitral	CE 29 CE 31	Leaflet destruction calcification	Streptococcus faecalis	Survived

8	M	58	HC 27 Aortic	BS 29	Leaflet destruction vegetations	Staphylococcus epidermidis	†
9	M	60	HC 25 Aortic	BS 23	Anular abscess	Proteus mirabilis	†
10	M	41	BS 25 Aortic* HC 33 Mitral HC 35 tricuspid	BS 33 BS 33 } BS 35 }	No pathologic changes leaflet destruction vegetations	Streptococcus viridans	Survived
11	F	44	HC 31 Mitral	BS 31	Leaflet destruction vegetations	Staphylococcus albus	Survived
12	M	36	HC 33 Mitral	HC 35	Paravalvular leak vegetations	Streptococcus anhaemolyticus	Survived
13	M	47	HC 33 Mitral	St.-J. 33	Paravalvular leak vegetations	Peptococcus (anaerobic)	Survived
14	M	47	HC 29 Aortic HC 31 Mitral	BS 29 BS 31	Leaflet destruction calcification	?	Survived

* HC: Hancock; CE: Carpentier-Edwards, BS: Björk-Shiley; St.-J.: St. Jude medical).

2. Bioprostheses should not be used in patients younger than 40 years of age (except when there is a clear contraindication for anticoagulation).
3. Bioprostheses or mechanical valves may be used in patients older than 40 years of age who have to have anticoagulants because of rhythm problems.
4. Bioprostheses or mechanical valves may be used in patients who have to be reoperated on because of endocarditis after valve replacement.
5. Mechanical valves should be used in patients who have to be reoperated on because of valve degeneration or calcification after bioprosthetic valve replacement.

Further careful studies of results after bioprosthetic valve replacement seem to be necessary to prove more clearly the long-term durability of these valves. Until then, there will remain a considerable number of patients in whom, based on our present knowledge, no precise decision can be made whether a bioprosthetic or mechanical valve should be implanted.

47

Clinical Analysis of the Hancock Porcine Bioprosthesis

P. E. Oyer, E. B. Stinson, D. C. Miller, S. W. Jamieson, B. A. Reitz, W. Baumgartner, N. E. Shumway

The Hancock glutaraldehyde-fixed porcine bioprosthesis has been used for replacement of the intracardiac valves at Stanford University Medical Center since 1971. Because of favorable results in the initial series of patients to receive this valve, it has been used virtually exclusively in patients undergoing valve replacement surgery at this center since 1974.[1,2] This report summarizes our experience with the Hancock bioprosthesis, specifically focusing upon the incidence of thromboembolism, infection, and reoperation in patients with this valve implanted, as well as experience regarding long-term clinical durability.

Patients and Methods

Eight hundred and fifty-eight adult patients (>15 years of age) who underwent aortic valve replacement (AVR) and 801 adult patients who underwent mitral valve replacement (MVR) were included in the analysis. In addition 10 children with MVR and 4 children with AVR were analyzed separately. This stratification of the patient group according to age was performed because of extensive previous documentation of a substantial difference in the clinical performance of bioprostheses in these 2 age groups.[3–5] Between 1971 and 1976, all AVR patients received standard orifice Hancock bioprostheses; since that time, all AVR patients received modified orifice prostheses of sizes 25 and smaller. The majority of patients in the analysis were older than 55 years of age at the time of operation (Fig. 1).

From the Department of Cardiovascular Surgery, Stanford University School of Medicine, Stanford, California.

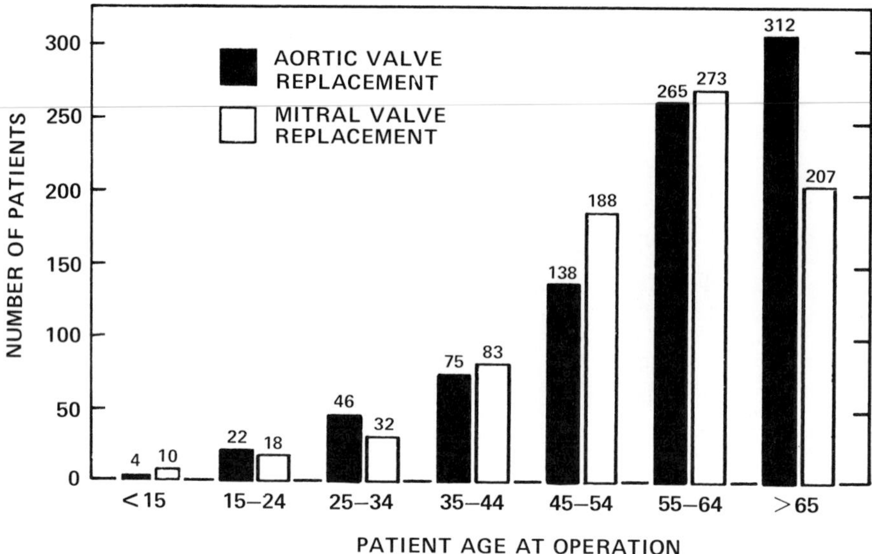

FIG. 1 Distribution of patient ages at the time of operation.

The cumulative duration of follow-up for adult patients undergoing AVR was 2,483 patient years and for adult patients undergoing MVR it was 2,484 patient years. The follow-up durations for children with AVR was 13 patient years and for children with MVR, 59 patient years. Figure 2 depicts the number of patients in each yearly postoperative follow-up interval at the time of analysis. Eighteen patients who underwent AVR (2.1%) and 7 patients who underwent MVR (0.9%) were lost to follow-up.

Meaningful comparison of data from various centers in regard to thromboembolic complications requires a clear definition of signs and symptoms considered to be of thromboembolic origin. For the purposes of this analysis, all new episodes of focal neurologic deficit, regardless of their transience or permanence, as well as all episodes of peripheral embolization were considered to be valve-related thromboembolic episodes, unless clearly established to be of separate origin. In addition, patients who failed to regain consciousness after valve replacement or who awoke with a neurologic deficit were included in this definition, unless such deficit clearly resulted from identifiable intraoperative complications. Since inclusion of such patients probably results in overestimation of the true incidence of valve-related thromboemboli, the incidence of thromboembolic complications reported herein should be considered to be maximal.

The criteria used to establish "overall valve failure" were similar to those used in previous publications from this institution. The occurrence of any of the following events were considered to constitute valve failure: 1) the

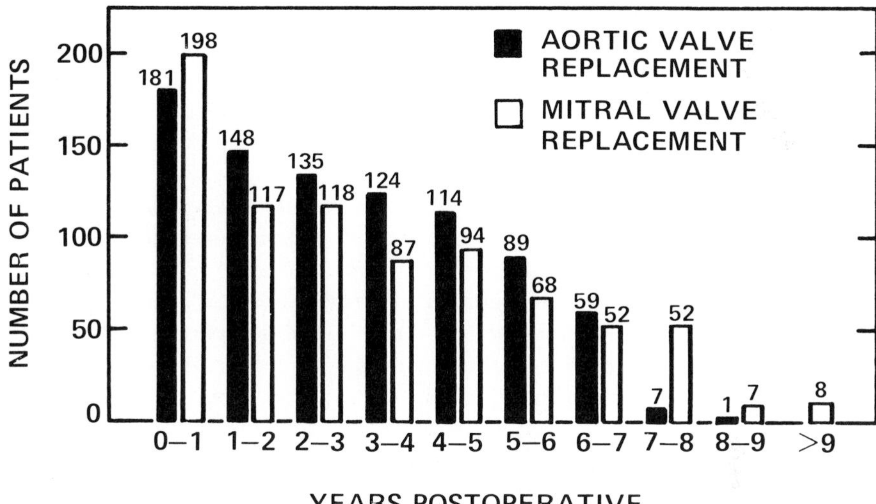

FIG. 2 Distribution of patients according to length of follow-up at the time of analysis.

postoperative development of a new regurgitant murmur unless proved by left ventricular angiography to result from a periprosthetic leak, 2) thromboembolic complications necessitating reoperation or resulting in death, 3) thrombotic valvular occlusion resulting in reoperation or death, 4) infective endocarditis that required reoperation or resulted in death, and 5) significant hemodynamic dysfunction resulting in reoperation or death.

"Primary tissue failure" is the term used to describe spontaneous degeneration of valve tissue, with or without calcification of the leaflets; patients with a previous history of endocarditis involving the bioprosthesis who were successfully treated medically but later required bioprosthesis replacement for hemodynamic dysfunction were not included in the "primary tissue failure" category. The term "intrinsic stenosis" was used to describe those bioprosthetic valves that required replacement because of large transvalvular pressure drops in symtomatic patients but at the time of removal appeared to have complete valve leaflet integrity and mobility.

The actuarial method of Kaplan and Meier[6] was used to describe various time-related data. Because of the nonlinearity of thromboembolism data and valve failure data, linearized rates over the entire follow-up time in this analysis were not employed to describe the frequency of these events. Rather, linearized rates were calculated over individual yearly postoperative intervals, since over the shorter periods of time the occurrence rates approximated a straight line. Such calculations were useful in assessing the relative risks of events during specific postoperative time intervals. Although several patients in this analysis have been followed for nearly 10 years, actuarial curves were not plotted beyond the time in which the standard errors of the associated data points exceeded ±5% because of the substantial uncertainty regarding the true value of data points with larger associated standard errors.

The anticoagulation policy for patients in this analysis was to administer warfarin sodium over a period of 6 weeks after AVR and for 12 weeks after MVR because the risk of thromboembolic complications was highest during these time frames. Anticoagulant therapy was thereafter discontinued, except in patients who exhibited abnormal intracardiac anatomy likely independently to increase the risk of late thromboembolic events. All patients who sustained postoperative thromboembolic complications were thereafter given indefinite anticoagulation therapy. The presence of atrial fibrillation alone was not considered sufficient to warrant long-term anticoagulation. Eight percent of patients who underwent AVR and 30% of patients with MVR received long-term anticoagulation.

Results

Bioprosthesis Failure

The types of bioprosthesis failure for aortic and mitral bioprostheses, along with the relative frequencies of such failures, are shown in Table I. A total of 60 valves (29 aortic, 31 mitral) failed among the 1,659 patients analyzed. Most failures of aortic bioprostheses were due to endocarditis, whereas most of the mitral bioprosthetic failures were accounted for by either primary tissue failure (spontaneous degeneration) or late-developing regurgitant murmurs of unknown etiology. It is noteworthy that bioprosthesis thrombosis was an exceedingly rare event, with only 5 cases observed in the entire series of patients.

The overall incidence of bioprosthetic failure calculated actuarially is shown in Fig. 3. The probability of valve failure from all causes was similar

TABLE I Modes of bioprosthesis failure

	AVR pts	MVR pts
Endocarditis	18 (62%)	6 (19%)
Primary tissue failure	5 (17%)	11 (35%)
Regurgitant murmur	3 (10%)	9 (29%)
Thrombosis	1 (4%)	4 (13%)
Intrinsic stenosis	2 (7%)	1 (4%)
Total failures	29	31

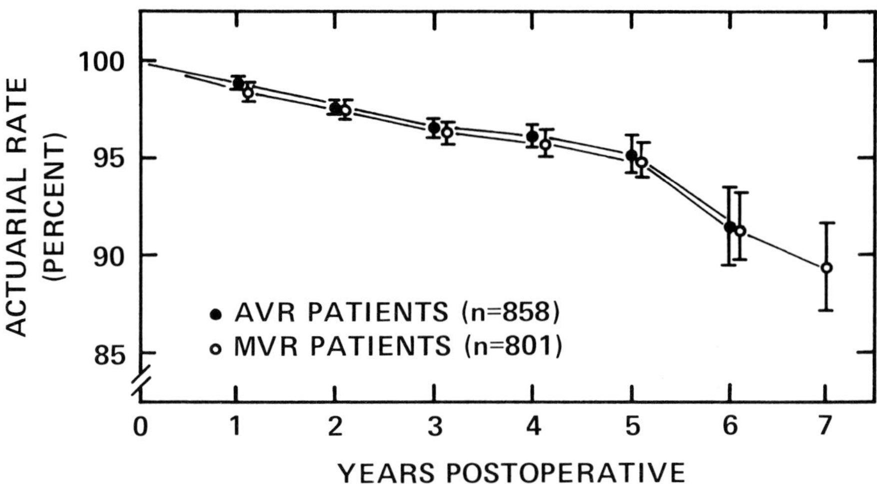

FIG. 3 Actuarial incidence of valve failure from all causes among adult AVR and MVR patients. Brackets denote 1 standard error of the mean (SE)

in both AVR and MVR patients, with 89.5% of patients free of any mode of failure after 7 years of follow-up. An acceleration in rate of valve failure was noted between 5 and 7 years after operation, reflecting the increased incidence of primary tissue failure observed during this interval.

The incidence of primary tissue failure is given according to actuarial calculations in Figs. 4 and 5 for AVR and MVR patients. In addition, the yearly linearized rates of this mode of failure are shown along with the actual number of events observed in each yearly postoperative interval. The acceleration in the rate of spontaneous degeneration of valve leaflet tissue is apparent after the 5th postoperative year. It is noteworthy that although an acceleration in the rate of degeneration occurs between the 5th and 6th postoperative year, no further acceleration in the rate was noted during the 6th and 7th postoperative year follow-up in the mitral patients. In spite of this increased rate of degeneration observed in the later follow-up intervals, nearly 95% of patients can be expected to remain free of this complication after 7 years of implantation.

As shown in Fig. 1, 14 children <15 years of age underwent valve replacement using bioprostheses; 4 received aortic valves and 10 received mitral valves. It has been necessary to reoperate on 3 of the 4 patients with aortic bioprostheses, 2 because of primary tissue failure and 1 because of bioprosthesis dysfunction resulting from an earlier bioprosthesis infection.

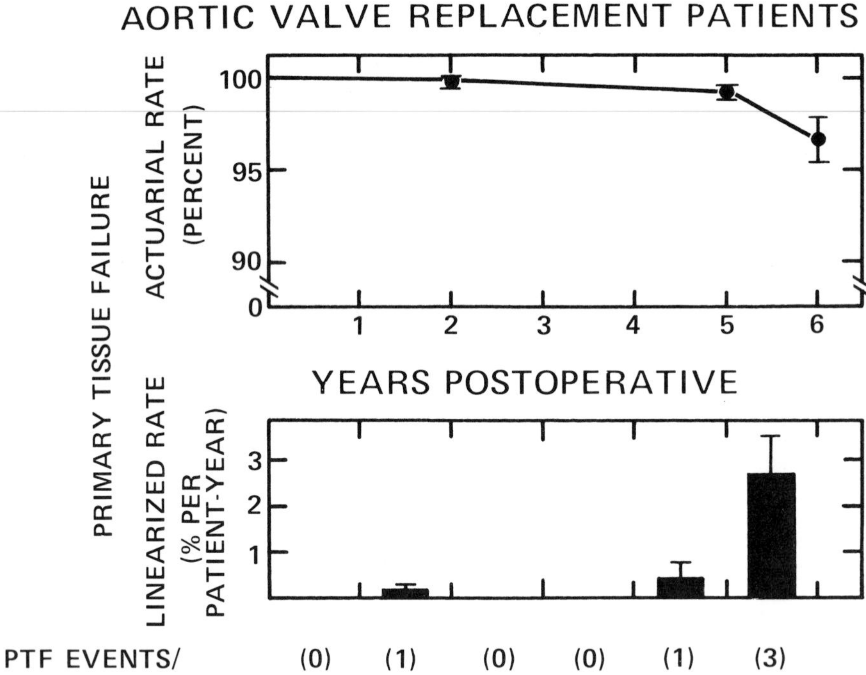

FIG. 4 Actuarial (upper panel) and interval linearized rates (lower panel) of primary tissue failure among adult AVR patients. Brackets denote 1 SE. The actual number of patients observed with primary tissue failure during each yearly interval are shown.

Likewise, a large proportion (70%) of the mitral bioprostheses implanted in children have been removed, all because of primary tissue failure. The average duration of implantation of the 3 aortic valves that required removal was 3.2 ± 1.2 years. That average implant duration for the 7 mitral bioprostheses that were removed was 5.5 ± 1.8 years. In all cases, the failed bioprostheses were replaced with new bioprosthetic valves. The reoperative mortality in this group of 10 children who required replacement of their bioprosthetic valves was 0. The number of children with bioprosthetic valves available for study was clearly too small to allow accurate projection of the risk of early bioprosthesis failure reliably by statistical methods. It is quite clear, however, that the incidence of this complication is substantially higher in these patients than in adults. A correlation between age and the incidence of primary tissue failure has not been noted in any age group >15 years in this series. In fact, no instances of primary tissue failure were observed in any patient between the age of 16 and 35 years. Thus, the suggestion by others that spontaneous degeneration occurs less frequently

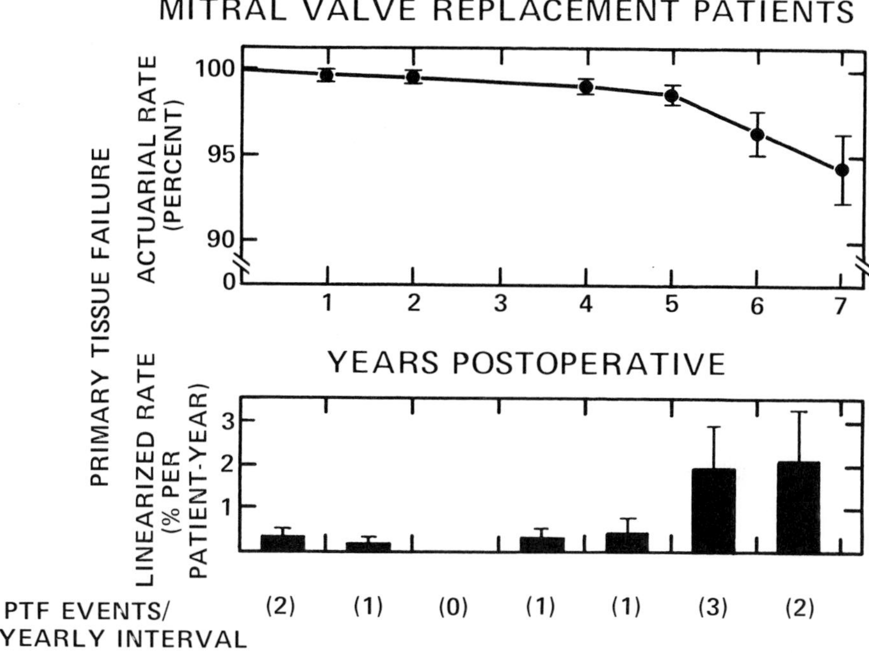

FIG. 5 Actuarial (upper panel) and interval linearized rates (lower panel) of primary tissue failure among adult MVR patients. Brackets denote 1 SE. The number of occurrences of this complications during each yearly postoperative interval are also shown.

with increasing age, even in the adult population, cannot be confirmed by these data.[7]

Thromboembolism

Figures 6 and 7 depict the incidence of thromboembolic complications observed in this series of patients, expressed both by the actuarial method and by linearized yearly interval risks. In addition, the actual number of such complications observed during each yearly interval are noted. The risk of this complication was clearly higher during the initial months after operation than during the later follow-up period, during which time the risk of thromboembolism was quite constant. Approximately one-half of all emboli that occurred were clustered in the first 6 postoperative weeks among AVR patients and the first 12 postoperative weeks among MVR patients. It should be pointed out again, however, that all new neurologic events occurring in the immediate postoperative period were considered to result from valve-related emboli, unless clearly the result of identifiable intraoperative

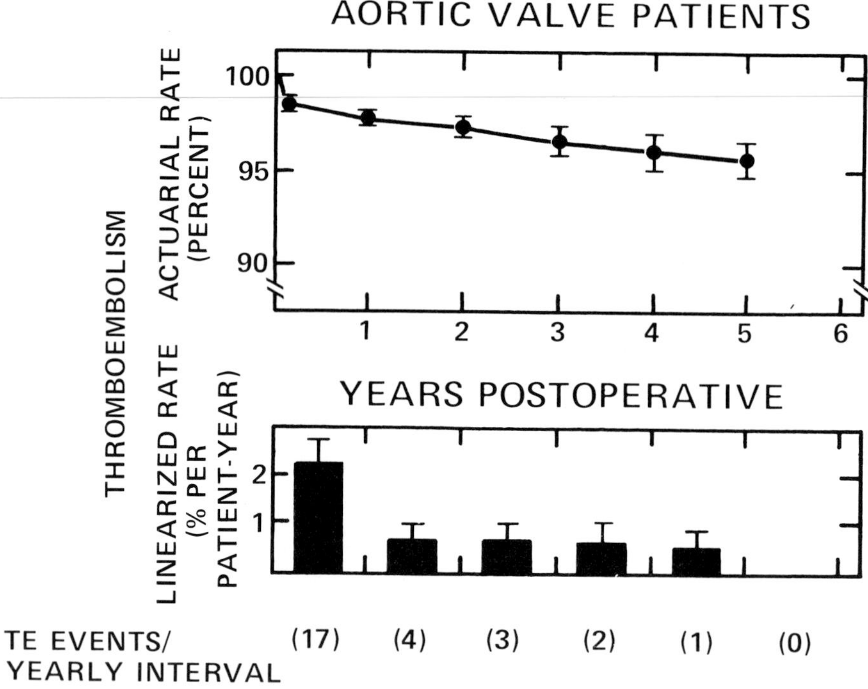

FIG. 6 Actuarial (upper panel) and yearly interval linearized rates (lower panel) of thromboembolism among adult AVR patients. Brackets denote 1 SE. The actual number of thromboembolic events observed as shown at the bottom.

complications. Since some of these immediately postoperative neurologic complications undoubtedly resulted from nonvalve-related causes, the true incidence of thromboemboli originating from the valves during the early postoperative interval was probably overestimated.

Endocarditis

A total of 39 instances of infection involving bioprosthetic valves was noted in this series of 1,659 adult patients. Twenty-seven involved aortic bioprostheses and 12 involved mitral prostheses. The actuarial incidence of bioprosthesis infection is shown in Fig. 8. The incidence of infection involving aortic bioprostheses was slightly higher than that observed among patients with mitral bioprostheses. As shown in Table I, 18 of the total of 27 aortic bioprosthesis infections resulted in valve failure; the remaining 9 patients (33%) were successfully treated with antibiotic therapy alone. Six of the 12 cases of mitral bioprosthesis infection resulted in valve failure; the

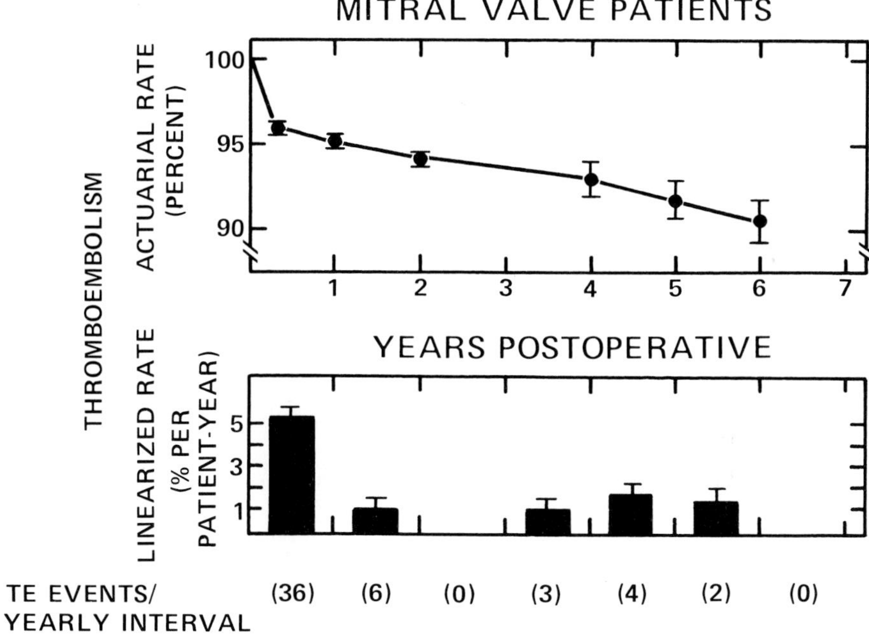

FIG. 7 Actuarial (upper panel) and yearly interval linearized rates (lower panel) of thromboembolism among adult MVR patients. Brackets denote 1 SE. Also shown are the number of such events observed during each yearly interval.

remaining 6 (50%) were likewise treated successfully without the need for operative intervention.

Patients who required reoperation because of active bioprosthesis infection sustained a high operative mortality. Thus, among the 21 patients in this series who came to operation because of active infection of their bioprosthesis, operatively mortality was 42%.

Perivalvular Leak

Perivalvular leaks were a rare complication among patients who received Hancock bioprostheses. Among the 858 adult patients receiving aortic valves, 6 (0.7%) developed perivalvular leaks that required reoperation. Among the 801 adult MVR patients, 5 (0.6%) required reoperation because of perivalvular leaks. Patients who developed leaks as a result of bacterial endocarditis were not included in these figures. The incidence of perivalvular leaks observed in this series may slightly underestimate the true incidence of such leaks because some of those patients who developed

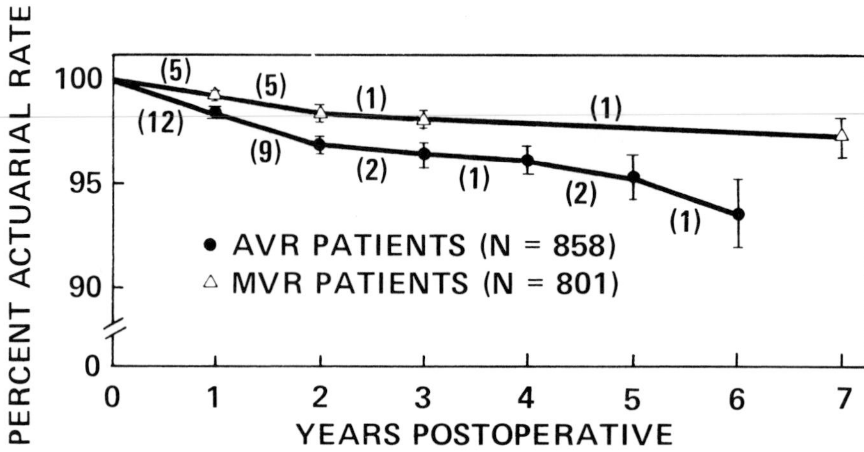

FIG. 8 Actuarial incidence of infections involving bioprosthetic valves observed in adult patients in the analysis. Brackets denote 1 SE.

valve failure due to new regurgitant murmurs may indeed have perivalvular leaks to account for the clinical findings.

Reoperation Among Patients with Bioprosthetic Valves

Reoperation was performed in a total of 28 adult AVR patients and 24 adult MVR patients in this series. The indications for reoperation, along with their relative frequencies, are shown in Table II. Endocarditis was the primary indication for reoperation among AVR patients, whereas primary tissue failure was the predominant indication in MVR patients. The actuarial rate of reoperation is given in Fig. 9. In addition, the actual number of reoperations that occurred during early yearly postoperative interval are listed. Three additional reoperations were performed (2 AVR and 1 MVR) that are not indicated on the actuarial curve because they occurred beyond the 6 and 7 year time points to which the respective curves can be accurately

TABLE II Indications for reoperation

	AVR pts		MVR pts	
Endocarditis	15	(54%)	6	(25%)
Primary tissue failure	4	(14%)	10	(42%)
Thrombosis	1	(4%)	2	(8%)
Intrinsic stenosis	2	(7%)	1	(4%)
Periprosthetic leak	6	(21%)	5	(21%)
Total reoperations	28		24	

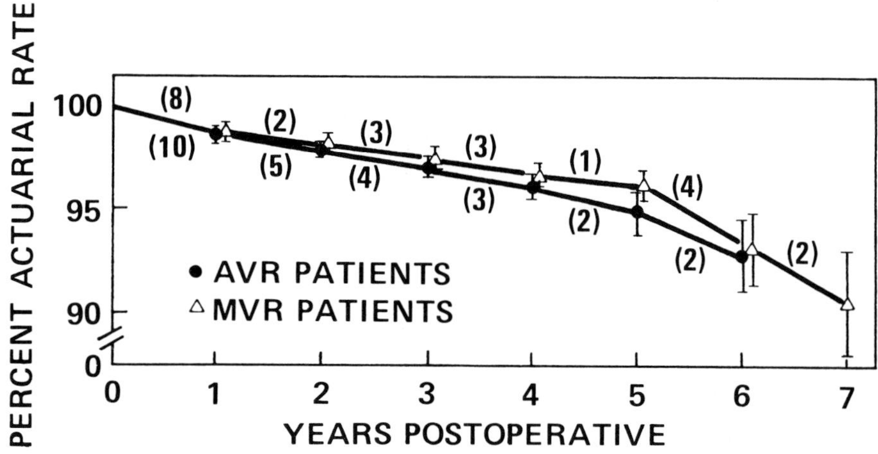

FIG. 9 Incidence of reoperation calculated actuarially for adult AVR and MVR patients. Brackets denote 1 SE.

drawn. Slight acceleration in the reoperation rates can be appreciated beyond 5 years, reflecting the increased incidence of primary tissue failure in this interval.

The linearized rates of reoperation were 1.1% per patient year for AVR patients and 0.97% per patient year for MVR patients calculated over the entire follow-up period.

Comment

The data reported herein allow firm, statistically based conclusions to be drawn regarding the performance of Hancock bioprosthetic valves through 7 years of follow-up. Furthermore, observations of the smaller numbers of patients with such valves implanted for longer periods of time suggest that satisfactory performance of the bioprosthetic valve may be expected through an even greater period of follow-up. The data presented confirm the fact that thromboembolic complications are distinctly unusual among patients with this valve, and bioprosthesis thrombosis is an exceedingly rare occurrence, without the use of long-term anticoagulation therapy.

The incidence of endocarditis observed among patients with bioprosthetic valves is likewise low and does not appear to differ from rates observed among patients with mechanical prostheses. Although the occurrence of infection on bioprosthetic valves was associated with a fatal outcome in a substantial proportion, as it is with any type of prosthetic valve, approximately 35% of such infections were managed successfully with antibiotic therapy alone.

The incidence of bland periprosthetic leaks not associated with valve infections has likewise been exceedingly low. This may relate in part to the surgical technique used for implantation, which consisted of interrupted horizontal mattress sutures in all cases, rarely with the use of Teflon pledgets. It may also result in part, however, from the construction of the Hancock bioprosthesis sewing ring, which cushions and conforms easily to friable and/or calcific and irregular valve anuli.

That the durability of the Hancock bioprosthesis remains fully satisfactory through at least 7 years of follow-up is confirmed by the data reported herein. Thus, only slightly more than 5% of patients experienced spontaneous degeneration of their valve leaflet tissue after this time interval. Although observations in patients in this series followed for more than 7 years suggest no further acceleration in the rate of tissue degeneration through these longer follow-up intervals, firm conclusions regarding extended durability cannot yet be made on a statistical basis.

It is noteworthy that the clinical features exhibited by patients with bioprosthetic tissue failure in all cases consisted of slowly progressive symptoms of valvular stenosis and/or regurgitation which developed over a period of weeks to months. Sufficient time was therefore available after the onset of symptoms of valve dysfunction to perform an orderly cardiologic evaluation and re-replacement. Sudden catastrophic failure of bioprosthetic valves due to spontaneous degeneration was not observed. In contrast, patients who developed bioprosthesis infections occasionally experienced sudden cardiac decompensation, in most cases because of valve dehiscence resulting from anular abscess formation or less commonly from rapid destruction of the valve leaflet tissue by bacterial organisms. Thus, sudden catastrophic dysfunction of a bioprosthetic valve strongly suggests the presence of infection.

The durability of bioprosthetic valves in children less than 15 years old is clearly inferior to that observed in adult patients. Therefore the advisability of using such valves in young patients remains controversial and is influenced heavily by individual considerations. Decisions in this regard must take into account not only the rate of spontaneous degeneration of porcine valves, but also the difficulties in anticoagulation in young patients, and the fact that sequential replacement of prosthetic valves in children may be required because of growth considerations, irrespective of what type valve is used. In addition, the cumulative risk of a series of valve replacements has undoubtedly been substantially reduced in recent years, inasmuch as newer modes of myocardial protection during operation have resulted in low reoperative morbidity and mortality rates. Since the relative impact of each of these factors on long-term patient survival cannot be determined at present, a decision as to the appropriate valve for use in children remains an individual judgment.

The rate of reoperation necessary among patients with prosthetic valves provides some insight into their long-term performance. The reoperation rate among patients with Hancock bioprostheses in this series was quite low through 7 years of follow-up. Interestingly, the rate of reoperation, was nearly identical to those reported for certain widely used mechanical prostheses.[8,9] Thus, although the indications for reoperation differ in patients with mechanical valves compared to those with bioprosthetic valves, a similar proportion of patients with both types of valvular prosthesis appears eventually to require reoperation, within the constraints of the follow-up period reported.

Conclusions

The Hancock bioprosthesis has now been shown to perform well in adult patients through at least 7 years of follow-up in terms of the major indices of valve performance. Among children, its durability is clearly less satisfactory, although this feature is difficult to quantify precisely because of the small number of children available for analysis. However, new developments in the preparation of biologic tissue for use in clinical heart valves, in particular low pressure fixation and processes aimed at inhibiting calcification, hold theoretic promise for improvement in the long-term results in young patients as well as in the adult population.

References

1. Oyer PE, Stinson EB, Reitz BA, Miller DC, Rossiter SJ, Shumway NE: Long-term evaluation of the porcine xenograft bioprosthesis. J Thorac Cardiovasc Surg 78:343, 1979.
2. Oyer PE, Miller DC, Stinson EB, Reitz BA, Moreno RJ, Shumway NE: Clinical durability of the Hancock porcine bioprosthetic valve. J Thorac Cardiovasc Surg 80:824, 1980.
3. Kutsche LM, Oyer PE, Shumway NE, Baum D: An important complication of Hancock mitral valve replacement in children. Circulation 60 (Suppl I): 98, 1979.
4. Geha AS, Laks H, Stansel HC Jr, Cornhill JF, Kilman JW, Buckley MJ, Roberts WC: Late failure of porcine heterografts in children. J Thorac Cardiovasc Surg 78:351, 1979.
5. Bachet J, Bical O, Goudot B, Menu P, Richard T, Barbagelatta M, Guilmet D: Early structural failure of porcine xenografts in young patients. In: Bioprosthetic Valves (F. Sebening, et al, Eds). Munich, Deutsches Herzzentraum, 1979.
6. Kaplan EL, Meier P: Non-parametric estimation from incomplete observations. Am J Statist Assoc 53:457, 1958.
7. Magilligan DJ, Lewis JW Jr, Jara FM, Lee MW, Alain M, Riddle JM, Stein PD: Spontaneous degeneration of porcine bioprosthetic valves. Ann Thorac Surg 30:259, 1980.
8. Björk VO, Henze A: Ten years experience with the Björk-Shiley tilting disc valve. J Thorac Cardiovasc Surg 78:331, 1979.
9. McManus Q, Grunkemeier GL, Lambert LE, Teply JF, Harlan BS, Starr A: Year of operation as a risk factor in the late results of valve replacement. J Thorac Cardiovasc Surg 80:834, 1980.

48

Valve Replacement in the Small Anulus Aorta: Performance of the Hancock Modified Orifice Bioprosthesis

V. J. DISESA, J. J. COLLINS, JR., L. H. COHN

The inherent problems of prosthetic valve surgery are magnified when aortic valve replacement must be accomplished in a patient with a small aortic anulus and ascending aorta.[1] The standard orifice porcine valve has a muscle bar at the base of the noncoronary cusp that may cause functional stenosis in the small diameter (19, 21, and 23 mm) valves. Because this functional stenosis has led to measured postoperative resting aortic valve gradients up to 33 mmHg and valve areas as low as 0.9 mm^2, the standard orifice porcine heterograft has not been recommended for use in sizes less than 25 mm.[2–4] A number of aortic anulus enlarging procedures have been devised to allow placement of a larger prosthesis in the small anulus aorta.[5–9] All have the disadvantage of increasing operative time and potential disruption of the aortic anulus and mitral valve apparatus.

The modified orifice porcine valve (Hancock) was designed to improve the flow characteristics and reduce postoperative gradients in small anulus prostheses. The obstructing noncoronary cusp of the native porcine valve is replaced by a muscle-free cusp from a second valve, reducing the inherent functional stenosis. This extra manipulation in the fabrication of this bioprosthesis raised questions regarding its long-term durability in patients. We performed the first clinical aortic valve replacement using the Hancock modified orifice (MO) valve at the Brigham and Women's Hospital in October 1976. We report here our 6 year experience with this valve.

Clinical Material

One hundred and eighty-five patients (112 M/73 F) with a mean age of 62 years (16–84 years) have undergone aortic valve replacement with the MO

From the Division of Cardiothoracic Surgery, Harvard Medical School, and the Brigham and Women's Hospital, Boston, Massachusetts.

prosthesis since late 1976. Preoperatively, 4 patients were in NYHA class II, 123 were in class III, and 58 were in class IV. One hundred and fifty-six patients had predominant aortic stenosis, whereas in 29, aortic regurgitation was the dominant lesion. Four patients with aortic insufficiency had active infective endocarditis at the time of valve replacement.

Sixty-six patients (36%) had concomitant operative procedures. These included coronary revascularization in 54 patients, mitral valve reconstruction in 7, ascending aortic aneurysmectomy in 3, and left ventricular outflow myomectomy and atrial septal defect repair in 1 each.

Operative technique employed cardiopulmonary bypass with profound local hypothermia, hyperkalemic cardioplegia (since October 1977), and either simple or horizontal mattress interrupted anular sutures. There were 82 of the 21 mm, 101 of the 23 mm, and 2 of the 25 mm MO valves implanted.

Results

There were 5 early deaths for an overall operative mortality of 2.7%. Causes of death included acute myocardial infarction (MI) in 3, arrhythmia in 1, and acute renal failure associated with preoperative endocarditis in 1 patient. Ten patients died late during a mean follow-up time of 24 months (1–60 months). The mean duration from initial valve replacement to death was 28 months with a range of 8–56 months. One patient died of a right ventricular infarct during reoperation for secondary valve dysfunction. One patient each died late from acute MI, cancer, chronic renal failure, noncardiac infection, and low cardiac output. Cause of late death was unknown in 4. The actuarial probability of survival calculated by the life table method is 88 ± 4% at 60 months (Fig. 1).

One hundred sixty-three surviving patients are in NYHA functional class I and II. There are 4 patients in class III and 3 are lost to follow-up. Nine patients are on long-term anticoagulation without hemorrhagic complications. Four patients have suffered nonfatal systemic emboli; 2 of these patients are in atrial fibrillation and on long-term anticoagulants. The actuarial probability of freedom from emboli at 60 months is 96 ± 2% (Fig. 2).

Four patients have been treated for prosthetic valve infection occurring 7–20 months (mean 14 months) after surgery. None of these patients had preoperative valve infections. Three have been treated with antibiotics alone. Two of the patients treated medically are in functional class III. The third patient treated without surgery died 3 months after presumed eradication of endocarditis. One patient with unsuspected endocarditis had an infected valve replaced at reoperation for recurrent aortic stenosis 12 months after initial aortic valve replacement. He is symptom-free 3 months after repeat valve replacement.

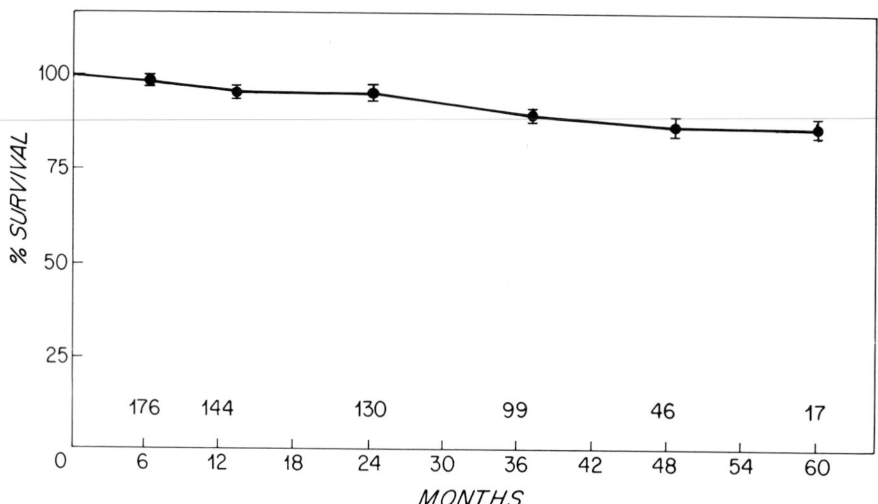

FIG. 1 Actuarial probability of survival of patients undergoing modified orifice Hancock aortic valve replacement.

Five other patients have required reoperation. There have been 4 perivalvular leaks occurring between 0 and 13 months (mean, 4.8 months) postoperatively and leading to replacement of the porcine valve. One patient with suspected primary valve dysfunction 25 months after initial replacement was found at reoperation to have a histologically normal valve that had eroded into her aortic wall, producing functional valve obstruction

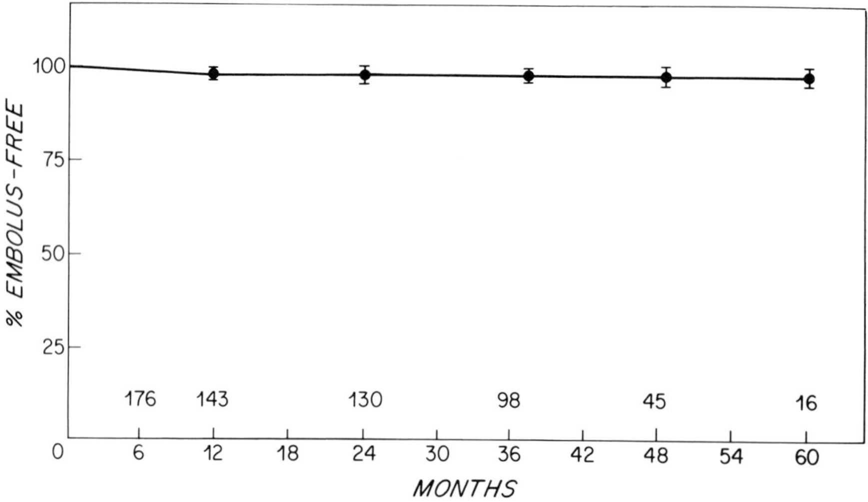

FIG. 2 Actuarial calculation of freedom from emboli after modified orifice aortic valve replacement.

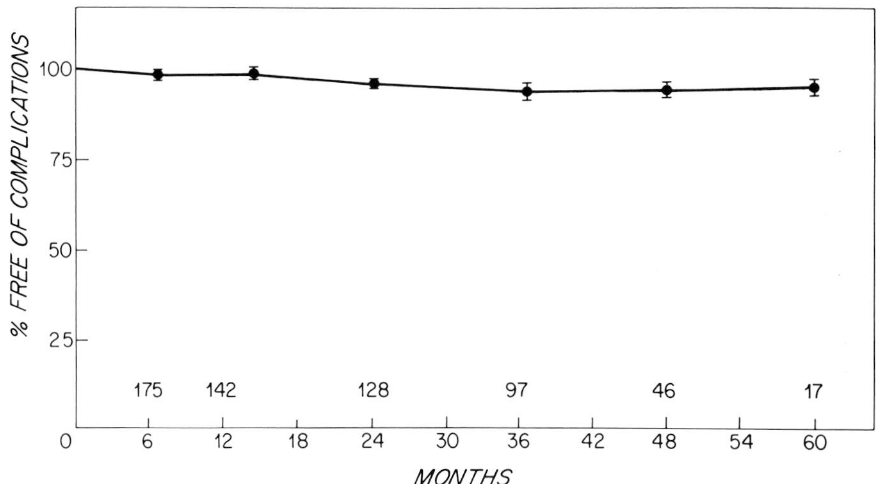

FIG. 3 Actuarial calculation of freedom from valve complications in patients undergoing modified orifice aortic valve replacement.

(stent "creep"). She died intraoperatively of a right ventricular infarct. There have been no cases of primary valve leaflet dysfunction noted during the study period. The actuarial probability of survival free of nonembolic valve-related complications (infection, perivalvular leak, stent "creep") is 93 ± 2% at 60 months (Fig. 3).

Four patients had repeat catheterization from 2–34 months after surgery (mean, 13 months) (Table I). Observed gradients at rest have been 0–19 mmHg (mean, 11 mmHg) with calculated valve areas of 1.3 and 1.4 cm².

Comment

The Hancock MO bioprosthesis has been effective in relieving symptoms of aortic valve disease in patients with small aortic anuli. We have observed a low incidence of thromboembolic complications without anticoagulation and the valves have shown acceptable durability thus far.

TABLE I Postoperative catheterization data

Pts	Months postoperative	Valve size (mm)	Gradient (mmHg)	Area (cm²)
1	8	23	15	1.3
2	5	23	12	1.4
	34		0	—
3	2	21	19	1.3
4	8	21	10	1.4

This is similar to our long-term results in patients receiving standard orifice porcine prostheses.[9] There is, as well, evidence suggesting that the small anular standard orifice porcine prosthesis has a functional gradient and valve area that are clinically acceptable and comparable to mechanical prostheses.[10,11] There is not widespread agreement on this point[2–4,12] and most groups have avoided using the standard orifice porcine valve in the patient with a small anulus. Measuring the valve gradient under conditions of enhanced cardiac output underlines the potential pitfalls of using the unmodified small diameter prosthesis. Gradients measured after exercise or isoproterenol infusion[11] have shown significant and unacceptable increases (up to 85 mmHg). Rare complications, such as strut compression (as in patients with stent "creep") and resultant valve thrombosis,[13] also illustrate the potential complications when too large a valve is placed in too small an aorta.

Our present experience and the early experience of others[14,15] document that the MO valves perform well clinically. Postoperative valve gradients greater than 20 mmHg have not been observed,[14–17] although some investigators[15] believe that the measurable hemodynamic differences between the standard and MO prostheses are small and inconclusive.

The MO valve shares with all porcine prostheses the incompletely defined risks of infection, stenosis, and late degeneration. Although prosthetic valve endocarditis remains a lethal complication,[18] 2 of our patients have survived late after medical treatment of valve infection and a third is asymptomatic after replacement of a stenotic, infected prosthesis.

Although calcific stenosis occurs mainly in children with porcine heterografts,[19] this complication can occur in the adult.[20] However, we observed no cases of calcific leaflet dysfunction. In fact, despite data predicting microscopic leaflet degeneration in all explanted valves,[21,22] there was not a single primary valve failure during our 5 year follow-up. This is consistent with the low incidence of primary valve dysfunction observed at 5 years with the standard porcine prosthesis[9,23–25] and suggests that the fabrication process itself does not lead to early failure of the MO valve. It is also consistent with other studies confirming the satisfactory clinical durability of porcine valve leaflets.

The MO porcine valve offers effective relief of severe aortic valve disease in patients with small aortic anuli. Our data document the fact that the MO valve shares the same acceptable long-term durability and low rate of thromboembolism of other tissue valves.

References

1. Hatcher CR Jr: Aortic valve replacement: The problem of the small aortic annulus. Ann Thorac Surg 22:400, 1976.

2. Jones EL, Craver JM, Morris DC, King SB III, Douglas JS Jr, Franch RH, Hatcher CR Jr, Morgan EA: Hemodynamic and clinical evaluation of the Hancock xenograft bioprosthesis of the aortic valve replacement (with emphasis on management of the small aortic root). J Thorac Cardiovasc Surg 75:300, 1978.
3. Cohn LH, Sanders JH Jr, Collins JJ Jr: Aortic valve replacement with the Hancock porcine xenograft. Ann Thorac Surg 22:221, 1976.
4. Morris DC, King SB, Douglas JS Jr, Wickliffe CW, Jones EL: Hemodynamic results of aortic valvular replacement with the porcine xenograft valve. Circulation 56:841, 1977.
5. Mori T, Kawashima Y, Kitamura S, Nakano S, Kawachi K, Nakata T: Results of aortic valve replacement in patients with a narrow aortic annulus: Effects of enlargement of the aortic annulus. Ann Thorac Surg 31:111, 1981.
6. Manouguian S, Seybold-Epting W: Patch enlargement of the aortic valve ring by extending the aortic incision into the anterior mitral leaflet. New operative technique. J Thorac Cardiovasc Surg 78:402, 1979.
7. Pupello DF, Blank RH, Ressone LN, Harrison E, Sbar S: Surgical management of the small aortic annulus. Hemodynamic evaluation. Chest 74:163, 1978.
8. Blank RH, Pupello DF, Bessone LN, Harrison E, Sbar S: Method of managing the small aortic annulus during valve replacement. Ann Thorac Surg 22:356, 1976.
9. Cohn LH, Mudge GH, Pratter F, Collins JJ Jr: Five to eight year follow-up of patients undergoing porcine heart valve replacement. N Eng J Med 304:258, 1981.
10. Angell WW, Angell JD: Porcine valves. Prog Cardiovasc Dis 23:141, 1980.
11. Borkon AM, McIntosh CL, Jones M, Lipson LC, Kent KM, Morrow AG: Hemodynamic function of the Hancock standard orifice aortic valve bioprosthesis. J Thorac Cardiovasc Surg 82:601, 1981.
12. Johnson A, Thompson S, Vieweg WV, Daily P, Oury J, Peterson K: Evaluation of the in vivo function of the Hancock porcine xenograft in the aortic position. J Thorac Cardiovasc Surg 75:599, 1978.
13. Salomon NW, Copeland JG, Goldman S, Larson DF: Unusual complication of the Hancock porcine heterograft: Strut compression in the aortic root. J Thorac Cardiovasc Surg 77:294, 1979.
14. Zusman DR, Levine FH, Carter JE, Buckley MJ: Hemodynamic and clinical evaluation of the Hancock Modified-Orifice aortic bioprosthesis. Circulation 64:189, 1981.
15. Rossiter SJ, Miller DC, Stinson EB, Oyer PE, Reitz BA, Moreno-Cabral RJ, Mace JG, Roberts EW, Tsasaris TJ, Sutton RB, Alderman EL, Shumway NE: Hemodynamic and clinical comparison of the Hancock Modified Orifice and standard orifice bioprostheses in the aortic position. J Thorac Cardiovasc Surg 80:54, 1980.
16. Cohn LH, Koster JK, Mee RB, Collins JJ Jr: Long-term followup of the Hancock bioprosthetic heart valve: A 6-year review. Circulation 60:87, 1979.
17. Levine FH, Carter JE, Buckley MJ, Daggett WM, Akins CW, Austen WG: Hemodynamic evaluation of Hancock and Carpentier-Edwards bioprostheses. Circulation 64:192, 1981.
18. Bortolotti U, Thiene G, Milano A, Panizzon G, Valente M, Gallucci V: Pathological study of infective endocarditis of Hancock porcine bioprostheses. J Thorac Cardiovasc Surg 81:934, 1981.
19. Curcio CA, Commerford PJ, Rose AG, Stevens JE, Barnard MS: Calcification of glutaraldehyde-preserved porcine xenografts in young patients. J Thorac Cardiovasc Surg 81:621, 1981.
20. Gordon MH, Walters MB, Allen P, Burton JD: Calcific stenosis of a

glutaraldehyde-treated porcine bioprosthesis in the aortic position. J Thorac Cardiovasc Surg 80:788, 1980.

21. Bloch WN Jr, Karcioglu Z, Felner JM, Miller JS, Symbas PN, Schlant RC: Idiopathic perforation of a porcine aortic bioprosthesis in the aortic position. Chest 74:579, 1978.
22. Ferrans VJ, Spray TL, Billingham ME, Roberts WC: Structural changes in glutaraldehyde-treated porcine heterografts used as substitute cardiac valves. Transmission and scanning electron microscopic observations in 12 patients. Am J Cardiol 41:1159, 1978.
23. Gallo JI, Ruiz B, Carrion MF, Gutierrez JA, Vesa JL, Duran CM: Heart valve replacement with the Hancock bioprosthesis: A 6-year review. Ann Thorac Surg 31:444, 1981.
24. Lakier JB, Khaja F, Magilligan DJ Jr, Goldstein S: Porcine xenograft valves. Long-term (60–80 months) followup. Circulation 62(Suppl II):313, 1980.
25. Oyer PE, Miller DC, Stinson EB, Reitz BA, Moreno-Cabral RJ, Shumway NE: Clinical durability of the Hancock porcine bioprosthetic valve. J Thorac Cardiovasc Surg 80:824, 1980.

49

Decreasing Incidence of Porcine Bioprosthetic Degeneration

D. J. MAGILLIGAN, JR, J. W. LEWIS, JR, P. D. STEIN, J. LAKIER, D. R. SMITH

The porcine xenograft bioprosthesis has been the prosthetic valve of choice at Henry Ford Hospital since October 1971. It was in 1976 that our first instance of spontaneous degeneration of a porcine bioprosthesis was seen. In 1978 we reported a total of 13 cases of spontaneous degeneration.[1] By 1980 this experience had increased to 23 valves and the incidence of spontaneous degeneration in our series was reported as 8% at 6 years and 16% at 7 years.[2] Since that time, degeneration has been reported in other large series occurring at a similar rate at 5 and 6 years.[3,4]

The interpretation of this experience by the medical and surgical community has been to predict that degeneration or primary failure was an inevitability in all patients with glutaraldehyde-treated bioprostheses and at a rate not much improved from previously used tissue valves. However, if this were the case, we would have expected to see a linear increase in the rate of degeneration as the number of valves at risk and the length of implantation increased. This has not been the case in our series. The following is a report of our experience with spontaneous degeneration of the porcine bioprosthesis with a maximum follow-up of 10 years, 4 months.

Patients and Methods

All patients who have had a porcine bioprosthetic valve inserted are followed by yearly visit or letter, if possible during the calendar month of implantation. All patients were accounted for in 1981 and follow-up was therefore 100% complete.

Patients were considered to have spontaneous degeneration of the por-

From the Henry Ford Hospital, Detroit, Michigan.

cine bioprosthesis if they were seen with valve incompetence or stenosis and if degenerative changes were confirmed on gross or histologic examination of the explanted valve. In addition, there could not be any clinical, bacteriologic, or histologic evidence of endocarditis.

Actuarial curves for valve survival without degeneration were constructed according to the method of Berkson and Gage.[5] Confidence limits were determined by the method described by Irwin.[6] Comparison between groups was determined by the chi-square test with matrix inversion.[7] The incidence of expected events was predicted using simple linear regression.

Results

Forty-one instances of valve degeneration have occurred in a follow-up period up to 124 months. Sixteen patients have been followed greater than 10 years. Valve survival without degeneration is depicted actuarially in Fig. 1. The earliest degenerated valve was seen at 14 months and then none until 40 months. The percentage of valve survival without degeneration was as follows: at 5 years, 96% ± 1.0 SE (standard error); at 6 years, 93% ± 1.5; at 7 years, 88% ± 2.0; at 8 years, 82% ± 2.9; at 9 years, 80% ± 3.4; and at 10 years, 69% ± 6.5.

There were 362 valves in male patients and 382 in female patients. The

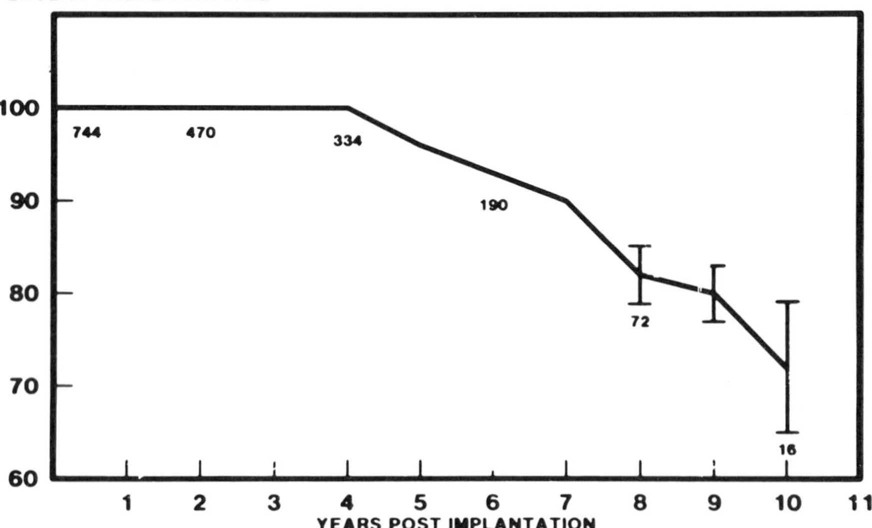

FIG. 1 Survival of valves without degeneration with longest follow-up at 10 years. Numbers refer to patients at risk.

survival of valves without degeneration plotted actuarially showed no significant difference between male and female patients (p = 0.30).

There were 284 aortic, 427 mitral, and 33 tricuspid valves at risk. Valve survival without degeneration plotted actuarially for aortic and mitral valves showed no significant difference (p = 0.77).

Survival without degeneration was calculated for 5 age groups: 0 to 20 years, 21 to 25 years, 26 to 30 years, 31 to 35 years, and older than 35 years. Degeneration was shown to be similar for all age groups equal to or below 35 years. However, the difference between all the age groups 35 years or less and those over 35 years was significant (p = 0.005; Fig. 2).

There was no significant difference when valve position was analyzed by sex (p = 0.69). When valve position and age groups ≤35 and >35 were analyzed, there was a significant difference only with respect to both aortic and mitral positions having a greater degeneration-free percentage in patients >35 years (Fig. 3; p = 0.03).

Prior to October 1974, the porcine bioprosthetic valves were immersed in a solution containing 1 g neomycin and 10,000 units of bacitracin in 100 ml of saline as outlined in the manufacturer's instructions.[8] This storage and handling information was revised October 1, 1974, with the warning that neomycin and bacitracin "will cause a chemical change tending to make the leaflets stiff."[9] Subsequently, in our institution, valves were rinsed only in

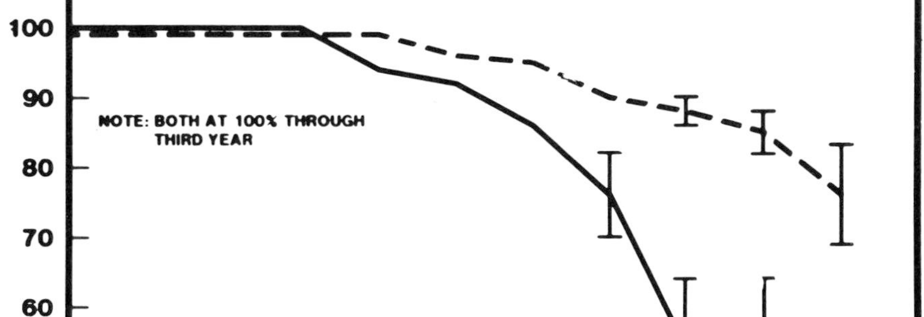

FIG. 2 Survival of valves without degeneration according to age <35 and >35 years. The difference was significant (p = 0.005).

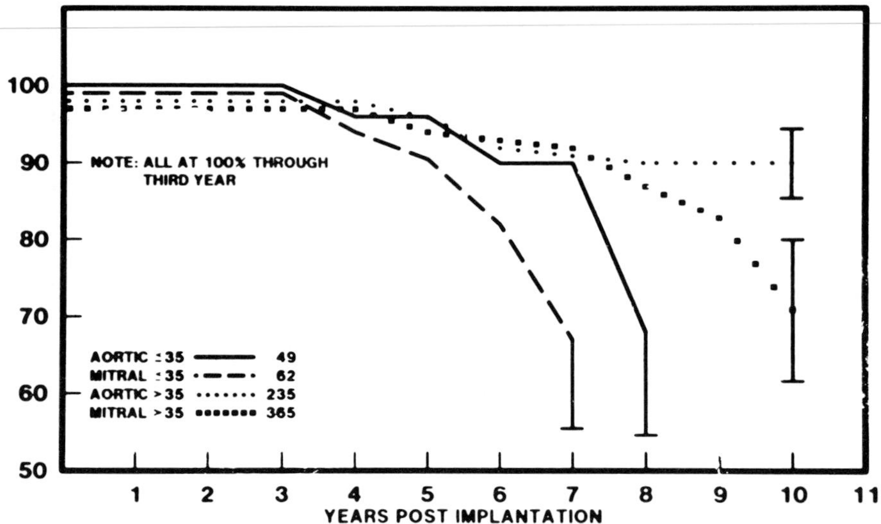

FIG. 3 Survival of valves without degeneration according to age <35 and >35 years and position. All patients <35 years fared worse than patients >35 years in both aortic and mitral positions.

lactated Ringer's solution. To determine whether antibiotic rinsing might play a part in degeneration, valves at risk implanted prior to October 15, 1974, ("early") were plotted against those implanted subsequently that did not undergo antibiotic rinsing ("late"). At 6 years, the survival for "early" valves was 93% ± 1.9 and for "late" valves was 94% ± 2.5 (p = 0.83).

Our 8 years of porcine bioprosthetic valve experience was reported in 1980 and it was during the year 1979 that 11 valves were removed for degeneration. As others, we expected the number of valves requiring removal for degeneration to increase linearly with the increasing number of valves at risk and increasing length of implantation. As seen in Fig. 4 this has not been the case. Whereas in 1977, 4 valves were removed for spontaneous degeneration, 8 in 1978, 11 in 1979, in 1980 only 5 valves were removed for degeneration, 10 in 1981, and thus far in 1982 the number has been 2. During this period of time, the total numbers of valves at risk has increased each year, and in October 1981 was 557. Similarly, the duration of implantation until degeneration has lengthened. Whereas the duration of implantation for degenerated valves was 56 months ± 11.8 SD in 1977 and 1978, it has increased above this figure in 1979 (71 months ± 14.4), 1980 (79 months ± 15.7), 1981 (77 months ± 19), and 1982 (113 months ± 1.4).

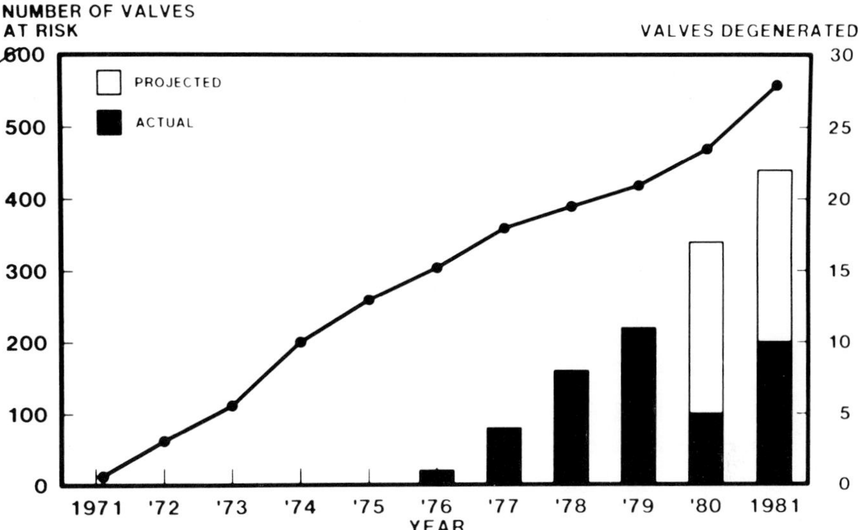

FIG. 4 It was expected that the number of valves degenerating in 1980 and 1981 would increase linearly as it had from 1976–79 and as the total number of valves at risk has increased. However, although the total number of valves at risk has increased in linear fashion to 557 in 1981, there has not been a similar linear increase in number of valves degenerating in years 1980 and 1981.

This is suggestive that degeneration is occurring at a frequency less than predicted in 1980. The duration of implantation for the 41 valves degenerated is depicted graphically in Fig. 5.

The data suggested that valves implanted early in the series might behave differently from valves implanted later, with the latter having a lower incidence of early degeneration. Analysis of the "early" and "late" groups with or without antibiotic rinsing did not show a difference. We then analyzed cohorts by year. Excluding the year 1971 when there were only 15 valves inserted, none of which degenerated, there are 3 cohorts that are available for analysis with at least a 7 year follow-up. At 7 year follow-up, the percent of valves free of degeneration is: 88% ± 4.4 SE for the 1972 cohort; 83% ± 4.8 for the 1973 cohort; 95% ± 2.6 for the 1974 cohort (Fig. 6). Although a difference is suggested between these 3 cohorts, it is not yet statistically significant ($p = 0.48$).

The lack of statistical significance may be due to the small numbers of degenerated valves. Looking graphically at the number of valves degenerated in each cohort year (Fig. 7), it is evident that the number of valves degenerated within 7 years appears less in the 1974 cohort compared to 1972 or 1973.

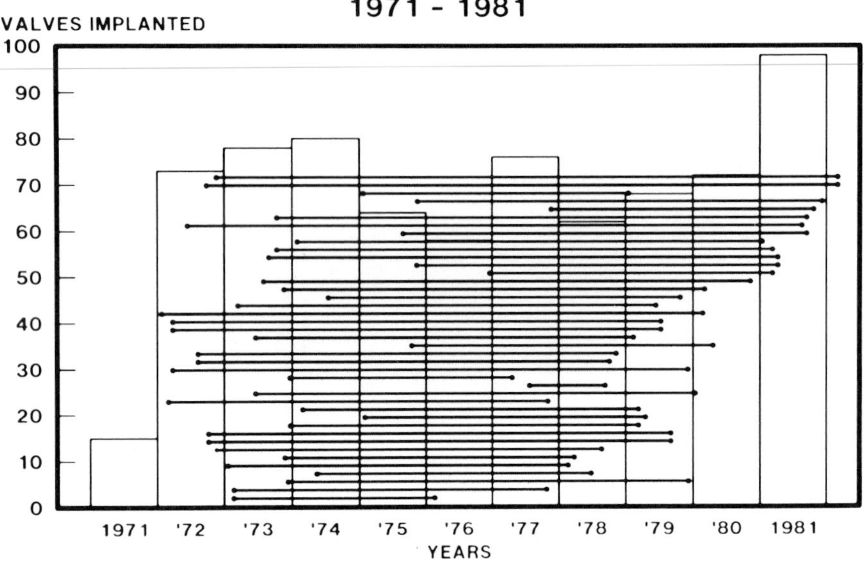

FIG. 5 The duration of implantation for the 41 degenerated valves is depicted by the horizontal lines. The vertical bars represent the number of valves implanted that particular year.

Comment

The overall valve survival without degeneration at 6, 7, and 8 years, is improved over our analysis published in 1980.[2] The reason is that as more valves have been followed for this length of time, the SE has decreased. For the 1980 report, the SE at 6 years was 2.4% and for 1982, 1.5%; in 1980 the SE at 7 years was 3.7% and for 1982, 2.2%; in 1980 the SE at 8 years was 11.7% and for 1982, 3.0%. This validates the contention that the leading edge of an actuarial curve does not lend itself to an accurate interpretation of events, since the large SE make this information unreliable for clinical judgment.[3] For this reason, we expect our 9 year data (SE = 3.4%) to be fairly accurate, but suspect that the 10 year data with 16 patients and a SE of 6.5% to be an overestimation of the incidence of degeneration.

As in 1980, we found no significant difference in the incidence of degeneration between males and females, aortic or mitral position, or whether the valves were rinsed in antibiotic solution or not.

As others have reported, we also have seen that the incidence of degeneration is greater in younger patients.[10,11] Although the age dividing line

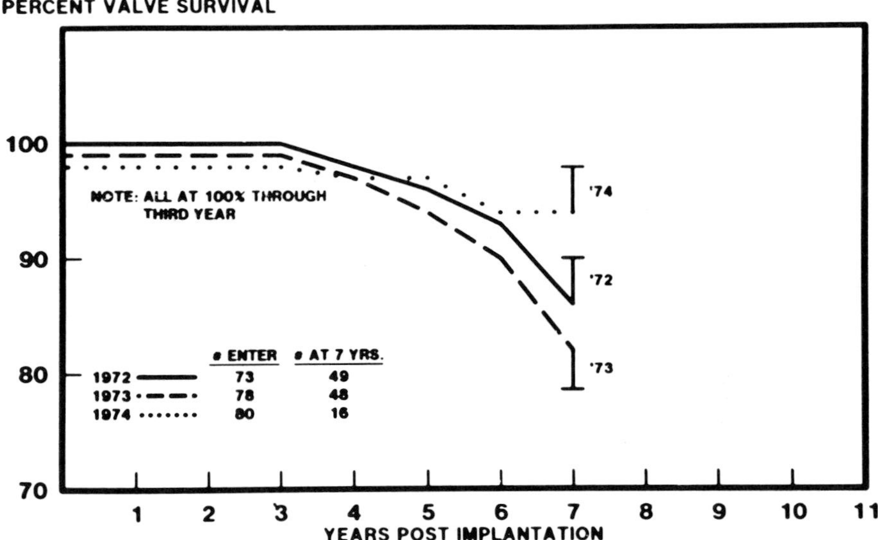

FIG. 6 Survival of valves without degeneration for the cohorts from years 1972, 1973, 1974, all of which have had at least 7 years follow-up. The percent free of degeneration at 7 years is: for 1972 = 88% ± 4.4; for 1973 = 83% ± 4.8; and for 1974 = 95% ± 2.6.

between better durability might be at 20 years, statistically this could not be shown. Rather, again, as in 1980 the only statistically significant grouping was patients ≤35 years and those >35 years (p = 0.005). If there is a trend to lowering the dividing age, statistical significance will only be reached with a larger number of young patients.

In 1980, our report of 23 cases of valve degeneration was followed by a response that varied from disbelief at the incidence to a dire prediction that primary valve failure was an inevitable event within 10 years for all glutaraldehyde-treated bioprostheses. As the experience lengthens in all large series, the incidence of degeneration has become similar. More importantly, the incidence of degeneration in the past 2 years has been less than predicted in 1980. In trying to analyze the data to determine the cause for the relative decrease in the incidence of degeneration, we could only find that the 1974 cohort of valves had a 7 year survival of 95% compared to 88 and 83% for 1972 and 1973, respectively. The only explanation appears to be that the increased experience with valve production accounted for better durability in 1974 compared to 1972 and 1973.

The small numbers of valves degenerating account for the failure to verify

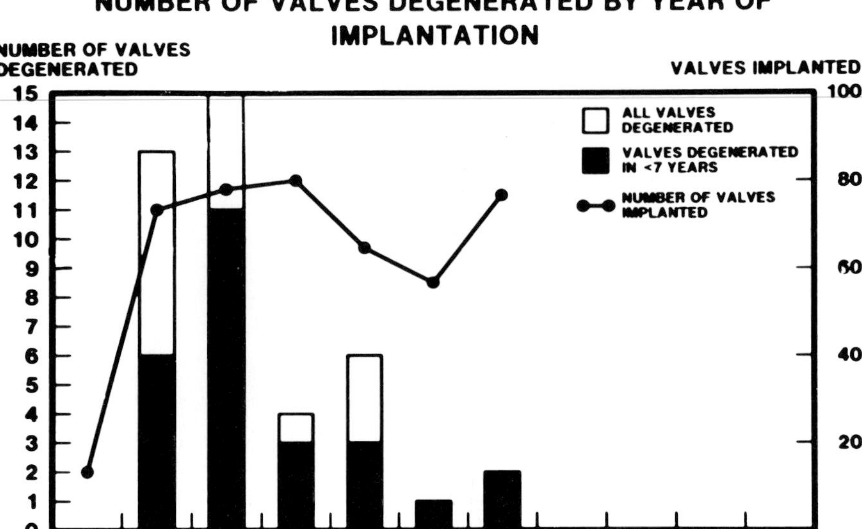

FIG. 7 Graphic representation of the number of valves degenerating by year implanted. The blackened portion of each bar represents experience within 7 years. For 1972, 1973, 1974 this experience was equal in duration and clearly the 1974 rate of degeneration was less than that in 1972 and 1973.

the trend toward a decline in the incidence of degeneration with statistical significance. However, the fact remains that in 1982 we are removing fewer porcine bioprosthetic valves for degeneration than even we predicted in early 1980.

Summary

The porcine bioprosthesis has been our prosthetic valve of choice since October 1971. By 1979, 23 cases of degeneration had been seen and the incidence reported as 16% at 7 years. We expected the incidence of degeneration to increase linearly as the number of valves at risk and length of implantation increased. Now, with 10 year follow-up, the number of valves degenerated is 41 and the percent free of degeneration is: 7 years, 88% ± 2 SE; 8 years, 82% ± 2.9; 9 years, 80% ± 3.4; 10 years, 69% ± 6.5. There was no difference in degeneration between males or females, aortic or mitral position, or whether the valves were rinsed in antibiotics or not. There was a significantly greater incidence of degeneration in patients younger than 35 years. The number of valves removed for degeneration has not increased linearly and has been: 1977, 4 valves; 1978, 8; 1979, 11; 1980, 5; 1981, 10. The number of valves at risk has continued to rise in linear fashion. The duration of implantation for degenerated valves has increased from 56 months ± 11 SD in 1977 and 1978 to 77 months ± 19 in 1981. Analysis of cohorts from 1972, 1973, and 1974 followed for 7 years reveals that at 7 years the percent free of degeneration is: 1972, 88% ± 4.4; 1973, 83% ± 4.8; 1974, 95% ± 2.6. Although a difference is suggested, it is not yet statistically significant ($p = 0.48$) due to the small number of valves degenerating. The incidence of porcine bioprosthetic degeneration appears to be decreasing. An explanation may be better durability of valves manufactured later in the series.

References

1. Magilligan DJ Jr, Lewis JW Jr, Davila JC, Goldstein S, Fine G: Spontaneous degeneration of the porcine xenograft valve. Circulation (Suppl II) 58:86, 1978.
2. Magilligan DJ Jr, Lewis JW Jr, Jara FM, Lee MW, Alam M, Riddle JM, Stein PD: Spontaneous degeneration of porcine bioprosthetic valves. Ann Thorac Surg 30:259, 1980.
3. Oyer PE, Miller DC, Stinson EB, Reitz BA, Moreno-Cabral RJ, Shumway NE: Clinical durability of the (Hancock) porcine bioprosthetic valve. J Thorac Cardiovasc Surg 80:824, 1980.
4. Cohn LH, Mudge GH, Pratter F, Collins JJ Jr: Five to eight-year followup of patients undergoing porcine heart-valve replacement. N Engl J Med 304:258, 1981.
5. Berkson J, Gage RP: Calculation of survival rates for cancer. Proc Staff Meet Mayo Clin 25:270, 1950.
6. Irwin JO: The standard error of an estimate of expectation of life with special reference of expectation of tumorless life in experiments with mice. J Hyg 47:188, 1949.
7. Mantel N, Hanszel W: Statistical aspects of analysis of data from retrospective studies of disease. J Natl Cancer Inst 22:719, 1959.
8. Hancock Laboratories: "Instruction," 1971.
9. Hancock Laboratories: "Storage and handling information," 1974.
10. Geha AS, Laks H, Stansel HC Jr, Cornhill JF, Kilman JW, Buckley MJ, Roberts WC: Late failure of porcine valve heterografts in children. J Thorac Cardiovasc Surg 78:351, 1979.
11. Silver MM, Pollock J, Silver MD, Williams WG, Trusler GA: Calcification in porcine xenograft valves in children. Am J Cardiol 45:685, 1980.

SECTION IX

SUMMING UP

50

A Cardiologist's Point of View and a Cardiac Surgeon's Point of View

S. H. Rahimtoola, L. H. Cohn

THE CARDIOLOGIST:

This symposium has been highly educational and a great success; we must thank 1) The University of Padova for sponsoring it. We must also recognize the great importance of the University of Padova in cardiology. The description of the circulation started with William Harvey who was educated at Padova more than 400 years ago. There have been many other cardiology "greats" from Padova—Dr. Morgagni, to name just one more. 2) The organizing committee of four illustrious individuals; we owe them a great deal of gratitude for putting together a superb symposium; 3) Hancock/Extracorporeal, for providing the funds and impetus for this symposium; and 4) last but not least, the participants, for without them there would not have been a symposium!

The good news that I must begin with is that *bioprostheses are here to stay.* Having said that, I hope all of you will relax; many of you have been talking about bioprostheses as though you were really having serious doubts about them. There has been great enthusiasm about the benefits of bioprostheses when perhaps some of these benefits had not been so obvious to me.

There are several other important issues to consider: *Data Analysis:* It was gratifying to see that a vast number of presenters used actuarial techniques which have not become routine. However, there are still areas in data analysis that cause concern. These include: comparing results in patients when the patients being compared are obviously different at time of entry into the study; ignoring the time factor in data analysis. For example,

---

From the Section of Cardiology, University of Southern California, Los Angeles, California (SHR) and the Department of Surgery, the Harvard Medical School, Brigham and Women's Hospital, Boston, Massachusetts (LHC).

patients operated upon and prostheses used were different in the 1960s from those used in the 1970s; some have compared bioprostheses to mechanical prostheses. Mechanical prostheses are very different and cannot be considered as a single homogeneous group; a comparison of survivors of valve replacement to the general population. I am unsure of what such a comparison means. One could potentially come to ridiculous conclusions by this technique; namely, life is prolonged by aortic valve replacement and therefore everybody should have it! This is absurd; and a survival curve represents in most instances an average, and thus must be presented with standard error or standard deviation or confidence limits.

Complications. My personal perception of the analysis of complications is that most likely *all* complications are underestimated. For example, emboli can be very difficult to evaluate, and mortality may be glossed over because there are emergency and nonemergency operations. Therefore, I would like to offer the hypothesis that when we look at data on complications, we are indeed looking at the lowest level of complications.

Thromboemboli occur even with bioprostheses, and it is important not to promise our patients that they will not have thromboemboli just because they will receive a bioprosthesis. Thromboemboli occur with about the same frequency as with mechanical prostheses and anticoagulant therapy. Select patients with bioprostheses do not need anticoagulant therapy and that is clearly an advantage. We have heard a very provocative group of papers with regard to a lack of need of anticoagulant therapy. In particular, the one from Naples suggested that maybe the risk of thromboemboli in patients with atrial fibrillation and mitral valve bioprosthesis is low. I think it is high; the problem here is one of perception. The important question is: does anticoagulant therapy make a different in patients with bioprostheses in the mitral position? This question must be answered. There are probably a variety of ways of doing that, one of which may be a randomized study. It has generally been accepted that a randomized study of prosthetic valves cannot be done. A large VA cooperative study in the United States is evaluating the Björk-Shiley valve versus the Hancock bioprosthesis; I believe there are two randomized studies also in progress in Europe.

Bioprosthetic Failure. This is obviously a very important issue. It occurs at an increased rate after five years. I made the point when Dr. Oyer's paper from Stanford was presented that when estimating the risk of bioprosthetic failure, one should look at the failure rate after five years in order to obtain a more realistic appraoch of what the risk is going to be at ten years.

A problem with detection of degeneration is that clinical and noninvasive evaluations are inadequate. Data from the NIH has shown that the porcine valve may undergo significant deterioration and the patients may be asymptomatic. Also, many patients with bioprosthetic valve degeneration do not have valve re-replacement. Thus, surgical evaluation of bioprosthetic failure by reoperation rate is inadequate. Data from Detroit presented by

Dr. Stein on orifice view angiography sounds interesting, but I am concerned whether it will be reliable in detecting bioprosthetic failure. A definitive study where one compares cross-sectional area by orifice view angiography to catheterization-proven valve area in the same patients at the same time seems appropriate. Perhaps the same information could be obtained by 2-dimensional echocardiography. However, we already know that 2-dimensional echocardiography is not a reliable technique for estimating the degree of obstruction in native aortic and mitral stenosis; whether it will be better with a prosthetic valve remains to be proven. Data from the Montreal Heart Institute showed that approximately 20% of patients had bioprosthetic valve regurgitation at angiography which was not detected by clinical means.

Improved Prosthesis. One makes improvements in prostheses in the expectation that benefit will result; however, past experience has repeatedly demonstrated that this may or may not occur. With an aim of obtaining a greater effective orifice area, the modified orifice Hancock bioprosthesis and a changed sewing ring of the Carpentier-Edwards valve were introduced. Data from Stanford, not presented at this meeting but already published, and data from the Montreal Heart Institute with the Carpentier-Edwards valve show that these changes have not resulted in any significant improvement in the effective orifice area in patients.

Re-operation. The most disturbing thing that I have heard repeatedly at this symposium is the downplay of the significance of reoperation. Many seem to think that reoperation is not that important, is something that can be done easily, and is no big deal. I would like to ask you a question: How many of you have had open heart surgery? I think I am correct in saying that not one person in the audience has had open heart surgery. Reoperation is very, very serious. Apart from the risks of mortality and morbidity, it can be extremely traumatic to the patient and the family. I would like to leave you with at least one message—*reoperation is indeed very serious!*

Improved Bioprosthesis. There is a great need for improvement in bioprostheses; there are at least two problems that we can identify which need correction. One is perforation. Dr. Victor Ferrans suggested very persuasively that perforation is probably an engineering problem and that if stress is taken into account we could possibly get rid of this problem. The second problem is that of the prevention of calcification; two papers sounded very promising. Data from Drs. Olsen on the effect of T-6 with Hancock bioprosthesis look enticing and need to be pursued. Dr. Alain Carpentier suggested that the use of polymers on bioprostheses may prevent calcification.

It has been suggested by many workers, including Carpentier, that maybe we should treat the patient. It is very difficult to change the calcium metabolism of most people unless it was abnormal to start with. A word of caution is appropriate; if we change calcium metabolism a lot, the bioprosthesis may or may not calcify, but the patient is at risk of developing pathologic fractures. If young children fracture their spine and are not able to walk, an extremely undesirable risk has been taken.

I would like to end by saying that it has been a pleasure, and I want to thank you once again.

THE CARDIAC SURGEON:

The important conclusions of this meeting, in my opinion, relate to: 1) the length of durability of cardiac bioprostheses; 2) the mechanisms of valve failure; 3) the risk of thromboembolism after implantation of these valves; 4) the use of bioprosthetic valves in right and left-sided congenital heart lesions; 5) new chemicals that may decrease the likelihood of mineralization of bioprosthetic valves; 6) new valve introduction heralding the second decade of bioprosthetic valves with improved bioengineering, and finally 7) an awareness of the need for better standardization of statistical analysis of all valve data.

The first generation bioprosthetic cardiac valves, either porcine or bovine pericardial, are reliable in terms of durability for at least 7 years. Data presented here these last three days from a number of centers have statistically documented that the probability of valve failure, within a 95% confidence limit, is less than 5% at that time period. These valves clearly do not "fall apart" at 5 years. In fact, at 5 years postimplantation, data from Stanford, Detroit, Europe, Boston, Munich, Leeds and others indicate that the probability of valve failure is less than 2%. Although not documented by every center, the mitral bioprosthetic valve seems to be more susceptible to degeneration, probably because 1) the cusps are exposed to systolic pressure, 2) there are different flow patterns due to supraventricular arrhythmias, and 3) possibly coexistent residual mild aortic valve disease. If there is bioprosthetic valve failure, the clinical course is usually slow and failure rarely catastrophic if the patients are followed adequately. Reoperation, though a very serious matter as Dr. Rahimtoola so correctly points out, is considerably safer now than during the 1960s because of improved myocardial protection and perfusion technology.

The papers on experimental pathology and bioengineering have yielded much important information at this meeting. Not only have biologic factors responsible for degeneration been elucidated, but bioengineering data have been reported in this same regard which has apparently already stimulated valve manufacturing companies to begin the second generation of bioprostheses based on some of these data.

The use of bioprostheses for congenital and acquired lesions in children was addressed by most of the major pediatric surgical groups in the world. In patients under 18, the data are incontrovertible that bioprostheses (porcine or bovine pericardial) are associated with accelerated calcification when placed on the left side of the heart. There is a markedly increased probability of failure within 5 years of implantation, over that seen in adults. This is not to say that this occurs in all patients; in some situations where reoperation is probable within 5 years on the basis of the primary lesion, these valves may still have a place. Right-sided conduits containing a bioprosthesis, though far from perfect, have allowed correction of extremely complex forms of congenital heart disease with reasonable long-term hemodynamic correction of these lesions. Graft thrombosis, excessive graft neointima and, rarely, valve calcification have here been described in a small percent of cases. Use of fresh antibiotic-treated homograft valves containing conduits were reported as an alternative to prosthetic graft bioprosthetic valve combination with success. Although many improvements are needed in these devices, they still have been revolutionary in allowing correction of complex congenital heart disease.

The risk of thromboembolism was a major area of interest at this meeting. Reduction of emboli without the morbidity and mortality of long-term anticoagulation was the prime reason for development of tissue valves in 1960. In the aortic position, the data are impressive: the risk of embolism without anticoagulation is low, approximately less than 3% at 7 years in the series presented. In the mitral area, the data are not so clear because of the presence of chronic atrial fibrillation in a large percentage of cases. However, a number of papers from Europe indicated that even with atrial fibrillation the risk of embolism without anticoagulants seemed about the same if they were used. High risk subgroups with atrial fibrillation were identified and all agreed that if atrial fibrillation is present, and a patient had experienced a prior embolism or an intraatrial clot with increased left atrial size is found, anticoagulation is indicated.

Experimental models in both large and small animals were discussed in detail and served as focal points in the discussion of new fabrication techniques for bioprostheses. The young sheep model of the National Institutes of Health is of particular importance and will be used extensively in the future to evaluate the new anticalcification agents presented by Olsen et al and Carpentier et al. In addition, totally new valve concepts were presented including a unileaflet pericardial valve and a totally flexible tricuspid valve.

Statistical presentation of the large amounts of data was, generally, very well done and reflects increasingly stringent requirements of medical societies and journals throughout the world that demand accurate, meaningful and standardized statistical data. The actuarial method seems basic to analysis of valve data but actuarial reporting with a small number of patients may be misleading. For example, if a curve is constructed for only 20 patients over a 5-year period, the number of patients at risk at each time interval is very small so that a single event will produce dramatic changes in actuarial percentage. Data points of significance should include a reasonably large number of patients with a small standard error of the mean so the specific data point is valid within a 95% confidence limit. In addition to making actuarial data more meaningful, there is still some confusion about the reporting of valve complications. Some units report primary tissue failure or infection while others lump all causes of valve failure under a single heading and construct an overall event-free probability curve. I think both have merit. The first evaluates the actual risk of a particular event occurring with a bioprosthesis, while the second method allows comparison of the total complication rate of bioprostheses to mechanical valves which have different risk factors but in sum may have either less or more event-free periods. There continues to be a need for worldwide standardization of statistical techniques with mechanical as well as bioprosthetic heart valves to improve and clarify data reporting. As the first conference on bioprostheses in Munich in 1979 codified tissue valve terminology, this conference will hopefully be noted for promulgation of increased accuracy in reporting of statistical data.

Author Index

Subject Index